AF293969

Rectal Cancer Surgery

Springer
Berlin
Heidelberg
New York
Barcelona
Budapest
Hong Kong
London
Milan
Paris
Santa Clara
Singapore
Tokyo

Odd Søreide   Jarle Norstein   (Eds.)

Rectal Cancer Surgery

Optimisation – Standardisation – Documentation

With 130 Figures and 92 Tables

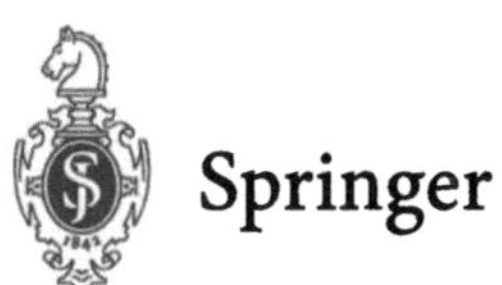 Springer

Professor Dr. Odd Søreide
Dr. Jarle Norstein

Surgical Department B
The National Hospital (Rikshospitalet)
University of Oslo
Pilestredet 32
0027 Oslo
Norway

CIP data applied for

Die Deutsche Bibliothek – CIP-Einheitsaufnahme
Rectal cancer surgery: optimisation – standardisation –
documentation; with tables/O. Søreide; J. Norstein (ed.). –
Berlin; Heidelberg; New York; Barcelona; Budapest; Hong
Kong; London; Milan; Paris; Santa Clara; Singapore;
Tokyo; Springer, 1997

NE: Søreide, Odd [Hrsg.]
ISBN-13: 978-3-642-64438-2

ISBN-13: 978-3-642-64438-2   e-ISBN-13: 978-3-642-60514-7
DOI: 10.1007/978-3-642-60514-7

© Springer-Verlag Berlin Heidelberg 1997
Softcover reprint of the hardcover 1st edition 1997

Cover Design: Design & Production GmbH, Heidelberg

Typesetting: Scientific Publishing Services (P) Ltd, Madras

SPIN: 10510099   24/3135/SPS – 5 4 3 2 1 0 – Printed on acid-free paper

Preface

Several studies worldwide have shown that results after surgery for cancer of the rectum are generally far from optimal. The major problem is locally recurrent disease which causes suffering and death in most patients. The exact incidence is difficult to determine, but it is now documented unequivocally that there are surgeon-related variances in outcome, not only in local recurrence but also in postoperative mortality and survival. Data are now accumulating that if surgeons apply identical surgical principles, they can achieve better results than those commonly reported. Comparison of results between surgeons or centers will, however, depend on a common understanding of anatomy, surgical dissection techniques, and reporting of results.

A group of international experts, renowned for their contribution to treatment of cancer of the rectum, met in Oslo, Norway, in June 1995 with the following objectives:

1. Define state-of-the-art treatment of cancer of the rectum;
2. Demonstrate the importance of surgical technique for recurrence rates, survival and functional outcome;
3. Agree on standards for evaluation and description of specimens; and
4. Formulate international standards for documentation and reporting.

The members of the meeting represented several disciplines (descriptive and clinical epidemiology, medical and radiation oncology, pathology, and surgery). Because of the rather unique collection of experts focusing on a single subject, the organiser felt justified in publishing the contributions to this meeting. Accordingly, this book represents the latest information from the world's authorities on cancer of the rectum. It is hoped that the approaches recommended in this work will provide the framework for standardisation and documentation and will guide clinical management of these patients.

Acknowledgements. The organizers wish to express their gratitude to Mr. R.J. Heald, Basingstoke, England, for his enthusiasm, contributions, and support prior to, during and after this meeting, and to Dr. Warren Enker, New York, USA for his interest and generous help during planning. We are also grateful for the substantial financial support from The Norwegian Society for Cancer (Den Norske

Kreftforening), Tannlege Olaf Aase og Frues Legat, and Auto Suture Norden. Finally our thanks and appreciation are due to Ms. Gabriele Schröder at Springer-Verlag, Heidelberg who has solved any problems and offered her help throughout the production of this book.

August 1996   O. Søreide
                        J. Norstein

Contents

Tumour Spread As a Basis for Rectal Cancer Surgery

Surgical Technique – Options

International Standardization and Research Strategies

List of Contributors

Kaoru Azekura
Surgical Department, Cancer Institute Hospital,
1-37-1 Kami-Ikebukuro, Toshima-ku, Tokyo, Japan

Anne Berger
Centre de Chirurgie Digestive, Hospital Saint-Antoine,
184 Rue du Fauburg Saint-Antoine, 75012 Paris, France

Paul Blomqvist
Department of Cancer Epidemiology, University of Uppsala,
75185 Uppsala, Sweden

Lynn Cawkwell
Department of Histopathology and Molecular Pathology,
Algernon Firth Institute of Pathology, Leeds General Infirmary,
University of Leeds, Leeds LS1 3EX, UK

Alfred M. Cohen
Colorectal Service, Department of Surgery,
Memorial Sloan-Kettering Cancer Center, 1275 York Avenue,
New York, NY 10021, USA

Milicent Cranor
Colorectal Service, Department of Surgery,
Memorial Sloan-Kettering Cancer Center, 1275 York Avenue,
New York, NY 10021, USA

Marco C. DeRuiter
Department of Surgery, Colorectal Service, Beth Israel Medical
Center, First Avenue and 16th Street, New York, NY 10003, USA

Graeme S. Duthie
Academic Surgical Unit, The University of Hull, Castle Hill Hospital,
Cottingham, North Humberside HU16 5JQ, UK

Tor J. Eide
Department of Pathology, The National Hospital, 0027 Oslo, Norway

Warren E. Enker
Department of Surgery, Colorectal Service, Beth Israel Medical
Center, First Avenue and 16th Street, New York, NY 10003, USA

Gernot Feifel
Department of General Surgery, University of Saarland,
66421 Homburg/Saar, Germany

L. Peter Fielding
University of Rochester School of Medicine and Dentistry,
Department of Surgery, The Genesee Hospital, 222 Alexander Street,
Rochester, NY 14607-4005, USA

Bengt Glimelius
Department of Oncology, University of Uppsala, 75185 Uppsala,
Sweden

Olof Hallböök
Department of Surgery, University Hospital, 58185 Linköping,
Sweden

John E. Hartley
Academic Surgical Unit, The University of Hull, Castle Hill Hospital,
Cottingham, North Humberside HU16 5JQ, UK

Klaas Havenga
Department of Surgery, Canisius Wilhelmina Ziekenhuis,
PO Box 9015, 6500 GS Nijmegen, The Netherlands

Richard J. Heald
Colorectal Research Unit, Department of Surgery,
The North Hampshire Hospital, Basingstoke,
Hampshire RG24 9NA, UK

Paul Hermanek
Department of Surgical Pathology, Chirurgische Universitatsklinik,
University of Erlangen, Krankenhausstrasse 12, 91054 Erlangen,
Germany

Ulrich Hildebrandt
Department of General Surgery, University of Saarland,
66421 Homburg/Saar, Germany

Werner Hohenberger
Department of Surgery, University of Erlangen, University Hospital,
Krankenhausstrasse 12, 91054 Erlangen, Germany

Tracy Hull
Department of Colorectal Surgery, The Cleveland Clinic Foundation,
9500 Euclid Avenue, Cleveland, OH 44195, USA

Frøydis Langmark
The Cancer Registry of Norway, Montebello, 0310 Oslo, Norway

Bernard Levin
Division for Cancer Prevention, M.D. Anderson Cancer Center,
University of Texas, 1515 Holcombe Boulevard, Box 203, Houston,
TX 77030, USA

C. Paul Maas
Department of Surgery, Academisch Ziekenhuis Leiden,
P.O. Box 9600, 2300 RC Leiden, The Netherlands

John MacFarlane
Department of Surgery, Faculty of Medicine,
St. Paul's Hospital, 1081 Burrard Street, Vancouver V6Z 1Y6,
Canada

Josep Rius Macias
Department of Colorectal Surgery, Cleveland Clinic Florida,
3000 West Cypress Creek Road, Ft. Lauderdale, FL 33309-1743,
USA

John L. McCall
Department of Surgery, Otago University Medical School,
P.O. Box 913, Dunedin, New Zealand

Katherine McDermott
Colorectal Service, Department of Surgery,
Memorial Sloan-Kettering Cancer Center, 1275 York Avenue,
New York, NY 10021, USA

Deborah A. Mhoon
Department of Surgery, The University of Chicago,
5841 South Maryland Avenue, Chicago, IL 60637, USA

Fabrizio Michelassi
Department of Surgery, The University of Chicago,
5841 South Maryland Avenue, Chicago, IL 60637, USA

John R.T. Monson
Academic Surgical Unit, The University of Hull, Castle Hill Hospital,
Cottingham, North Humberside HU16 5JQ, UK

Yoshihiro Moriya
Department of Surgery, National Cancer Center Hospital,
1-1 Tsukiji 5-Chome, Chuo-ku, Tokyo 104, Japan

Jarle Norstein
Department of Surgery, The National Hospital, Pilestredet 32,
0027 Oslo, Norway

Olof Nyrén
Department of Cancer Epidemiology, University of Uppsala,
75185 Uppsala, Sweden

Hirotoshi Ota
Surgical Department, Cancer Institute Hospital,
1-37-1 Kami-Ikebukuro, Toshima-ku, Tokyo, Japan

Philip B. Paty
Colorectal Service, Memorial Sloan-Kettering Cancer Center,
1275 York Avenue, New York, NY 10021, USA

Tatyana Polyak
Epidemiology and Biostatistics Department,
Memorial Sloan-Kettering Cancer Center, 1275 York Avenue,
New York, NY 10021, USA

Lars Påhlman
Department of Surgery, Akademiska Sjukhuset,
University of Uppsala, 75185 Uppsala, Sweden

Rolland Parc
Centre de Chirurgie Digestive, Hospital Saint-Antoine,
184 Rue du Fauburg Saint-Antoine, 75012 Paris, France

Philip Quirke
Department of Histopathology and Molecular Pathology,
Algernon Firth Institute of Pathology, Leeds General Infirmary,
University of Leeds, Leeds LS1 3EX, UK

Kenji Sato
Department of Basic Medical Sciences, School of Allied Health
Sciences, Tokyo Medical and Dental University,
1-5-45 Yushima 1-Chome, Bunkyo-Ku, Tokyo 113, Japan

Tatsuo Sato
2nd Department of Anatomy, Tokyo Medical and Dental University,
1-5-45 Yushima 1-Chome, Bunkyo-Ku, Tokyo 113, Japan

William Silen
Harvard Medical School, 320 Brookline Avenue, Boston, MA 02215,
USA

Rune Sjödahl
Department of Surgery, University Hospital, 58185 Linkøping,
Sweden

Willem-Hans Steup
Department of Surgery, Hospital Leyenburg, The Hague,
The Netherlands

Odd Søreide
Department of Surgery, University of Oslo, The National Hospital,
Pilestredet 32, 0027 Oslo, Norway

Carlo W. Taat
Academical Medical Center, Amsterdam, The Netherlands

Takashi Takahashi
Surgical Department, Cancer Institute Hospital,
1-37-1 Kami-Ikebukuro, Toshima-ku, Tokyo, Japan

Howard T. Thaler
Epidemiology and Biostatistics Department,
Memorial Sloan-Kettering Cancer Center, 1275 York Avenue,
New York, NY 10021, USA

Emmanuel Tiret
Centre de Chirurgie Digestive, Hôpital Saint-Antoine,
184 Rue du Fauburg Saint-Antoine, 75012 Paris, France

Masashi Ueno
Surgical Department, Cancer Institute Hospital,
1-37-1 Kami-Ikebukuro, Toshima-ku, Tokyo, Japan

Cornelis J. van de Velde
Department of Surgery, Academisch Ziekenhuis Leiden,
P.O. Box 9600, 2300 RC Leiden, The Netherlands

David A. Wattchow
Gastrointestinal Surgical Unit, Flinders Medical Centre, Adelaide,
Australia

Kees Welvaart
Department of Anatomy and Embryology, University of Leiden,
Academisch Ziekenhuis Leiden, 2300 RC Leiden, The Netherlands

Steven D. Wexner
Department of Colorectal Surgery, Cleveland Clinic Florida,
3000 West Cypress Creek Road, Ft. Lauderdale, FL 33309-1743, USA

Johan N. Wiig
Department of Surgery, The Radium Hospital, Oslo, Norway

Rectal Cancer – Natural History of the Disease

Cancer of the Rectum: Epidemiology, Improvement in Survival and the Role of a National Cancer Registry

Frøydis Langmark

The Norwegian Cancer Registry – Organization and Reporting

The Norwegian Cancer Registry was established in 1951 and is based on obligatory reporting of all cancer cases and precancerous conditions. All hospitals in Norway report clinical data on every patient discharged with a diagnosis of neoplasia. The registry also receives copies of all working documents from pathologists (cytology, surgical specimens, autopsy). The pathology laboratory connections are a particularly important basis for the quality control and completeness of the registry. Each year, the registry receives information on approximately 20 000 new cancer patients plus follow-up information on those previously diagnosed. Close to 100% of all rectal cancers are reported. A sine qua non for the quality of the data is the unique national eleven-digit personal identification number which allows any individual to be traced from birth to death. Thus follow-up data with respect to survival is 100% [1].

Epidemiologic Background in Rectal Cancer

Colorectal cancer is a disease of the Western world (Table 1) [2]. It is the most prevalent cancer in USA, comprising 14% of the total cancer burden, with rectal cancer alone comprising 5% [3]. The descriptive data in Table 1 support the hypothesis that it is the lifestyle pattern in the Western world rather than any ethnic-genetic predisposing factors that explain the contrast in incidence between US whites and Japanese in Japan, since Japanese who have emigrated to USA have an incidence more similar to that of US whites than that of their country of origin.

Table 1. The incidence of cancer of the colon and rectum in various populations (Data abstracted from [2])

Country	Incidence (per 100 000 males per year)	
	Colon	Rectum
Nigeria	0.4	0.4
Japan	8.3	9.2
India	3.5	4.5
China	6.7	9.0
Colombia	4.5	3.4
Spain	6.6	6.2
Denmark	19.0	17.0
Poland-Urban	11.6	9.4
Romania	5.5	6.8
Canada	21.5	14.9
USA - White	25.6	14.6
USA - Black	28.4	6.7
USA - Japanese	26.7	15.3
USA - Chinese	25.8	17.9
USA - Spanish	18.8	11.4
Australia	21.5	12.8
New Zealand - Maori	9.0	9.8
New Zealand - Non Maori	25.5	16.1

Rectal cancer is more common among men than women, except in the youngest age group, where they are affected equally (Fig. 1) [4]. This supports the notion that risk factors for colorectal cancer in young patients include a much stronger component of genetic vulnerability than in the elderly, where different lifestyle patterns between the genders probably are the explanation

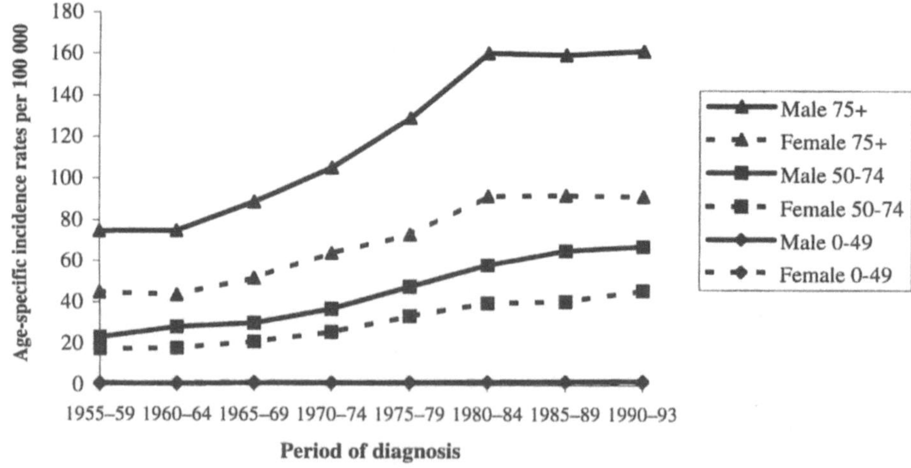

Fig. 1. Age-specific annual incidence rates of rectal cancer in Norway [4]

Table 2. Age-adjusted cancer incidence rates in Mormons and non-Mormons, Utah 1971–1985 (Data abstracted from [5])

Cancer site	Males				Females			
	Mormons	SE	Non-Mormons	SE	Mormons	SE	Non-Mormons	SE
Colon	23.6	0.7	39.0	1.5	19.4	0.5	29.2	1.1
Rectum	11.6	0.5	20.4	1.1	8.4	0.4	12.2	0.7

for the differing pattern in the incidence of rectal cancer. The data presented in Table 2 [5] lend further support to the important connection between lifestyle and rectal cancer, in that Mormons have a substantially lower incidence of colorectal cancer than non-Mormons.

In Norway, there was a 150% increase in the incidence of rectal cancer between the mid-1950s and the early 1990s (Fig. 2) [4]. This time trend also supports the lifestyle hypothesis. The increase in incidence of all cancers together was 50% during the same period, and the incidence of stomach cancer was even reduced by 50% [4].

Many risk factors, both genetic and acquired, have been identified which promote the development of colorectal cancer [6]. Although hereditary forms are important for many reasons, most colorectal cancers develop without any known risk factors except that they are most prevalent in societies that have a high intake of fat and calories as well as alcohol and tobacco consumption. In Norway, rectal cancer below the age of 50 years is rare and accounts for less than 1% of the total rectal cancer group [4].

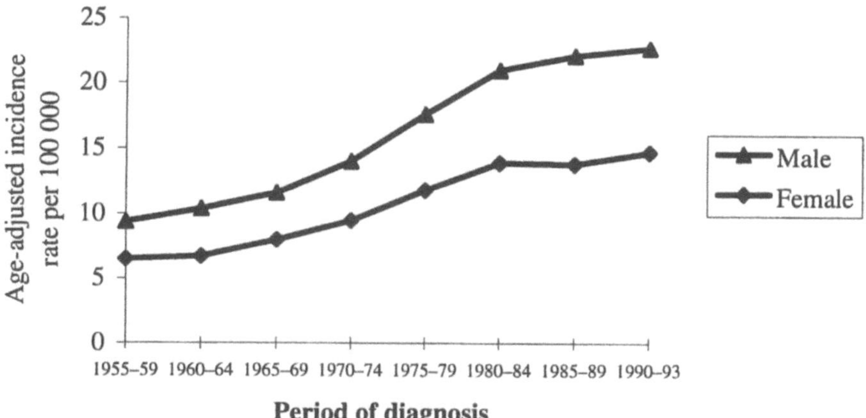

Fig. 2. Age-adjusted annual incidence rates of rectal cancer in Norway by sex and period of diagnosis (age-adjusted to the World Standard Population) [4]

Cancer Registry Data As a Basis for Survival Analyses

European Data

The International Agency for Research on Cancer (IARC) has recently published a comparative analysis of cancer outcome based on data from several European cancer registries [7]. The National Finnish and Danish Cancer Registries participated from the Nordic region. Most other countries represented in this study have more than one cancer registry, and each registry participated on its own. The publication contains the incidence and survival figures according to gender, age groups and time periods for most cancer forms.

Table 3 [7] shows the country-specific survival figures for rectal cancer. Even in a fairly homogeneous European population, we observe a marked difference in rectal cancer survival between countries, from more than 50% 5-year relative survival in Switzerland to around 20% in Poland. There are several explanations for such marked variations apart from the effects of treatment. Overall, data retrieval was incomplete with only a limited number of patients included from each country; for rectal cancer a total of approximately 45 000 patients were included for the entire study period (1978–1985). The basis for diagnosis varied, for instance 93% of colon cancers were verified microscopically in patients aged above 65 years in Switzerland compared with 40% in Poland. The basis for diagnosis for rectal cancer was not given. The availability of endoscopy, the aggressiveness in perfection of staging, the autopsy rates, and the verification of "Death Certificate Only" cases, all vary and may have contributed to the considerable differences observed (Fig. 3) [7]. Death certificate analysis was done for colon cancer and not for rectal cancer. In addition we must realize that marked differences exist between the Eastern and the Western part of Europe with regard to national death rates, from around

Table 3. Rectal cancer: average 5-year relative survival (diagnostic period 1978–1985; data abstracted from [7])

European countries (average)	Male (%)	Female (%)
	36	40
Switzerland	50	57
Finland	43	46
The Netherlands	41	47
Germany	40	42
France	39	45
Denmark	37	41
England	36	36
Spain	35	36
Italy	35	36
Estonia	30	39
Scotland	31	35
Poland	15	26

Fig. 3. The effect of tracing back Death Certificate Only cases and including them in Survival Computations. Data from Berrino et al. [7]

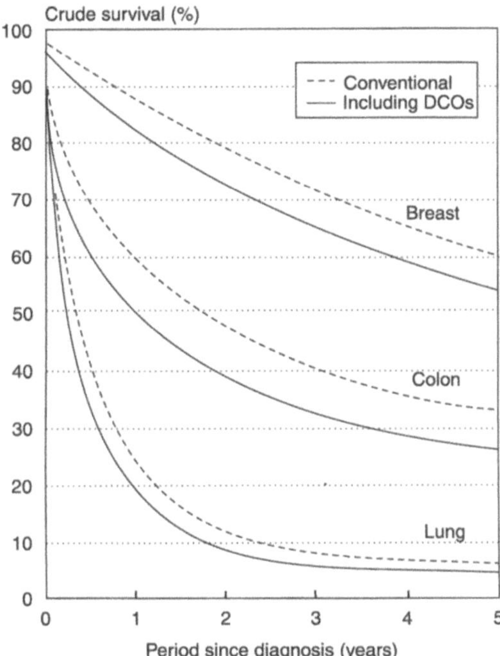

700 per 100 000 in Switzerland to approximately 1100 per 100 000 in Poland (sex- and age-standardized) [7].

A common problem in rectal cancer studies is the influence of anatomical subsite, i.e. whether or not cancer of the rectosigmoid is included, a location which lacks precise anatomical definition. Table 4 [7] illustrates this point; the proportion of rectosigmoid cancers varies from 5.3% to 28.9% of all colorectal cancers. Furthermore, in Estonia rectal cancer represents 49% of all colorectal cancers compared with 34.5% in Scotland (Table 4). Such site classification

Table 4. Rectum cancer by anatomical site in the European Study (Data abstracted from [7])

Site (ICD – 9 code)	Denmark		Estonia		Italy		Scotland		France	
	n	%[a,b]	n	%	n	%	n	%	n	%
Rectum, Total (154.0–154.8)	9440	(43.6)	1171	(49.1)	1132	(37.7)	4260	(34.5)	2345	(44.0)
Rectosigmoid junction (154.0)	1341	14.2	62	5.3	327	28.9	553	13.0	503	21.5
Rectum, NOS (154.1)	7766	82.3	1069	91.3	745	65.8	3578	84.0	1065	45.4
Other parts of rectum (154.8)	44	0.5	2	0.2	11	1.0	21	0.5	673	28.2

[a](within brackets): Percentage over the total number of colon and rectum cases (153.0–153.9 & 154.0–154.8)
[b]without brackets: Percentage over the total number of specified anatomic subcategories (153.0–153.8 and, respectively, 154.0–154.8)

problems will certainly influence treatment results [7]. Therefore, before we can confidently compare national survival figures we must know the basis for the data.

Nordic Data

The Nordic region is a much more homogeneous area than Europe, and the registries certainly operate more similarly to each other. The five Nordic cancer registries have recently published data on prediction of cancer incidence and prediction of cancer mortality in the Nordic countries [8, 9]. These predictions are based on trends in incidence and mortality up till 1988 plus population forecasts up to the period 2008–2012. Possible effects of recent preventive or therapeutic interactions are not included.

At the start of the study period, Denmark had the highest incidence rates for rectal cancer, but with time, a decreasing trend can be seen (Figs. 4 and 5) [8]. The incidence in Sweden, Finland and Iceland is increasing slightly, while Norway experienced a steep increase from 1960 to 1988. The predictions mirror this picture.

As to survival, Denmark has the worst survival rates the last 20 years (Figs. 6 and 7) [9]. The contrasts between the countries are remarkable considering the supposedly homogeneous geographic area and populations. Is the risk for developing rectal cancer higher in Norway or are variations in clinical practice (endoscopic activities, differing histopathological criteria) causing the differ-

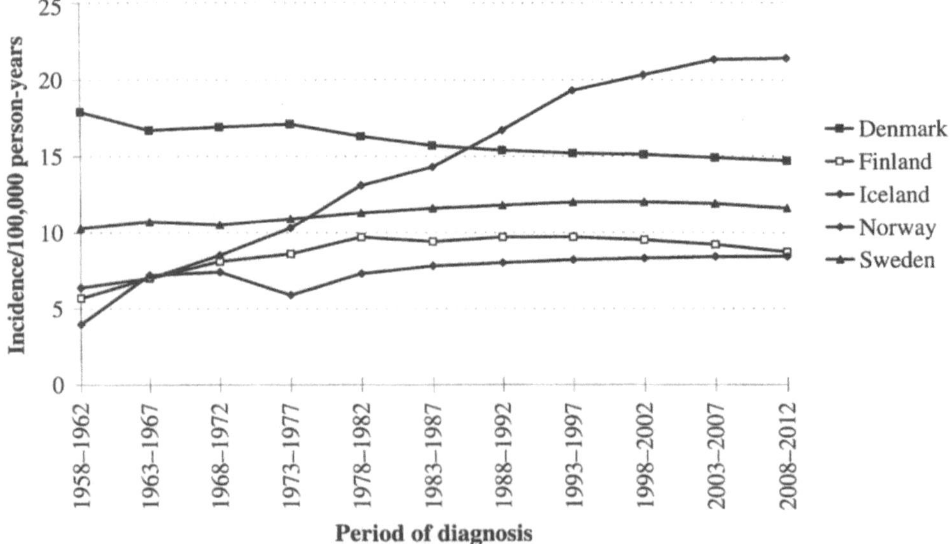

Fig. 4. Actual and predicted incidence trends in rectal cancer in men in the Nordic countries 1958–2012. Data from Engeland et al. [8]

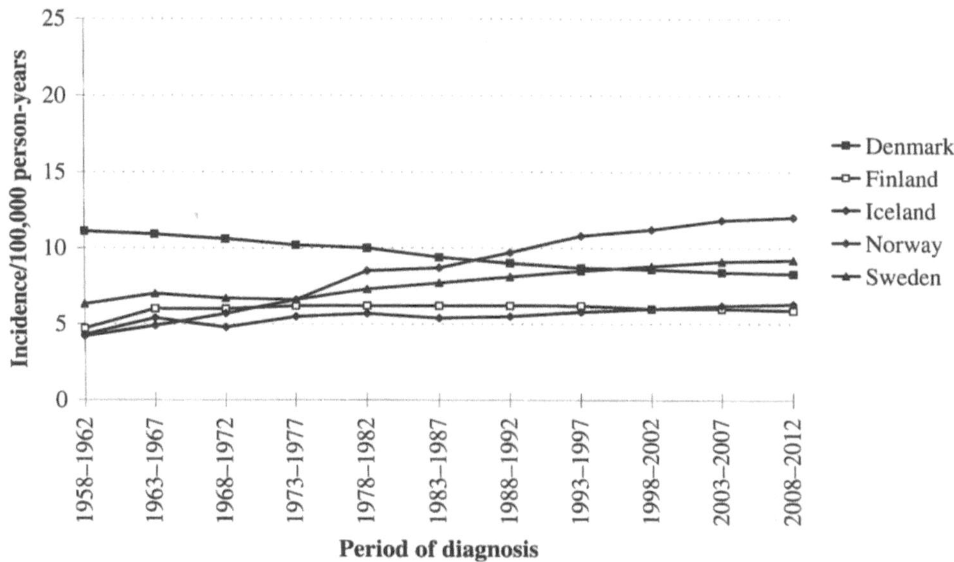

Fig. 5. Actual and predicted incidence trends in rectal cancer in women in the Nordic countries 1958–2012. Data from Engeland et al. [8]

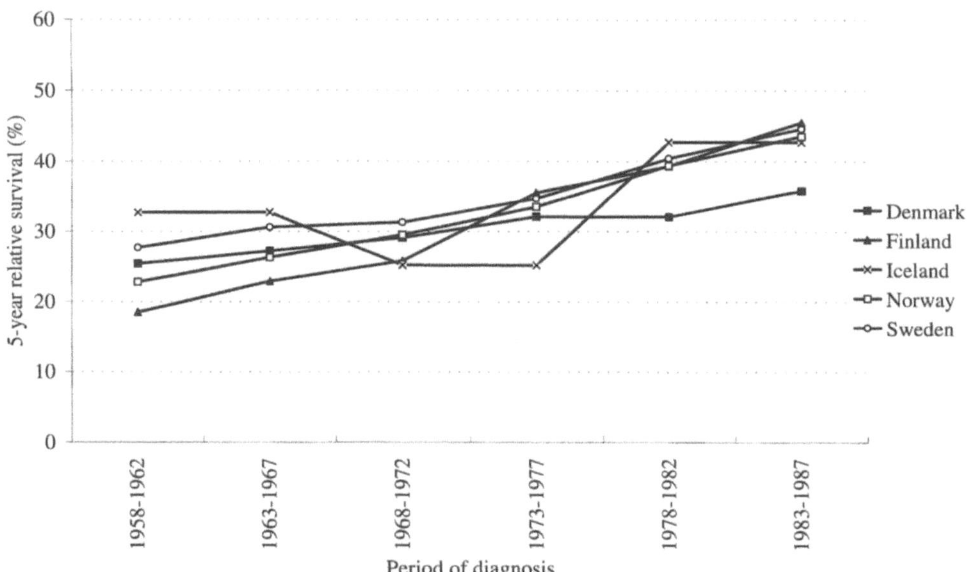

Fig. 6. Age-adjusted 5-year relative survival rates in rectal cancer in men in the Nordic countries 1958–1987. Data from Engeland et al. [9]

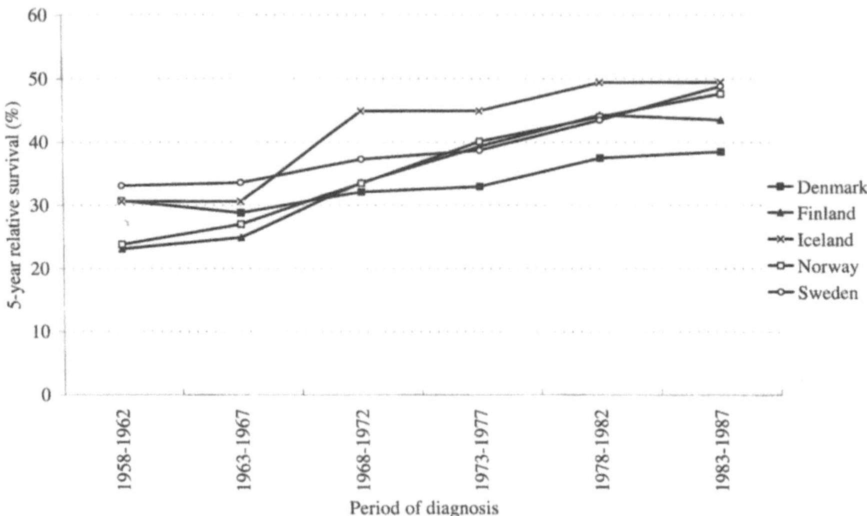

Fig. 7. Age-adjusted 5-year relative survival rates in rectal cancer in women in the Nordic countries 1958–1987. Data from Engeland et al. [9]

ences? Why has Denmark the worst survival for most cancers including rectal cancer? Do lifestyle patterns not only influence the risk and development of cancer but prognosis as well? We do not know for certain at this stage.

The Norwegian Cancer Registry and Research in Colorectal Cancer

Norway has a population of 4.5 million, and is divided into 20 counties, 450 municipalities, and 5 health regions. There are 4 medical schools, 6 university

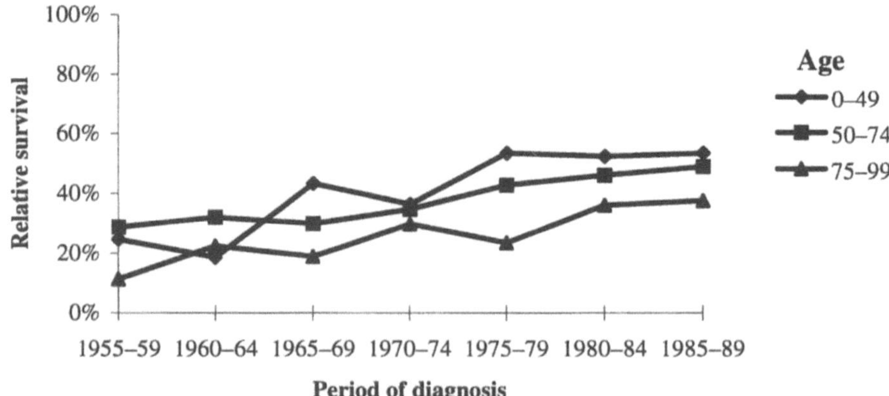

Fig. 8. Age-specific 5-year relative survival rates in rectal cancer according to period of diagnosis in men in Norway [4]

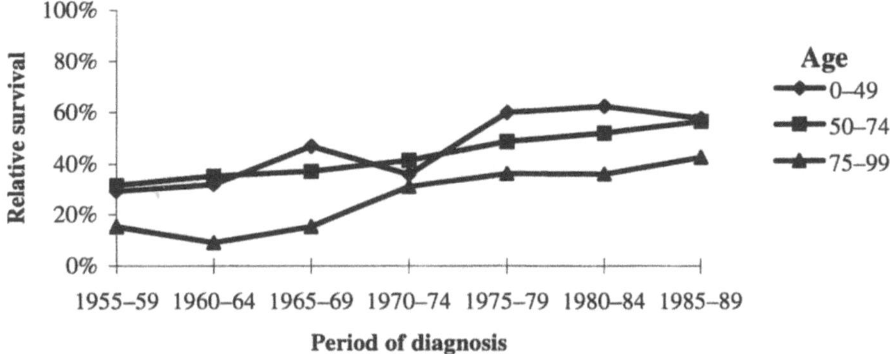

Fig. 9. Age-specific 5-year relative survival rates in rectal cancer according to period of diagnosis in women in Norway [4]

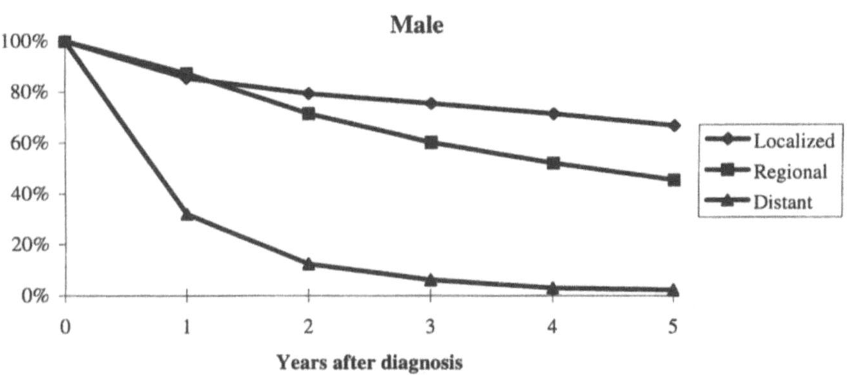

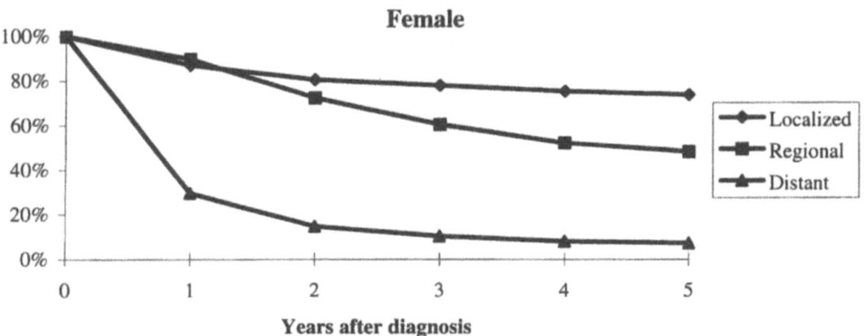

Fig. 10. Relative survival rates of male and female rectal cancer patients diagnosed in 1985–1989 by stage at diagnosis (For staging system, see text)[4]

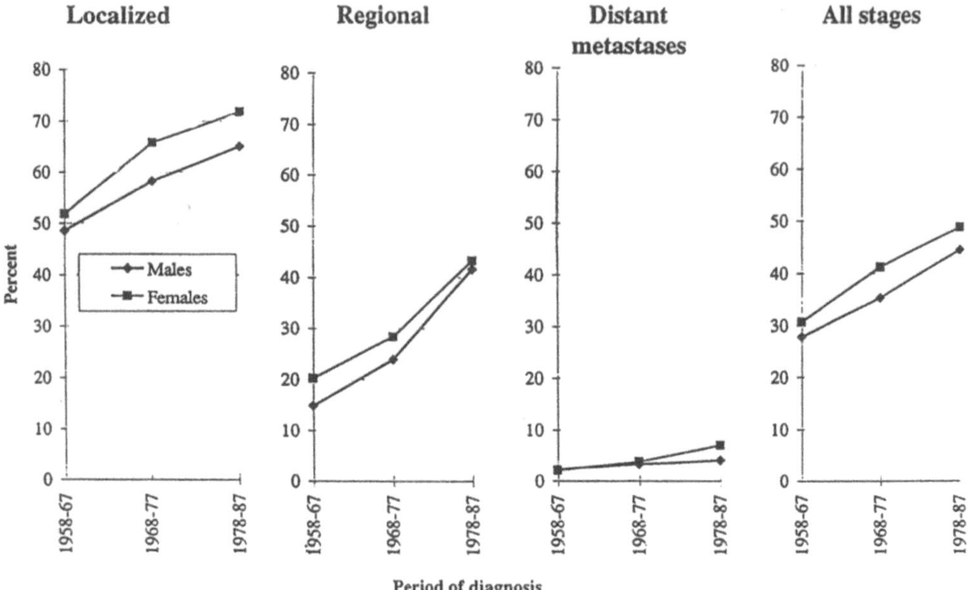

Fig. 11. Five-year relative survival rates in rectal cancer by stage and period of diagnosis in Norway [4]

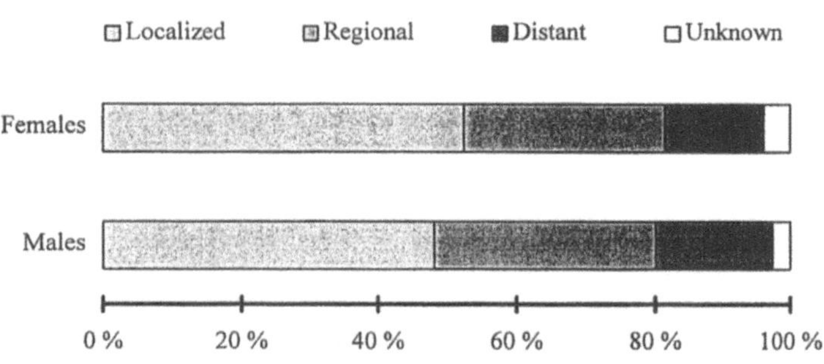

Fig. 12. Stage distribution of rectal cancer in Norway, 1989–1993 [4]

Table 5. Operative mortality and survival after curative surgery according to stage of disease (national data 1983–1987 [4])

Stage	Total	Perioperative *n*	Death %	Alive after 1 year	Relative survival 1 year	Alive after 5 years	Relative survival 5 years
Localized	1456	11	0.8	1320	94.8	885	78.1
Regional	1502	16	1.1	1272	88.3	543	45.7
Distant	385	8	2.1	165	44.6	17	5.5
All	3369	35	1.0	2777	86.1	1453	54.9

hospitals, and 60 county hospitals with surgical departments. Rectal cancer is the fourth most frequent cancer form among women (422 cases in 1992) and the fifth among men (535 cases in 1992), totalling 5% of all cancers in Norway in 1992 [1]. Colon cancer is twice as frequent as rectal cancer and does not occur more frequently in men than in women, as is typically observed for rectal cancer. However this gender contrast has become less apparent in the past few years. In 1992, rectal cancer accounted for 319 (1.4%) of all deaths among men, and 226 (1.3%) among women in Norway [10]. Among cancer deaths, rectal cancer mortality ranks high.

In Norway, 5-year relative survival in rectal cancer patients has improved from around 20% in the 1950s to around 50% in recent years for both men and women (Figs. 8 and 9) [4]. Several factors may explain this improvement such as earlier diagnosis through endoscopy, improved surgical techniques and better pre-, peri- and postoperative care, more precise diagnostic criteria and staging, and a better health of the population in general. However, the relative proportion of each factor cannot be assessed.

In the Norwegian Cancer Registry, the following stage definitions are used:

- *Localized.* Tumour confined to organ of origin without invasive growth in adjacent organs or regional lymph nodes
- *Regional.* Tumour with invasion of adjacent organs and/or regional lymph node metastasis
- *Distant.* Tumour spread to distant organs and/or distant lymph node metastasis [1].

The 5-year relative survival rates according to this staging system (Fig. 10) [4] is around 75% for localized disease, and around 5% for disease with distant metastases. When time periods are compared for each stage, we can demonstrate significant improvements in survival over time for localized and regional tumors, but not for distant spread of disease (Fig. 11) [4]. The stage distribution of rectal cancer for the last period (1989–1993) shows that fortunately relatively few patients have distant metastases at diagnosis (Fig. 12) [4].

The Norwegian Cancer Registry also records whether potentially radical surgery has been performed (Fig. 13) [4]. While less than 50% of the patients underwent radical surgery in the 1950s, more than 70% had such treatment in the 1990s. Table 5 [4] gives the distribution of patients according to tumour stage and perioperative deaths (defined as less than 1 month after surgery) and includes only those patients who actually underwent potentially local curative surgery (irrespective of whether distant spread was present). The proportion of patients with histological verification has improved from approximately 70% in the 1950s, to close to 100% in the 1990s (Fig. 14) [4]. Further analyses demonstrate that the improvement in verification is most pronounced in the oldest age group (Fig. 15) [4]. Long-term survival analyses up to 15 years show that patients who are still alive after 5 years have a survival rate a little below but close to the average for the population (Fig. 16) [4].

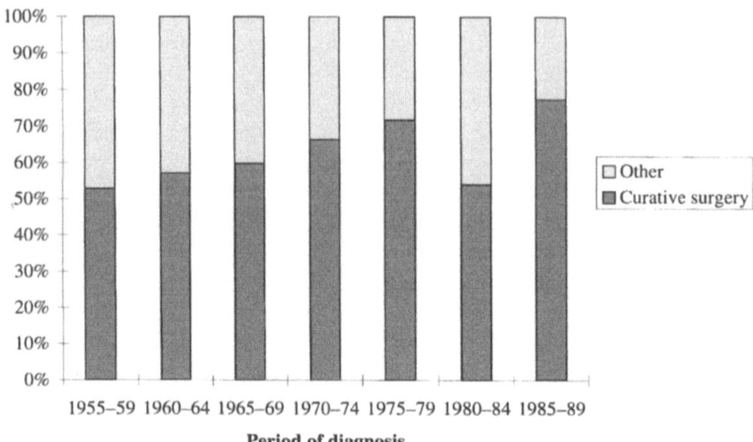

Fig. 13. Treatment of rectal cancer patients by period of diagnosis in Norway [4]

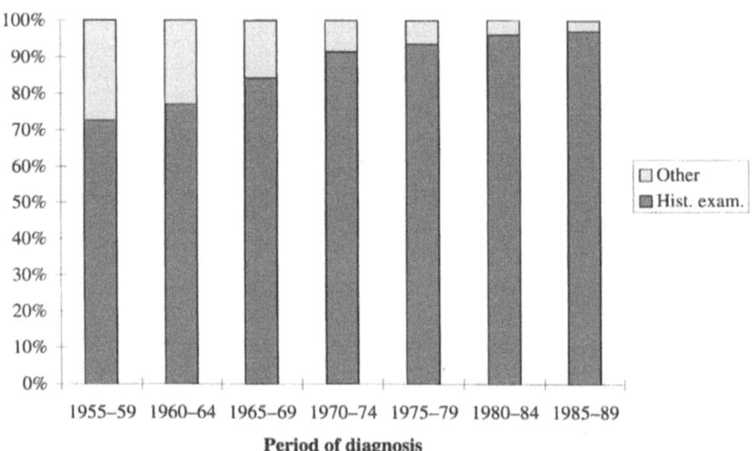

Fig. 14. Diagnostic basis by period of diagnosis in rectal cancer patients in Norway [4]

Can a Cancer Registry Contribute to Quality Control of Clinical Care?

End points other than death (e.g. local recurrence), knowledge of somatic adverse effects of therapy (e.g. leakage), knowledge of patients' quality of life (e.g. sexual functioning) and reliable and reasonable follow-up control methods are some of the important topics that should be included in "clinical care".

Since traditional registry data are based on diagnostic and therapeutic heterogeneity and insufficient follow-up, The Norwegian Cancer Registry started a National Colorectal Cancer Project in 1985 in close collaboration with surgeons, radiologists, pathologists and other health professionals, with the

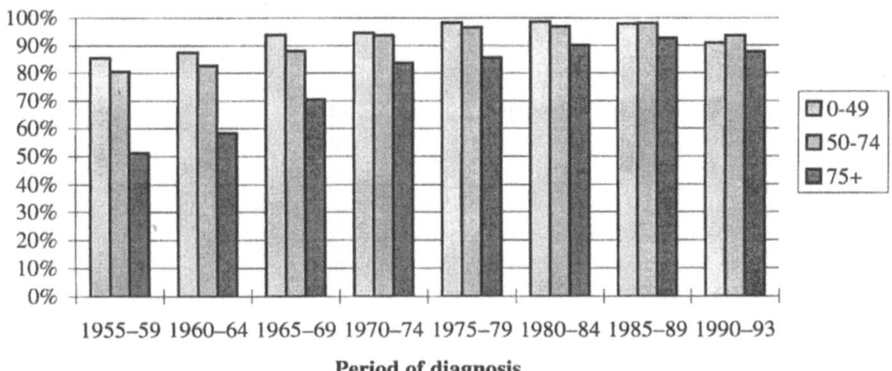

Fig. 15. Histological verification in rectal cancer patients by age and period in Norway [4]

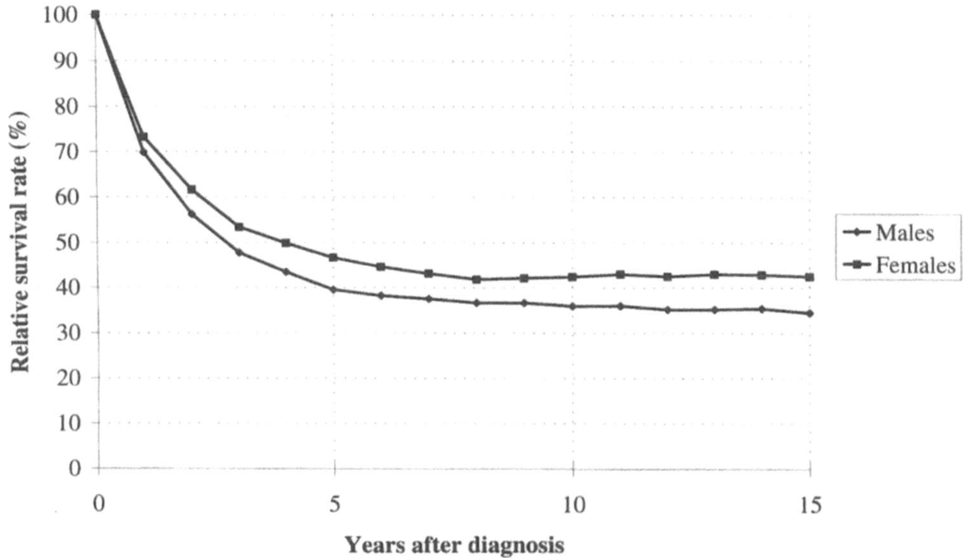

Fig. 16. Relative survival rates 0–15 years after diagnosis in rectal cancer patients from 1973 to 1977 in Norway [4]

purpose of improving diagnostics and treatment in colorectal cancer, including follow-up and surveillance. The concrete actions were aimed at earlier diagnosis of the primary cancer, identification of synchroneous tumours of the large intestine, improved primary treatment, earlier diagnosis and treatment of local recurrences, metachroneous new cancers in the bowel, and distant metastases in the liver or lung in supposedly curatively treated patients. The key factors for the success of this project were the inclusion in the registry of obligatory reporting, complete and high-quality data, efficient communication with the collaborators, good computer systems, and a scientifically competent interdisciplinary team, including medical and statistical expertise in the registry. Some of the data from this project are presented in Chap. 2 in this book.

Comments

Experience from The Norwegian Cancer Registry as well as from the EURO-CARE program leads us to conclude that cancer registries should be important collaborators in clinical cancer research.

References

1. The Cancer Registry of Norway (1992) Cancer in Norway. The Cancer Registry of Norway, Oslo
2. Hill MJ (1989) Aetiology of colorectal cancer: current concepts. Bailliere's Clin Gastroenterol 3:567–592
3. Steele Jr. G, Tepper BTM, Bruckner HW (1993) Adenocarcinoma of the colon and rectum. In: Holland JF et al (eds) Cancer Medicine 1993, 3rd edn, vol 2. pp 1493–1522
4. The Cancer Registry of Norway, Oslo (1996) Cancer in Norway 1993
5. Lyon JL, Gardner K, Gress RE (1994) Cancer incidence among Mormons and non-Mormons in Utah (United States) 1971–85: Cancer Causes Control 5:149–156
6. Cohen AM, Shank B, Friedman MA (1989) Colorectal cancer. In: DeVita et al (eds) Cancer principles and practice of oncology 3rd edn. pp 895–964
7. Berrino F,, Sant M, Verdecchia A, Capocaccia R, Hakulinen T, Estève J (1995) Survival of cancer patients in Europe. IARC Scientific Publications (No. 132), Lyon
8. Engeland A, Haldorsen T, Tretli S et al (1993) Prediction of cancer incidence in the Nordic countries up to the years 2000 and 2010. APMIS 101 [Suppl. 38]
9. Engeland A, Haldorsen T, Tretli S et al (1995) Prediction of cancer mortality in the Nordic countries up to the years 2000 and 2010. APMIS 103 [Suppl. 49]
10. Central Bureau of Statistics (1994) Causes of death. Statistics Norway

CHAPTER 2

Results of Rectal Cancer Treatment: A National Experience

Jarle Norstein and Frøydis Langmark

Introduction

Data from the Norwegian Cancer Registry demonstrate that survival following rectal cancer treatment in Norway has been poor, particularly in patients with lymph node metastases (Chap. 1). Local recurrences and distant metastases were responsible for deaths, but the relative importance of these two patterns of failure were unknown. Reports published in the early 1980s [19, 21] indicated that secondary surgery for recurrences and metastases could result in a survival benefit for individual patients. Carcinoembryonic antigen (CEA) guided second look surgery in asymptomatic patients seemed to be particularly beneficial [19, 21, 33].

A Norwegian prospective multicenter cohort study (Norwegian Colorectal Cancer Project, NCCP) of curatively treated colorectal cancer patients less than 75 years of age was designed in 1985 to evaluate the impact of specific surveillance methods on the ability to detect and treat recurrences and metachronous metastases at an asymptomatic stage. The study included 279 patients with curatively treated rectal cancer from 40 hospitals during a 2-year period. In this carefully followed cohort, 31.5% of patients who underwent curative operations eventually developed local recurrences after a median observation time of 8 years (Norstein et al., manuscript in preparation).

The participating hospitals in the NCCP cohort study were predominantly small and intermediate-sized community and district general hospitals, with only one of seven university hospitals in Norway participating. Although the referral structure in Norway is such that individual hospitals with few exceptions treat all rectal cancer patients in a defined geographic area, we could not eliminate the possibility that selection bias contributed to the poor results. We therefore retrieved information from all Norwegian hospitals (n=64) on all rectal cancer patients treated in a 2-year period in order to obtain completely unselected data on recurrences and survival.

National Data on Patients with Cancer of the Rectum

During the inclusion period of the NCCP from September 1986 to August 1988, a total of 1049 patients less than 75 years of age were diagnosed with invasive rectal cancer in Norway (population 4.3 million). Invasive rectal cancer was defined as carcinoma invading at least the submucosa [31]. The curative resection rates were 70.0% in women and 73.6% in men (Table 1). Extensive clinical information on *all* curatively operated rectal cancer patients ($n=757$) was retrieved by The Norwegian Cancer Registry and stored in separate files. This was possible due to the obligatory reporting to the Cancer Registry of all diagnosed cancer patients in Norway (Chap. 1). There is a dual reporting system, with independent notification from both the pathologist and by the clinician treating the patient. All patients are identified by a unique 11-digit national identification number.

The retrieved information comprised clinical notifications from the hospitals with information on diagnosis, staging, and treatment of all rectal cancer patients. Photocopies of all pathology reports were available. Follow up results on the 279 patients included in the prospective NCCP study were also available. In 1993 and 1994, the Norwegian Cancer Registry mailed letters to all hospitals with name lists of the 478 additional patients that had been registered by the Cancer Registry, but not included in the prospective study, to provide follow up information on local recurrences and distant metastases. A 100% response rate was achieved.

All Norwegian hospitals treating rectal cancer were owned by the government or the municipialities. No rectal cancer treatment was offered by private hospitals. Patients were generally treated at hospitals defined by their residence. Patients who received preoperative radiotherapy at regional radiotherapy units due to primary irresectability were generally operated upon at their primary hospital. The university departments did not generally serve as referral centers for rectal cancer, but had defined primary catchment areas.

Table 1. Proportion of curative and palliative resections in patients less than 75 years of age diagnosed with invasive cancer of the rectum in Norway during the 2-year period September 1986–August 1988

	Women		Men		All	
	n	%	*n*	%	*n*	%
Curative procedures	284	70	473	74	757	72
Palliative resections	61	15	91	14	152	15
No tumor-directed surgery	61	15	79	12	140	13
All patients diagnosed	406	100	643	100	1049	100

An important difference exists between patients included in the prospective NCCP study and the other patients; in the former study patients were included on the basis of the information available on the day of primary surgery, without any knowledge of results of pathology evaluations, thus including ten patients in whom the specimen later proved to have positive resection margins.

Photocopies of the operative reports were retrieved for all but two patients, in whom sufficient information was collected from the pathology report. No operative report mentioned the mesorectum or stated that this structure was removed. A large number of operative reports specifically mentioned that a manual dissection was carried out. We were not able to identify any patient where the operative report suggested that the total mesorectal excision (TME) technique had been used [7, 10, 11, 17].

The pathology reports described the distal intramural margin in specimens from major rectal resections. The distal margin was measured by the surgeon or by the pathologist in 371 of 391 patients who had undergone an anterior resection. The circumferential margin [2, 26] was described in a minority of cases as the "deep resection margin", particularly if this margin was grossly invaded by tumor. Information on this parameter was too incomplete for inclusion in further analyses.

Hospitals were categorised by treatment volume (annual caseload) into hospitals treating less than ten cases per year ($n=53$) and hospitals treating ten cases or more per year ($n=11$). Hospitals were also divided into university clinical departments ($n=7$), district general hospitals ($n=11$), and community hospitals ($n=46$). Operating surgeons ($n=291$) were divided into three groups, namely, specialists in surgical gastroenterology (who had fulfilled a 3-year fellowship following residency, $n=44$), consultant general surgeons without specialist status in surgical gastroenterology ($n=88$), and surgeons in training ($n=159$). The attendance of a specialist in surgical gastroenterology or a general surgeon during the operation was noted. Seven of 64 hospitals had a "documented interest in rectal cancer surgery", i.e., those arranging post-graduate courses in colorectal cancer surgery ($n=2$), and/or those with a documented research interest in rectal cancer surgery (publication of articles or theses on rectal cancer surgery) ($n=5$).

According to the criteria set by the Norwegian Cancer Registry, patients with tumors less than 20 cm from the anal verge as measured with a rigid procto-scope were classified as rectal. In order to allow comparison with other studies, we subdivided the rectum into four parts: Lower rectum (0–5 cm from the anal verge), mid-rectum (6–10 cm), upper rectum (11–15 cm), and rectosigmoid (16–19 cm from the anal verge).

Local recurrence was defined as recurrent tumor in the pelvis, perineum or the abdominal scar [18]. The diagnosis was based on histologic confirmation or undisputable clinical evidence of recurrent disease. Distant metastases were defined as metastases outside the pelvis, exclusive of implantation metastases in the abdominal scar. Tumors were staged according to the original Dukes' staging system [5] and later restaged by the principal author to the TNM system [12, 31, 32].

Adjuvant radiation therapy was administered to 52 patients (6.9%), pre-operatively to 16 patients, postoperatively to 35 patients, and both pre- and postoperatively to one patient.

Statistics

Univariate analyses were performed using contingency tables and chi-square statistics. In time-to-event analyses risk of local recurrence was calculated by the product-limit method according to Kaplan and Meier [15]. Failures were local recurrences. Patients dying from cancer without local recurrence or death from other causes were censored. Differences between recurrence curves were tested for statistical significance by the generalised Wilcoxon test as modified by Tarone and Ware [30]. Cox proportional hazard regression analyses were performed utilising a backward-stepping procedure. Significant variables from the univariate analysis were selected for the multivariate analysis. In addition, statistically nonsignificant variables thought to be clinically significant such as degree of tumor differentiation, the volume (caseload) variable, and distal margin length were included in the initial model.

National Results

Primary Surgical Management of Rectal Cancer

Anterior resection was performed in 391 patients (52%), including one patient who received subtotal colectomy. A local resection of tumor was done in 35 patients (5%). Seventeen patients (2%) received a Hartmann's resection. An abdominoperineal resection (APR) was done in 314 patients (41%).

Local Recurrences

Local recurrences were diagnosed in 215 patients (28.4%) after a follow-up of 6.5–8.5 years (Fig. 1). Local recurrences without evidence of distant metastases

Table 2. Local recurrences alone and local recurrences in combination with distant recurrences

	Local recurrences alone		Local and distant recurrences		All	
	n	%	n	%	n	%
Dukes' stage A (TNM stage I)	26	72.2	10	27.8	36	100
Dukes' stage B (TNM stage II)	42	52.5	38	47.5	80	100
Dukes' stage C (TNM stage III)	45	45.5	54	54.5	99	100
All stages	113	52.6	102	47.4	215	100

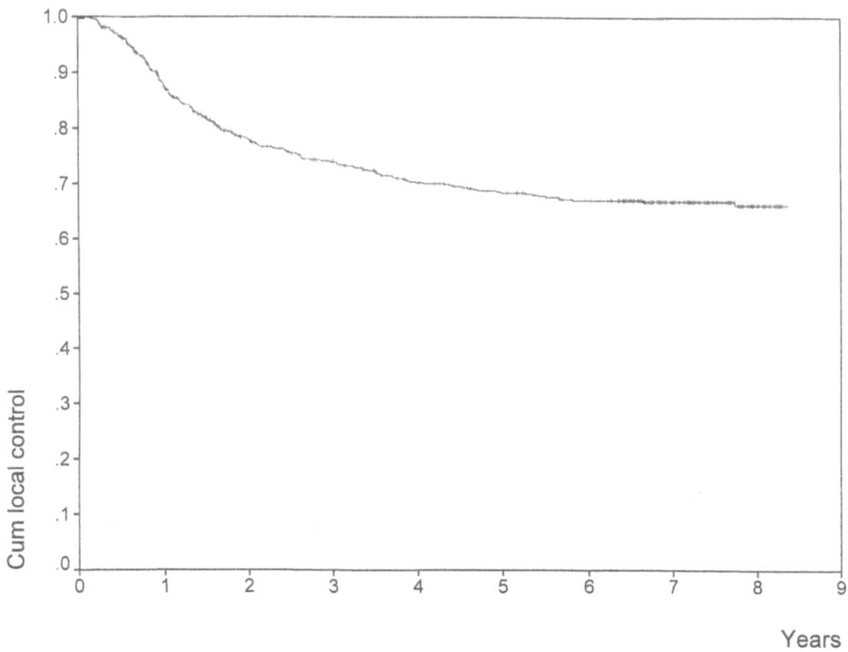

Fig. 1. Time to local recurrence ($n=757$)

Table 3. Local recurrence (%) by Dukes' (UICC/TNM) stage and tumor distance from the anal verge ($n=757$)

	Distance from anal verge (cm)			
	0–5 cm	6–10 cm	11–15 cm	16–19 cm
Dukes' stage A (TNM stage I)	24.1	18.1	4.3	0.0
Dukes' stage B (TNM stage II)	41.4	32.1	20.4	14.3
Dukes' stage C (TNM stage III)	36.5	41.6	42.1	31.8

were found in 53% of patients with local recurrence (Table 2). Subdivison by distance from the anal verge and Dukes' (TNM) stage demonstrated a distinctive pattern of recurrences (Table 3). In patients with Dukes' stage A and B tumors (TNM stage I and II), the recurrence rate was dependent on distance from the anal verge, with a diminishing frequency of local recurrences with increasing tumor distance from the anal verge, from 24.1% in the lower rectum to 0% in the rectosigmoid in Dukes' A cases ($p<0.01$), and from 41.4% to 14.3% in Dukes' B cases ($p<0.01$). There was no significant relation between local recurrence rate and distance from the tumor to the anal verge in patients with Dukes' C tumors (TNM stage III) ($p=0.8$; n.s.).

There was no significant relationship between operative procedure and local recurrence. Local procedures, anterior resections and APR (analyzed together with Hartmann's resections) had local recurrence rates of 31.5%, 25.8%, and 31.1%, respectively ($p=0.3$; n.s.).

Perforation of the rectum during the operation occurred in 43 patients. A local recurrence later developed in 19 patients (44%). Patients with a distal margin of less than 1 cm, but no infiltration in the distal margin, had a local recurrence rate of 31.3% (26 of 83). In patients with a distal resection margin of more than 1 cm, no relation existed between local recurrence rate and the length of distal margin.

Local recurrence rate was unrelated to age or sex and there was no relation to hospital treatment volume. In univariate analysis a significant relation existed between hospital type and local recurrence rate ($p<0.05$). University hospitals had a local recurrence rate of 22%, while district general hospitals had a local recurrence rate of 34%, and community hospitals had 30% local recurrences. Hospitals with a documented interest in rectal cancer surgery (see definition above), had a local recurrence rate of 14%, while hospitals without such an expressed interest had a recurrence rate of 33% ($p<0.0001$).

The median number of patients operated on per year per surgeon was *one*. Three surgeons performed five or more procedures per year, no individual surgeon had done more than seven procedures per year. A relationship between caseload per surgeon and local recurrence rate could therefore not be determined. Local recurrence rate was unrelated to the attendence during the operation of a consultant surgeon or a surgeon specialized in surgical gastroenterology. Patients who were operated upon by surgeons in training had a significantly lower local recurrence rate (24.1%) than patients who were operated upon by a consultant surgeon (33.6%) or a surgeon specialised in surgical gastroenterology (30.6%; $p<0.05$). The difference was most marked in patients with Dukes' stage A (TNM stage I); 6.2% of patients operated on by a surgeon in training had local recurrence, while patients operated on by consultants or surgical gastroenterologists had 22.1% and 25.5% local recurrences ($p<0.002$).

Patients who had received radiotherapy preoperatively had a local recurrence rate of 40.0%, and patients who had postoperative radiotherapy had 39.1% local recurrences. One patient who received pre- and postoperative radiotherapy was recurrence-free.

Within 2 years after the primary operation 151 (70%) of the local recurrences were diagnosed. Only 36% of recurrences eventually developing in patients with Dukes' A (TNM stage I) primaries were diagnosed within 2 years and median time from the primary operation to the diagnosis of local recurrence was 29 months. In Dukes' B (TNM stage II) tumors, 70% of local recurrences were diagnosed at 2 years (median time to local recurrence 15 months) and 82% of Dukes' C (TNM stage III) tumor recurrences were diagnosed within 2 years (median time to local recurrence 12 months).

If only high-risk patients were considered, as defined by Krook and Moertel [16] and MacFarlane and Heald [17] comprising patients with transmural growth or lymph node metastases (Dukes' stage B and C, TNM stage II and III),

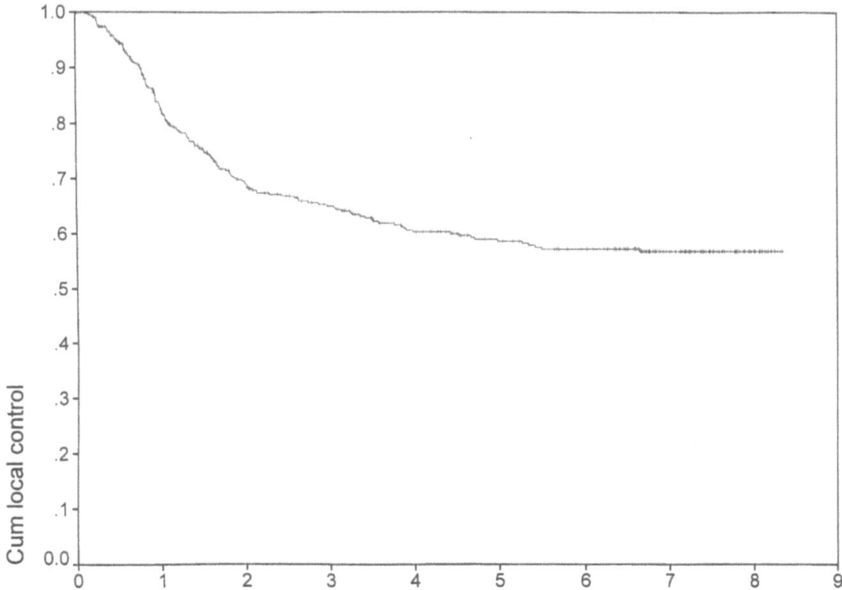

Fig. 2. Time to local recurrence in high-risk cases (n=475)

a subgroup of 475 patients could be defined with such tumors located less than 16 cm from the anal verge. In this patient group, 167 local recurrences (34.6%) were found. Analysis by actuarial method, censoring for patients dying of metastases or other causes (thus no longer at risk for local recurrence) showed an estimated local recurrence rate of 41.3% in this high-risk group (Fig. 2), and 52.2% in Dukes stage C (TNM stage III) patients.

Multivariate Analysis of Risk Factors for Local Recurrence

Only stage (Dukes'; TNM), distance from the anal verge, and the training level of the operator emerged as significant variables in the multivariate analysis (Table 4). Hospital type, a significant risk factor for local recurrence in the univariate analysis, was not an independent risk factor in the multivariate analysis. The variable "documented interest in rectal cancer surgery", however, when substituted for hospital type in the model, had a significant independent effect. The relative risk of local recurrence in hospitals without an expressed interest in rectal cancer surgery as compared with hospitals with such an interest was 2.6 (95% CI 1.7–4.0).

Survival

Operative mortality within 30 days was 1.6%, within 60 days 2.0%. Crude 5-year survival was 55.2 per cent (95% confidence interval, CI, 51.7–58.7%). The

Table 4. Multivariate analysis: independent risk factors for local recurrence of rectal cancer

Variable	Relative risk	95% Confidence interval
Stage		
Dukes' stage A (TNM stage I)	1[a]	
Dukes' stage B (TNM stage II)	2.4	1.6–3.6
Dukes' stage C (TNM stage III)	4.1	2.9–6.2
Distance from anal verge		
<6 cm	2.5	1.3–4.6
6–10 cm	2.1	1.1–3.9
11–15 cm	1.5	0.8–2.7
>16 cm	1[a]	
Surgeon's training level		
In training	1[a]	
Consultant	1.5	1.1–2.1
Surgical gastroenterologist	1.3	0.9–2.0

[a]Reference value

5-year survival rate was 77% in Dukes' stage A (TNM stage I), 48% in Dukes' stage B (TNM stage II), and 35% in Dukes' stage C (TNM stage III) (Fig. 3). Five-year survival in high risk cases was 44% (Fig. 4).

The estimated 5-year survival survival rate after diagnosis of local recurrence was 7.7% (95% CI 3.9–11.6%); nine patients have lived more than 5 years

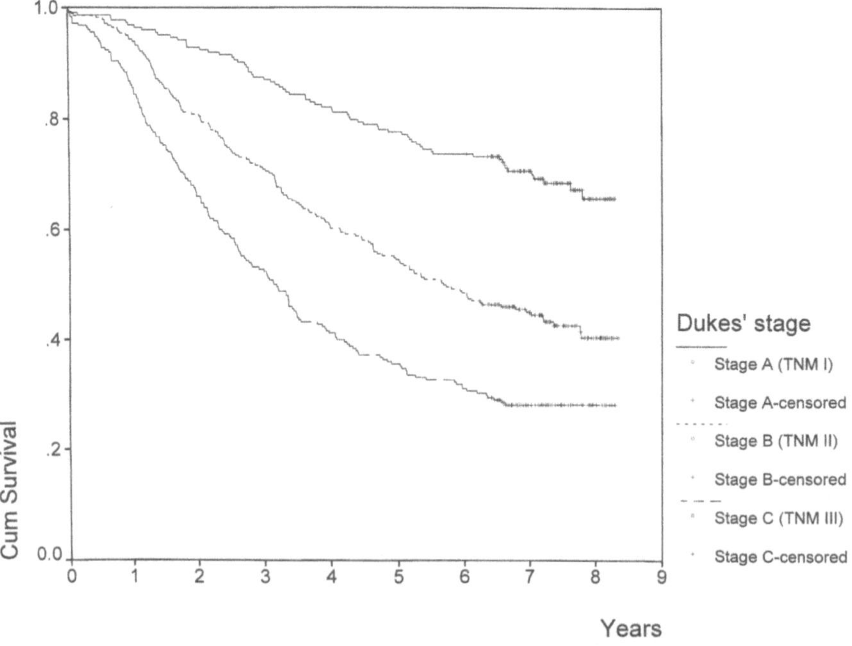

Fig. 3. Survival by stage (*n*=757)

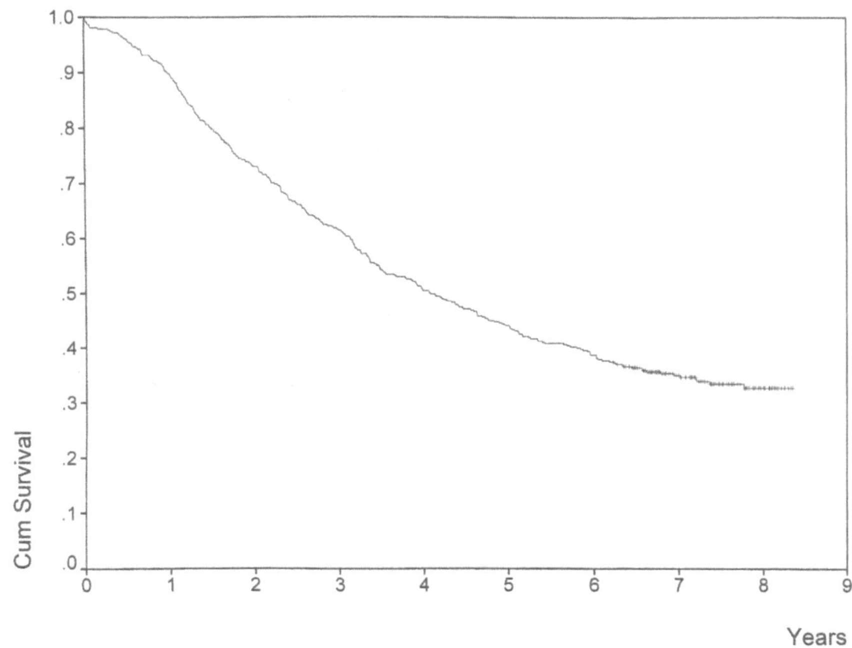

Fig. 4. Survival in high-risk cases (n=475)

after diagnosis of a local recurrence. In the 113 cases with local recurrence and no evidence of distant metastases the 5-year survival rate was 13.7% (95% CI 6.7–20.7%). In the remaining 102 patients with evidence of local recurrence and metastatic disease, the projected 5-year survival rate was 2.0%, with one observed 5-year survivor.

Comments

The results of this population-based national study confirms data published by others on conventional surgery for rectal cancer [3, 4, 22, 23, 25], documenting a high rate of local recurrences. The favorable operative mortality rate of 1.6% within 30 days of surgery indicated that the general surgical management was excellent. In spite of the low operative mortality, 5-year survival rates were poor.

A high local recurrence rate in Dukes' stage A patients (TNM stage I), is highly suggestive of suboptimal surgical technique. The length of the distal margin of the specimen, when the margin was not infiltrated with cancer, did not predict outcome. This is in accordance with the results from the Large Bowel Cancer Project [23]. The data on circumferential margin involvement, shown in other studies to be of great prognostic importance [2], could not be analyzed due to incomplete data.

The majority of local recurrences, in particular in Dukes' stage A cases (TNM stage I), was localised in the pelvis with no evidence of distant metastases. In spite of this, the results of treatment of the recurrences were generally unfavorable, in accordance with results summarized by Abulafi and Williams [1]. Gagliardi et al. recently published a study showing an 18% 5-year survival rate after resection of rectal cancer recurrence [8]. The potential benefits of improved radicality of the primary operative procedure are evident.

Radiotherapy was used infrequently and in selected patients only. The few patients receiving radiotherapy in the present study had advanced disease or doubt about the radicality of the surgical treatment. The poor results in irradiated patients in the present study do not allow any conclusions to be drawn with regard to the efficiency of adjuvant therapy in unselected, high-risk patients (Dukes' stage B and C, TNM stages II–III).

Our attempt to account for the surgeon variable, shown in previous studies to be of prognostic importance [13, 24], was precluded by the large number of surgeons performing the procedures, resulting in a median number of procedures per surgeon of one curative rectal cancer operation per year. Only three surgeons performed five or more procedures per year, and no individual surgeon did more than seven procedures per year. The finding that experienced surgeons as a category did not influence the outcome favorably may be regarded as a consequence of the lack of adequate training and specialized interest.

A selection feature may be responsible for the finding that surgeons in training actually had a lower recurrence rate than their more experienced colleagues, even though this finding persisted in a multivariate analysis adjusting for case severity. Hospital caseload or hospital type was unrelated to outcome. The variable "documented interest in rectal cancer surgery" came out as a highly significant predictor of local recurrence. This finding leads us to believe that competence specific to the technical features of rectal cancer surgery is of importance for the outcome. However, the use of this post-hoc variable may be criticized due to its subjectivity, and its validity would have been greater if hospitals were preassigned to "interest" categories.

There was no significant difference in local recurrence rate in the population that was investigated retrospectively and the population followed up prospectively with a rigorous regimen. This indicates that retrospective studies may give acceptable results if follow-up is complete, when the outcome parameters are limited to survival and local recurrence rates. Local recurrences will rarely remain undiagnosed due to their severity of symptoms.

The frequency and pattern of recurrence in the present study closely mirrors the results from Memorial Sloan-Kettering Cancer Center from the time period 1968–1976 as described by Pilipshen et al. [25] and Enker et al. [6], following conventional resection or extended pelvic lymphadenectomy. The Memorial Sloan-Kettering series showed an extremely low survival rate of 3.8% in patients with local recurrence in spite of intensive treatment of recurrences, comparable to the 7.7% survival rate for patients with local recurrence in the present study. Long-term survival in patients with local recurrence was almost confined to patients without distant metastases.

How can the results be improved? In Norway, we have chosen to reorganize rectal cancer surgery and train experienced surgeons with workshops and demonstration operations by experts [9, 29]. The auditing of this initiative is organized as a population-based prospective follow-up cohort, and concomitant controls with patients operated on by conventional methods. This design is weaker than a randomized study, but retains some of its virtues; in particular, there are no exclusions. The advancement of knowledge in surgery should not be paralyzed by the inability to perform randomized trials. Alternatives to randomization do exist which may be used to evaluate surgical problems and controversies [14, 20]. The alternatives to randomized studies as described in the present paper are not readily available in most countries, and this may in part be the reason why such designs have been sparsely discussed in the literature of clinical research methods [27, 28]. The Scandinavian countries, and in particular Norway, with a very clinically oriented cancer registry, may serve as a clinical research laboratory to the international surgical community.

References

1. Abulafi AM, Williams NS (1994) Local recurrence of colorectal cancer: the problem, mechanisms, management and adjuvant therapy (Review). Br J Surg 81:7–19
2. Adam IJ, Mohamdee MO, Martin IG, Scott N, Finan PJ, Johnston D, Dixon MF, Quirke P (1994) Role of circumferential margin involvement in the local recurrence of rectal cancer. Lancet 344:707–711
3. Athlin L, Bengtsson NO, Stenling R (1988) Local recurrence and survival after radical resection of rectal carcinoma. Acta Chir Scand 154:225–229
4. Carlsson U, Lasson Å, Ekelund G (1987) Recurrence rates after curative surgery for rectal carcinoma, with special reference to their accuracy. Dis Colon Rectum 30:431–434
5. Dukes CE (1932) The classification of cancer of the rectum. J Pathol 35:323–332
6. Enker WE, Pilipshen SJ, Heilweil ML, Stearns MWJ, Janov AJ, Hertz REL, Sternberg SS (1986) En bloc pelvic lymphadenectomy and sphincter preservation in the surgical management of rectal cancer. Ann Surg 203:426–433
7. Enker WE, Thaler HT, Cranor ML, Polyak T (1995) Total mesorectal excision in the operative treatment of carcinoma of the rectum. J Am Coll Surg 181:335–346
8. Gagliardi G, Hawley PR, Hershman MJ, Arnott SJ (1995) Prognostic factors in surgery for local recurrence of rectal cancer. Br J Surg 82:1401–1405
9. Heald RJ (1995) Total mesorectal excision is optimal surgery for rectal cancer: a Scandinavian consensus. Br J Surg 82:1297–1299
10. Heald RJ, Husband EM, Ryall RD (1982) The mesorectum in rectal cancer surgery-the clue to pelvic recurrence? Br J Surg 69:613–616
11. Heald RJ, Ryall RD (1986) Recurrence and survival after total mesorectal excision for rectal cancer. Lancet I:1479–1482
12. Hermanek P, Sobin LH (1987) TNM classification of malignant tumours. Edited by Union Internationale Contre le Cancer. Springer, Berlin Heidelberg New York, p 197
13. Hermanek P, Wiebelt H, Staimmer D, Riedl S (1995) Prognostic factors of rectum carcinoma-experience of the German Study Group Colo-Rectal Carcinoma SGCRC. Tumori 81[Suppl]:60–64
14. Hu X, Wright JG, McLeod RS, Lossing A, Walters BC (1996) Observational studies as alternatives to randomized clinical trials in surgical clinical research. Surgery 119:473–475
15. Kaplan EL, Meier P (1958) Nonparametric estimation from incomplete observations. J Am Stat Assoc 53:457–481

16. Krook JE, Moertel CG, Gunderson LL, Wieand HS, Collins RT, Beart RW, Kubista TP, Poon MA, Meyers WC, Mailliard JA et al (1991) Effective surgical adjuvant therapy for high-risk rectal carcinoma. N Engl J Med 324:709–715
17. MacFarlane JK, Ryall RD, Heald RJ (1993) Mesorectal excision for rectal cancer. Lancet 341:457–460
18. Marsh PJ, James RD, Schofield PF (1995) Definition of local recurrence after surgery for rectal carcinoma. Br J Surg 82:465–468
19. Martin EW Jr, Minton JP, Carey LC (1985) CEA-directed second-look surgery in the asymptomatic patient after primary resection of colorectal carcinoma. Ann Surg 202:310–317
20. McLeod RS, Wright JG, Solomon MJ, Hu X, Walters BC, Lossing Al (1996) Randomized controlled trials in surgery: issues and problems. [Review]. Surgery 119:483–486
21. Minton JP, Hoehn JL, Gerber DM, Horsley S, Connolly DP, Salwan F, Fletcher WS, Cruz AB Jr., Gatchell FG, Oviedo M, Meyer KK, Leffall LD Jr., Berk RS, Stewart PA, Kurucz SE (1984) Results of a 400-patient carcinoembryonic antigen second-look colorectal cancer study. Cancer 55:1284–1290
22. Påhlman L, Glimelius B (1984) Local recurrences after surgical treatment for rectal carcinoma. Acta Chir Scand 150:331–335
23. Phillips RK, Hittinger R, Blesovsky L, Fry JS, Fielding LP (1984) Local recurrence following 'curative' surgery for large bowel cancer: II. The rectum and rectosigmoid. Br J Surg 71:17–20
24. Phillips RK, Hittinger R, Blesovsky L, Fry JS, Fielding LP (1984) Local recurrence following 'curative' surgery for large bowel cancer: I. The overall picture. Br J Surg 71:12–16
25. Pilipshen SJ, Heilweil M, Quan SH, Sternberg SS, Enker WE (1984) Patterns of pelvic recurrence following definitive resections of rectal cancer. Cancer 53:1354–1362
26. Quirke P, Durdey P, Dixon MF, Williams NS (1985) Local recurrence of rectal adenocarcinoma due to inadequate surgical resection. Histopathological study of lateral tumour spread and surgical excision. Lancet II:996–999
27. Solomon MJ, Laxamana A, Devore L, McLeod RS (1994) Randomized controlled trials in surgery. Surgery 115:707–712
28. Solomon MJ, McLeod RS (1995) Should we be performing more randomized controlled trials evaluating surgical operations? Surgery 118:459–467
29. Søreide O, Norstein J (1996) Local recurrence after rectal cancer surgery - a strategy for change. J Am Coll Surg (in press)
30. Tarone RE, Ware J (1977) On distribution-free tests for equality of survival distributions. Biometrika 64:156–160
31. UICC (1992) TNM classification of malignant tumours. Springer, Berlin Heidelberg
32. UICC (1993) TNM Supplement 1993. A commentary on uniform use. Springer, Berlin Heidelberg
33. Wanebo HJ, Stearns M, Schwartz MK (1978) Use of CEA as an indicator of early recurrence and as a guide to a selected second-look procedure in patients with colorectal cancer. Ann Surg 188:481–493

CHAPTER 3

Failure After Curative Surgery Alone

John L. McCall and David A. Wattchow

Introduction

Many changes have occurred in the surgical treatment of rectal cancer this century. Improvements in surgical technique, anaesthesia and postoperative care all contributed to a marked reduction in mortality during the first half of the century [42, 84]. The trend towards sphincter preservation, which had begun decades before, accelerated through the 1980s due to the widespread availability and use of modern stapling devices and the recognition that 2 cm was adequate distal clearance on the rectal wall in most cases [101]. Consequently, the ratio of abdominoperineal resections (APR) to anterior resections (AR) for rectal cancer has been reversed in the last two decades. However, this trend has not been accompanied by significant reductions in disease recurrence and death over the same period [41, 60, 101, 127].

Local recurrence (LR) is an important clinical problem which afflicts one in five patients with rectal cancer treated surgically for "cure" and an even higher proportion of patients treated for palliation. LR is not often cured, produces debilitating symptoms which are difficult to palliate [10, 17, 43, 100, 109] and, in some patients, is the only site of tumour recurrence [38, 43, 109]. LR is much more common following surgery for rectal cancer than colon cancer [35, 69], and reported pelvic recurrence rates vary widely, from 3% to 50% [58, 91]. A major factor may be related to the surgical technique [73, 98], but differences in case selection, follow-up, definition and diagnosis of LR may also be relevant [2, 72].

Numerous approaches have been used in an attempt to reduce LR rates in rectal cancer. These include complete excision of the mesorectum [5, 8, 11, 16, 18, 22, 27, 48, 56, 60, 67, 78, 119], lateral pelvic lymph node dissection [26, 40, 54, 76, 80, 129], flush ligation of inferior mesenteric artery (IMA) [19, 96, 117], the "no touch" isolation technique [126], rectal stump washout with cytocidal agents [124], pre- and postoperative adjuvant radiotherapy [10, 20, 34, 37, 71, 85, 89, 116, 122] and adjuvant chemotherapy [33, 36, 62].

In a meta-analysis of randomised controlled trials of adjuvant radiotherapy in rectal cancer, completed prior to 1989, Twomey et al. [123] showed that LR was reduced by up to 40% with pre- or postoperative adjuvant radiotherapy given in doses of 3000 cGy or more. Subsequent randomised controlled trials have confirmed that preoperative radiotherapy alone [34, 71] or postoperative radiotherapy combined with chemotherapy both effectively reduce LR rates after surgery for Dukes' B and C (Astler-Coller B2 and C) disease [36, 62]. However, the absolute improvement in local control expected from radiotherapy is dependent on the underlying LR risk with surgery alone. To date, all trials demonstrating improved local control with adjuvant radiotherapy, with or without chemotherapy, have recorded LR rates in control patients treated with surgery alone in excess of 18% [2, 94].

In 1986, Quirke et al. demonstrated the importance of adequacy of rectal excision by showing that involvement of radial resection margins after surgery for rectal cancer was highly predictive of LR [102]. Utilising the technique of total mesorectal excision (TME), Heald reported LR rates through the 1980s of around 3% [50]. Some observers have attributed these results to selection bias [55]; however, other surgeons have also reported favourable results with TME [5, 8, 11, 16, 18, 22, 56, 60, 78]. Extended pelvic lymphadenectomy (EPL), which adds en bloc removal of internal iliac lymph nodes to complete excision of the mesorectum [45], has also been reported to reduce LR in some series when compared with historical controls [26, 54].

The question of whether surgery alone for rectal cancer can achieve acceptable LR rates has remained controversial. There have been no randomised trials examining key issues of surgical technique in rectal cancer and, although desirable [108], there are potential difficulties in a surgeon randomly adopting different surgical techniques [32]. In 1992, in lieu of randomised trials, we undertook a systematic review of the surgical literature over the preceding decade to try to objectively evaluate the available data regarding failure rates after surgery alone for rectal cancer [74]. A systematic review differs from a standard review in that criteria for selecting papers and the methods of analysis are prospectively determined to avoid the selection and interpretation bias inherent to traditional reviews [86, 115]. These criteria should be evenly applied and transparent enough for the findings to be independently verified [86]. The findings of this study, supplemented by more recently published data, form the basis of the present chapter.

Selection of Papers and Analysis

Selection of Papers

A Medline-based search was undertaken for papers published in English between January 1982 and December 1992 reporting the results of surgical treatment for rectal cancer. The list of papers was supplemented by extensive cross-checking of reference lists. Those papers reporting follow-up on at least 50 patients surviving rectal excision with curative intent were selected from the ensuing list. The patients who survived a curative operation, and were therefore at risk of developing LR, were selected from each paper for inclusion in the analysis. As the primary aim was to document the results of surgery alone for rectal cancer, papers were excluded if adjuvant therapy was used in more than 10% of cases. Control patients in adjuvant therapy trials, randomised to receive surgery alone, were included. Clear information regarding treatment intent (curative or palliative) and LR rate were mandatory requirements for inclusion. Duplication was avoided by including only the most recent complete report from the same surgical series.

Definition of Terms

"Curative" operation was taken to mean removal of all macroscopic disease, whether or not this was histologically confirmed. Although this definition can be criticised in the light of knowledge about microscopically involved margins [3, 16, 88, 102], it remains the most widely accepted and utilised interpretation. Few studies appear to have confined the selection of potentially curative cases to those in which histologically documented tumour-free margins were obtained.

LR was defined as recurrent tumour within the pelvis or perineum, with or without distant metastases. LR and pelvic recurrence are taken to mean the same thing. Marsh et al. [72] showed that wide variations in LR rates can be demonstrated, even using the same data, depending on the definition of LR used. All patients with LR should be included and not just those with recurrent disease isolated to the pelvis [2].

Disease stage was defined according to the original Dukes' classification [24]. This was chosen to allow re-classification of all patients to one standard system which has stood the test of time. Patients staged by the Modified Dukes', Astler-Coller, TNM, Australian Clinicopathological Staging System (ACPS) or Japanese Research Society systems were re-classified according to the matrix for staging system conversion established by the 1990 World Congress of Gastroenterology Working Party on Clinicopathological Staging [31].

Definitions of rectal cancer vary. Some authors have excluded lesions beyond 12 cm from the anal verge, whereas others include all upper rectal and rectosigmoid tumours. For the purposes of our study, rectal cancer was categorised according to distance from the anal verge on rigid sigmoidoscopy.

Other morphological definitions were re-categorised as follows: the lower two thirds of the rectum and below the peritoneal reflection were categorised as "within 12 cm", and below the sacral promontory and rectosigmoid as "within 20 cm".

The method (prospective versus retrospective) and length of follow-up were recorded. Average follow-up was defined as either mean or median follow-up or, if neither of these were given, the mid-point of the follow-up range.

Analysis

Data extracted from each paper was entered on a standard form and then transferred into a computerised database. LR rates were determined for patients with Dukes' A, B and C disease and for patients undergoing APR and AR. Over the last decade, a great deal of interest has centred around the techniques of EPL and TME [30, 111]. LR rates were therefore determined for patients undergoing EPL and TME. Patients were assumed to have undergone these procedures when it was explicitly stated in the methods of the paper. Case mix, according to Dukes' classification, was determined for each category and for series in which the reported LR rate was 10% or less.

Descriptive analysis was used to summarise the data. The diverse nature of series included meant that quantitative comparative statistical analysis, or meta-analysis, would have been inappropriate [44, 86]. Data obtained by combining patients from different series has been prefixed as "pooled". Other data are described by median (range) values, and the Spearman's rank correlation (r_s) was used to test for association between follow-up time and LR.

No attempt was made to collate survival data because of wide variations in reporting of survival figures [110].

Local Failure

Overall Local Failure

A total of 52 papers were included in the study (Table 1), reporting data on 10 640 patients. The median LR rate for all series was 18.5%, with a range of 3%–50%. The pooled LR rate for all series combined was 18.8%. Nine series, involving 1176 patients, reported total LR rates of 10% or less. Of these, 695 patients underwent TME and 64 had EPL; surgical technique was not specified for the other 417 patients.

Length and method of follow-up may influence observed LR rates. Sixteen papers reported prospective follow-up with median LR of 20% (range, 3%–38%); 26 papers reported retrospective follow-up with 17.5% (range, 4%–38%) LR; and no information was given regarding the nature of follow-up in ten papers with 19.5% (range, 4%–50%) LR. The median average duration of follow-up for the 52 series was 60 months (range, 24–256 months), and minimum follow-up was 24 months (range, 6–216 months). For the nine series

Table 1. List of papers included in the study (reproduced by permission)

First author	Year	Reference	Patients (n)	LR rate (%)	Surgical technique
Adloff	1984	[4]	113	32	NS
Amato	1991	[6]	147	11	EPL
Athlin	1988	[9]	99	37	NS
Balslev	1986 (controls)	[10]	247	18	NS
Belli	1988	[11]	72	4	TME
Braun	1992	[12]	119	14	NS
Carlsson	1987	[14]			
Series I			100	24	NS
Series II			231	38	NS
Cawthorn	1990	[16]	122	7	TME
Colombo	1987	[18]	89	11	TME
Dahl	1990 (controls)	[20]	128	21	NS, "minimal touch"
Danzi	1986	[21]	83	10	NS
Dixon	1991	[22]	227	4	TME
Domergue	1989	[23]	58	25	NS
Feil	1988	[28]	90	20	NS
Fick	1990	[29]	58	14	NS
Fisher NSABP R-01	1988 (controls)	[33]	184	25	NS
Gerard (EORTC)	1988 (controls)	[37]	175	28	NS (early IMA ligation)
Gillen	1986	[39]	66	20	NS
GITSG	1985 (controls)	[36]	58	24	NS
Glass	1985	[40]	73	14	EPL
Heimann	1986	[51]	320	16	NS
Hojo	1989	[54]			
Extended			192	14	EPL
Standard			245	19	NS
Jatzko	1992	[56]	249	13	TME, "no touch"
Karanjia	1990	[58]	152	3	TME
Kennedy	1985	[59]	90	24	NS
Kirwan	1989	[60]	67	4	TME
Lasson	1984	[63]	102	16	NS
Leff	1985	[64]	128	14	NS
Localio	1983	[65]	360	13	NS
Malmberg	1986	[70]	83	19	NS
McDermott	1985	[75]	934	20	NS
Michelassi	1988	[76]	83	16	NS
			64	9	EPL
Moran	1992	[78]	55	7	TME
Neville	1987	[87]	373	19	NS
Nilsson	1984	[91]	68	50	NS
Påhlman	1984	[93]	197	38	NS
Pheils	1983	[97]	193	10[b]	NS
Phillips	1984	[99]	848	15	NS
Pollett	1983	[101]	334	7	NS

Table 1 (*Contd.*)

First author	Year	Reference	Patients (*n*)	LR rate (%)	Surgical technique
Reed	1988	[104]	78	31	NS
Rich	1983	[105]	142	30	NS
Rosen	1985	[106]	119	23	NS
Rubbini	1990	[107]	183	24	NS
Secco	1989	[113]	90	22	NS
Stockholm	1987 (controls)	[116]	274	20	NS
Sweeney	1989	[118]	84	18	NS
Tagliacozzo[a]	1992	[119]	175	19	TME
Theile	1982	[120]	210	12	NS
Tonak	1982	[121]	224	23	NS
Treurniet-Donker	1991 (controls)	[122]	84	33	NS
Williams	1985	[128]	148	17	NS
Zirngibl	1990	[130]	1153	23	NS

EPL, extended pelvic lymphadenectomy; NS, not specified; TME, total mesorectal excision; LR, local recurrence; IMA, inferior mesenteric artery; NSABP, National Surgical Adjuvant Breast and Bowel Project; EORTC, European Organization for Research and Treatment of Cancer; GITSG, Gastrointestinal Tumor Study Group.
[a]Omitted from the initial study [74].
[b]Isolated LR only.

with LR of 10% or less, average follow-up was 68 months (range, 32–156 months) and minimum follow-up 24 months (range, 12–60 months). The nine TME series had a slightly shorter average follow-up time of 53 months (range, 32–78 months), with minimum follow-up of 29 months (range, 6–72 months). The correlation between minimum (r_s, 0.25; $p=0.09$) and average (r_s, 0.2; $p=0.25$) follow-up times and LR rate were not statistically significant. This is perhaps because around 80% of all LR are evident within 2 years [2, 119] and average follow-up times exceeded 2 years in all series, as do minimum follow-up times in 50% of the series.

Tumour Stage and Definition

Dukes' stage was determined for 7544 patients, of whom 25% had Dukes' A, 40% Dukes' B and 35% Dukes' C lesions. LR according to Dukes' stage was able to be determined for 6158 patients. The pooled LR rates increased with increasing stage of disease (Fig. 1). For the nine series with LR of 10% or less, the case mix according to Dukes' stage was similar to the case mix for all series combined (Fig. 2).

For rectal cancer defined as a lesion lying within 12 cm ($n=1156$), 16 cm ($n=1225$) and 20 cm ($n=4385$) of the anal verge, the pooled LR rates were 18%, 16.9% and 18.3%, respectively. When rectal cancer was not defined ($n=3874$), the pooled LR rate was 20%. Thus the inclusion of upper rectal and rectosigmoid tumours did not appear to influence reported LR rates.

Fig. 1. Local recurrence rates according to Dukes' stage. Pooled data on 6158 patients (reproduced by permission)

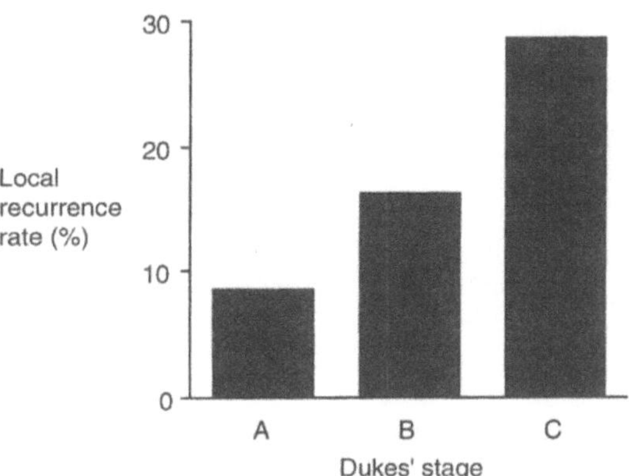

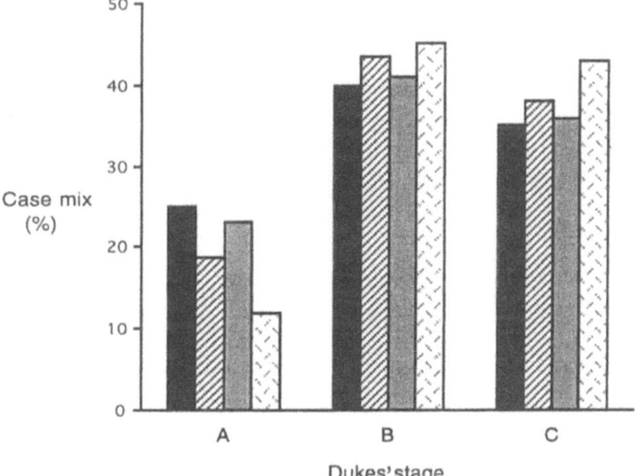

Fig. 2. Case mix, defined by Dukes' stage. Pooled data for all series combined (*black bars*), nine series with a local recurrence (LR) rate of 10% or less (*hatched bars*), nine series of total mesorectal excision (TME) (*grey bars*), and four series of extended pelvic lymphadenectomy (EPL) (*mottled bars*) (reproduced by permission)

Restricting the selection of "curative" cases to those with histologically clear margins introduces a potential source of bias. However, there was no association between a histological definition of curative resection and lower LR rates. In the nine papers reporting LR rates of 10% or less, six defined curative surgery macroscopically [11, 16, 22, 58, 60, 101], three did not define it [21, 40, 79] and none defined curative surgery histologically. Similarly, curative surgery was defined macroscopically in six [11, 16, 18, 22, 58, 60] and not defined in three [56, 78, 119] of the nine series of TME.

Surgical Procedure (Anterior Resection and Abdominoperineal Resection)

Specific information regarding surgical procedure, AR or APR, was available for 6188 patients. Hartmann's resections were included with AR. Transanal excisions were not included. The pooled LR rate for 3577 patients (derived from 30 papers) who underwent AR was 16.2%, and for 2601 patients (derived from 24 papers) who underwent APR was 19.3%.

The higher LR rate after APR than AR may reflect the higher risk of LR with low-lying lesions [4, 9, 75, 76, 113, 120]. Risk factors for recurrence, such as inadvertent tumour perforation [103, 114, 130] and a large surgical wound for tumour implantation [66], are increased with APR, and lateral lymph node involvement is more common with distal-third lesions [53, 82].

Surgical Technique

Total Mesorectal Excision

Of the 52 series, 1208 patients from nine series were identified as having undergone TME [11, 16, 18, 22, 56, 58, 60, 78, 119]. The pooled LR rate for the TME series was 8.8%, with a range of 3%–19% (Fig. 3). Seven of nine TME series [11, 16, 18, 22, 58, 60, 78] and two of the 43 remaining series [21, 101] reported LR rates of 10% or less. The median 30-day mortality rate in the TME series was 2.5% (range, 1.6%–5.4%).

Since LR risk increases with disease stage (Fig. 1), it is important to determine whether or not case mix or selection bias could account for these results [1, 55]. The case mix of patients treated in series of TME and the case mix of all of the series combined were almost identical (Fig. 2). Studies published since 1992 reinforce this observation. In Heald's series, 135 consecutive patients with Dukes' B and C (Astler-Coller B2 and C) disease underwent AR or APR with TME and were prospectively followed for a median of 7.5 years. The cumulative LR rate, independently verified, was 5% [67]. The patients did not

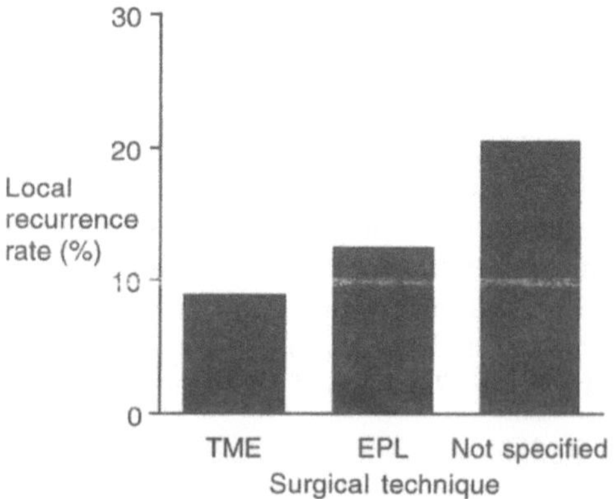

Fig. 3. Local recurrence (LR) rates according to surgical technique. Pooled data for total mesorectal excision (*TME*; *n*=1208), extended pelvic lymphadenectomy (*EPL*; *n*=476) and others (*n*=8956)

receive adjuvant therapy. In another consecutive series of 246 Dukes' B and C patients treated by TME, with long-term prospective follow-up, Enker et al. [27] reported LR in 7.3%. Peri-operative radiotherapy was given to 28% of patients with no apparent advantage. The case mix, methods and length of follow-up in these two series were comparable to the North Central Cancer Treatment Group's trial of postoperative adjuvant therapy, in which LR rates were 25% for surgery plus radiotherapy and 13.5% for surgery plus chemo-radiotherapy [62]. However, these studies are not comparable with respect to the number and experience of the contributing surgeons, which in itself is likely to influence LR [98].

While the list of individual surgeons reporting good results with TME continues to grow [5], interest is now focusing on whether these results can be reproduced on a wider scale [48]. Arbman et al. [8] have reported results before and after TME was adopted as the standard surgical technique for rectal excision in a region of Sweden serving a stable population of 370 000. Consecutive patients from each period were studied without exclusion. Surgical expertise was also consolidated to some degree, but despite this some eight surgeons performed an average of only five resections each annually. Following the introduction of TME, the actuarial LR rate at 4 years was reduced by almost two thirds to under 10% [8]. Adjuvant therapy was used in three patients only.

The clinical results of TME have been corroborated by pathological studies examining lateral and distal mesorectal spread. In two very similar studies, detailed histological evaluation of the circumferential resection margin was undertaken following conventional resection [3, 88]. Adam et al. [3] studied 141 patients undergoing curative resection with an overall LR rate of 25%. Microscopic tumour involvement at or within 1 mm of the circumferential margin was associated with a 78% LR risk compared with 10% risk if the margin was not involved. Ng et al. [88] studied 65 patients undergoing curative resection with an overall LR of 20%. The LR rate was 60% when tumour extended to within 1 mm of the circumferential margin histologically. Circumferential margin involvement is therefore a major risk factor for LR after conventional surgery.

The same methods of evaluating circumferential margins have been applied to specimens in which TME was undertaken [15, 112]. After TME, positive circumferential margins occur less frequently, in keeping with a lower risk of LR, and are more predictive of systemic rather than local recurrence [15]. Furthermore, the mesorectum harbours disease beyond the distal extent of intramural spread in 25% of cases [112]. This disease may be discontinuous [49, 57] and is often not evident to the surgeon [3, 102]. It follows that failure to adequately excise the mesorectum routinely risks leaving residual disease behind in a significant percentage of patients.

Extended Pelvic Lymphadenectomy

Of the 10 640 patients, 476 underwent EPL (four series). Two papers reported separate series of patients undergoing EPL and conventional surgery [54, 76].

The pooled LR rate for EPL was 12.4%, despite a higher proportion of Dukes' B and C patients (Fig. 2).

EPL should incorporate en bloc excision of the mesorectum [45]. The crucial difference between this technique and TME alone is the addition of an aorto-iliac lymph node dissection, including dissection lateral to the internal iliac artery. Lymph node dissection lateral to the internal iliac vessels may be oncologically equivalent to flush ligation of the inferior mesenteric artery, which has not been associated with significant improvements in LR or survival in non-randomised studies [19, 96, 117]. Similarly the "no touch" technique, combining early high ligation of the inferior mesenteric vessels with isolation of the tumour-bearing segment by tapes, failed to demonstrate a significant improvement in LR or survival rates in a randomised trial [126].

The overall incidence of metastasis to lateral pelvic lymph nodes is in the order of 10% in rectal cancer [53, 81], but is higher for lower- than for middle- and upper-third tumours [53, 82]. Most patients with positive lateral nodes die of systemic disease despite radical node clearance [53]. The prognosis associated with positive lateral pelvic lymph nodes is in fact similar to that associated with histologically positive circumferential margins following TME. Cawthorn et al. [16] found that patients with positive lateral margins after TME usually died of systemic disease before developing symptomatic LR, and Scott et al. [112] found that three of four patients with circumferential margin involvement after TME developed distal recurrence.

The benefits of lateral pelvic node dissection are unproven in terms of disease control [45, 80, 111]. However, the technique results in a high incidence of urinary and sexual dysfunction [54, 129]. Surgeons practising a less radical lateral dissection, confined within the internal iliac vessels, sacral nerve roots and inferior pelvic plexus, have reported single-figure LR rates combined with good functional results [25, 83]. Few major differences appear to exist between the latter type of pelvic node dissection and that accomplished by TME [25, 47]. The key feature of both procedures is sharp dissection, under direct vision, within the fascial planes encompassing the mesorectum [46].

Cytocidal Irrigation

Surgical wounds are a fertile medium for implantation metastasis [66, 124]. Irrigating the rectal stump with a cytocidal solution may prevent implantation of viable exfoliated tumour cells into the wound or anastomosis [124]. Although widely practiced, the hypothesis that irrigating with cytocidal agents reduces LR has not been formally tested in humans.

Of the 52 series studied, rectal washout with a cytocidal agent (water, povidine-iodine, cetrimide or mercuric perchloride) was reported to have been undertaken routinely in ten series, involving 1364 patients. The pooled LR rate in these series was 12.2%. A total of 41% of the patients underwent TME, and 11% EPL. When separated according to TME, EPL or other, the pooled LR rates for patients having cytocidal washout were only 1%–2% less than pooled LR for the groups as a whole. This implies that the LR rate in patients having cytocidal irrigation reflected the resection technique more than the use of cytocidal irrigation per se.

Studies detailing patterns of local recurrence, combined with more recent pathological studies, strongly suggest that LR is usually due to residual disease rather than implantation [3, 43, 52, 57, 88, 100, 102, 112]. Nevertheless, irrigating with a cytocidal agent may confer a small additional benefit, even after optimal surgery, by preventing implantation metastasis from occurring.

Distant Failure

In 22 of the 52 series studied, both isolated LR (no evidence of disseminated disease) and total LR rates were reported. Pooled LR for these 3838 patients was 11.3% and 21.5% for isolated and total LR, respectively. Thus 52% of patients with LR had no evidence of disseminated disease. This figure may be an over-estimate, given variations in the extent to which evidence for metastatic disease was sought and the limitations of all diagnostic modalities.

The fact that adjuvant radiotherapy can reduce LR without improving survival, except with the addition of chemotherapy [36, 62], goes against the concept of survival being enhanced by prevention of LR alone. Nevertheless, complete surgical excision of LR is associated with 20%–40% long-term survival rates in selected patients [17, 68, 109]. This indicates that a percentage of patients with LR have either no metastatic disease or have micrometastases which remain quiescent for long periods.

Adjuvant radiotherapy alone has no effect on survival, but it seems that the surgeon does. McArdle and Hole [73] demonstrated a four-fold difference in survival after surgery for colorectal cancer contingent on the surgeon. It has been postulated that surgery which minimises pelvic recurrences may also enhance survival [30], and there is some circumstantial evidence to support this [8, 27, 67]. However, comparing survival figures between different series is even more difficult than comparing LR rates, due to greater variation in the way in which survival is measured and reported [110]. Without randomised trials, progress towards resolving these issues can only be made by using standardised criteria for selecting, treating, staging and reporting outcomes. There is also a need for high-quality multi-surgeon studies, preferably population based [8], to augment the evidence gained from single-surgeon series.

Conclusions

There is considerable evidence implicating incomplete removal of tumour as the major cause of local treatment failure following surgery for rectal cancer [3, 43, 52, 57, 88, 100, 102, 112]. In a systematic review of 52 published results of surgery for rectal cancer over a 10-year period, the technique associated with the least risk of LR risk was TME [11, 16, 18, 22, 56, 58, 60, 78, 119] (Fig. 3). More recently published work corroborates these findings [5, 8, 27, 67].

TME may reduce the risk of leaving behind microscopic deposits, especially discontinuous spread harboured within the distal mesorectum [49, 57, 102,

112], and insures against the tendency to "cone down" on the mesorectum when approaching the rectal wall below the tumour [7]. Careful sharp dissection, rather than blunt extraction, also offers the potential benefits of reduced transfusion requirements [13, 95], preservation of autonomic nerves [25, 125] and avoidance of inadvertent tumour perforation [103, 114, 130].

All series of TME reported in the literature to date, with one exception [119], have achieved equally good or better local control than conventional surgery combined with postoperative adjuvant chemo-radiotherapy [36, 62]. Furthermore, the results of TME have for the most part been achieved without pelvic radiotherapy. The postoperative adjuvant chemo-radiotherapy regimen currently recommended by the NIH [90] approximately doubles total treatment-related mortality [62] and has a long-term detrimental effect on bowel function [61]. Such treatments may be best reserved for patients with inadequately excised tumours, as judged clinically and pathologically, rather than all tumours penetrating beyond the bowel wall. Preoperative radiotherapy is less morbid [34] and may be beneficial in more advanced disease [34, 71] identified with the aid of endorectal ultrasound [77, 92]. Lateral pelvic node dissection results in urinary and sexual dysfunction and has not yet been shown to improve disease control [45, 80, 111] over and above that achieved by nerve-sparing procedures incorporating complete excision of the mesorectum [25, 83].

The wide range of LR rates with surgery alone indicates that rectal cancer should be treated by surgeons with a special interest and training in the management of this disease. In expert hands, LR rates of 10% or less can be achieved with surgery alone. Although some surgeons have argued that LR is merely a manifestation of systemic disease [55], this idea propagates a dangerously nihilistic approach to prevention and treatment of LR, and the evidence suggests that it is false as far as rectal cancer is concerned [109]. Biological factors do play an inevitable role in determining outcome, but LR and survival are both significantly influenced by the surgeon [73, 98]. Surgeons must therefore assume some responsibility for treatment failure, rather than ascribing it all to the disease, and must strive to emulate the excellent results being achieved by a growing number of colleagues. Optimal surgery for rectal cancer needs to be complemented by optimal pathological evaluation of the resected specimen. The prognostic significance of circumferential margin involvement has been demonstrated [3, 16, 102], and future studies need to address the role of adjuvant therapy in this subset of patients, for whom the risk of recurrence remains high [16, 112].

References

1. Abcarian H (1992) Operative treatment of colorectal cancer. Cancer 70:1350–1354
2. Abulafi AM , Williams NS (1994) Local recurrence of colorectal cancer: the problem, mechanisms, management and adjuvant therapy. Br J Surg 81:7–19
3. Adam IJ, Mohamdee MO, Martin IG et al (1994) Role of circumferential margin involvement in the local recurrence of rectal cancer. Lancet 344:707–711

4. Adloff M, Arnaud JP, Schloegel M et al (1985) Factors influencing local recurrence after abdominoperineal resection for cancer of the rectum. Dis Colon Rectum 28:413–415
5. Aitken RJ (1996) Mesorectal excision for rectal cancer. Br J Surg 83:214–216
6. Amato A, Pescatori M, Butti A (1991) Local recurrence following excision and anterior resection for rectal carcinoma. Dis Colon Rectum 34:317–322
7. Anderberg B, Enblad P, Sjodahl R et al (1983) Recurrent rectal carcinoma after anterior resection and rectal stapling. Br J Surg 70:1–4
8. Arbman G, Nilsson E, Hallbook O et al (1996) Local recurrence following total mesorectal excision for rectal cancer. Br J Surg 83:375–379
9. Athlin L, Bengtsson NO, Stenling R (1988) Local recurrence and survival after radical resection of rectal carcinoma. Acta Chir Scand 154:225–229
10. Balslev IB, Pedersen M, Teglbjaerg PS et al (1986) Postoperative radiotherapy in Dukes' B and C carcinoma of the rectum and rectosigmoid. A randomized multicentre study. Cancer 58:22–28
11. Belli L, Beati CA, Frangi M et al (1988) Outcome of patients with rectal cancer treated by stapled anterior resection. Br J Surg 75:422–424
12. Braun J, Pfingsten F, Schippers E et al (1992) Rectal cancer. Results of continence-preserving resections. Leber Magen Darm 22:59–66
13. Busch ORC, Hop WCJ, Hoynck van Papendrecht MAW et al (1993) Blood transfusion and prognosis in colorectal cancer. N Engl J Surg 328:1372–1376
14. Carlsson U, Lasson A, Ekelund G (1987) Recurrence rates after curative surgery for rectal carcinoma, with special reference to their accuracy. Dis Colon Rectum 30:431–434
15. Cawthorn SJ, Gibbs NM, Marks CG (1986) Clearance technique for the detection of lymph nodes in colorectal cancer. Br J Surg 73:58–60
16. Cawthorn SJ, Parums DV, Gibbs NM et al (1990) Extent of mesorectal spread and involvement of lateral resection margin as prognostic factors after surgery for rectal cancer. Lancet 335:1055–1059
17. Cohen AM, Minsky BD (1990) Aggressive surgical management of locally advanced primary and recurrent rectal cancer. Dis Colon Rectum 33:432–438
18. Colombo PL, Foglieni CLS, Morone C (1987) Analysis of recurrence following curative low anterior resection and stapled anastomoses for carcinoma of the middle third and lower rectum. Dis Colon Rectum 30:457–464
19. Corder AP, Karanjia ND, Williams JD et al (1992) Flush aortic tie versus selective preservation of the ascending left colic artery in low anterior resection for rectal carcinoma. Br J Surg 79:680–682
20. Dahl O, Horn A, Morild I et al (1990) Low-dose preoperative radiation postpones recurrences in operable rectal cancer. Cancer 66:2286–2294
21. Danzi M, Ferulano GP, Abate S et al (1986) Survival and locations of recurrence following abdomino-perineal resection for rectal cancer. J Surg Oncol 31:235–239
22. Dixon AR, Maxwell WA, Thornton Holmes J (1991) Carcinoma of the rectum: a 10-year experience. Br J Surg 78:308–311
23. Domergue J, Rouanet P, Daures JP et al (1989) Multivariate analysis of prognostic factors for curative resectable rectal cancer. Eur J Surg Oncol 15:93–98
24. Dukes C (1932) The classification of cancer of the rectum. J Pathol 35:323–332
25. Enker WE (1992) Potency, cure, and local control in the operative treatment of rectal cancer. Arch Surg 127:1396–1402
26. Enker WE, Pilipshen SJ, Heilweil ML et al (1986) En bloc pelvic lymphadenectomy and sphincter preservation in the surgical management of rectal cancer. Ann Surg 203:426–433
27. Enker WE, Thaler H, Cranor M et al (1995) Total mesorectal excision in the operative treatment of carcinoma of the rectum. J Am Coll Surg 181:335–346
28. Feil W, Wunderlich M, Kovats E et al (1988) Rectal cancer: factors influencing the development of local recurrence after radical anterior resection. Int J Colorect Dis 3:195–200
29. Fick TE, Baeten CGMI, von Meyenfeldt MF et al (1990) Recurrence and survival after abdominoperineal and low anterior resection for rectal cancer, without aduvant therapy. Eur J Surg Oncol 16:105–108

30. Fielding LP (1993) Colorectal carcinoma. Mesorectal excision for rectal cancer (editorial). Lancet 341:471–472
31. Fielding LP, Arsenault PA, Chapuis PH et al (1991) Working party report to the World Congress of Gastroenterology, Sydney, 1990. Clinicopathological staging for colorectal cancer: an International Documentation System (IDS) and an International Comprehensive Anatomical Terminology (ICAT). J Gastroenterol Hepatol 6:325–344
32. Fielding LP, Stewart-Brown S, Dudley HAF (1987) Surgeon-related variables and the clinical trial. Lancet II:778–779
33. Fisher B, Wolkman N, Rockette H et al (1988) Postoperative adjuvant chemotherapy or radiation therapy for rectal cancer: results from NSABP protocol R-01. J Natl Cancer Inst 80:21–29
34. Frykholm GJ, Glimelius B, Påhlman L (1993) Preoperative or postoperative irradiation in adenocarcinoma of the rectum: final treatment results of a randomized trial and an evaluation of late secondary effects. Dis Colon Rectum 36:564–572
35. Galandiuk S, Wieand HS, Moertel CG et al (1992) Patterns of recurrence after curative resection of carcinoma of the colon and rectum. Surg Gynecol Obstet 174:27–32
36. Gastrointestinal Tumor Study Group (1985) Prolongation of the disease-free interval in surgically treated rectal carcinoma. N Engl J Med 312:1465–1472
37. Gerard A, Buyse M, Nordlinger B et al (1988) Preoperative radiotherapy as adjuvant treatment in rectal cancer. Ann Surg 208:606–614
38. Gilbert JM, Jeffrey I, Evans M et al (1984) Sites of recurrent tumour after 'curative' colorectal surgery: implications for adjuvant therapy. Br J Surg 71:203–205
39. Gillen P, Peel AL (1986) Comparison of the mortality and incidence of local recurrence in patients with rectal cancer treated by either stapled anterior resection or abdominoperineal resection. Br J Surg 73:339–341
40. Glass RE, Ritchie JK, Thompson HR et al (1985) The results of surgical treatment of cancer of the rectum by radical resection and extended abdomino-iliac lymphadenectomy. Br J Surg 72:599–601
41. Goligher JC (1979) Recent trends in the practice of sphincter saving exision for rectal cancer. Ann R Coll Surg Eng 61:169–173
42. Goligher JC (1980) Treatment of carcinoma of the rectum. In: Surgery of the anus, rectum, and colon, 4th edn. Bailliere Tindall, London, pp 502–666
43. Gunderson LL , Sosin H (1974) Areas of failure at reoperation (second or symptomatic look) following "curative surgery" for adenocarcinoma of the rectum. Cancer 34:1278–1292
44. Halvorsen KT (1986) Combining results from independent investigations. Meta-analysis in medical research. In: Bailar JC, Mosteller F (eds) Medical uses of statistics. NEJM Books, Waltham, pp 392–416
45. Harnsberger JR, Vernava AM, Longo WE (1994) Radical abdominopelvic lymphadenectomy: historical perspective and current role in the surgical management of rectal cancer. Dis Colon Rectum 37:73–87
46. Havenga K, De Ruiter MC, Enker WE et al (1996) Anatomical basis of autonomic nerve-preserving total mesorectal excision for cancer. Br J Surg 83:384–388
47. Heald RJ (1995) Rectal cancer: the surgical options. Eur J Cancer 31A:1189–1192
48. Heald RJ (1995) Total mesorectal excision is optimal surgery for rectal cancer: a Scandinavian consensus. Br J Surg 82:1297–1299
49. Heald RJ, Ryall RDH (1982) The mesorectum in rectal cancer surgery – the clue to pelvic recurrence? Br J Surg 69:613–616
50. Heald RJ, Ryall RDH (1986) Recurrence and survival after total mesorectal excision for rectal cancer. Lancet I:1479–1482
51. Heimann TM, Szporn A, Bolnick K et al (1986) Local recurrence following surgical treatment of rectal cancer. Comparison of anterior and abdominoperineal resection. Dis Colon Rectum 29:862–864
52. Hohenberger P, Liewald F, Schlag P et al (1990) Lectins and immunohistochemistry of colorectal cancer, its recurrences and metastases. Eur J Surg Oncol 16:289–297
53. Hojo K, Koyama Y, Moriya Y (1982) Lymphatic spread and its prognostic value in patients with rectal cancer. Am J Surg 144:350–354

54. Hojo K, Sawada T, Moriya Y (1989) An analysis of survival and voiding, sexual function after wide iliopelvic lymphadenectomy in patients with carcinoma of the rectum, compared with conventional lymphadenectomy. Dis Colon Rectum 32:128–133
55. Isbister WH (1990) Basingstoke revisited. Aust N Z J Surg 60:243–246
56. Jatzko G, Lisborg P, Wette V (1992) Improving survival rates for patients with colorectal cancer. Br J Surg 79:588–591
57. Joyce W, Dolan J, Hyland J (1993) The mesorectum: re-appraisal of its morphology and its unique importance in rectal cancer. (abstract) Int J Colorectal Dis 8:235
58. Karanjia ND, Schache DJ, North WRS et al (1990) 'Close shave' in anterior resection. Br J Surg 77:501–512
59. Kennedy HL, Langevin JM, Goldberg SM et al (1985) Recurrence following stapled coloproctostomy for carcinomas of the mid portion of the rectum. Surg Gynecol Obstet 160:513–516
60. Kirwan WO, O'Riordan MG, Waldron R (1989) Declining indications for abdominoperineal resection. Br J Surg 76:1061–1063
61. Kollmorgen CF, Meagher AP, Pemberton JH et al (1994) The long-term effect of adjuvant postoperative chemoradiotherapy for rectal carcinoma on bowel function. Ann Surg 220:676–682
62. Krook JE, Moertel CG, Gunderson LL et al (1991) Effective surgical adjuvant therapy for high-risk rectal carcinoma. N Engl J Med 324:709–715
63. Lasson ALL, Eklund GR, Lindstrom CG (1984) Recurrence risk after stapled anastomosis for rectal carcinoma. Acta Chir Scand 150:85–89
64. Leff EI, Shaver JO, Hoexter B et al (1985) Anastomotic recurrences after low anterior resection. Stapled vs hand-sewn. Dis Colon Rectum 28:164–167
65. Localio SA, Eng K, Coppa GF (1983) Abdominosacral resection for midrectal cancer. Ann Surg 198:320–324
66. Long RT, Edwards RH (1989) Implantation metastasis as a cause of local recurrence of colorectal cancer. Am J Surg 157:194–201
67. MacFarlane JK, Ryall RDH, Heald RJ (1993) Mesorectal excision for rectal cancer. Lancet 341:457–460
68. Maetani S, Nishikawa T, Iijima Y et al (1992) Extensive en bloc resection of regionally recurrent carcinoma of the rectum. Cancer 69:2876–2883
69. Malcolm AW, Perencevich NP, Olson RN et al (1981) Analysis of recurrence patterns following curative resection for carcinoma of the colon and rectum. Surg Gynecol Obstet 152:131–136
70. Malmberg M, Graffner H, Ling L et al (1986) Recurrence and survival after anterior resection of the rectum using the end to end anastomotic stapler. Surg Gynecol Obstet 163:231–234
71. Marsh PJ, James RD, Schofield PF (1994) Adjuvant preoperative radiotherapy for locally advanced rectal carcinoma. Dis Colon Rectum 37:1205–1214
72. Marsh PJ, James RD, Schofield PF (1995) Definition of local recurrence after surgery for rectal carcinoma. Br J Surg 82:465–468
73. McArdle CS, Hole D (1991) Impact of variability among surgeons on postoperative morbidity and mortality and ultimate survival. BMJ 302:1501–1505
74. McCall JL, Cox MR, Wattchow DA (1995) Analysis of local recurrence rates after surgery alone for rectal cancer. Int J Colorectal Dis 10:126–132
75. McDermott FT, Hughes ESR, Pihl E et al (1985) Local recurrence after potentially curative resection for rectal cancer in a series of 1008 patients. Br J Surg 72:34–37
76. Michelassi F, Block GE, Vannucei L et al (1988) A 5- to 21-year follow-up and analysis of 250 patients with rectal adenocarcinoma. Ann Surg 208:379–389
77. Milsom JW, Graffner H (1990) Intrarectal ultrasonography in rectal cancer staging and in the evaluation of pelvic disease. Ann Surg 212:602–606
78. Moran BJ, Blenkinsop J, Finnis D (1992) Local recurrence after anterior resection for rectal cancer using a double stapling technique. Br J Surg 79:836–838
79. Moran MR, Rothenberger DA, Gallo RA et al (1993) Multifactorial analysis of local recurrences in rectal cancer, including DNA ploidy: Predictive model. World J Surg 17:801–805

80. Moreira LF, Hizuti A, Iwagaki H et al (1994) Lateral lymph node dissection for rectal carcinoma below the peritoneal reflection. Br J Surg 81:293–296
81. Morikawa E, Yasutomi M, Shindou K et al (1994) Distribution of metastatic lymph nodes in colorectal cancer by the modified clearing technique. Dis Colon Rectum 37:219–223
82. Moriya Y, Hojo K, Sawada K et al (1989) Significance of lateral node dissection for advanced rectal carcinoma at or below the peritoneal reflection. Dis Colon Rectum 32:307–315
83. Moriya Y, Sugihara K, Akasu T et al (1995) Patterns of recurrence after nerve-sparing surgery for rectal adenocarcinoma with special reference to loco-regional recurrence. Dis Colon Rectum 38:1162–1168
84. Moynihan B (1926) Abdominal operations. 4th edn. Saunders, London
85. MRC Working Party (1984) The evaluation of low dose pre-operative X-ray therapy in the management of operable rectal cancer, results of a randomly controlled trial. Br J Surg 71:21–25
86. Mulrow CD (1994) Rationale for systematic reviews. BMJ 309:597–599
87. Neville R, Fielding LP, Amendola C (1987) Local tumor recurrence after curative resection for rectal cancer. A ten-hospital review. Dis Colon Rectum 30:12–17
88. Ng IOL, Luk ISC, Yuen ST et al (1993) Surgical lateral clearance in resected rectal carcinomas. Cancer 71:1972–1976
89. Niebel W, Schulz U, Ried M et al (1988) Five-year results of a prospective and randomised study: experience with combined radiotherapy and surgery of primary rectal carcinoma. In: Schlag P, Hohenberger P, Metzger U (eds) Combined modality therapy of gastro-intestinal tract cancer. Springer, Berlin Heidelberg New York, pp 111–113 (Recent results in cancer research, vol 110)
90. NIH Consensus Conference (1990) Adjuvant therapy for patients with colon and rectal cancer. JAMA 264:1444–1450
91. Nilsson E, Gregersen N-P, Hartvig B et al (1984) Carcinoma of the colon and rectum. Acta Chir Scand 150:177–182
92. Orrom WJ, Wong WD, Rothenberger DA et al (1990) Endorectal ultrasound in the preoperative staging of rectal tumors. Dis Colon Rectum 33:654–659
93. Påhlman L, Glimelius B (1984) Local recurrences after surgical treatment for rectal carcinoma. Acta Chir Scand 150:513–516
94. Påhlman L, Glimelius B (1992) Pre-operative and post-operative radiotherapy and rectal cancer. World J Surg 16:858–865
95. Parrott NR, Lennard TW, Taylor RM et al (1986) Effect of perioperative blood transfusion on recurrence of colorectal cancer. Br J Surg 73:970–973
96. Pezim ME, Nichols RJ (1984) Survival after high or low ligation of the inferior mesenteric artery during curative surgery for rectal cancer. Ann Surg 200:729–733
97. Pheils MT, Chapuis PH, Newland RC et al (1983) Local recurrence following curative resection for carcinoma of the rectum. Dis Colon Rectum 26:98–102
98. Phillips RKS, Hittinger R, Blesovsky L et al (1984) Local recurrence following 'curative' surgery for large bowel cancer: I. The overall picture. Br J Surg 71:12–16
99. Phillips RKS, Hittinger R, Blesovsky L et al (1984) Local recurrence following 'curative' surgery for large bowel cancer. II. The rectum and rectosigmoid. Br J Surg 71:17–20
100. Pilipshen SJ, Heilweil M, Quan HQ et al (1984) Patterns of pelvic recurrence following definitive resections of rectal cancer. Cancer 53:1354–1362
101. Pollett WG, Nicholls RJ (1983) The relationship between the extent of distal clearance and survival and local recurrence rates after curative anterior resection for carcinoma of the rectum. Ann Surg 198:159–163
102. Quirke P, Dixon MF, Durdey P et al (1986) Local recurrence of rectal adenocarcinoma due to inadequate surgical resection. Lancet II:996–999
103. Ranbarger KR, Johnson WD, Chang JC (1982) Prognostic significance of surgical perforation of the rectum during abdominoperineal resection for rectal carcinoma. Am J Surg 143:186–188
104. Reed WJ, Garb JL, Park WC et al (1988) Long-term results and complications of pre-operative radiation in the treatment of rectal cancer. Surgery 103:161–167

105. Rich T, Gunderson LL, Lew R et al (1983) Patterns of recurrences of rectal cancer after potentially curative surgery. Cancer 52:1317–1329
106. Rosen CB, Beart RWJ, Ilstrup DM (1985) Local recurrence of rectal carcinoma after hand-sewn and stapled anastomosis. Dis Colon Rectum 28:305–309
107. Rubbini M, Vellorello GF, Guerrera C et al (1990) A prospective study of local recurrence after resection and low stapled anastomosis in 183 patients with rectal cancer. Dis Colon Rectum 33:117–121
108. Russell I (1995) Evaluating new surgical procedures. BMJ 311:1243
109. Sagar PM, Pemberton JH (1996) Surgical management of locally recurrent rectal cancer. Br J Surg 83:293–304
110. Schofield PF, Walsh S, Tweedle DEF (1986) Survival after treatment of carcinoma of the rectum. Br Med J 293:496–497
111. Scholefield JH, Northover JMA (1995) Surgical management of rectal cancer. Br J Surg 82:745–748
112. Scott P, Jackson T, Al-Jaberi MF et al (1995) Total mesorectal excision and local recurrence: a study of tumour spread in the mesorectum distal to rectal cancer. Br J Surg 82:1031–1033
113. Secco GB, Fardelli R, Campora E et al (1989) Factors influencing local recurrence after curative surgery for rectal cancer. Oncology 46:10–13
114. Slanetz CA (1984) The effect of inadvertent intraoperative perforation on survival and recurrence in colorectal cancer. Dis Colon Rectum 27:792–797
115. Stocker M, Coates A (1993) What have we learned from meta-analysis? Med J Aust 159:291–293
116. Stockholm Rectal Cancer Study Group (1987) Short-term preoperative radiotherapy for adenocarcinoma of the rectum. Am J Clin Oncol 10:369–375
117. Surtees P, Ritchie JK, Phillips RKS (1990) High versus low ligation of the inferior mesenteric artery in rectal cancer. Br J Surg 77:619–621
118. Sweeney JL, Ritchie JK, Hawley PR (1989) Resection and sutured peranal anastomosis for carcinoma of the rectum. Dis Colon Rectum 32:103–106
119. Tagliacozzo S, Accordino M (1992) Pelvic recurrence after surgical treatment of rectal and sigmoid cancer. Int J Colorectal Dis 7:135–140
120. Theile DE, Cohen JR, Evans EB et al (1982) Pelvic recurrence after curative resection for carcinoma of the rectum. Aust N Z J Surg 52:391–394
121. Tonak J, Gall FP, Hermanek P et al (1982) Incidence of local recurrence after curative operations for cancer of the rectum. Aust N Z J Surg 52:23–27
122. Treurniet-Donker AD, van Putten WLJ, Wereldsma JCJ et al (1991) Postoperative radiation therapy for rectal cancer. Cancer 67:2042–2048
123. Twomey P, Burchell M, Strawn D et al (1989) Local control in rectal cancer. A clinical review and meta-analysis. Arch Surg 124:1174–1179
124. Umpleby HC, Williamson RCN (1987) Anastomotic recurrence in large bowel cancer. Br J Surg 74:873–878
125. Walsh PC, Schlegel PN (1988) Radical pelvic surgery with preservation of sexual function. Ann Surg 208:391–400
126. Wiggers T, Jeekel J, Arendst JW et al (1988) No-touch isolation technique on colon cancer: a controlled prospective trial. Br J Surg 75:409–415
127. Williams NS (1986) Changing patterns in the treatment of rectal cancer. Br J Surg 76:5–6
128. Williams NS, Durdey P, Johnston D (1985) The outcome following sphincter-saving resection and abdomino-perineal resection for low rectal cancer. Br J Surg 72:595–598
129. Yasutomi M, Shindo K, Mori N et al (1991) Does the pelvic nodes dissection for the rectal cancer patients make any contribution to the end-results of surgery? Gan To Kagaku Ryoho 18:541–546
130. Zirngibl H, Husemann B, Hermanek P (1990) Intraoperative spillage of tumor cells in surgery for rectal cancer. Dis Colon Rectum 33:610–614

Tumour Staging

CHAPTER 4

Staging Systems – A Review

Paul Hermanek

Introduction

Staging is defined as the assessment and description of the anatomical extent of cancer at certain points in its natural history, as a rule at diagnosis or first treatment. Its significance is based on the fact that, for most solid tumours, anatomical extent is the best predictor of outcome. The purposes of staging are to assist in the planning of treatment, to estimate prognosis and to enable meaningful evaluation of treatment results.

The first widely used staging system dates from the beginning of this century, when C.F. Steinthal introduced clinical staging of breast cancer in 1905 [42]. In 1930, Cuthbert Dukes introduced a pathological stage classification for rectal cancer [6], and staging of gynaecological tumours started in 1937 with the publication of the *Annual Reports* by the League of Nations Health Organization [30]. Based on the pioneer work of Pierre Denoix at the Institute Gustav Roussy, Villejuif, France, in the 1950s the TNM system was developed by the International Union Against Cancer (UICC) and the American Joint Committee for Cancer Staging and End Results Reporting (AJC; the name was changed in 1980 to American Joint Committee on Cancer, AJCC) as a system applicable to most tumour sites and entities and following uniform general rules [45].

Types of Staging Systems

The aim of staging is to assist in the planning of treatment by assessing the anatomical extent of cancer before treatment. After treatment, the residual tumour status is assessed to evaluate the results of treatment, to guide additional therapy (e.g. adjuvant treatment after surgery) and to estimate prognosis.

Staging may be based on clinical findings (clinical classification) or on findings from surgery and pathological examinations (pathological classification).

Various categories of staging may be distinguished depending on the time of assesment and the methods used:

1. *Clinical staging systems.* These involve assessment of the anatomical extent of cancer before treatment by clinical examination and other investigative methods.
2. *Pathological staging systems.* These involve assessment of the anatomical extent before treatment by pathological methods.
3. *Clinico-pathological staging systems.* These involve a combination of pathological staging with residual tumour status after treatment.
4. *Comprehensive staging systems.* These are systems which provide a clinical and a pathological staging system as well as a residual tumour classification.

History of Staging of Colorectal Carcinoma

All four types of staging systems have been developed and refined during the last 70 years for colorectal carcinoma (Fig. 1).

The first attempt at classification can be traced back to the differentiation between curative and non-curative treatment at the Mayo Clinic in 1926 [37]. In the subsequent decades, the focus was changed to pathological staging.

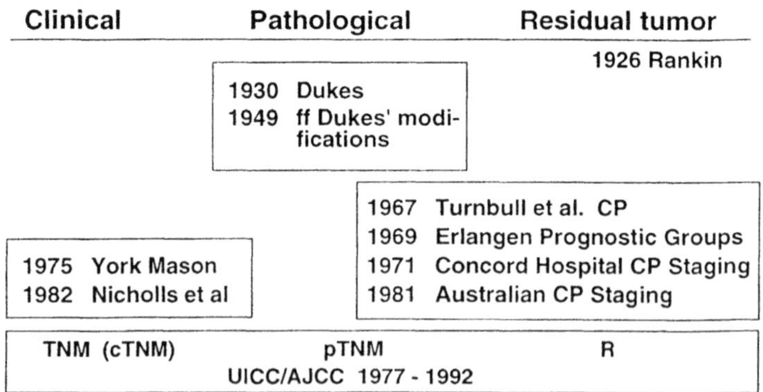

Fig. 1. History of staging of colorectal carcinoma. *CP*, clinico-pathological

Dukes' classification proposed for rectal carcinoma in 1932 [7] is generally referred to as the "original" Dukes' system, although an earlier variant had been published in 1930 [6]. The Dukes' system combines depth of invasion and regional lymph node metastasis status to define three stages:

1. *Stage A.* Invasion not beyond the muscularis propria, no lymph node metastasis
2. *Stage B.* Invasion beyond the muscularis propria, no lymph node metastasis
3. *Stage C.* Regional lymph node metastasis

In 1936, an expansion of this system was proposed by the Dukes' group, by the subdivision of stage C into C1 and C2, i.e. without or with apical node involvement [11]. The Dukes' system has been further applied to colonic carcinoma since 1945 [8].

In the subsequent years, the pathological Dukes' system was repeatedly modified. The most frequently used modifications are those of Kirklin et al. [28], Astler-Coller [3], Gunderson and Sosin [12], the Gastrointestinal Tumour Study Group (GITSG) [41] and the National Surgical Adjuvant Breast and Bowel Project (NSABP) [49]. These modifications include different categorization of depth of invasion, different subclassifications of lymph node metastasis status, different definitions of the A, B and C classes and different subdivisions of B and C. The multitude of "Dukes' modifications" resulted in considerable confusion, which was illustrated by Kyriakos [29] in the light of the public discussion of president Reagan's disease.

In the late 1960s, the residual tumour situation (remaining distant metastasis and loco-regional residual tumour) was combined with pathological staging. As such staging systems include clinical findings (e.g. diagnosis of liver or lung metastasis), the combinations of pathological staging and residual tumour assessment were designated *clinico-pathological staging.* Turnbull et al. [43] were the first to publish this concept. Refinements were later introduced in 1969 in Erlangen, Germany, by the Erlangen Prognostic Groups [19] and in 1971 in Australia as the Concord Hospital Clinicopathologic Staging System [35]. The condensed revision of the latter was puplished in 1981 as Australian Clinicopathological Staging (ACPS) System [4].

In the 1970s, a *clinical staging system* based on digital rectal examination was described by York Mason [50] and refined by inclusion of imaging methods [36]. In the 1980s, the findings of endorectal ultrasonography were designated as uT and uN [24], although such symbols for a special type of clinical staging were not approved by the UICC or AJCC.

The first *TNM Staging* for colorectal cancer was published in October 1966 [44] and included both a clinical and a pathological classification. An alternative TNM classification by the AJCC appeared in 1977, together with the introduction of a residual tumour (R) classification to describe the residual tumour status. Subsequently, the UICC and the AJC/AJCC worked fairly independently for a number of years, despite similar objectives. The principal difference was the method used for staging. Murray Copeland, a surgeon and the first chairman of the AJC, recognised early the need for more precision by adding the pathological to the clinical classification.

In November 1979, the so-called Peace Talks of Toronto promoted the co-operation of the AJC and UICC. The decision was made to formulate a single TNM staging system at the 13th International Cancer Congress in 1982. The result was the unification of the UICC and AJCC system with the publication of the fourth edition of TNM in 1987 (for references and details, see [21]).

Present Standard of Staging

In 1995, the international standard for staging is given by the TNM system, as edited by the UICC in *TNM Classification of Malignant Tumours* [45] and *TNM Atlas* [46], the most recent versions being published in 1992. This classification corresponds exactly to the fourth edition of the AJCC's *Manual for Staging of Cancer* [1]. These publications are supplemented by the *TNM Supplement 1993* [47], a commentary on uniform use. The current TNM system (Table 1) was

Table 1. Present TNM system [1, 45] for invasive colorectal carcinoma

---

Regional lymph node
The regional lymph nodes are the pericolic and perirectal and those located along the ileocolic, right colic, middle colic, left colic, inferior mesenteric, superior rectal and internal iliac arteries.

TNM Clinical Classification
T – Primary tumour
TX   Primary tumour cannot be assessed
T0   No evidence of primary tumour
T1   Tumour invades submucosa
T2   Tumour invades muscularis propria
T3   Tumour invades through muscularis propria into subserosa or into non-peritonealized pericolic or perirectal tissues
T4   Tumour directly invades other organs or structures and/or perforates visceral peritoneum

N – Regional lymph nodes
NX   Regional lymph nodes cannot be assessed
N0   No regional lymph node metastasis
N1   Metastasis in one to three pericolic or perirectal lymph nodes
N2   Metastasis in four or more pericolic or perirectal lymph nodes
N3   Metastasis in any lymph node along the course of a named vascular trunk and/or metastasis to apical node(s) (when marked by the surgeon)

M – Distant metastasis
MX   Presence of distant metastis cannot be assessed
M0   No distant metastasis
M1   Distant metastasis

pTNM Pathological Classification
The pT, pN and pM categories correspond to the T, N and M categories.

Residual Tumour (R) Classification
RX   Presence of residual tumour cannot be assessed
R0   No residual tumour
R1   Microscopic residual tumour
R2   Macroscopic residual tumour

Intra-epithelial and intramucosal carcinoma (Tis, pTis) is not considered.

Table 2. National TNM committees

Committee	Abbreviation
American Joint Committee on Cancer	AJCC
British Isles Joint TNM Classification Committee	BIJC
Canadian National TNM Committee	CNC
Comité National Uruguayo TNM	CNU-TMN
Deutschsprachiges TNM-Komittee	DSK-TNM
French TNM Group	FTNM
Italian Committee for TNM Cancer Classification	ICC
Japanese Joint Committee	JCC

agreed upon by all national TNM Committees (Table 2) and is the most widely used "common language" to describe the anatomical extent of cancer. Although the Japanese TNM Committee has agreed to use the UICC-TNM staging system of 1987 and 1992, a modified N classification and stage grouping is often used in Japan [25].

The general principles of the TNM system may be summarized in four points as follows:

1. Local spread of the primary tumour (T), regional lymph node metastasis (N) and distant metastasis (M) are assessed and classified separately.
2. T, N and M are condensed to stage groups.
3. Two classifications are provided for each site: a clinical TNM (cTNM) and a pathological classification (pTNM).
4. While TNM and pTNM describe the anatomical extent of cancer in general without considering treatment, the supplementary R (residual tumour) classification describes the tumour situation after treatment.

TNM Versus Dukes

Several authors prefer the original Dukes' classification or modifications. The main reason for *not* using the Dukes' classification is the considerable confusion introduced by the numerous modifications. Further arguments can be added: in the Dukes' classifications, early carcinoma (limited to the submucosa) cannot be identified; the Dukes' C stage is prognostically not homogeneous and in the various modifications it is subdivided according to different rules; the orginal Dukes' classification does not consider distant metastasis. Thus the National Institutes of Health (NIH), in its consensus conference on adjuvant treatment of colorectal carcinoma in 1990 [34], stated that "the TNM system, based on a complete pathological description, can effectively describe risk groups for recurrence and should be used in clinical trials, research and clinical practice." In both the United States and Germany, the TNM system was also introduced for quality management in oncology.

Anatomical Extent and Prognosis

Review

In the TNM system, prognosis is estimated from pT, pN, M or pM and R. There are correlations between these categories, as shown schematically in Fig. 2. With increasing pT, the possibility of R0 resection decreases. In most patients with distant metastasis, an R0 resection is not possible. Prognosis is independently influenced by the R classification as well as by pT, pN and M or pM (for references, see [22]).

Residual Tumour Classification

The most important prognostic factor is the residual tumour status, as defined by the residual tumour (R) classification [16, 20]. In this classification, not only is loco-regional residual tumour considered, but also distant metastasis. Figure 3 illustrates the prognostic influence of the R classification. These data (as well as all the following) orginate from a German prospective multicentre study by the Study Group on Colorectal Carcinoma (SGCRC), in which 2347 unselected patients with invasive colorectal carcinoma were recruited from seven departments of surgery [15, 23].

Prognosis of Patients with Residual Tumour

The prognosis of the patients who have had R1,2 resection is predominantly influenced by the absence or presence of distant metastasis. In the SGCRC study, the median survival time was 21.4 months for M0 (n=48) and 11.4 months for M1 patients (n=118). The 2-year survival rates were 44% and 16%, and the 95% confidence intervals (CI) 30%–58% and 10%–23%, respectively; the 5-year survival rates were 23% (95% CI, 10%–36%) and 3% (95% CI, 0%–6%), respectively. Local tumour spread (pT) and lymph node metastasis (pN) have no major prognostic significance in this patient group.

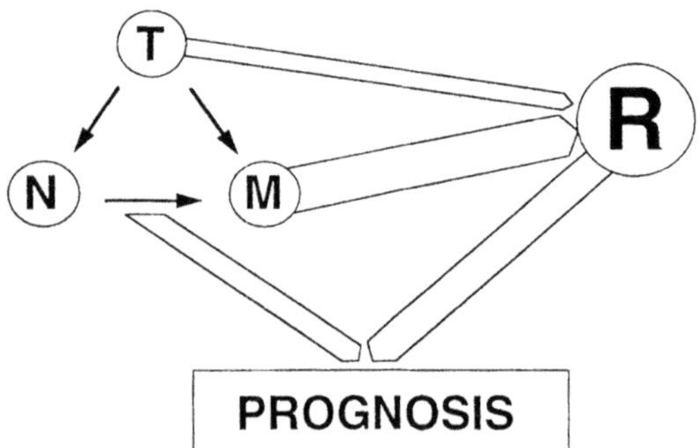

Fig. 2. Components of the TNM system influencing prognosis. *T*, primary tumour; *N*, regional lymph node metastasis; *M*, distant metastasis; *R*, residual tumour

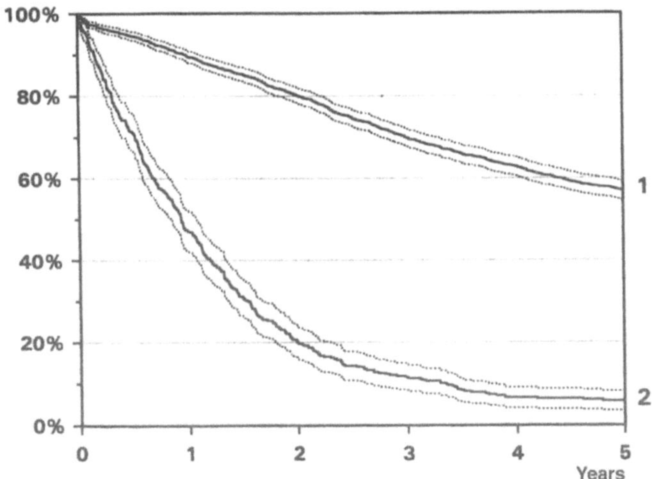

Fig. 3. R classification and prognosis. Observed 5-year survival rates with 95% confidence interval, surgical mortality not excluded. 1, R0 (no residual tumour) (n=887); 55 ± 3%. 2, (macroscopic or microscopic residual tumour) (n=231); 7 ± 4%; < p 0.001. In 166 out of 231 R1,2 patients, the tumour was resected without achieving a R0 status; 65 patients were treated without tumour resection. Data from the SGCRC study [23]

Prognosis of Patients Without Residual Tumour

The prognosis of patients resected for cure (R0) varies widely and depends predominantly on pTNM. Table 3 shows survival in relation to pT and pN.

Prognosis in Relation to Stage Grouping

In rectal carcinoma there are four T/pT categories, four N/pN categories and two M/pM categories, resulting in 32 TNM categories. For purposes of tabulation and analysis, except in very large series, it is necessary to condense these categories into a convenient number of TNM stage groups (Table 4). The prognosis of R0 patients related to the UICC stage grouping is shown in Fig. 4. The differences in survival between the four stages are highly significant. It is important to note that UICC stage III is not homogeneous with respect to survival. There is a significant difference between pN1 and the more advanced categories pN2 and pN3 in stage III, as demonstrated in Fig. 5.

Further Development of Staging

For the TNM system, as for other classification systems in medicine, there are two problems which arise from contradictory requirements:

1. The classification needs to be stable so that data can be accumulated in an orderly way over reasonable periods of time. On the other hand, major

Table 3. Prognosis following R0 resection of rectal carcinoma depending on pT and pN (data of the German Multicenter Study Group for Colorectal Carcinoma; from [23])

Category	Patients (*n*)	5-year survival rates[c] (%)	(95% CI)	Median survival time (months)
pT[a]				
pT1	80	74.3	64.1–84.5	n.d
pT2	231	70.9	64.8–77.0	n.d.
pT3	518	48.7	44.2–53.2	56.6
pT4	58	24.1	12.9–35.3	25.1
pN[b]				
pN0	464	68.1	63.7–72.5	n.d.
pN1	160	46.6	38.6–54.6	53.7
pN2	74	31.1	20.3–41.9	38.8
pN3	132	32.7	24.3–41.1	36.2

The presence or absence of lymph node metastasis could not be assessed (pNX) in 57 patients treated by local resection.
CI, confidence interval; n.d., not determined.
[a]Three statistically different classes: pT1,2/pT3/pT4 ($p<0.001$).
[b]Three statistically different classes: pN0/pN1/pN2,3 ($p<0.001$).
[c]Observed rates, Surgical mortality not included; calculation according to Kaplan-Meier.

Table 4. Stage grouping according to UICC [45] and AJCC [1]

Stage	T	N	M
I	(p)T1,2	(p)N0	(p)M0
II	(p)T3,4		
III			
(A)	Any (p)T	(p)N1	(p)M0
(B)	Any (p)T	(p)N2,3	
IV	Any (p)T	Any (p)N	(p)M1

advances in diagnosis or treatment must be considered and may lead to changes in the classification [45].

2. The classification should be simple enough for universal use in both highly developed and developing countries and sufficiently uncomplicated so that medical professionals are not discouraged from using it. On the other hand, for specialized institutions and for investigative purposes, a relatively simple staging system is inadequate and runs the risk of not being used [47].

With respect to stability, the UICC and AJCC have adopted the policy of not publishing new editions of the system before experience has been accumulated over a period of 10 years. Thus the fifth edition of TNM classification system is planned for 1997.

Optional proposals for so-called *telescopic ramifications*, i.e. subdivisions of the existing T, N and M categories, were presented in *TNM Supplement 1993* [47]. This telescoping enables further specifications for specialized institutions and accommodates the collection of additional data without altering the definitions of the existing TNM categories. In this way, data for future changes can

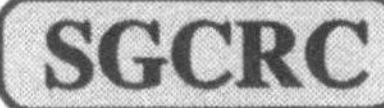
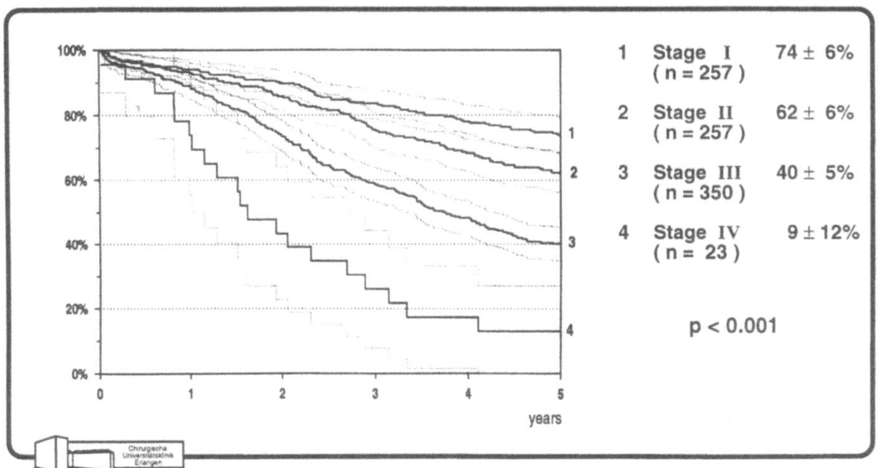

Fig. 4. Stage grouping and prognosis. Tumour resection for cure (R0). For details, see legend to Fig. 3

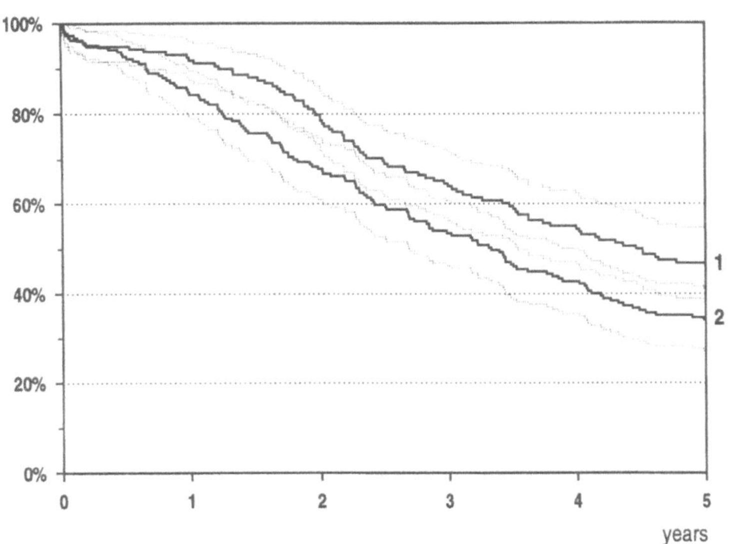

Fig. 5. Inhomogeneity of prognosis in stage III. Tumour resection for cure (R0). *1*, stage III/ pN1 (*n*=159); observed 5-year survival rate (surgical mortality not included), 47% (95% confidence interval, 39%–55%). *2*, stage III/pN2,3 (*n*=191); 34% (27%–41%); *p*<0.01

be obtained; such data are needed because of the principle that changes made to the TNM system should be based on data, and not on philosophy.

The same purpose can be achieved by *optional descriptors*, also presented in *TNM Supplement 1993*. Table 5 shows the respective proposals relevant to the staging of colorectal carcinoma.

An alternative proposal for a future M classification comes from the results of an UICC field study on liver metastasis [17]:

- M1: metastasis in non-regional lymph nodes only
- M2: liver metastasis only
- M3: lung metastasis only
- M4: bone metastasis only
- M5: metastasis in more than one site or at sites other than those listed under M1–4

Standardization of Staging

The results of staging according to a specific system are comparable only if the rules are uniformly applied and the methods used for assessment are largely similar or identical. Thus standardization of staging is crucial to achieve the goal of comparability.

Standardization includes definition of the data which are to be included in the clinical and pathological staging reports. For clinical staging, the methods used have to be standardized. Standardization of pathological staging includes specimen handling, information on the pathologist, gross description, dissection and sampling and histological work-up.

Table 5. Proposals for further development of the TNM system; telescopic ramifications and new descriptors (from [47])

Telescopic ramifications
  pT3 According to the extent of histologically measured perimuscular invasion:
      pT3a (minimal)   1 mm or less
      pT3b (slight)   > 1–5 mm
      pT3c (moderate)   >5–15 mm
      pT3d (extensive)   >15 mm
  pT4 pT4a Invasion of adjacent organs or structures without perforation of visceral peritoneum
      pT4b Perforation of visceral peritoneum
  M1 M1a Metastasis in nonregional lymph nodes only
      M1b Metastasis in viscera (excluding peritoneal and pleural metastasis)
      M1c Peritoneal or pleural metastasis
  pM1 As M1

New descriptors
  (mi) To identify micrometastasis, i.e. no metastasis larger than 0.2 cm, in regional lymph nodes, e.g. pN1 (mi), or in viscera or bone marrow, e.g. pM1 (mi)
  (i) To designate the finding of isolated tumour cells in bone marrow, e.g. by immunohistology, which is classified M1 (i)

There have been various national and international initiatives in recent years, focused on standardization of staging, both generally and specifically for colorectal carcinoma (Table 6).

The work of the International Working Party on Clinicopathological Staging for Colorectal Cancer was a milestone in this respect [9]. Its aim was not only to contribute to standardization of staging, but also to identify other non-anatomical variables of prognostic significance and thus to create a documentation system, i.e. a standard format for clinical and pathology features which should be prospectively documented in all patients treated for colorectal cancer.

Staging and Prognostic Systems

The axis of classification used in staging is the anatomical extent of cancer. There is no doubt that additional non-anatomical factors may independently influence outcome.

Table 6. National and international activities on standardization of staging

Year	Standardization	Author
1979	Standardized histopathological reporting	Hermanek and Gall [18]
1981	Manual of surgical pathology gross procedures	Rosai [38]
1983	General rules for clinical and pathological studies on cancer of the colon, rectum and anus	Japanese Research Society for Cancer of the Colon and Rectum [25]
1983	Pathology reporting of tumours	Hermanek [14]
1989	Handbook for the clinico-pathological assessment and staging of colorectal cancer	UKCCR [48]
1991	Synoptic surgical pathology reporting	Markel and Hirsch [31]
1992	Association of Clinical Pathologists Broadsheet: gross examination of large intestine	Sheffield and Talbot [40]
1992	Checklists for surgical pathology reports	Frable et al. [10] Kempson [27] Rosai et al. [39]
1993-96	Tumour documentation in clinic and practice (four volumes)	ADT (Working Group of German Cancer Centers) [2]
1994	Protocol for examination of specimens removed from patients with colorectal carcinoma	Henson et al. [13]
1995	Diagnostic standards in oncology	DKG (German Cancer Society) [5]

In 1987, Jass et al. [26] published a new prognostic classification of rectal carcinoma with an expansion of pathological staging (local tumour spread and lymph node metastasis) by additional consideration of the pattern of invasive margin and degree of peri-tumoural lymphocytic infiltration. Although this expansion is sometimes referred to as a staging system, it is actually an example of the integration of anatomical extent with two additional histological prognostic factors.

Another example of this type of prognostic classification system is that presented by Michelassi et al. [32, 33], although it was incorrectly designated as a clinico-pathological staging system by the authors. In addition to anatomical extent, it considers race, gross tumour morphology (exophytic versus non-exophytic) and lymphatic and/or vascular micro-invasion.

The identification of independent prognostic factors requires careful methods of investigation, including modern multifactorial biometric analysis (for references, see [22]) because of the multitude of interactions among the different prognostic factors.

The UICC has published a compilation of prognostic factors for the most common tumour sites [22], which is intended to aid in portraying the scope of this field and to stimulate further studies of prognostic factors.

The identification of independent prognostic factors other than TNM/pTNM and R (Fig. 6) opened up the way for the creation of so-called prognostic systems, i.e. the integration of multiple independent prognostic factors, with TNM and R remaining intact. In such prognostic systems it will be possible to calculate a so-called prognostic index which predicts outcome for the individual patient based on all relevant information of prognostic significance. According to their prognostic index, patients may be assigned to various prognostic groups.

In this way, the present staging systems based on anatomical extent of cancer will be replaced by a prognostic system using not only anatomical extent, but also other relevant prognostic information. Such systems will facilitate the estimation of prognosis, the selection of appropriate treatment and the analysis of treatment results. It will also enable a better design of future clinical trials by appropriate stratification and consideration of all relevant prognostic factors [22].

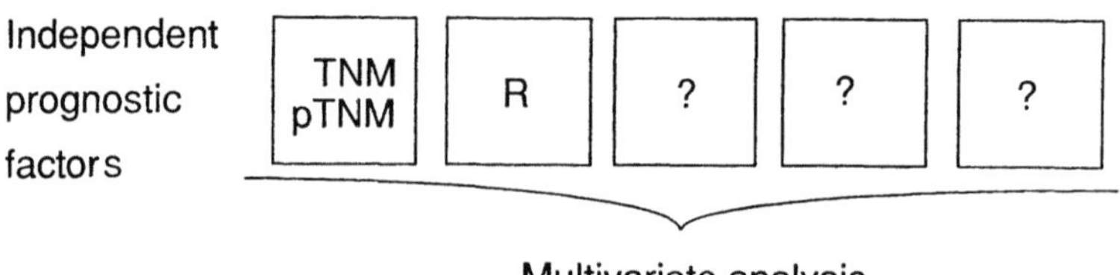

Fig. 6. Development of prognostic systems

References

1. American Joint Committee on Cancer (AJCC), Beahrs OH, Henson DE, Hutter RVP, Kennedy BJ (eds) (1992) Manual for staging of cancer, 4th edn. Lippincott, Philadelphia
2. Arbeitsgemeinschaft Deutscher Tumorzentren (ADT), Wagner G, Dudeck J, Grundmann E, Hermanek P (eds) (1993–1996) Tumordokumentation in Klinik und Praxis, 4 vols. Springer, Berlin Heidelberg New York
3. Astler VB, Coller FA (1954) The prognostic significance of direct extension of carcinoma of the colon and rectum. Ann Surg 139:846–851
4. Davis NC, Newland RC (1982) The reporting of colorectal cancer: the Australian clinicopathological staging system. Aust NZ J Surg 52:395–397
5. Deutsche Krebsgesellschaft (DKG) (1995) Qualitätssicherung in der Onkologie 3.1. In: Hermanek P (ed) Diagnostische Standards Lungen-, Magen-, Pankreas- und Kolorektales Karzinom. Zuckerschwerdt, Munich
6. Dukes CE (1930) The spread of cancer of the rectum. Br J Surg 17:643–648
7. Dukes CE (1932) The classification of cancer of the rectum. J Pathol Bacteriol 35:323–332
8. Dukes CE (1945) Discussion on the pathology and treatment of carcinoma of the colon. Proc R Soc Med 38:381–384
9. Fielding LP, Arsenault PA, Chapuis PH, Dent O, Gatright B, Hardcastle JD, Hermanek P, Jass JR, Newland RC (1991) Clinicopathological staging for colorectal cancer: an International Documentation System (IDS) and an International Comprehensive Anatomical Terminology (ICAT). J Gastroenterol Hepatol 6:325–344
10. Frable WJ, Kempson RL, Rosai J (1992) Quality assurance and quality control in anatomic pathology: standardization of the surgical pathology reports. Mod Pathol 5:102a,b
11. Gabriel WB, Dukes C, Bussey HJ (1935) Lymphatic spread in cancer of the rectum. Br J Surg 23:395–413
12. Gunderson LL, Sosin H (1974) Areas of failure found at operation (second or symptomatic look) following "curative surgery" for adenocarcinoma of the rectum. Cancer 34:1278–1292
13. Henson DE, Hutter RVP, Sobin LH, Bowman HE for the members of the Cancer Committee, College of American Pathologists, and the Task Force for Protocols on the Examination of Specimens From Patients with Colorectal Cancer (1994) Protocol for the examination of specimens removed from patients with colorectal carcinoma. Arch Pathol Labor Med 118:122–125
14. Hermanek P (1983) Pathohistologische Begutachtung von Tumoren. Perimed, Erlangen
15. Hermanek P (1993) Long-term results of a German prospective multicenter study on colorectal cancer. In: Takahashi T (ed) Recent advances in management of digestive cancers. Springer, Berlin Heidelberg New York
16. Hermanek P (1995) pTNM and residual tumor classifications: problems of assessment and prognostic significance. World J Surg 19:184–190
17. Hermanek P (1997) Classification of distant metastasis (in preparation)
18. Hermanek P, Gall FP (1979) Grundlagen der klinischen Onkologie. Witzstrock, Baden-Baden
19. Hermanek P, Gall FP, Altendorf A (1980) Prognostic grouping in colorectal carcinoma. J Cancer Res Clin Oncol 98:185–193
20. Hermanek P, Wittekind C (1994) Residual tumor (R) classification and prognosis. Semin Surg Oncol 10:12–20
21. Hermanek P, Sobin LH, Hayat M (1995) Staging classifications. In: Peckham M, Pinedo B, Veronesi U (eds) Oxford textbook of oncology. Oxford University Press, Oxford
22. Hermanek P, Gospodarowicz MK, Henson DE, Hutter RVP, Sobin LH (eds) (1995) Prognostic factors in cancer. Springer, Berlin Heidelberg New York
23. Hermanek P, Wiebelt H, Staimmer D, Riedl S, German Study Group Colo-Rectal Carcinoma (SGCRC) (1995) Prognostic factors of rectum carcinoma. Experience of the German multicentric study SGCRC. Tumori 81 [Suppl]:60–64
24. Hildebrandt U, Feifel G (1985) Preoperative staging of rectal cancer by intrarectal ultrasound. Dis Colon Rectum 28:42–46

25. Japanese Research Society for Cancer of the Colon and Rectum (1983) General rules for clinical and pathological studies on cancer of the colon, rectum, and anus. Jpn J Surg 13:557–598
26. Jass JR, Love SB, Northover JMA (1987) A new prognostic classification of rectal cancer. Lancet I:1303–1306
27. Kempson EL (1992) The time is now. Checklists for surgical pathology reports. Arch Pathol Lab Med 116:1107–1108
28. Kirklin JW, Dockerty MB, Waugh JM (1949) The role of the peritoneal reflection in the prognosis of carcinoma of the rectum and sigmoid colon. Surg Gynecol Obstet 88:326–331
29. Kyriakos M (1985) The president's cancer, the Dukes classification and confusion. Arch Pathol Lab Med 109:1063–1066
30. League of Nations Health Organisation, Heyman J (ed) (1937) Annual report on the results of radiotherapy in cancer of the uterine cervix. First volume. League of Nations Publications no CH 1225, Geneva
31. Markel SF, Hirsch SD (1991) Synoptic surgical pathology reporting. Hum Pathol 22:807–810
32. Michelassi F, Block GE, Vannucci L, Montag A, Chappell R (1988) A 5- to 21-year follow-up and analysis of 250 patients with rectal adenocarcinoma. Ann Surg 208:379–389
33. Michelassi F, Ayala JJ, Balestracci T, Goldberg R, Chappell R, Block GE (1991) Verification of a new clinicopathologic staging system for colorectal adenocarcinoma. Ann Surg 214:11–18
34. National Institute of Health (NIH) (1990) Consensus conference adjuvant therapy for patients with colon and rectal cancer. JAMA 264:1444–1445
35. Newland RC, Chapuis PH, Pheils MT, MacPherson JG (1981) The relationship of survival to staging and grading of colorectal cancer: a prospective study of 503 cases. Cancer 47:1424–1429
36. Nicholls RJ, York Mason A, Morson BC, Dixon AK, Kelsey Fry I (1982) The clinical staging of rectal cancer. Br J Surg 69:404–409
37. Rankin FW (1926) Surgery of the colon. Appleton, New York
38. Rosai J (1983) Manual of surgical pathology gross room procedures. University of Minnesota Press, Mineapolis
39. Rosai J, Bonfiglio TA, Corson JM, Fechner RE, Harris NL, LiVolsi VA, Silverberg StG (1992) Standardization of the surgical pathological report. Mod Pathol 5:197–199
40. Sheffield JP, Talbot IC (1992) Gross examination of large intestine. ACP Broadsheet 132. J Clin Pathol 42:751–755
41. Steele G Jr, Ellenberg S, Ramming K, O'Connell M, Moertel C, Lessner H, Bruckner H, Horton J, Schein P, Zamcheck N, Novak J, Holyoke ED (1982) CEA monitoring among patients in multiinstitutional adjuvant G.I. therapy protocols. Ann Surg 196:162–169
42. Steinthal CF (1905) Zur Dauerheilung des Brustkrebses. Beitr Klin Chir 47:226–239
43. Turnbull RB Jr, Kyle K, Watson FR, Spratt J (1967) Cancer of the colon: the influence of no-touch isolation technic on survival rates. Ann Surg 166:420–427
44. UICC Committee on TNM Classification (1966) Malignant tumours of the oesophagus, stomach, colon, and rectum. UICC, Geneva
45. UICC, Hermanek P, Sobin LH (eds) (1992) TNM classification of malignant tumours, 4th edn, 2nd rev. Springer, Berlin Heidelberg New York
46. UICC, Spiessl B, Beahrs OH, Hermanek P, Hutter RVP, Scheibe O, Sobin LH, Wagner G (eds) (1992) TNM atlas. Illustrated guide to the TNM/pTNM classification, 3rd edn, 2nd rev. Springer, Berlin Heidelberg New York
47. UICC, Hermanek P, Henson DE, Hutter RVP, Sobin LH (eds) (1993) TNM supplement 1993. A commentary on uniform use. Springer, Berlin Heidelberg New York
48. United Kingdom Co-ordinating Commission on Cancer Research (UKCCCR) (1989) Handbook for the clinico-pathological assessment and staging of colorectal cancer. UKCCCR, London
49. Wolmark N, Fisher B, Wieand HS (1986) The prognostic values of the modifications of the Dukes' C class of colorectal cancer. An analysis of the NSABP clinic trials. Ann Surg 203:115–122
50. York Mason A (1975) Local excision. Clin Gastroenterol 4:582–593

Limitations of Existing Systems of Staging for Rectal Cancer: The Forgotten Margin

Philip Quirke

Introduction

Good staging is central to the logical management of patients with rectal cancer since the choice of future treatment is frequently based upon the stage of the tumour. Before one can describe the limitations of existing staging systems, the best method must be considered. The ideal staging system would be clinicopathological, however, there are two disadvantages of such methods. Firstly, clinical impressions can be inaccurate with false-positive and negative diagnoses, e.g. radiological imaging of metastases, surgeon's impression of adequacy of resection, and secondly, communication and cooperation must be high between the surgeon and his specialist pathologist, which may not always be the case. With improved imaging, more specialisation of both surgeons and pathologists, and the realisation of the importance of the close relationship between the pathologist and surgeon, it should be possible to move towards a clinicopathological system.

The ideal staging system should be simple, reproducible, and have a high predictive value for the chosen end points for the individual patient.

For me an ideal staging system would:

1. Identify those patients who had undergone a palliative resection and the site(s) of residual disease and if possible predict the type of treatment required for that pattern of residual disease.
2. Identify cured patients with 100% success.
3. Predict the site of recurrence whether local, peritoneal, liver or other distal sites or a combination of these sites with 100% success and thus predict the type of treatment.

Any additional information such as the quality of the surgical resection would be a bonus. Where possible there should be the minimum possible number of groups to answer the important clinical questions or alternatively an accurate percentage risk of recurrence could be given.

The ideal grading system would predict the biological aggressiveness, e.g. rate of growth, the ability of the tumour to spread and, if possible, its response to the therapeutic armamentarium available for treatment.

Current Methods of Staging

The *Dukes'* [15] *classification* is the basis of many of the subsequent systems. Dukes' A carcinomas have invaded through the muscularis mucosa, but have not penetrated the whole thickness of the muscularis propria. Dukes' B carcinomas have invaded through the muscularis propria and out into the subserosa or mesorectum; they do not involve lymph nodes. Dukes' C carcinomas have metastasized to lymph nodes. These were subsequently divided [17] into those cases in which the lymph node at the high surgical tie was involved (Dukes' C2) and those where it was not involved (Dukes' C1). A further stage has come into popular usage after its description by Turnbull et al. [37]. This is frequently used to indicate the presence of hepatic metastases.

The *Astler-Coller modification* [3] *of the Kirklin, Dockerty and Waugh* [26] *classification* is still based on the depth of penetration of the tumour and lymph node involvement, but has more subdivisions within it. It is confusing as it uses A, B and C but these are different from Dukes' description. Astler-Coller stage A tumours had mucosal involvement only, i.e. under Dukes' these were not invasive cancers. Stage B1 carcinomas have invaded into the submucosa or the muscularis propria, but not through the muscularis propria, and there is no lymph node involvement. Stage B2 carcinomas have invaded through the muscularis propria with no lymph node involvement. Stage C1 carcinomas are not through the muscularis propria, but have lymph node involvement. Stage C2 carcinomas are through the muscularis propria with lymph node metastases but the site of the metastases, e.g. apical lymph node involvement, are unimportant.

The *TNM classification* [4, 13, 19, 20, 38, 39] looks at direct spread (T) through the wall, into adjacent organs and the presence of involvement of the peritoneal surface. Lymph node involvement (N) of one to three nodes (N1), four nodes or more (N2), or nodal involvement along named vascular trunks or of the apical lymph node (N3). Liver metastases are classified as present (M1) or absent (M0). If the data is purely pathological then it should be prefixed by a 'p', e.g. pT2 pN2 pM1. There is also a classification for a curative excision (R0), microscopic involvment of the margin(s) (R1) or macroscopic residual disease (R2). The TNM classification accurately describes the stage of the tumour but leads to over 30 possible combinations, even without the addition of the R staging. To be clinically useful it needs to be fused into a smaller number of stages (see below).

The major strength of the *Australian Clinico-Pathological correlation* [9, 11, 12, 30] is that it is a clinicopathological system and that it is easy to use compared with TNM since it has only nine groups.

The *system devised by Jass* et al. [24, 25] is unusual in that it utilises both staging information such as depth of penetration and lymph node involvement and grading information such as the type of invasive border and the nature of the lymphocytic reaction. It has been criticised for the subjective nature of the grading variables and has not been widely adopted.

All staging systems combine an assessment of depth of penetration with lymph node involvement as well as additional factors such as adequacy of resection, type of border, degree of inflammatory reaction and presence of metastases.

Dukes, Astler-Coller and TNM are the major classifications in international usage. Each has advantages and disadvantages, and there is no ideal system. Dukes' stage is simple and used in many countries. Astler-Coller is used in the United States, and TNM is used widely in Europe and is gaining ground elsewhere, especially in the United States. All predict prognosis to a greater or lesser extent, but no one system predicts it with 100% accuracy. These systems have been used extensively to predict the survival of a group of patients but not for their accuracy in predicting death or cure, let alone the site of failure for an individual patient. The nearest anyone has got to assessing the accuracy of prediction is Nathanason et al. [29]. Their data are set out in Table 1. Whilst there are reasonable criticisms of this paper, it is an interesting way to compare classifications. It is clear that no single classification in their hands was greatly superior to Dukes' classification, and it is obvious that all the systems can be improved, especially with respect to accuracy in identifying individually those patients who will die and more importantly the site of failure.

Other disadvantages are that all have multiple categories and that the numbers of cases in a category can be small, e.g Dukes's stage A's corresponding to T1 N0 M0 (Group 1) or Astler-Coller A/B1 frequently do not exceed 15% of cases seen. TNM staging provides the most information and is easy to use, but ends up with multiple different categories that frequently have to be amalgamated as they may have a similar prognosis. The 33 variables can, however, be amalgamated into five stages. The 5-year survival ranges from Stage I 71%–74%, Stage II 57%–62%, Stage III 25%–40% to Stage IV 7%–9% [22, 41]. Considering the level of complexity of the classification, does it ac-

Table 1. The sensitivity and specificity of a staging system in predicting death from colorectal cancer from Nathanson et al. [29]

Staging method	Sensitivity (%)	Specificity (%)	Correct (%)
Dukes'	50.6	82.1	68.2
Kirklin et al.	50.6	82.1	68.2
Astler-Coller	50.6	82.1	68.2
GI Tumour Study Group	46.2	91.3	71.3
pTNM	64.7	76.0	71.0

tually help more than a simple modified Dukes' classification once it has been re-amalgamated into stages I–IV?

Blenkinsop et al. [5] showed that in routine practice even the simple Dukes' system suffered from wide interobserver variation amongst pathologists. Therefore, more complex systems must demonstrate their reproducibility in a routine setting. Audit of the large bowel cancer project showed the frequency of Dukes' A's varied from 5% to 30% in different hospitals and the mean number of lymph nodes detected per case from 1 to 11.2 nodes [5]. The larger the number of factors that need to be collected, the less likely that they will be accurately recorded and that the variability between pathologists will be increased.

In rectal cancer all the systems currently fail to place as much significance as is required on involvement of the circumferential resection margins (CRM) [1, 14, 31, 32, 36]. The TNM and the Australian system can incorporate CRM involvement, but we do not know how it would affect the prognostic value of the classifications as there are as yet no prospective evaluations of these systems with and without CRM involvement.

What Staging Method Should We Use?

Work needs to continue on improving current systems including new factors such as the assessment of CRM and peritoneal involvement. However, in the absence of one universal staging system it is relatively easy to use both Dukes' and TNM. It is sensible to ascertain whether the data which are common to most of the systems can be easily and reproducibly collected routinely by pathologists, if possible on a proforma basis which could be used in all clinical trials. Examples are shown in Fig. 1. The Royal College of Surgeons form is a routine reporting form containing the minimum data set developed by Professors Williams and Talbot and myself. This is based on a form used in Yorkshire developed by Yorkshire pathologists. The second form of this is a modification of the original UKCCCR colorectal cancer form [40] by myself and Dr. N. Shepherd. It is probably naive to imagine that there will ever be a single staging system, but ways must exist for comparison of the clinicopathological data in major trials, especially for meta-analysis.

Local Recurrence

In this section, I would like to explore more fully the factors involved in local recurrence and suggest that recurrence can be predicted by simple pathological methods. The current method by which we examine our specimens will be described as well as the value of the careful pathological examination of the specimen with respect to the quality of surgery.

RCS National Guidelines Minimum Data Set
Colorectal Cancer Histopathology Report

Patient Name: ....   Date of Birth: ....

Hospital: ....   Hospital No: ....

Histology No: ....   Surgeon: ....

Gross Description

Site of Tumour ....

Maximum tumour diameter................................... cm

Distance of tumour to nearest margin .... cm

For rectal tumours

Peritoneal reflection

    Above ☐   At ☐   Below ☐

Distance from pectinate line .... cm

Histology
Type

	Yes	No
Adenocarcinoma	☐	☐

If No, Other ....

Differentiation by predominant area

    Poor ☐   Other ☐

Local Invasion

Submucosa (pT1)   ☐

Muscularis propria (pT2)   ☐

Beyond Muscularis propria (pT3)   ☐

Tumour cells have reached the serosal surface   ☐
    or invaded adjacent organs (pT4)

Margins

Tumour involvement	Yes	No
doughnut	☐	☐
margin	☐	☐
circumferential margin	☐	☐

    (rectal cancer only – involved if ≤1mm)

Histological measurement

from tumour to circumferential margin................... mm

Metastatic Spread

No of lymph nodes examined......................................

No of positive lymph nodes ....
    (pN1 1-3 nodes pN2 ≥4 nodes involved
    pN3 nodes along named vascular trunk)

	Yes	No
Apical node positive (C2)	☐	☐
Extramural vascular invasion	☐	☐

Background Abnormalities

	Yes	No
Adenoma(s)	☐	☐
Synchronous carcinoma(s)	☐	☐
Ulcerative colitis	☐	☐
Crohn's	☐	☐
Familial adenomatous polyposis	☐	☐

Complete a separate form for each cancer

Pathological Staging

	Yes	No
Complete resection at all margins	☐	☐

TNM

T ☐   N ☐   M ☐

Dukes

Dukes A ☐   (Growth limited to wall, nodes negative)

Dukes B ☐   (Growth beyond M. propria, nodes negative)

Dukes C1 ☐   (Nodes positive and apical node negative)

Dukes C2 ☐   (Apical node positive)

	Yes	No
Histologically confirmed liver metastases	☐	☐

Signature ....

Date ....

Fig. 1. Possible colorectal cancer histopathology request form

UKCCCR Clinico-pathological Reporting of Colorectal Cancer

Patient Name: .... Date of Birth: ....

Hospital: .... Hospital No: ....

Histology No: .... Surgeon: ....

Preoperative assessment

Date

Day	Month	Year

Distance of lower edge of tumour from anal verge
by rigid sigmoidoscopy .... cm   NA ☐

Quadrants:

Anterior ☐   Left Lateral ☐
Posterior ☐   Right Lateral ☐
NA ☐

Fixity

Mobile ☐   Tethered ☐
Fixed (immobile) ☐   NA ☐

Rectal Biopsy

Primary adenocarcinoma ☐   Other ☐
(specify other ....)
Differentiation   Poor ☐   Other ☐
Synchronous lesions   Yes ☐   No ☐
(please specify..)

Chest X-ray

Metastases present ☐   Meatstases absent ☐

Liver Metastases

Present ☐   Equivocal ☐
Symptoms ☐   Absent ☐

Type of Scan

CT ☐   US ☐   Isotope ☐

Established liver metastases

Solitary: Right lobe ☐   Left lobe ☐
Multiple: Unilobar ☐   Bilobar ☐

Serum CEA

Normal ☐   Raised ☐   Not Measuerd ☐
If Raised, state level ....

Operative Assessment

Date of operation

Day	Month	Year

Operating surgeon

Name:..
Grade: ....

Surgery

Elective ☐   Emergency ☐
If emergency, state reason ....

Presence of: Yes   No
synchronous carcinoma   ☐   ☐
adenomas   ☐   ☐

Site

Caecum ☐   Ascending colon ☐
Hepatic flexure ☐   Transverse colon ☐
Splenic flexure ☐   Descending colon ☐
Sigmoid colon ☐
Rectum, above peritoneum ☐
Rectum, stradles peritoneal reflexion ☐
Rectum, below peritoneum ☐

Fixity

Mobile ☐   Tethered ☐   Fixed ☐
If fixed, state to which structures ....

Complications

Obstruction   Yes ☐   No ☐
Spontaneous perforation   Yes ☐   No ☐
Local Abscess   Yes ☐   No ☐
Operative perforation   Yes ☐   No ☐

Clinical evidence of metastases

Peritoneum   Yes ☐   No ☐
Para-aortic lymph nodes   Yes ☐   No ☐
Liver: None ☐   1 ☐   2 ☐
3 ☐   4 ☐   Multiple ☐
Lobes   Right ☐   Left ☐
Both ☐   NA ☐
Replacement   <25% ☐   25-50% ☐
>50% ☐   NA ☐

Biopsy of distant metastases
Yes ☐   No ☐   NA ☐

Excision of tumour

Complete ☐   Indefinite ☐   Incomplete ☐
Is surgery considered curative?   Yes ☐   No ☐
Biopsy taken from tumour bed?   Yes ☐   No ☐

Additional data   Yes   No

Pre-op radiotherapy   Short course   ☐   ☐
Long course   ☐   ☐
Previous local excision   ☐   ☐

UKCCCR Clinico-pathological Reporting of Colorectal Cancer

Patient Name: .... Date of Birth: ....

Hospital: .... Hospital No: ....

Histology No: .... Surgeon: ....

Gross Description

Operation ....

Site of Tumour ....

   Rectum: Peritoneal reflection

      Above ☐   At ☐   Below ☐

Specimen length .... cm

Tumour length .... cm

Tumour width........................... cm

Perforation?   Tumour ☐   Bowel ☐

Distance of tumour to nearest margin .... cm

Which?   Distal ☐   Proximal ☐

Histology
Grading

Type	Yes	No
Adenocarcinoma NOS	☐	☐
Mucinous (>50% of tumour)	☐	☐

Other ....

Differentiation by predominant area

	Poor ☐	Other ☐
Margin	Pushing ☐	Infiltrating ☐
Lymphocytic reaction	Dense ☐	Sparse ☐

Local Invasion

Submucosa (pT1) ☐

Muscularis propria (pT2) ☐

Beyond Muscularis propria (pT3) ☐

   Maximum distance beyond .... mm

   (measured macroscopically)

Penetrates peritoneum with tumour cells on ☐

   surface/tumour ulceration of serosa (pT4)

Invades adjacent organs (pT4) ☐

Which organ ....

Margins

Tumour involvement	Yes	No
distal doughnut	☐	☐
distal margin	☐	☐
proximal doughnut	☐	☐
proximal margin	☐	☐
circumferential margin	☐	☐

(rectal cancer/caecal only tumour <1mm from margin)

Histological measurement

from tumour to circumferential margin................... mm

Metastatic Spread

No of lymph nodes examined ....

No of positive lymph nodes ....

   (pN1 1-3 nodes pN2 ≥4 nodes involved

   pN3 nodes along named vascular trunk)

	Yes	No
Apical node positive (C2/pN3)	☐	☐
Lymph node along named vascular trunk positive (pN3)	☐	☐
Extramural vascular invasion	☐	☐
Histologically proven distant metastases	☐	☐

   Site ....

Metastasis completely resected	☐	☐

Other pathology

	Yes	No
Adenoma(s)	☐	☐

   Number .... Site ....

Synchronous carcinoma(s)*	☐	☐

   Number .... Site ....

   *Complete a separate form for each cancer

Ulcerative colitis	☐	☐
Crohn's	☐	☐
Familial adenomatous polyposis	☐	☐

Other (specify)...

Clinico–Pathological Staging

	Yes	No
Complete resection at all margins	☐	☐

pTNM

pT ☐   pN ☐   pM ☐   R0 ☐   R1 ☐   R2 ☐

   (see guidance notes)

Dukes A ☐   (Growth limited to wall, nodes negative)

Dukes B ☐   (Growth beyond M. propria, nodes negative)

Dukes C1 ☐   (Nodes positive and apical node negative)

Dukes C2 ☐   (Apical node positive)

Stage D ☐   (Liver metastases)

Signature ....

Date ....

Evidence of CRM Involvement and Local Recurrence

Involvement of the proximal bowel margin is very unusual, and involvement of the distal margin infrequent. The most important margin is the CRM. A relationship between the degree of local spread and the frequency of local recurrence was shown by Dukes and Bussey [16], but they did not investigate involvement of the CRM. We commenced a prospective study in 1982 to investigate this problem [32]. Chan et al. [7] in 1985 published a method of transverse slicing which was similar to ours to assess CRM involvement but reported no survival data. In our first series, 52 cases were followed prospectively for a median of 23 months. The specimens were opened, the tumours sliced transversely and totally embedded with the preparation of whole mount sections on glass slides. This was time-consuming but meant that the whole tumour could be reviewed. These were assessed for CRM involvement, which was present in 27%. Local recurrence developed in 23% of all patients. Eleven of 13 patients with CRM involvement, who survived to be assessed, subsequently developed local recurrence. This gave a sensitivity of 92%, a specificity of 95%, and a positive predictive value of 85%. Five of 39 patients (14%) in the curative group had CRM involvement, of which four recurred. At that time we did not investigate the lymph node chain above the tumour for CRM involvement. We subsequently modified the method from embedding and sectioning of the whole tumour in favour of transverse slicing of the tumour followed by careful visual inspection and selective histological sampling of the slices, with subsequent examination of the posterior mesorectum above the tumour for CRM involvement. This was routinely adopted in the department and has proved robust in practice.

Between 1986 and 1990 we prospectively followed 194 patients [1]. Sixty-nine of 194 patients (36%) had involvement of the CRM, of which 44 recurred. Thus CRM status predicted local recurrence in 64%. Of the 141 patients who underwent a curative operation, 35 (25%) had involvement of the CRM. Of these 35 patients 23 (66%) recurred locally. For all CRM-positive patients, 64% recurred locally as opposed to 9% in the CRM-negative group. In the curative group, 66% recurred locally as opposed to 8%, indicating that the technique was equally effective in predicting local recurrence in both groups. For patients with a clear CRM and a potentially curative resection ($n=106$), 90% (95% CI 84%–96%) avoided local recurrence, whereas only 22% (95% CI 6%–38%) of patients with CRM involvement at 5 years did so. The risk of local recurrence in CRM-positive patients was 12-fold (95% CI 4–34) that of CRM-negative patients and their risk of death three times higher (95% CI 1.6–6.5) than CRM-negative patients. The overall survival in the potentially curative resection group was 74% for CRM-negative patients as opposed to 24% for CRM-positive patients. Overall, patients who were CRM-positive had a 15% 5-year survival.

The importance of CRM involvement has been confirmed by Ng et al. [31] on 80 patients, de Haas-Kock et al. [14] on 248 patients, and Shepherd et al. [36], on 209 patients. Cawthorne et al. [6] did not confirm its value with respect to local recurrence but this study stripped the fat from the rectum before examining the CRM. This would have made assessment of involvement of the

CRM much more difficult. However, in this study patients with CRM involvement had a very poor prognosis.

CRM involvement has thus emerged as a powerful predictor of local recurrence and is a valuable new addition to staging rectal cancer. The involvement of the upper rectal peritoneal surface by tumour with ulceration of the peritoneum or free tumour cells on the surface [36] should also be added, but there are far fewer data available especially of its relative importance as compared to CRM involvement. Shepherd et al. [36] found 13/209 (6.2%) cases to have CRM involvement, but the impact on the surgically curative group could not be ascertained, as all such cases were classified as palliative. Importantly, they also found peritoneal involvement in 54/209 (25.8%) of cases. The relative importance of peritoneal involvement as a predictor of local recurrence would probably increase with a reduction in the frequency of CRM involvement which would be obtained by better surgery. The local recurrence rate in Shepherd et al.'s study was 13% at 30 months [36]. The surgeon involved in the study practised total mesorectal excision. This study indicates that pathological assessment of peritoneal involvement with between two and six histological blocks merits further attention. It does, however, demonstrate that peritoneal ulceration by tumour cells, or the presence of tumour cells on the surface of the peritoneum are required for local recurrence. The presence of tumour cells abutting the peritoneum but not penetrating it did not lead to local recurrence.

From our latest study, CRM involvement and the presence of involved lymph nodes were the only independent predictors of survival and were better than Dukes' stage. De Haas-Kock et al. [14] in 248 patients showed CRM status and T stage to be independent predictors of local recurrence and CRM status and N stage to be independent prognostic factors for distant metastases. Ng et al. [31] showed CRM status, lymph node involvement and grade of differentiation predicted survival. The predictors of local recurrence alone were not stated.

The current staging systems are geared to providing the surgeon with a percentage likelihood of the patient surviving. This is of less value than a staging system that can accurately predict cure or relapse and the site of that relapse. We now have a routine method for the prediction of patients likely to develop local recurrence (64% versus 9%) that adds little time to the dissection of a specimen (5–10 min). It is easily performed by any histopathologist and adds less than 5% to the cost of the examination.

The method to use to predict distant relapse is less certain. In our series of an average local recurrence rate of 25% in curative cases, CRM status and lymph node involvement were the best predictors of distant recurrence. This is confirmed by de Haas-Kock et al. [14]. Shepherd et al. [36] found lymph node involvement, the type of invasive margin and extent of local spread to predict distant recurrence. The lesser importance of local spread was probably due to the low rate of local recurrence observed in this series, probably due to good surgery. It is now clear that we should move to the routine assessment of *all* margins and reassess the other prognostic factors required. Lymph node status is important but how many other factors do we need to add, especially when intra- and interobserver variation will increase with the rise in the number of variables assessed. Current staging systems need to be reassessed.

The Quality of Rectal Surgery

Additional information is gathered by visual inspection and full thickness slicing of the tumour. Visual inspection gives a clear indication of the quality of specimens. Slicing the tumour as well as the posterior mesorectum above the tumour allows a good assessment of the adequacy of excision and the regularity of the circumferential/mesorectal margin which is an indictor of the quality of the resection. Specimens vary widely between surgeons. Most pathologists only receive resections from three or four surgeons and, therefore, are unable to gain enough experience of the wide range of specimens of different quality that are being resected. Figures 2a–d show resections of varying quality. Inadequate specimens demonstrate the CRM very close to or at the muscularis propria (Fig. 2a). Figure 2d is a total mesorectal excision resection by Mr. R.J. Heald. With experience the macroscopic visual inspection of the specimen allows the pathologist to gauge the quality of the resection and thus the surgeon.

Examples of transverse slices through rectal carcinoma specimens of differing quality of resection are shown in Figs. 3a–d. In the worst resections (Figs. 3a,b) it is possible to see the muscularis propria forming the CRM and, as such, the recurrence of Dukes' A tumours can be explained. The most frequent problem is the irregular margin where the surgeon has accidentally left an area of mesorectum behind or lost the plane and cut inwards towards the muscularis propria before finding the correct plane again. The ideal resection should have a smooth circumferential margin as far as possible away from the muscularis propria. Figure 3d shows a reasonable resection.

The routine measurement of the maximum depth of penetration of the tumour and the frequency of local recurrence in that surgeon's practice allows comparison of the quality of surgery between surgeons. If surgeon A had a high proportion of tumours extending out less than 5 mm from the muscularis propria and a high recurrence rate, then the quality of his/her surgery must be investigated. If surgeon B has a high recurrence rate but is routinely operating on cases where the tumour extends out 25–30 mm, then advanced tumours, not poor surgery, is probably the key factor responsible for recurrence. Measurement of the extent of local spread is an important factor when considering the degree of responsibility the surgeon should bear for local recurrence.

Fig. 2a–d. Photographs of resections by different surgeons showing a varying degree of removal of the mesorectum. **a** It is possible to see muscularis propria over large areas of the specimen. **b** More tissue is removed but the specimen surface is very irregular. Mesorectal fat has either not been removed (*thin arrows*) or the plane of excision has been lost (*fat arrow*). **c** This is a better resection as the mesorectal surface is smooth. It does not, however, show the same amount of tissue removed as in **d**, a resection by Mr. Heald

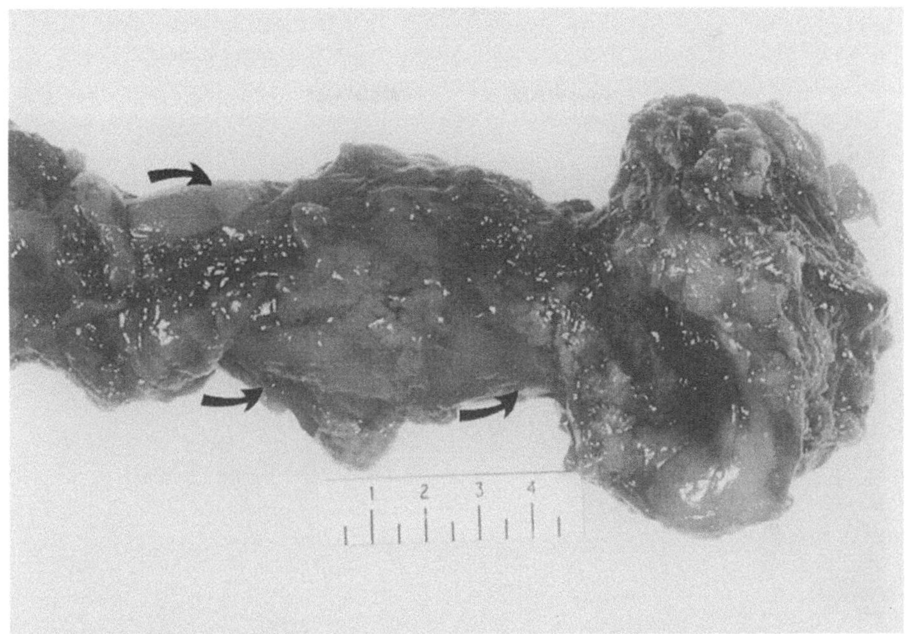

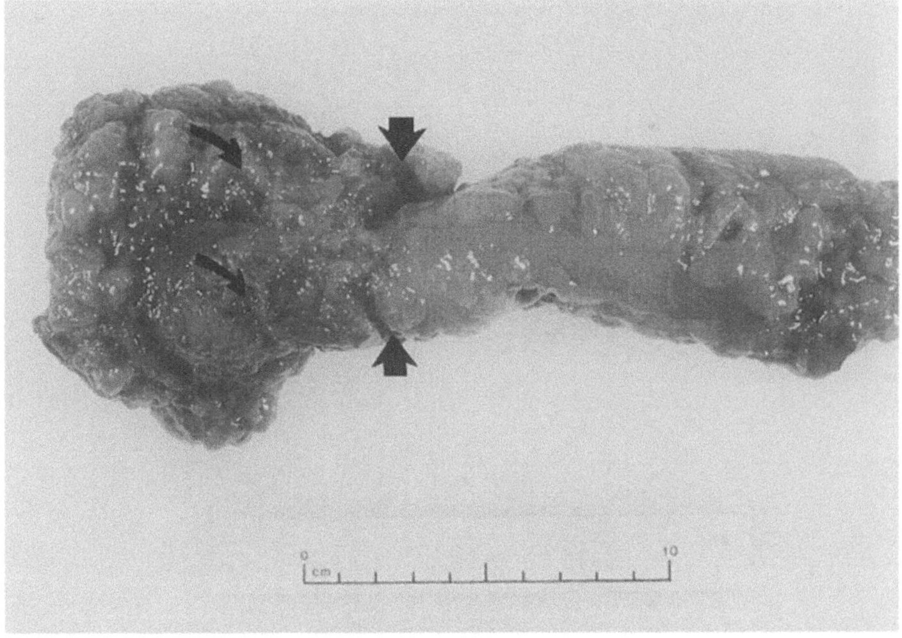

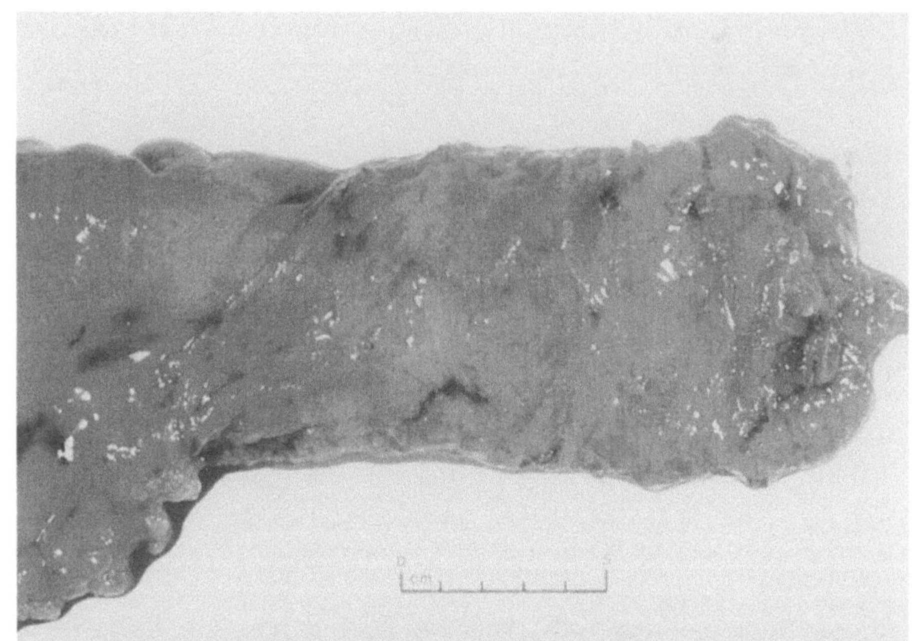

c

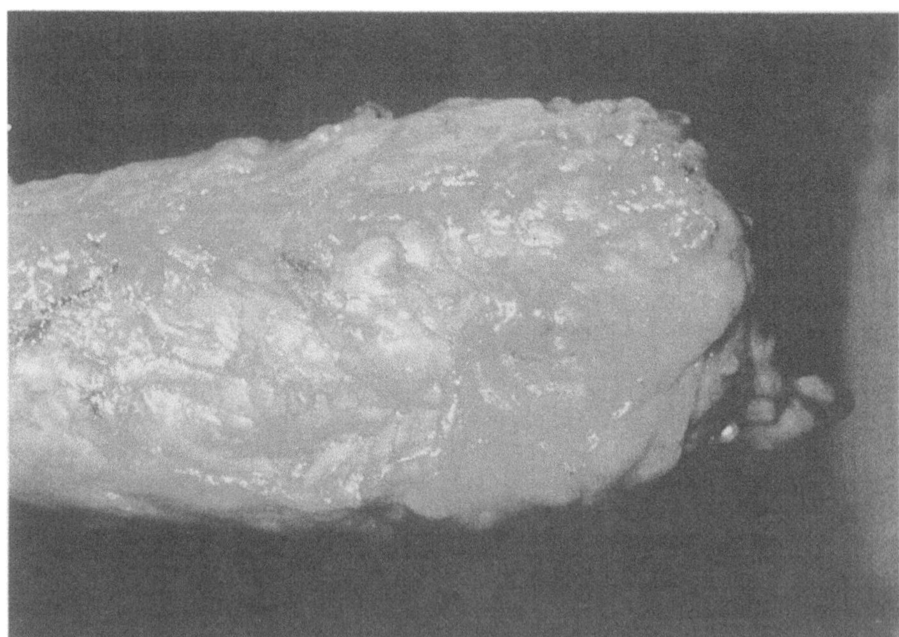

d

Since (a) the resection specimen varies so much between surgeons, (b) survival differs dramatically between surgeons [18, 22, 23, 27, 28] and (c) it has been shown that the adoption of total mesorectal excision can improve local recurrence rates and survival [2], we should surely concentrate on the skill of the surgeon as an important prognostic factor. Should we not classify surgeons as well as the stage of the tumour? We might use groups like those laid out below, preferably based on the external audit of data:

Group 1. Those with a 5-year survival for all cases of more than 60% and a local recurrence rate below 10%.

Group 2. Those with a 5-year survival for all cases of 40%–60% and a local recurrence rate between 10% and 25%.

Group 3. Those with a 5-year survival for all cases of less than 40% and a local recurrence rate of more than 25%.

Group 4. Those who do not have sufficient experience to provide outcome data.

The aim should be to fully utilise those surgeons in Group 1 and to improve the performance or exclude those surgeons in Group 3 from rectal surgery. Surgeons in Group 2 should receive educational visits from Group 1 surgeons. Such a proposal would be highly controversial, but would set standards which could be aimed at. Moving surgeons in Group 3 to Group 1 would yield a major improvement in prognosis, probably greater than that from adjuvant chemotherapy. Changing surgical practice could yield as much as a 20% 5-year survival advantage for patients with rectal cancer.

The Optimum Specimen

The optimum specimen consists of an adequate proximal margin and an adequate distal margin ideally greater than 5 cm but usually at least 2 cm. It is, however, possible to get away with 1 cm in many situations if there is no coning [18]. Ideally, such short margins should be avoided since distal mesorectal metastases do occur [35]. Coning of the distal mesorectum must be avoided since it can bring the CRM much closer to the tumour, especially when the tumour lies in close proximity to the distal margin. A good clearance circumferentially around the tumour with as much tissue removed as possible is important. The mesorectum above the tumour should also be removed intact since it contains lymph nodes which may harbour metastatic tumour. Involvement of the CRM can occur from this source. The surgeon should routinely obtain at least 2 cm circumferential clearance posteriorly and at least 0.5 cm anteriorly from the muscularis propria, and frequently it should be 3–3.5 cm and 1 cm, respectively. The margin should be even with a consistent distance from the muscularis propria without dipping in towards it. This is shown in Fig. 3d. This is especially important with respect to the sacro-coccygeal raphe where the margin is frequently reduced to 0–1 cm from the muscularis propria. Anteriorly there is much less tissue to remove. In females this can be ameliorated to some extent by the removal of the posterior wall of

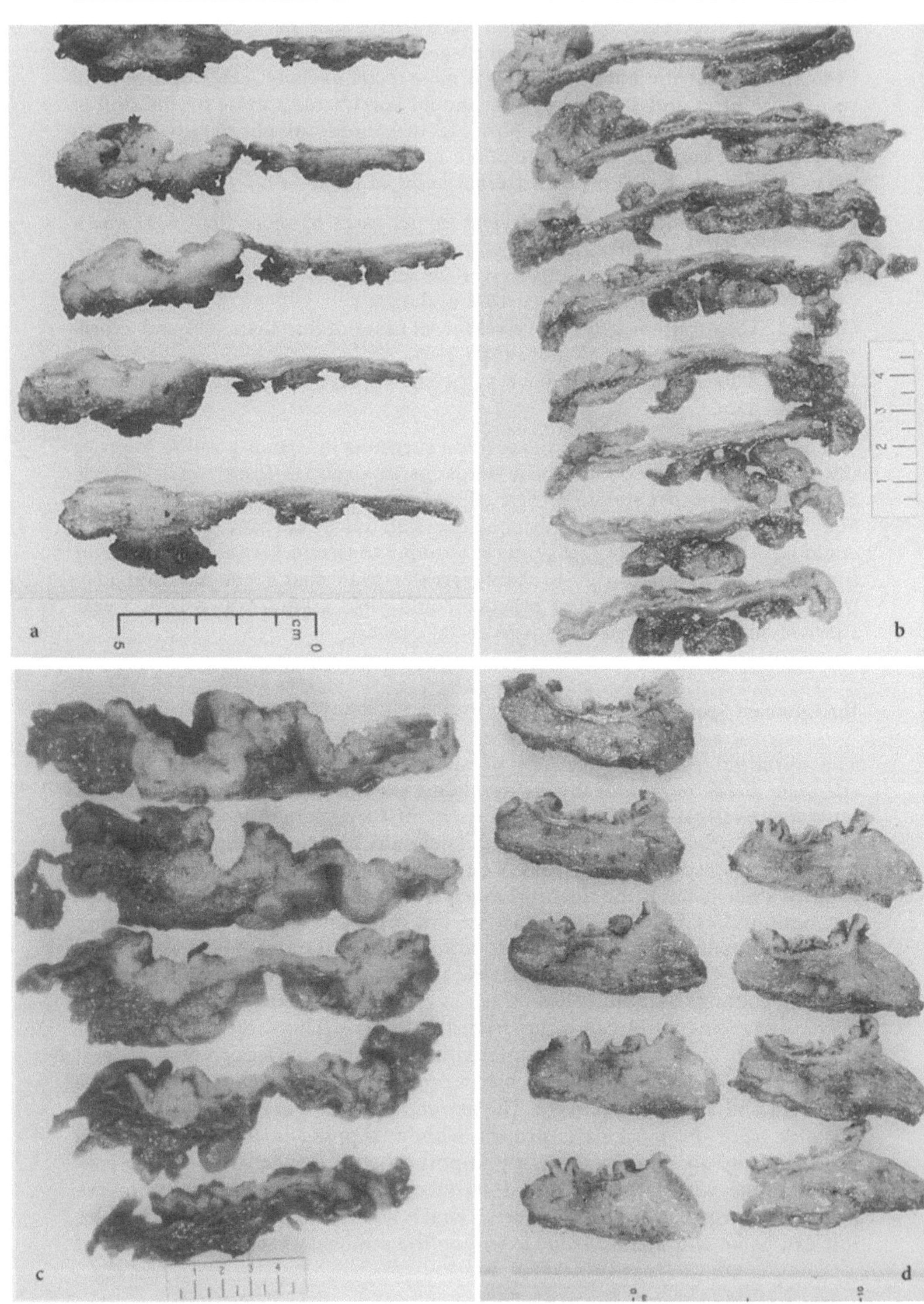
a
cm
5
0
b
1
2
3
4
c
1
2
3
4
d

the vagina, but in men the area of the prostate makes anterior tumours more difficult to resect. Recently quantitative studies (Payne and Quirke, unpublished data) have shown that there is 2.5 times more tissue posteriorly than anteriorly. It is important for the surgeon to consistently achieve the distances away from the muscularis propria stated above, for the specimen to have a smooth surface preferably with some mesorectal fascia of the holy plane on the surface to indicate that the surgical plane is correct (Fig. 4). The posterior aspect will frequently appear bilobed but again the indentation in the posterior midline should not be pronounced and should remain at least 2 cm from the muscularis propria. The plane should be consistent all the way up the posterior aspect of the specimen, since involvement of the CRM can occur from involved lymph nodes which lie against the CRM in this area as well as the primary tumour.

Pathological Assessment of a Rectal Cancer Specimen

The pathological assessment of a rectal cancer specimen has been described previously [33, 34], but minor modifications are presented here. Where possible, specimens should be received fresh and be opened by the pathologist. If this is not possible, then the surgeon should open the bowel in the way described below and pin it out on a cork board for fixation. If neither of these are possible, then the specimen should be placed in an adequate volume of formalin, usually 20 times the volume of the specimen. We now open the rectum anteriorly apart from the area 1–2 cm above and below the tumour where the anterior part of the rectum is left intact. This change is because of the importance of the anterior quadrant with respect to local spread. Below the peritoneal reflection, the surgeon can only usually remove between 0.5 and 1.0 cm anteriorly, thus tumours involving this area are at greater risk of CRM involvement.

In tumours above the peritoneal reflection, involvement of the peritoneal surface can occur, and it is best not to destroy this area during opening by avoiding opening the site of the tumour. If the surgeon or the pathologist is interested in the quality of the resection then macroscopic photographs of the posterior and anterior sides of the specimen are warranted as an audit record. The opened specimen should then be pinned to a cork board and fixed for at least 48 h, preferably more if possible. After fixation the specimen should be

---

Fig. 3a–d. Photographs of transverse sections of the area of the tumour after fully opening the lumen of the rectum. **a,b** Poor resections with the circumferential margins lying on the muscularis propria in places and relatively little mesorectum excised around the tumour. **c** A slightly better resection but the margin is again uneven, close to the muscularis propria and this case shows CRM involvement 1.5 cm from the muscularis propria. **d** A much better resection with a smooth, even CRM. Note the lymph nodes in the mesorectal fat and the mesorectal metastatic deposits. It is easy to see how they could be left behind by operations such as shown in **a, b,** and **c**

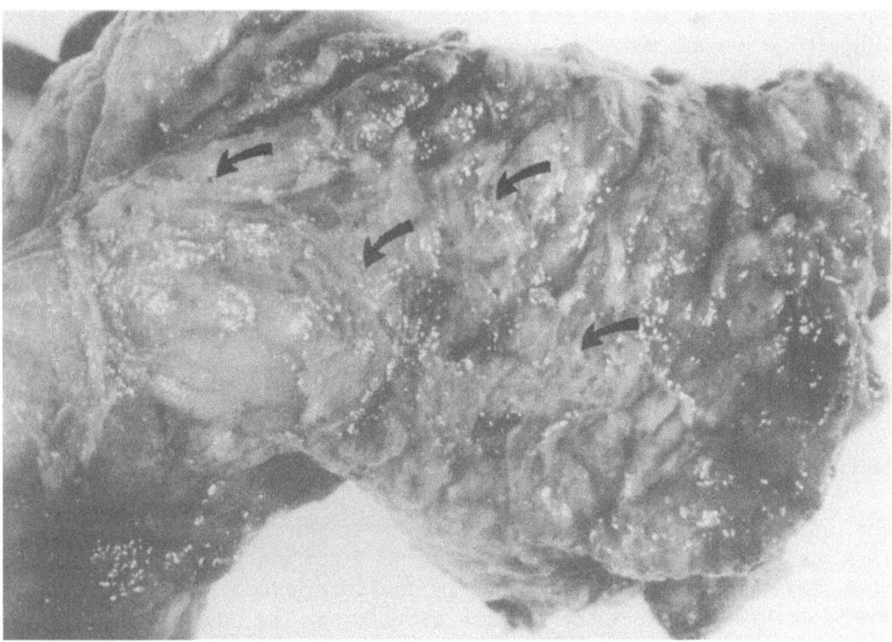

Fig. 4. A good mesorectal excision (TME) performed by Mr. Heald. The surface of the mesorectum is smooth with areas of fascia adherent to the surface (*thin arrows*). These are remnants of the 'holy plane'

removed from the board and the non-peritonealised surfaces painted with ink by the method in use locally. We wash the surface with alcohol, then paint with black india ink, and then apply Bouin's fixative. The macroscopic description of the specimen is then performed. Failing to open the specimen does cause a problem with recording the tumour characteristics but the length, width, area and macroscopic appearances of the tumour are not prognostic whereas CRM and peritoneal involvement are.

The area of the tumour that has been left intact is now sectioned transversely as thinly as possible. It is feasible to slice the specimen at 0.3–0.5 cm intervals. If the specimen is not well-fixed (i.e. at least 48 h in formalin) then this process is more difficult. The fixed slices are laid out under a good light and inspected macroscopically. The maximum depth of extension of the tumour from the muscularis propria is measured as is the distance from the CRM to the tumour. If the tumour is within 1 mm on histological sections, then CRM involvement is said to have occurred. This distance was chosen by analysis of previous studies [1, 32]. If any lymph nodes abut the CRM, then these should be taken in continuity with the CRM so that involvement by this route can be identified, similarly if there is any evidence of isolated deposits or thickening/fibrosis in this area it should be sampled. Any peritumoral lymph nodes will be collected at this time. If the tumour approaches the peritoneal surface this must also be sampled to exclude malignant cells on the surface or ulceration of the serosa by tumour [36].

Four blocks of the primary tumour must be taken to assess tumour characteristics. These may be the same blocks as those for the CRM if there is adequate tumour represented. After assessing the primary tumour, attention should be turned to the lymph nodes. Starting at the vascular resection margin the lymph nodes should be visualised by cross cutting the vessels and mesorectum. Vessels along the inferior mesenteric or superior rectal artery should be identified and embedded separately (pN3) as should the highest lymph node (Dukes' C2/pN3). All other lymph nodes should be identified and embedded. If any lymph nodes lie against the circumferential margin then they should be taken in continuity with the margin to exclude CRM involvement. The distal margin should then be sampled and the doughnuts embedded. The proximal margin does not need to be examined unless within 5 cm of the tumour. Any mucosal lesions seen should be sampled. The status of the background mucosa can be obtained from the distal margin or the doughnuts.

Standard histological examination of the haematoxylin and eosin sections should then be performed. If tumour is within 1 mm of the CRM, then it should be deemed to be involved. This measurement should be made on the glass slide using the Vernier scale. If tumour is close to the margin but greater than 1 mm then deeper levels should be cut to exclude involvement. If fibrosis has led to a mistaken impression of the depth of invasion from the muscularis propria, then this measurement should be corrected from the slide.

Conclusions

The ideal staging system does not yet exist. Reporting using Dukes' and TNM is recommended, together with careful examination of the CRM.

The quality of surgical resection varies widely and this can be audited by careful macroscopic examination of the specimen. Areas to pay special attention to for CRM involvement are anteriorly, the posterior sacrococcygeal raphe and above the tumour where spread can occur from lymph nodes containing metastatic tumour.

References

1. Adam IJ, Mohamdee MO, Martin IG, Scott N, Finan PJ, Johnston D, Dixon MF, Quirke P (1994) Role of circumferential margin involvement in the local recurrence of rectal cancer. Lancet 344:707–711
2. Arbman G, Nilsson E, Hallböök O, Sjödahl R (1996) Can total mesorectal excision reduce the local recurrence rate in rectal cancer surgery? Br J Surg 83:375–379
3. Astler VB, Coller FA (1954) The prognostic significance of direct extension of carcinoma of the colon and rectum. Ann Surg 139:846–852
4. Beahrs OH, Myers MD (1983) American Joint Committee on Cancer. Manual for staging cancer, 2nd edn. Lippincott, Philadelphia
5. Blenkinsopp WK, Stewart-Brown S, Blesovsky L, Kearney G, Fielding LP (1981) Histopathology reporting in large bowel cancer. J Clin Pathol 34:598–613

6. Cawthorne SJ, Gibbs NM, Marks CG (1986) Clearance techniques for the detection of lymph nodes in colorectal cancer. Br J Surg 73:58–60
7. Chan KW, Boey J, Wong SKC (1985) A method of reporting radial invasion and surgical clearance of rectal carcinoma. Histopathology 9:1319–1327
8. Chapuis PH, Fisher R, Dent OF, Newland RC, Pheils MT (1985) The relationship between different staging methods and survival in colorectal carcinoma. Dis Colon Rectum 28:158–161
9. Chapuis PH, Dent OF, Fisher R, Newland RC, Pheils MT, Smyth E, Colquhoun K (1985) A multivariate analysis of clinical and pathological variables in prognosis after resection of large bowel cancer. Br J Surg 72:698–702
10. Chapuis PH, Dent OF, Newland RC, Bokey EL, Pheils MT (1986) An evaluation of the American Joint Committee pTNM staging method for cancer of the colon and rectum. Dis Colon Rectum 29:6–10
11. Davis NC, Newland RC (1982) The reporting of colorectal cancer. The Australian clinico-pathological staging system. Aust NZ J Surg 53: 211–221
12. Davis NC, Newland RC (1983) Terminology and classification of colorectal adenocarcinoma: The Australian Clinico-pathological Staging System. Aust NZ J Surg 53:211–221
13. Denoix PF (1954) French Ministry of Public Health. National Institute of Hygiene Monograph No. 4, Paris
14. de Haas-Kock D, Baeten C, Jager J, Langendijk J, Schouten L, Arends J (1995) The prognostic significance of the lateral resection margin in rectal cancer. Proceedings of the conference "Colorectal Cancer: From Gene to Cure", Amsterdam, December 1995. Abstract P43
15. Dukes CE (1932) The classification of cancer of the rectum. J Pathol Bacteriol 35:323–332
16. Dukes CE, Bussey HJR (1958) The spread of rectal cancer and its effect on prognosis. Br J Cancer 12:309–320
17. Gabriel WB, Dukes CE, Bussey HJR (1935) Lymphatic spread in cancer of the rectum. Br J Surgery 23:395–413
18. Heald RJ, Karanjia ND (1992) Results of radical surgery for rectal cancer. World J Surg 16:848–857
19. Hermanek P (1986) Problems of pTNM classification of carcinoma of the stomach, colorectum and anal margin. Pathol Res Pract 181:296–300
20. Hermanek P, Giedl J, Dworak O (1989) Two programmes for examination of regional lymph nodes in colorectal carcinoma with regard to the new pN classification. Path Res Pract 185:867–873
21. Hermanek P, Wittekind C (1994) The pathologist and the residual tumour (R) classification. Path Res Pract 190:115–123
22. Hermanek P (1995) Interdepartmental variability in long time survival for surgical therapy for colonic cancer – results of the German Study Group for Colorectal Carcinoma (SGCRC). Proceedings of the conference "Colorectal Cancer: From Gene to Cure", Amsterdam, December 1995. Abstract P40
23. Hermanek P, Wiebelt H, Staimmer D, Riedl S (1995) Prognostic factors of rectum carcinoma – experience of the German Multicentre Study SGCRC. Tumori 81:60–64
24. Jass JR, Atkin WS, Cuzick J, Bussey HJR, Morson BC, Northover JMA, Todd IP (1986) The grading of rectal cancer: historical perspectives and a multivariate analysis of 447 cases. Histopathology 10:437–459
25. Jass LR, Love SB, Northover JMA (1987) A new classification of rectal cancer. Lancet I:1303–1306
26. Kirklin JW, Dockerty MB, Waugh JM (1949) The role of the peritoneal reflection in the prognosis of carcinoma of the rectum and sigmoid colon. Surg Gynecol Obstet 88:326–331
27. McArdle CS, Hole D (1991) Impact of variability among surgeons on post-operative morbidity and mortality and ultimate survival. Br Med J 302:1501–1505
28. MacFarlane JK, Ryall RD, Heald RJ (1993) Mesorectal excision for rectal cancer. Lancet 341:457–460
29. Nathanson SD, Schultz L, Tilley B, Kambouris A (1986) Carcinomas of the colon and rectum. A comparison of staging classifications. Am Surg 52:429–433

30. Newland RC, Chapuis PH, Smyth EJ (1987) The prognostic value of substaging colorectal carcinoma: a prospective study of 1117 cases with standardised pathology. Cancer 60:852–857
31. Ng IOL, Luk ISC, Yuen ST, Lau PWK, Pritchett CJ, Ng M, Poon GP, Ho J (1993) Surgical lateral clearance in resected rectal carcinomas. A multivariate analysis of clinicopathological features. Cancer 71:1972–1976
32. Quirke P, Durdey P, Dixon MF, Williams NS (1986) The prediction of local recurrence of rectal adenocarcinoma due to inadequate surgical resection. Histopathological study of lateral tumour spread and surgical excision. Lancet II:996–999
33. Quirke P, Dixon MF (1988) How I do it: the prediction of local recurrence in rectal adenocarcinoma by histopathological examination. Int J Colorect Dis 3:127–131
34. Quirke P, Scott N (1992) The pathologist's role in the assessment of local recurrence in rectal carcinoma. Surg Oncol Clin N Am 1:1–17
35. Scott N, Jackson P, Al-Jaberi T, Dixon MF, Quirke P, Finan PJ (1995) Total mesorectal excision and local recurrence: a study of tumour spread in the mesorectum distal to rectal cancer. Br J Surg 82:1031–1033
36. Shepherd NA, Baxter KJ, Love SB (1995) Influence of local peritoneal involvement on pelvic recurrence and prognosis in rectal cancer. J Clin Pathol 48:849–855
37. Turnbull RB, Kyle K, Watson FR, Spratt J (1967) Cancer of the colon: the influence of the no touch isolation technique on survival rates. Ann Surg 166:420–427
38. UICC (1993) TNM supplement. A commentary on uniform use. Hermanek P, Henson DE, Hunter RVP, Sobin L (eds) Springer, Berlin Heidelberg New York
39. United Kingdom Coordinating Committee for Cancer Research Colorectal Cancer Subcommittee (1987) Handbook for the clinicopathological assessment of colorectal cancer. Medical Research Council, London
40. Wood DA, Robins GF, Zipin C, Lum D, Stearns M (1979) Staging of cancer of the colon and cancer of the rectum. Cancer 43:961–968

CHAPTER 6

Preoperative Staging: A Critical Analysis

Ulrich Hildebrandt and Gernot Feifel

Introduction

> No two patients with rectal cancer are ever exactly alike. It must follow, there-
> fore, that no single orthodox standard operation can be the best treatment for
> every patient with carcinoma of the rectum. York Mason 1976 [60].

The decision as to the best surgical technique for treatment of a patient with
rectal cancer depends on several factors: tumour location, penetration of bowel
wall, lymph node status, tumour grading, and, last but not least, the surgeon's
experience and preference.

Miles' [42] radical abdominoperineal resection is no longer the gold standard for rectal cancer surgery, and the choice of operation must be made on
the basis of preoperative staging. The preoperative clinical staging should
provide information which closely matches the postoperative pathology staging. The TNM system is the only one which can be used for preoperative
clinical staging indicated by adding the prefix "c". For preoperative staging
with ultrasound the prefix "u" is used and for postoperative pathological
staging the prefix "p" is added.

From a historical and practical point of view rectal digital examination will
be discussed first.

Clinical Staging

Rectal Digital Examination

For low tumours within reach of the finger, rectal digital examination has been the traditional method for assessing local invasion by characterization of size, the level and the extent of the cancer, the number of quadrants involved and the degree to which it is tethered or fixed within the pelvis.

This information is used in the decision making as to what can be achieved technically and oncologically, including the choice between a restorative, sphincter-saving resection or an abdominoperineal resection (APR) or to identify patients suitable for local treatment. From an oncological point of view digital examination may identify those at high risk for local recurrence in whom preoperative radiotherapy can be considered.

York Mason [60] proposed a clinical staging system (CS) based on assumed rectal invasion according to digital examination. The examiner moves the tumour to asses the degree of local invasion. This allows staging in four clinical groups, which have different survival and local recurrence rates (Table 1).

Some years later Nicholls and coworkers [43] in collaboration with York Mason redefined the clinical staging system and tested its potential limitations and reproducibility in 70 patients. In this system four stages were defined, as outlined in Table 2.

Clinical findings were compared with the results of pathological examination of the resected specimen. Gross tumour spread was accurately predicted by digital examination in around 80% of cases. Invasion within the rectal wall and early local spread were more difficult to identify. In 67%–83% of patients with different degrees of extent of local spread four stages of tumour could be recognized by digital examination by expert clinicians. Not surprisingly, the less experienced examiners were less accurate (44%–78%). Clinical assessment of extrarectal spread also correlated reasonably well with survival. Understaging was a more common error than overstaging.

Table 1. Description of local extent based on digital examination as suggested by York Mason in 1976 [60]

CS I:	Freely mobile: tumour has not invaded the muscularis propria
CS II:	Mobile: Invasion into muscularis propria but still confined to rectal wall
CS III:	Tethered mobility: invasion into perirectal tissuses
CS IV:	Fixed: Tethered fixation to pelvic organs: levator, vagina, bladder, etc.

CS, clinical staging.

Table 2. Local extent assessed by digital examination as proposed by Nicholls and coworkers [43]

Stage 1: Confined to rectum
Stage 2: Confined to rectum or slight extrarectal spread
Stage 3: Moderate or extensive extrarectal spread
Stage 4: Involvement of other organs or unresectability

These figures are considerably better than those of other published series [5, 58] and represent probably the optimal of what digital examination can achieve. Nicholls et al. found that fixity is associated with a poorer prognosis [43]. However, fixation of the rectum can be caused by both local invasion and inflammation. In the study of Durdey and Williams [18] 26% of tumours were tethered by inflammation only. Bonfanti et al. [8] also found a significant percentage of inflammatory fixation, which did not, however, influence prognosis. Another problem with simple clinical examination is that some 20%–30% of rectal tumours are inpalpable and that imaging studies have not been conducted.

Despite its limitations, digital examination is the first step in staging for rectal cancer. Since the goal is to achieve the highest degree of certainty in preoperative staging, simple clinical examination must be supplemented by imaging techniques.

Imaging Modalities

Computed Tomography

Pelvic computed tomography (CT) is used to detect local spread of rectal cancer. Its accuracy depends on the thickness of the "cuts" (5–12 mm), the skill and technique of the operator and the standard of the available equipment. It is tempting to regard the CT image as a transverse anatomical cut through the tumour. CT scan is still unable, however, to distinguish the various layers of the rectal wall. The rectal wall between the rectal lumen distended with air or water and the perirectal fat appears as one layer on CT. Differentiation between T1 and T2 tumours is impossible. Furthermore, the anal canal cannot be differentiated from the external anal sphincter; therefore tumour infiltration into the anal sphincters cannot be detected. Apart from very small tumours and those close to the anal canal, though, nearly all rectal cancers can be demonstrated on CT.

In 1981 Thoeni and coworkers [54] proposed a classification system dividing rectal tumours into four stages based on CT imaging (Table 3). A somewhat similar system was suggested the same year by Dixon and associates [15] (Table 4). Lymph nodes were classified as "enlarged" and "not enlarged". None of these two systems corresponds directly with the TNM staging system. Therefore direct comparison with TNM staging after resection and assessment of the specimens is of questionable value.

The early results published in the literature [56, 58, 61] were optimistic and indicated a satisfactory correlation of more than 90% between CT staging and the final histopathologic assessment. A critical analysis of these first reports reveals limitations in stage definitions and demonstrates that, commonly, only advanced lesions were investigated by CT. More recent studies [4, 21] indicate that results have improved due to clearer stage definitions, with an accuracy ranging from 47% to 75%. Angelelli et al. reported an accuracy of 83% comparing CT imaging with Dukes' classification of resected specimens [3]. In this

Table 3. Staging system based on computed tomographic imaging introduced by Thoeni and coworkers [54]

Stage I:	Intraluminal polypoid mass without thickening of the bowel wall
Stage II:	Thickening of the bowel wall (> 0,5 cm) without invasion of surrounding tissue
Stage III A:	Invasion of surrounding tissue but no extension to the pelvic side walls
Stage III B:	Extension to the pelvic side walls
Stage IV:	Pelvic tumour and distant metastases

Table 4. Staging system based on computed tomographic imaging after Dixon et al. [15]

Stage I:	No spread or slight spread (< 1 cm)
Stage II:	Moderate spread (1–2 cm)
Stage III:	Extensive spread (> 2 cm)

series only 10% of the patients had Dukes' A lesion; the remaining patients had more advanced disease. Several authors have reported a high accuracy for CT in predicting local malignant extension beyond the bowel wall [23, 47, 58]. A review of the literature demonstrates a sensitivity ranging from 53% to 72% and specificity from 57% to 92% (Table 5). A problem is that infiltration of a few millimeters is not detectable by CT and that perirectal inflammation may mimic invasion.

Resectability can also be predicted by CT. When planning resection of rectal cancer it is important to know the relation between perirectal infiltration and the perirectal fascia. The perirectal fascia constitutes an important barrier to tumour invasion into the pararectal connective tissue. Grabbe, Lierse and Winkler have demonstrated that, normally, the perirectal fascia cannot be detected because of limited spatial resolution [23]. Only pathologic changes in the perirectal fat, such as tumour infiltration or inflammation, cause perirectal fascial thickening. Under such circumstances tumour growth beyond the fascia may be detectable, indicating unresectability. With the exception of one publication only [58], all authors agree that differentiation between inflammation and tumour infiltration is not possible.

Enlarged lymph nodes (LN) can be visualized on CT but it is not possible to ascertain whether the enlargement is due to malignant infiltration. Some authors have tried to define LN metastases by node size. Applying different definitions of "affected nodes" ranging from 5 to 15 mm the results vary extremely. As indicated in Table 5 specificity ranges from 64% to 96% and the sensitivity from 22% to 88%. It is well known from histologic examinations that small nodes may harbour metastases. Such findings reduce the clinical value of CT imaging as an investigative tool for the detection of occult LN metastases.

Thus the usefulness of CT for staging rectal cancer is disappointing. Tumours within the rectal wall and slight invasion through the wall cannot be assessed. Despite some enthusiastic reports [4, 61] the results of evaluation of

Table 5. Correlation between computed tomographic imaging and tumour infiltration and lymph node status at histopathologic examination

Study	Year	Patients (*n*)	Infiltration	Lymph nodes	Tumour stage
Dixon et al. [15]	1981	47	sens. 79% sens. 39%	spec. 96%	
Thoeni et al. [54]	1981	34	acc. 92%		
Zaunbauer et al. [61]	1981			acc. 100%	acc. 100%
van Waes et al. [56]	1983	21			acc. 80%
Grabbe et al. [23]	1983	155	spec. 92% sens. 74% acc. 79%	spec. 92% sens. 34% acc. 56	
Adalsteinsson et al. [2]	1983	150	acc. 60%		
Romano et al. [47]	1985	23	acc. 83%		
Freeny et al. [21]	1986	80	spec. 80% sens. 61%	spec. 96% sens. 26%	acc. 47%
Thompson et al. [55]	1986	25	spec. 57% sens. 77% acc. 70%	spec. 75% sens. 22% acc. 35%	acc. 60%
Hodgman et al. [36]	1986	30		spec. 90% sens. 40% acc. 65%	acc. 90%
Rifkin et al. [46]	1989	81	spec. 53% sens. 53%	spec. 88% sens. 27%	acc. 40%
Rotte et al. [49]	1989	30	acc. 76%		
Beynon et al. [7]	1989	50		spec. 91% sens. 25% acc. 57%	
Shank et al. [52]	1990	85			acc. 51%
Angelelli et al. [3]	1990	42	acc. 98%	spec. 65% sens. 88% acc. 79%	acc. 83%
Bech-Shriver et al. [4]	1992	22	acc. 84%	acc. 75%	acc. 75%
Herzog et al. [27]	1993	87			spec. 86% sens. 68% acc. 74%

spec.=specificity; sens. = sensitivity; acc.= accuracy.

LN with CT are still unacceptable. Accurate assessment of local spread can only be achieved in advanced tumours. CT may thus be helpful in monitoring the effects of preoperative radiotherapy. However, the distinction between malignant or inflammatory fixation is still questionable. Staging of rectal cancers with CT is therefore not recommended although it may be helpful for advanced lesions [21, 55].

Magnetic Resonance Imaging

A potentially superior imaging technique is magnetic resonance imaging (MRI). A variety of scanning techniques can be used which map the hydrogen nuclei density and molecular environment. It was hoped that this technique would demonstrate lesions that otherwise would be below the threshold for anatomical resolution using CT. Few studies on rectal cancer have been performed within the last 10 years and the number of patients studied is small. Using conventional MRI technique the rectal wall appears as one layer; distinctive, anatomical rectal wall layers are not discernable.

Substantial problems were encountered in preliminary in vivo studies because of extensive motion artefacts [12]. With high-resolution endorectal surface coil MRI it is now possible to develop criteria for staging of rectal cancer, as the coil technique allows the identification of multiple layers. These layers consist of an inner layer of high signal intensity (the mucus and fluid between the coil and the rectal wall), a layer of low signal intensity (mucosa and muscularis mucosae), a middle layer of high signal intensity (the submucosa), a second layer of low signal intensity (the muscularis propria), and an outer layer of high signal intensity (the perirectal fat).

Based on such findings Schnall et al. [51] have defined criteria for MRI staging of rectal cancer (Table 6). Using the MRI staging criteria given above prospective MR imaging staging correlated with the pathologic stage in 29 of 36 patients (81%). The extent of invasion was overestimated in seven cases. The criterion "irregularity of nonluminal surface" led to substantial overstaging of T2 lesions. Lymph nodes were differentiated by the criterion "non-fat-containing". Non-fat-containing nodes were identified as N1. Based on this definition sixteen patients had N1 lesions and 20 had N0 lesions. The accuracy in differentiating N1 from N0 disease was 78%, with a sensitivity of 81%.

In other studies, summarized in Table 7, different layers of the rectal wall could not be demonstrated by MRI. Even in very recent studies [40, 41] it has been impossible to differentiate T1 from T2 tumours.

MRI is therefore of limited value. Even in the study of Schnall and coworkers [51], which is the only one in which layers of the rectal wall could be distinguished, these layers are only identified in parts of the circumference. Criteria used for identification of metastatic lymph nodes are vague (fat-containing). It is generally accepted that inflammatory nodes cannot be differentiated from metastatic nodes on the basis of size or signal intensity only.

Endosonography

Endosonography (ES) was introduced into clinical practice in 1983 [16, 30]. Using low frequency probes of 3.5 and 4.0 MHz the rectal wall could be demonstrated as a two- or three-layer structure. Initially it was attempted to stage rectal cancer according to the TNM classification and the prefix "u" for ultrasound was introduced [28]. With the introduction of 7.5 MHz transducers five different layers of the rectal wall could be identified (Fig. 1). The physical and anatomical description of the two hypoechoic and three hyperechoic layers is extensively discussed elsewhere [9, 31, 33]. The uT-staging definition of 1985 was later accepted by Saitoh and associates [50], Yamashita and coworkers [59] and many others.

Table 6. Staging criteria of rectal cancer with magnetic resonance imaging (Schnall and coworkers [51])

Tl:	Mucosal thickening, preservation of submucosa at lesion centre
T2:	Disruption of submucosa off centre, disruption of submucosa at lesion centre with partial preservation of muscularis propria
T3:	Irregularity of nonluminal surface, disruption of muscularis propria

Table 7. Correlation of magnetic resonance imaging with tumour infiltration at histopathology, tumour stage, and lymph node status

Study	Year	Patients (n)	Infiltration	Lymph nodes	Tumour stage
Butch et al. [11]	1986	16			acc. 93%
Hodgman et al. [36]	1986	27		spec. 88% sens. 13% acc. 39%	acc. 60%
Guinet et al. [24]	1990	21	acc. 76%		
De Lange et al. [13]	1990	29	acc. 87%	acc. 78%	acc. 65%
Chan et al. [12]	1991	12	acc. 90%	acc. 57%	
Waitzer et al. [57]	1991	13	acc. 76%		
Okizuka et al. [44]	1993	33	spec. 89% sens. 64% acc. 79%		
Mc Nicholas et al. [40]	1994	20	acc. 95%	acc. 95%	
Schnall et al. [51]	1994	36		spec. 72% sens. 81% acc. 78%	acc. 81%
Meyenberger et al. [41]	1995	6	acc. 80%		acc. 40%

The accuracy for staging of tumour penetration by ultrasound (uT) ranges from 64% to 94% [1, 37], with an average of 84% (Table 8; Figs. 2–10). A common error is overstaging of T2 lesions. This is due to peritumoural inflammation which appears hypoechoic on the sonogram and mimics invasion where there is none (Fig. 10). Overstaging, however, is a minor clinical problem because undertreatment will not be the consequence. Stenosis of the rectal lumen preventing the insertion of the ultrasound probe occurs in about 5%. Such advanced lesions must be assessed by CT.

Before treatment is started it may be of interest to know whether LN metastases are present. The absolute number of involved nodes is, on the other hand, largely irrelevant. Using ES, LN appear with different echopatterns. Two main groups can be discerned: hyperechoic and hypoechoic LN. Between these distinctive groups are nodes which are both hypo- and hyperechoic. On the basis of different echopatterns LN can be differentiated as follows: By definition hyperechoic nodes represent nonspecific inflammation (Figs. 11, 12). Hypoechoic nodes or nodes with mixed echopattern represent lymph node metastases (Figs. 13, 14). These criteria of differentiation have been applied by

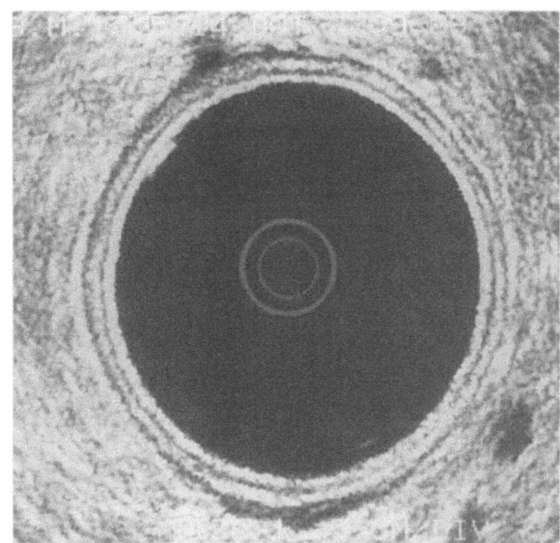

Fig. 1. Sonogram of the normal rectal wall demonstrating three hyperechoic and two hypoechoic layers. Inner hyperechoic layer, water filled balloon; Inner hypoechoic layer, mucosa; middle hyperechoic layer, submucosa; outer hypoechoic layer, muscularis propria; outer hyperechoic layer, reflection line at perirectal fat

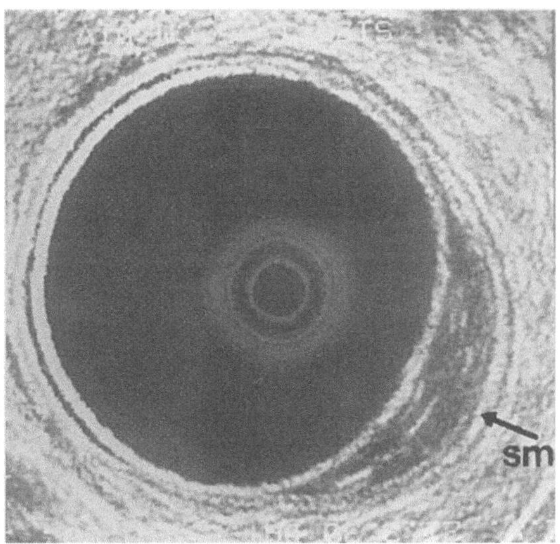

Fig. 2. Sonogram of a tumour stage uT1. The submucosa (*sm*) is not interrupted

most investigators [7, 22, 27, 35] and give an accurracy rate of 73%–83% (Table 8). Criteria such as size, shape or outer borderlines of a lymph node were not characteristic [29].

Potential of CS, CT, MRI and ES

For years the Dukes' classification was the most widely accepted staging system because it is simple and easy to remember. Unfortunately it is a posttreatment

Fig. 3. Sonogram of a tumour stage uT1 as demonstrated by the intact submucosa (*arrows*)

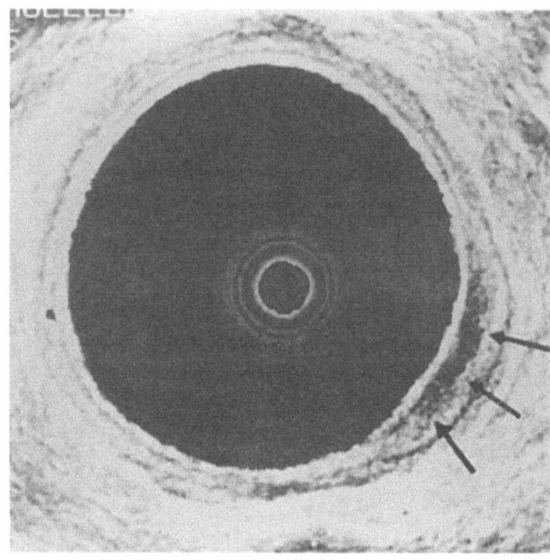

Fig. 4. Sonogram of a tumour stage uT2. The submucosa is interrupted by tumour invasion (*arrows*)

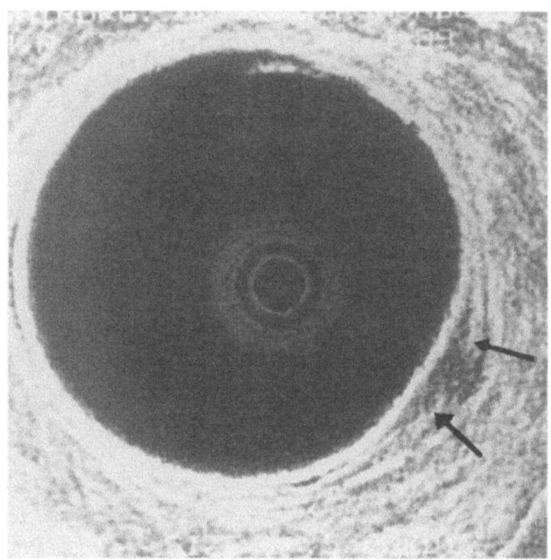

classification for colorectal cancer and is applied after surgery has been performed.

In 1976 York Mason published his clinical staging system, which is used before a surgical decision is made [60]. He showed that useful information can be obtained by digital examination of tumours lying within 10 cm of the anal verge, a part of the rectum where the surgeon is likely to be faced with a choice of treatment. The reliability of this system formed the basis of local excision of rectal cancer. Mason's clinical staging system is fairly accurate because the stages CS I–III correspond exactly with T1–3 of the TNM classification.

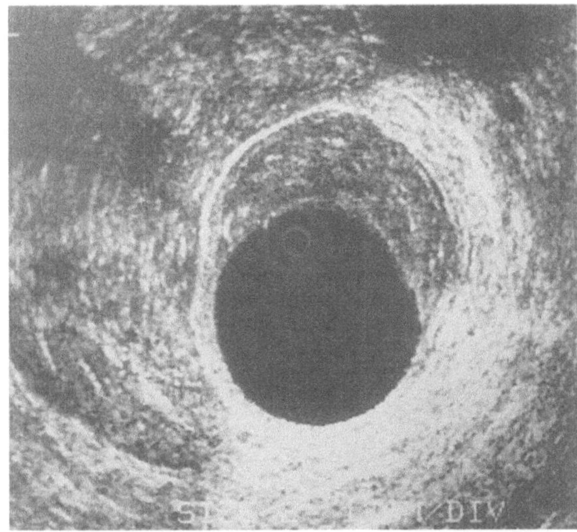

Fig. 5. Sonogram of a tumour stage uT2. The muscle layer is infiltrated. The sharp outer confinement by the hyperechoic line demonstrates that the tumour does not penetrate into the perirectal fat

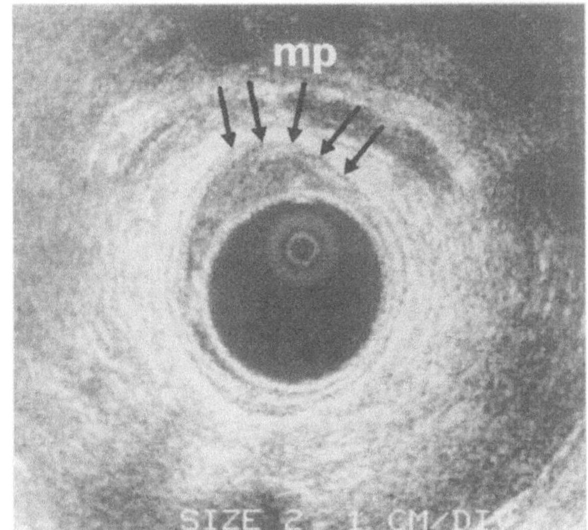

Fig. 6. Sonogram of a uT2 tumour. Tumour invasion (*arrows*) is confined to the muscularis propria (*mp*)

The modification by Nicholls and coworkers [43] does not differentiate tumours within the rectal wall (T1, T2) and those confined to rectum or with slight extrarectal spread (T2, T3). It is apparent that this staging modality does not conform with the TNM system (Fig. 15).

The introduction of CT in 1981 later led to an accuracy rate of 92% compared with the Dukes' classification. The accuracy of pooled data is lower, despite improvement in the imaging technology. The reason for this is that many investigators try to use the TNM system for the evaluation of tumour penetration depth. It is not surprising that the inability of CT to demonstrate single layers of the rectal wall makes it a useless tool for small lesions. CT is

Fig. 7. Sonogram of a tumour stage uT3. The tumour interrupts the muscularis propria (*mp*) and penetrates into perirectal fat

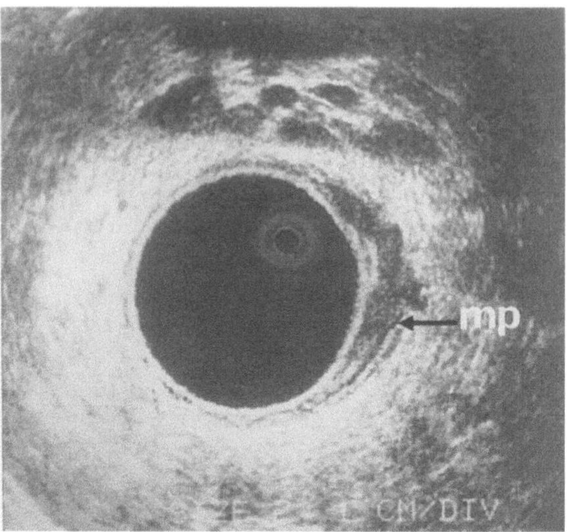

Fig. 8. Sonogram of a tumour stage uT3. *sm*, submucosa; *mp*, muscularis propria; *f*, infiltration of perirectal fat

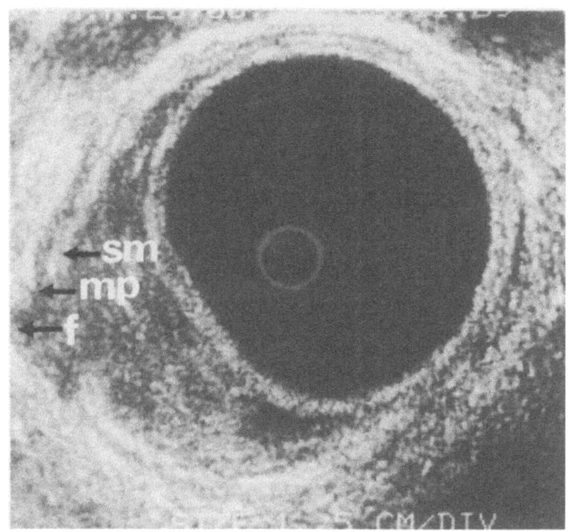

very effective in predicting extensive spread and pelvic wall infiltration, however.

Technical advances in the field of MRI, especially the intrarectal use of small coils, have increased the precision of the MR images and may give a higher resolution. Demonstration of single layers is rare and incomplete. Consequently, small tumours cannot be staged. Further improvement of the MR technique will probably not be required in the future since less expensive, time-consuming and more effective tumour assessment can be obtained with ES.

ES is said to have one disadvantage that other imaging modalities do not have – it is operator-dependent. This is true and may in part explain the low

Fig. 9. Sonogram of a tumour stage uT3. The dentated muscle layer indicates tumour penetration into the mesorectum

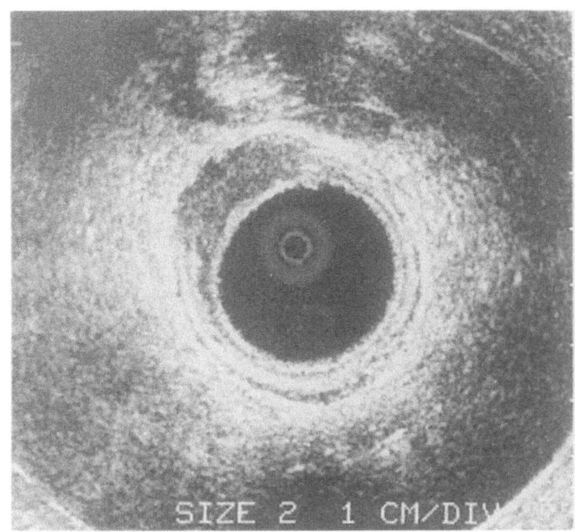

Fig. 10. Sonogram of a tumour stage uT3. Peritumoral inflammation mimics invasion where there is none histologically (pT2)

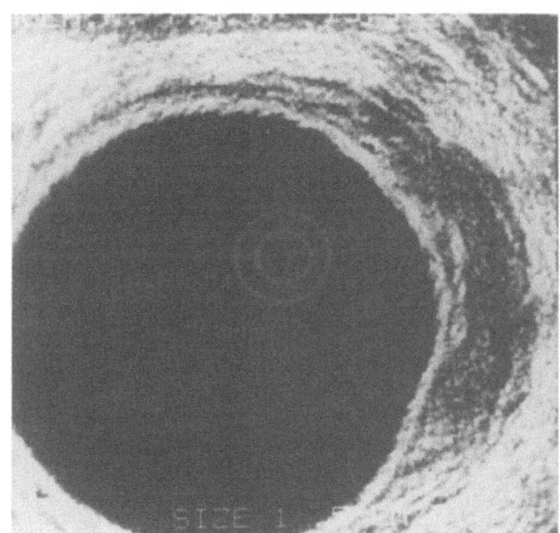

accuracy rate in series with few patients. The advantages are well known: low cost, availability, short examination time, minimal discomfort for the patient and highest accuracy for tumour staging.

Today ES is the best imaging modality which, with some skill, demonstrates the single layers of the rectal wall in nearly all cases. Thus ultrasound (u) predicts tumour penetration and correlates well with the T stage of the TNM classification (Fig. 16).

LN metastases are predicted with an accuracy of 75%, which is not accurate enough but still better than CS, CT and MRI. In our opinion pretreatment knowledge of LN metastases has only limited influence on treatment decisions.

Fig. 11. Hyperechoic lymph node (*arrow*) representing nonspecific inflammation

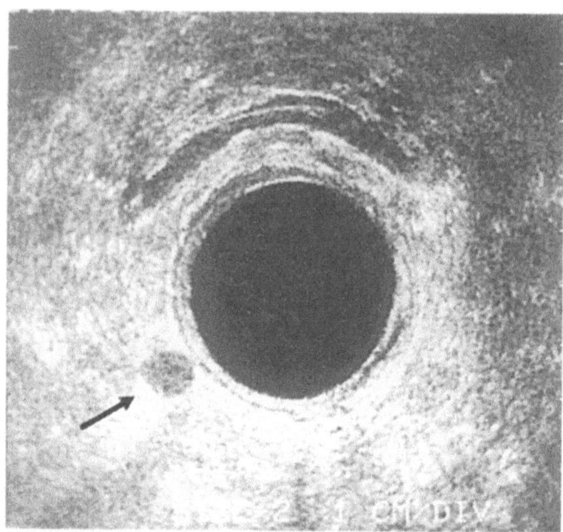

Fig. 12. Hyperechoic lymph node (*ln*) and blood vessel (*v*)

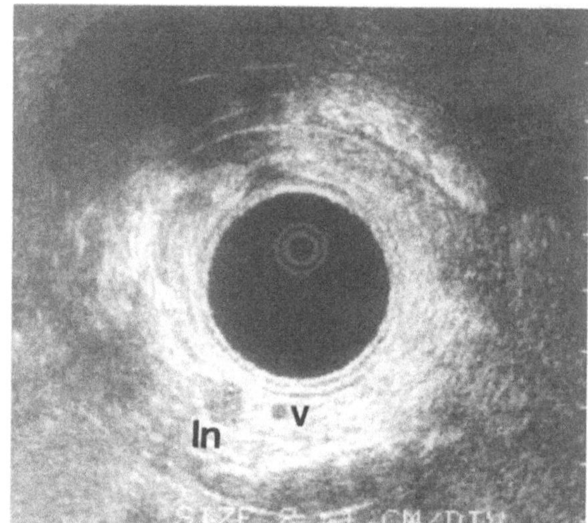

Implications for Treatment

Despite all efforts to stage a rectal tumour prior to surgery, the decisive step is surgery itself. Even with the best staging system a poorly trained surgeon will do little to minimize the disability that rectal cancer so commonly causes. It has been clearly demonstrated by Heald [25] that total mesorectal excision is an important step in order to improve results of rectal cancer surgery. This principle, together with autonomic nerve-preserving dissection [19], optimizes the chances for cure with preservation of sexual and urinary functions. In-tersphincteric rectal excision is restricted to tumours which are confined to the

Fig. 13. Hypoechoic lymph node (*ln*) representing metastatic involvement

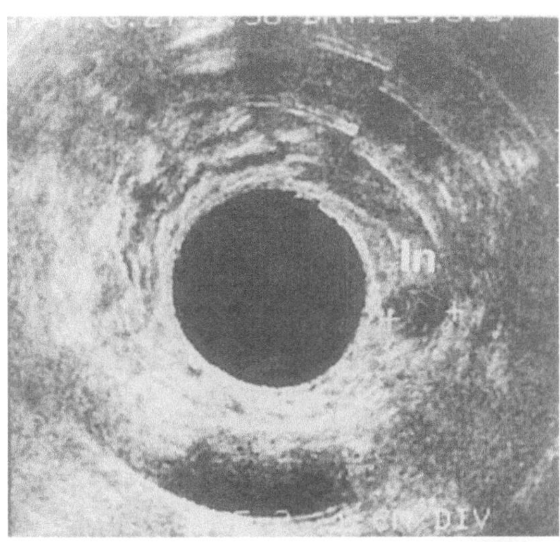

Fig. 14. Hypoechoic lymph node (*ln*)

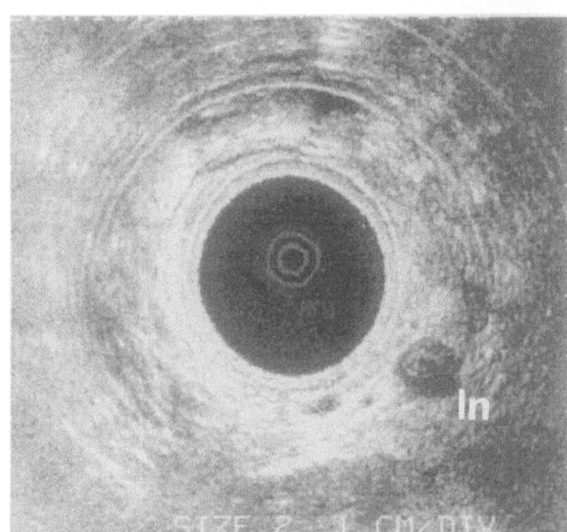

muscularis propria and which do not infiltrate the sphincter [35]. For T1 lesions local excision of rectal cancer is an option in selected cases.

Based on preoperative ultrasound staging our treatment policy for rectal cancer can be summarized as follows:

Upper third of rectum:
Anterior resection for all tumour stages

Middle third of rectum:
uT1 NO: Transanal endoscopic microsurgery for "low risk" carcinomas
uT1-2: Anterior resection

Table 8. Correlation of endosonography with tumour stage (pT) and lymph node status (pN)

Study	Year	Patients (n)	Tumour stage accuracy (%)	Lymph node accuracy (%)
Hildebrandt and Feifel [29]	1985	25	92	
Saitoh et al. [50]	1986	88	90	73
Di Candio et al. [14]	1987	55	91	
Accarpio et al. [1]	1987	54	94	
Beynon et al. [6]	1988	89	92	
Hildebrandt et al. [31]	1988	98	89	
Yamashita et al. [59]	1988	122	78	
Beynon et al. [7]	1989	95		83
Rifkin et al. [46]	1989	102	60	82
Buess et al. [10]	1989	56	86	
Glaser et al. [22]	1990	86	88	76
Heintz et al. [26]	1990	86	88	
Konishi et al. [39]	1990	47	78	
Orrom et al. [45]	1990	77	75	81
Roseau et al. [48]	1990	31	87	
Hildebrandt et al. [33]	1990	113		79
Herzog et al. [27]	1992	118	89	80
Katsura et al. [38]	1992	120	92	
Feifel et al. [20]	1992	204	92	
Hulsmans et al. [37]	1994	55	64	
Thaler et al. [53]	1994	37	88	80

uT3: Anterior resection with total mesorectal excision, reconstruction with coloanal pouch

Lower third of rectum:
uTl NO: Transanal endoscopic microsurgery for "low risk" carcinomas
uTl-2: Anterior or intersphincteric resection with total mesorectal excision, reconstruction with colonic pouch
uT3: Within mesorectum: resection with total mesorectal excision, colonic pouch
uT3: Outside mesorectum: abdominoperineal excision

Conclusion

Digital rectal examination, CT and MRI are less accurate than ES in predicting local invasion of T1 and T2 tumours. If an experienced rectal endosonographer has carried out the examination and the scan is correct for depth of invasion, ES will help select tumours suitable for local excision or for a sphincter-saving procedure. More advanced tumour stages (T3 and T4) can be assessed with a comparable accuracy by CT. Currently, the role of MRI, including MRI using intrarectal coils, is probably limited and should be assessed in further comparative studies.

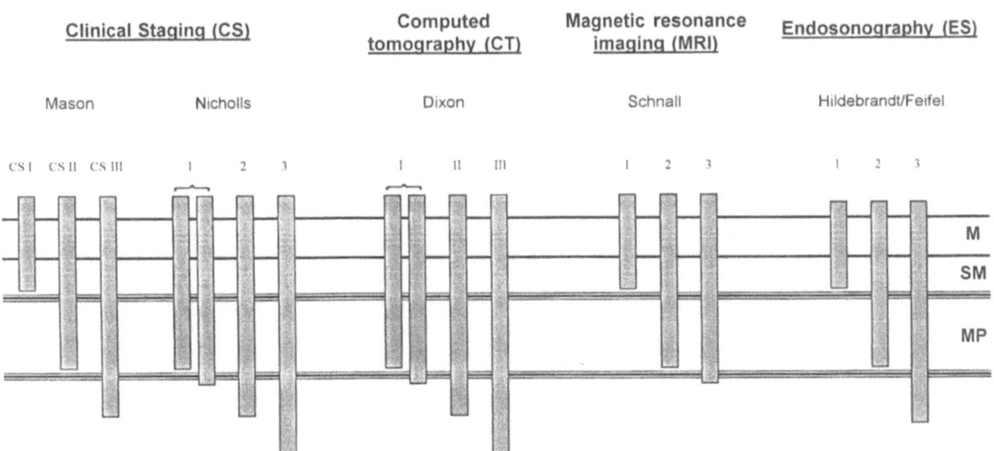

Fig. 15. Comparison of CS, CT, MRI and ES in the assessment of the tumor penetration depth (*M, mucosa; SM, submucosa; MP, muscularis propria*)

Fig. 16. Tumour penetration corresponding to T stage 1-4 evaluated with ultrasound

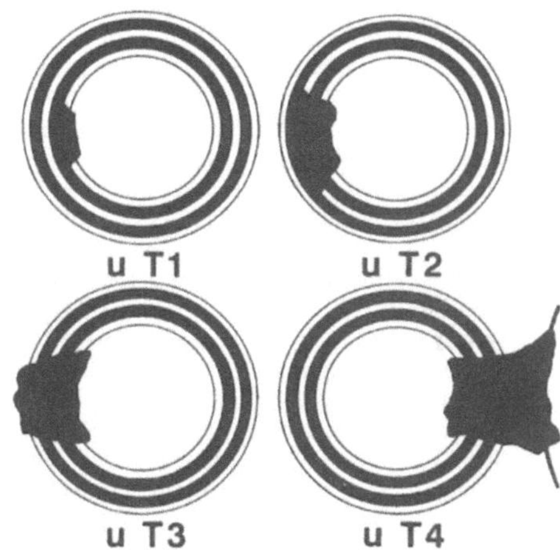

References

1. Accarpio G, Scopinaro G, Claudiani F, Davini D, Mallarini G, Saitta S (1987) Experience with local rectal cancer excision in light of two recent preoperative diagnostic methods. Dis Colon Rectum 30:297–298
2. Adalsteinsson B, Glimelius B, Graffman S, Hemmingsson, Pählman L (1985) Computed tomography in staging of rectal carcinoma. Acta Radiol 26:45–55
3. Angelelli G, Macarini L, Lupo L, Caputi-Jambrenghi O, Pannarale O, Memeo V (1990) Rectal carcinoma: CT staging with water as contrast medium. Radiology 177:511–514
4. Bech-Shriver E, Bachmann-Nielsen M, Qvitzan S, Christiansen J (1992) Comparison of precontrast, postcontrast and delayed scanning for the staging of rectal carcinoma. Gastrointest Radiol 17:267–270

5. Beynon J, Mortensen NJMcC, Foy DMA, Channer JL, Virjee J, Goddard P (1986) Preoperative assessment of local invasion in rectal cancer: digital examination, endoluminal sonography or computed tomography. Br J Surg 73:1015–1017

6. Beynon J, Mortensen NJMcC, Rigby HS (1988) Rectal endosonography, a new technique for the preoperative staging of rectal carcinoma. Eur J Surg Oncol 14:297–309

7. Beynon J, Mortensen NJMcC, Channer JL, Rigby H, Virjee J (1989) Preoperative assessment of mesorectal lymph node involvement in rectal cancer. Br J Surg 76:276–279

8. Bonfanti G, Bozetti F, Doci R, Baticci F, Marolda R. Bignami P, Gennari L (1982) Results of extended surgery for cancer of the rectum and sigmoid. Br J Surg 69:305–307

9. Boscaini M, Montori (1986) Transrectal ultrasonography: interpretation of normal intestinal wall structure for the preoperative staging of rectal cancer. Scand J Gastrointerol 21(Suppl. 123):87–98

10. Buess G, Mentges B, Manncke K, Starlinger M, Becker HD (1992) Technique and results of transanal endoscopic microsurgery in early rectal cancer. Am J Surg 163:63–70

11. Butch RJ, Stark DD, Wittenberg J, Tepper JE, Saini S, Simeone JF, Müller PR, Ferruci JT (1986) Staging rectal cancer by MR and CT. Am J Roentgenol 146:1155–1160

12. Chan TW, Kressel HY, Milestone B, Tomachefski J, Schnall M, Rosato E, Daly J (1991) Rectal carcinoma: staging at MR imaging with endorectal surface coil. Radiology 1181:461–467

13. De Lange EE, Fechner RE, Edge JB, Spaulding CA (1990) Preoperative staging of rectal carcinoma with MR imaging: surgical and histopathologic correlation. Radiology 176:623–628

14. Di Candio G, Mosca F, Campatelli A, Cei A, Ferrari M, Basolo F (1987) Endosonographic staging of rectal carcinoma. Gastrointest Radiol 12:289–295

15. Dixon AK, Kelsey Fry I, Morson BC, Nicholls RJ, York Mason A (1981) Preoperative computed tomography of carcinoma of the rectum. Br J Radiol 54:655–659

16. Dragsted J, Gammelgaard J (1983) Endoluminal ultrasonic scanning in the evaluation of rectal cancer. Gastrointest Radiol 8:367–369

17. Dukes CE (1932) The classification of cancer of the rectum. J Pathol Bacteriol 54:655–659

18. Durdey P, Williams NS (1984) The effect of malignant and inflammatory fixation of rectal carcinoma on prognosis after rectal excision. Br J Surg 71:787–790

19. Enker WE (1992) Potency, cure and local control in the operative treatment of rectal cancer. Arch Surg 127:1396–1402

20. Feifel G, Hildebrandt U (1992) New diagnostic imaging in rectal cancer: endosonography and immunoscintigraphy. World J Surg 16:841–847

21. Freeny PC, Marks WM, Ryan JA, Bolen JW (1986) Colorectal carcinoma evaluation with CT: preoperative staging and detection of postoperative recurrence. Radiology 158:347–353

22. Glaser F, Schlag P, Herfarth C (1990) Endorectal ultrasonography for the assessment of invasion of rectal tumors and lymph node involvement. Br J Surg 77:883–887

23. Grabbe E, Lierse W, Winkler R (1983) The perirectal fascia: morphology and use in staging of rectal carcinoma. Radiology 149:241–246

24. Guinet C, Ghossain M, Buy JN, Sezeur A, Bigot JM. Malbec L, Vadrot D, Ecoiffier J (1990) Comparative study of MRI and x-ray computed tomography in the preoperative evaluation of rectal carcinoma. J Radiol 71:357–363

25. Heald RJ (1988) The "holy plane" of rectal surgery. J R Soc Med 81:503–508

26. Heintz A, Buess G, Junginger T (1990). Endorektale Sonographie zur präoperativen Beurteilung der Infiltrationstiefe von Rektumtumoren. Dtsch Med Wochenschr 115:1083–1087

27. Herzog U, von Flue M, Tondelli P, Schuppiser JP (1993) How accurate is endorectal ultrasound in the preoperative staging of rectal cancer? Dis Colon Rectum 36:127–134

28. Hildebrandt U, Feifel G (1985) Preoperative staging of rectal cancer by intrarectal ultrasound. Dis Colon Rectum 28:42–46

29. Hildebrandt U, Feifel G (1993) Endosonography in the diagnosis of lymph nodes. Endoscopy 25:243–245

30. Hildebrandt U, Feifel G, Zimmermann FA, Goebbels R (1983) Significant improvement in clinical staging of rectal carcinoma with a new intrarectal ultrasound scanner. J Exp Clin Cancer Res [Suppl] 2:53

31. Hildebrandt U, Feifel G, Schwarz HP, Scherr O (1986) Endorectal ultrasound: instrumentation and clinical aspects. Int J Colorect Dis 1:203–207
32. Hildebrandt U, Feifel G, Dhom G (1988) The evaluation of the rectum by transrectal ultrasonography. Ultrasound Q 6:167–179
33. Hildebrandt U, Feifel G, Ecker KW (1989) Rectal endosonography. Baillieres Clin Gastroenterol 3:531–541
34. Hildebrandt U, Klein T, Feifel G, Schwarz HP, Koch B, Schmitt RM (1990) Endosonography of pararectal lymph nodes. In vitro and in vivo evaluation. Dis Colon Rectum 33:863–868
35. Hildebrandt U, Lindemann W, Kreipler-Haag D, Feifel G (1995) Die intersphinctere Rektumresektion mit colosphincterem Pouch. Chirurg 66:377–384
36. Hodgman CG, Maccarty RL, Wolff BG, May GR, Berquist TH, Scheedy PF, Beart RW, Spencer RJ (1986) Preoperative staging of rectal carcinoma by computed tomography and 0,15 T magnetic resonance imaging. Dis Colon Rectum 29:446–450
37. Hulsmans JH, Tio TL, Fockens P, Bosma A, Tytgat GNJ (1994) Assessment of tumour infiltration depth in rectal cancer with transrectal sonography: caution is necessary. Radiology 190:715–720
38. Katsura Y, Yamada K, Ishizawa T, Yoshinaka H, Shimazu H (1992) Endorectal ultrasonography for the assessment of wall invasion and lymph node metastasis in rectal cancer. Dis Colon Rectum 35:362–368
39. Konishi F, Ugajin H, Ito K, Kanazawak K (1990) Endorectal ultrasonography with a 7.5 MHz linear array scanner for the assessment of invasion of rectal carcinoma. Int J Colorect Dis 5:15–20
40. McNicholas MMJ, Joyce WP, Dolan J, Gibney RG, MacErlaine DP, Hyland J (1994) Magnetic resonance imaging of rectal carcinoma: a prospective study. Br J Surg 81:911–914
41. Meyenberger C, Huch Böni RA, Bertschinger P, Zala GF, Klotz HP, Krestin GP (1995) Endoscopic ultrasound and endorectal magnetic resonance imaging: a prospective, comparative study for preoperative staging and follow-up of rectal cancer. Endoscopy 27:469–479
42. Miles WE (1923) Cancer of the rectum. Trans Med Soc 46:127
43. Nicholls RJ, York Mason A, Morson BC, Dixon AK, Kelsey Fry I (1982) The clinical staging of rectal cancer. Br J Surg 69:404–409
44. Okizuka H, Sugimura K, Ishida T (1993) Preoperative local staging of rectal carcinoma with MR imaging and a rectal balloon. J Magn Reson Imaging 3:329–335
45. Orrom WJ, Wong WD, Rothenberger DA, Jensen LL, Goldberg SM (1990) Endorectal ultrasound in the preoperative staging of rectal tumours. A learning experience. Dis Colon Rectum 33:654–659
46. Rifkin MD, Ehrlich SM, Marks G (1989) Staging of rectal carcinoma: prospective comparison of endorectal US and CT. Radiology 120:319–320
47. Romano G, de Rosa P, Vallone G, Rotondo A, Grassi R, Santangelo ML (1985) Intrarectal ultrasound and computed tomography in the pre- and postoperative assessment of patients with rectal cancer. Br J Surg 72 [Suppl]:117–119
48. Roseau G, Palazzo L, Amonyal G, Gayet B, Pousot P, Paolaggi JA (1990) L' échoendoscopie dans le bilan préoperatoire de cancer. Presse Med 19:1450–1453
49. Rotte KH, Kluhs L, Kleinau H, Kriedemann E (1989) Computed tomography and endosonography in the preoperative staging of rectal carcinoma. Eur J Radiol 9:187–190
50. Saitoh N, Okui K, Sarashina H, Suzuki M, Avai T, Nunomura M (1986) Evaluation of echographic diagnosis of rectal cancer using intrarectal ultrasonic examination. Dis Colon Rectum 29:234–242
51. Schnall MD, Furth EE, Rosate EF, Kressel HY (1994) Rectal tumour stage: correlation of endorectal MR imaging and pathologic findings. Radiology 190:709–714
52. Shank B, Dershaw DD, Caravelli J, Barth J, Euler W (1990) A prospective study of the accuracy of preoperative computed tomographic staging of patients with biopsy proven rectal carcinoma. Dis Colon Rectum 33:285–290
53. Thaler W, Watzka S, Martin F, La Guardia G, Psenner K, Bonatti G et al. (1994) Preoperative staging of rectal cancer by endoluminal ultrasound vs. magnetic resonance

imaging. Preliminary results of a prospective, comparative study. Dis Colon Rectum 37:1189–1193
54. Thoeni RF, Moss AA, Schnyder P, Margulis AR (1981) Detection and staging of primary rectal and rectosigmoid cancer by computed tomography. Radiology 141:135–138
55. Thompson WM, Halvorsen RA, Foster WL, Roberts L, Gibbons R (1986) Preoperative and postoperative CT staging of rectosigmoid carcinoma. Am J Roentgenol 146:703–710
56. Van Waes PF, Koehler PR, Feldberg MA (1983) Management of rectal carcinoma: impact of computed tomography. Am J Roentgenol 140:1137–1142
57. Waizer A, Powsner E, Russo I, Hadar S, Cytron S, Lombrozo R, Wolloch Y, Antebi E (1991) Prospective comparative study of magnetic resonance imaging versus transrectal ultrasound for preoperative staging and follow-up of rectal cancer: preliminary report. Dis Colon Rectum 34:1068
58. Williams NS, Durdey P, Quirke P, Robinson PJ, Deyson JED, Dixon MF, Bird CC (1985) Preoperative staging of rectal neoplasm and its impact on clinical management. Br J Surg 72:868–874
59. Yamashita Y, Machi J, Shircuzu K, Morotomi T, Isomoto H, Kakegawa T (1988) Evaluation of endorectal ultrasound for the assessment of wall invasion of rectal cancer. Dis Colon Rectum 31:617–623
60. York Mason A (1976) Rectal cancer: the spectrum of selective surgery. Proc R Soc Med 69:237–244
61. Zaunbauer W, Haertel M, Fuchs WA (1981) Computed tomography in the carcinoma of the rectum. Gastrointest Radiol 6:79–84

CHAPTER 7

Potential of Molecular Biology in Preoperative Evaluation

Philip Quirke and Lynn Cawkwell

Introduction

Molecular biological knowledge will only be used if it can replace or complement current knowledge. It must be able to do this more rapidly and ideally at lower cost than current methods. A large number of studies will mature in the next 3–5 years and will make claims for the value of using a particular method in clinical practice. Prior to adopting them in clinical usage, they should be carefully evaluated, since it is relatively easier to publish positive series than negative series. It is only when several retrospective and preferably prospective studies have been performed and compared against the gold standards for prognosis derived from the histopathological staging and grading of rectal cancer that the newer techniques should be adopted.

In other situations it is immediately apparent that a new method or molecular discovery is of great importance. Excellent examples of this are the discovery of the APC gene [1–4], which causes familial adenomatous polyposis (FAP) and the DNA repair genes hMSH2 [5, 6], hMLH1 [7, 8], hPMS1 [9], hPMS2 [9] and GTBP [10–12], which are responsible for most cases of hereditary non-polyposis colorectal cancer (HNPCC).

The current methods of preoperative evaluation are improving all the time. Endorectal ultrasound and more powerful and technically advanced types of computed tomography (CT) and magnetic resonance imaging (MRI) will make a major contribution, but as yet they are unable to answer all the important preoperative questions of the surgeon. Standard histopathological techniques will continue to add to our knowledge, but it is in the field of molecular biology that new opportunities await. In this chapter, the potential value of molecular biology in the preoperative evaluation of rectal cancer will be discussed.

Summary of Our Understanding of the Molecular Basis of Sporadic Colorectal Cancer

Types of Gene Involved

Several types of gene are thought to be involved.

Proto-oncogenes

Proto-oncogenes are normal cellular genes which stimulate proliferation and other key cellular processes and are abnormally switched on by mutation, amplification or translocation. This class of genes can be looked upon as the accelerator pedal of the cell. When they become activated, the cell accelerates and can go out of control.

Tumour Suppressor Genes

Tumour suppressor genes are normal cellular genes which suppress cell growth and other important cellular processes. Classically, one copy (or allele) of the gene becomes inactivated by mutation and the other allele is subsequently deleted, leading to complete loss of function [13, 14]. The latter process is called loss of heterozygosity (LOH). Inactivation of function can also occur at the protein level. Tumour suppressor genes can be likened to the brake pedal in that they control important cellular processes. If you lose the brakes, the cell can go out of control.

DNA Repair Genes

DNA repair genes control the repair of specific types of induced and endogenous DNA damage. Inactivation of a particular repair mechanism (the DNA mismatch repair system) is known to occur in colorectal cancer and is responsible for most cases of HNPCC. The mismatch repair system corrects small regions of mismatched bases in DNA. Microsatellites are short, repetitive, two- to five-base DNA sequences such as CA or GTT repeats [15], and these regions are prone to mismatches during DNA replication. Thus the inactivation of the mismatch repair mechanism leads to the appearance of changes within large numbers of microsatellite sequences (a phenomenon known as microsatellite instability [16]), some of which affect the function of important genes, e.g. type-2 transforming growth factor (TGF)-β receptor [17]. To continue the motoring analogy, if a car needed continuous maintenance because it was continually going wrong, then failure of the repair system would lead to an accumulation of defects which after a while would affect key elements involved in control of the car, e.g. the brakes. It has been postulated [18] that the immune response system may recognise such defective cells, leading to the removal of "dangerous cars" from the streets by the police.

Other Genes

Other genes such as *Bcl-2* [19] are involved in the pathways controlling cell suicide (apoptosis; see [20, 21]). In addition, the *nm23* gene [22] and a cell adhesion molecule named CD44 [23] are factors which may affect the metastatic process.

Molecular Changes in Sporadic Colorectal Cancer

A summary of the changes seen in colorectal cancer is shown in Fig. 1.

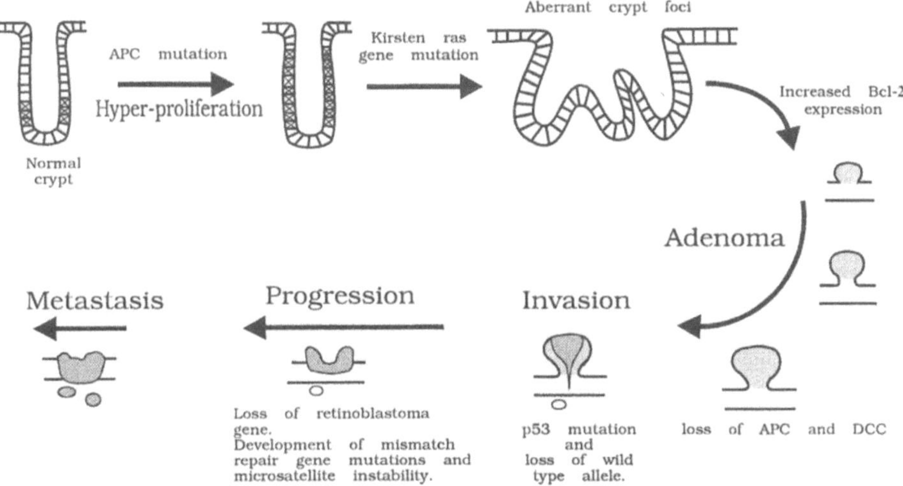

Fig. 1. Postulated timing of occurrence of the main molecular alterations which have so far been described in sporadic colorectal cancer. *APC*, adenomatous *DCC*, deleted in colorectal cancer gene. *Crosses* indicate proliferative zones. For more details, see text. Polyposis coli gene

Aberrant Crypt Foci

Aberrant crypt foci are microscopic lesions that may precede adenoma formation.

In the progression to sporadic colorectal cancer, one of the earliest lesions is thought to be a point mutation in the APC tumour suppressor gene [24]. The APC gene is responsible for FAP, and thus mutations of this gene may give rise to hyperproliferation of the colonic crypts. Mutations of APC have been detected in aberrrant crypt foci [25]. The APC protein interacts with the catenins [26, 27], which in turn are associated with E cadherin, a cell surface protein, but the mechanism by which a point mutation in APC affects the colonic crypt is unknown. Mutations in the Kirsten *ras* (K-*ras*) oncogene have been detected in aberrrant crypt foci, and the reported frequency of alterations at codon 12 or 13 ranges from 58% to 100% [28, 29]. Mutations in *ras* lead to abnormally increased signal transduction from cell surface receptors through to the nucleus [30].

Adenomas

K-*ras* mutations reportedly occur in up to 75% of adenomas [31]. Bcl-2 is usually only expressed in the base of the crypt [32], but with the onset of dysplasia, as demonstrated in very early adenomas, marked nuclear Bcl-2 expression is seen throughout the crypt. The abnormal expression of this protein may confer the ability on the cell to escape apoptosis and contribute to the excess local cell proliferation and development of dysplasia. As adenomas grow, loss of other tumour suppressor genes occur. In addition to loss of heterozygosity of APC, there are deletions of the deleted in colorectal cancer gene (DCC), which functions at the cell surface [33–35].

Carcinomas

At the adenoma–carcinoma interface, point mutations and loss of heterozygosity of the *p53* tumour suppressor gene are seen [36–38]. Less frequently, over-expression of the protein occurs without point mutation. Changes in *p53* are linked to the development of major changes in chromosome number such as DNA aneuploidy. At least 40% of carcinomas will have *ras* mutations [33, 39]. A subset of approximately 20% of sporadic colorectal cancer patients exhibit microsatellite instability (MI) in their carcinomas. Most of these patients are probably not HNPCC individuals, but may have developed somatic mutations in their DNA mismatch repair genes. In HNPCC families, microsatellite instability occurs earlier since it is present in 57% of HNPCC adenomas versus 3% of sporadic adenomas [40]. As the carcinoma progresses, other genes are inactivated, including the retinoblastoma gene (RB1), as well as genes on 1p [41, 42], 8p [43, 44], 11q [45] and 14q [46].

Metastases

It has been suggested that the onset of metastasis is associated with loss of *nm23* [47], and altered expression of CD44 [48]. However, further work is required in this area.

Molecular Changes in Ulcerative Colitis-Associated Cancer

The sequence of molecular events that occur in ulcerative colitis are much less studied and have been performed on smaller series of cases than sporadic colorectal cancer. The same spectrum of genetic lesions appears to occur in both sporadic and ulcerative colitis-associated cancer [49, 50], and the frequency of microsatellite instability is also the same [51]. There are, however, some apparent differences in the timing and frequency of some events. Mutations in K-*ras* are reported to occur at a lower frequency in ulcerative colitis-associated carcinomas [52]. A more significant finding is that *p53* lesions occur earlier than in the sporadic pathway and can be detected during the development of dysplasia [53]. Whether the finding of *p53* or other abnormalities in mucosa adjacent or at a distance from the cancer will help in the decision to remove a colon earlier in this condition and/or will reduce colonoscopy rates is unclear.

Potential Areas Where Molecular Biology Can Help Preoperative Evaluation

There are several areas where preoperative evaluation using molecular biological techniques could be of value. Tests could be carried out on somatic tissue or biopsy specimens.

Screening

While screening for colorectal cancer is not directly related to preoperative evaluation, molecular biology could help in the identification of colorectal tumours. Importantly, for screening FAP and HNPCC kindreds, the causative genes have now been isolated and molecular tests based on these are being devised. Current methods such as faecal occult blood screening appear to be helpful in identifying patients at risk of colorectal cancer. It is now possible to identify *ras* mutations in the faeces of individuals bearing colorectal cancers [54]. Newer, more sensitive and rapid tests are becoming available, and it is likely that such work will bear fruit in the next 5 years.

Biological Aggressiveness and Patient Prognosis

The grade of a tumour has been, and still is, used to identify patients who should be treated more radically (for example, by an abdominoperineal resection or perhaps radiotherapy). This is in spite of the inter-observer variation seen on tumour grading [55]. If it were possible to grade a tumour more accurately by an assessment of molecular changes, then it might be valuable. It might also be possible to stage a tumour in this manner if genetic lesions restricted to tumours which have metastasised are identified. Help in predicting the outcome for an individual patient may also be possible from molecular studies. The grade of a tumour predicts the future biological aggressiveness of a tumour. The stage of a tumour is where it currently appears to be in its natural history. Tumour grade should be predictable by molecular methods. It may also be possible to identify tumour stage if certain molecular events only occur at specific stages of the disease, such as metastasis. The identification of tumour stage by molecular biological methods would also be extremely useful, since other modalities such as radiology may not be able to identify whether a tumour has metastasised. This section will therefore deal with potential molecular grading and staging parameters.

Ideally, the ability to identify both mutations and loss of heterozygosity should be available to the molecular pathologist; however, current methods of identification of point mutations are time consuming unless the likely site of the lesion is known. This will improve in the future, with many methods holding out much promise, including the multiplex oligonucleotide ligase detection test [56], which can detect 28 known point mutations simultaneously, and methods using DNA repair enzymes to identify point mutations on pieces of DNA up to 0.5 Kb long [57]. Methods such as single-strand conformation polymorphism (SSCP) analysis and chemical cleavage mismatch analysis are being used to screen for mutations, but at present DNA sequencing is the most reliable method for the identification of unknown point mutations.

The exception to the rule that large-scale assessment of point mutations is difficult are the point mutations in K-*ras*. At least 40% of colorectal cancers harbour K-*ras* mutations, of which 84% occur in the first two bases of codon 12. These can be rapidly identified by polymerase chain reaction (PCR)-based tests such as SSCP, allele-specific PCR (ASPCR), and restriction enzyme cleavage methods. To date, there has been one report that the type of K-*ras* mutation in colorectal cancer is of prognostic importance [58]. While point mutations and small deletions play an important role in inactivating many tumour suppressor genes, their detection is still too difficult to be used in a large routine service.

A method which can be used for the assessment of lesions of tumour suppressor genes is measurement of loss of heterozygosity. This can be performed either using restriction fragment-length polymorphisms or microsatellite sequence polymorphisms. The latter are the current method of choice as they are more frequently distributed throughout the genome, are more informative, and are easier to use. The value of microsatellites lies in their polymorphic nature, i.e. they are frequently different from one chromosome to the other and thus the two copies of a gene can be distinguished from each other in terms of the length of the repeated sequence. This allows study of loss of heterozygosity, linkage analysis and microsatellite instability. The latter is manifest as an increase or decrease in the number of repeat sequences in the microsatellite.

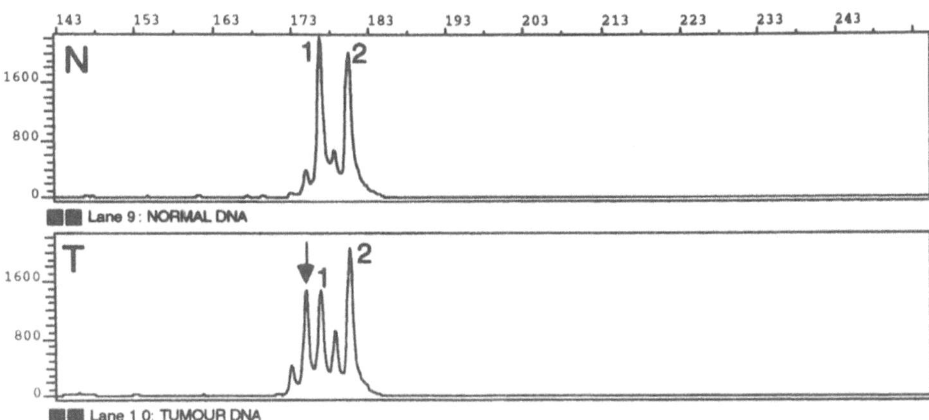

Fig. 2. A colorectal cancer specimen showing microsatellite instability, which indicates that a mutation may have occurred in a DNA mismatch repair gene. This microsatellite assay was performed using fluorescent polymerase chain reaction (PCR), and the products were electrophoresed on a polyacrylamide gel in an Applied Biosystems automated DNA sequencer. Genescan software (Applied Biosystems) was used to automatically assess the size (in base pairs), height and area of each fluorescently labelled product. The *upper trace* shows the two alleles (peaks labelled *1* and *2*), distinguished by their sizes, of a microsatellite marker in the DNA extracted from normal (*N*) tissue. The *minor peaks* are PCR artefacts known as stutter bands. In the corresponding tumour (*T*) DNA (*lower trace*), the same constitutional alleles (labelled *1* and *2*), as determined by their size, are seen, but a novel allele (*arrow*) is also apparent that is not present in the normal DNA. Also see Table 1

Microsatellites can either be identified by the use of PCR with the incorporation of radioactive or fluorescent nucleotides or by labelling of the primers. Fluorescence offers the advantages of multiple markers, sensitivity and the avoidance of the hazards of radioactivity, but requires a DNA sequencer [59, 60]; examples are shown in Figs. 2 and 3.

A number of studies have appeared trying to link molecular lesions to prognosis. As is often the case, they are contradictory. Several suggest that lesions of *p53* and DCC may increase the aggressiveness of the tumour. Our study of K-*ras* mutation and *p53* over-expression showed a poor prognosis in cases which showed abnormalities in both *ras* and *p53* [61]. This series consisted of 100 colorectal cancer patients, but when the study was repeated on a second series this observation was not confirmed. This is the major problem in this area, since small numbers of cases and different methods used for analysis can limit comparability between studies.

One of the largest series on 100 patients failed to show any relationship between the common molecular alterations and prognosis [62]; however, a relationship between DCC loss and prognosis has been reported by others [63]. Thus it seems that, with regard to loss of heterozygosity, much larger series are required. Patients with colorectal cancer showing microsatellite instability seem to have a good prognosis in several series, including our own [64].

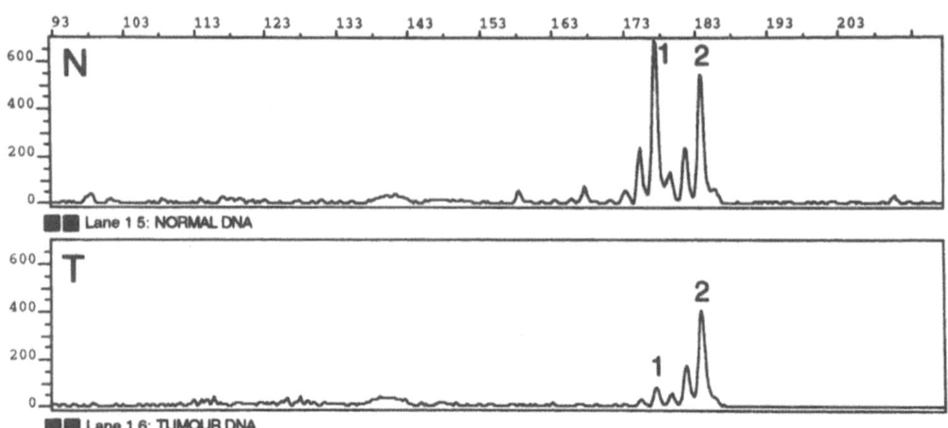

Fig. 3. This figure shows the outcome of a fluorescent polymerase chain reaction (PCR) assay using microsatellites to reveal allele loss (loss of heterozygosity) close to the location of a tumour suppressor gene (APC). The fluorescent PCR products were electrophoresed on a polyacrylamide gel in an Applied Biosystems automated DNA sequencer. In the *upper trace*, the normal (*N*) DNA is shown with the two alleles labelled *1* and *2*. The *lower trace* shows the corresponding tumour (*T*) DNA; the amount of allele *1* has obviously decreased, which is indicative of allele loss. A calculation based on the area under each allele peak, which is calculated automatically by the Genescan software (Applied Biosystems), can be used to quantify the change in allele ratios between the normal and the tumour DNA

Table 1. Size, type, height and area of each peak for the specimen shown in Fig. 2

Peak	Peak type	Size (bp)	Peak height	Peak area
N				
1	Stutter	174.50	410	2792
2	Allele 1	176.47	2328	19814
3	Stutter	178.42	663	4748
4	Allele 2	180.36	2235	20531
T				
1	Stutter	172.51	415	3115
2	Novel allele	174.42	1542	12352
3	Allele 1	176.32	1621	11958
4	Stutter	178.35	931	7176
5	Allele	180.36	2112	18188

Other gene products which have been investigated by imunocytochemistry, such as over-expression of c-*myc*, *bcl-2* and *p53*, have shown that only c-*myc* relates to prognosis [32].

Detection of Occult Metastases

Many patients die after potentially curative operations due to occult metastases not detected at the time of surgery. If molecular markers could be found which indicate the presence of metastases, and if exfoliated malignant cells circulating in the blood could be used to screen for such markers, then this assay could aid in preoperative evaluation. It is also worth noting that it has been reported that molecular biological techniques are more sensitive in the detection of occult lymph node metastases than histopathological examination [65]. If this is confirmed and could be used as a peri-operative procedure, it could have implications for both prognosis and prediction of recurrence.

Response to Therapy

A major question which would be helpful to answer is the likelihood of the tumour responding to preoperative radiotherapy, chemotherapy or both. If it was known that the tumour would significantly decrease in volume, then a delay prior to surgery would be worthwhile. If molecular markers could be discovered that identified patients who would not respond to particular types of chemotherapy, then it would be possible to avoid exposing the patient to such an agent. This is as yet a relatively unexplored area.

Since a normally functioning p53 molecule will push a cell which has been damaged into apoptosis, it may be true that cells which have been damaged by radio- or chemotherapy may be more likely to survive if they have aberrant p53 function than if they have a normal p53. The opposite may be true of DNA repair gene lesions. These tumours may be less likely to repair minor DNA damage than those tumours with normal DNA repair mechanisms. The *bcl-2* gene or other genes involved in apoptosis might also be of great interest in this context. Expresssion of this gene is usually lost in moderately and poorly differentiated tumours but retained in well-differentiated cancers. Other methods that might be of interest are the identification of gene products which interact with chemotherapeutic agents. An example of this is thymidylate synthase, which is the target enzyme for 5-fluorouracil. The level of expression of this enzyme, which can be assessed using immunohistochemical staining, appears to have a significant bearing on response to 5-fluorouracil therapy [66].

Radical or Local Resection

A small subgroup of patients who have small carcinomas or malignant polyps can be difficult to manage. With small rectal carcinomas which could be resected locally, there is a 10% risk of local metastatic spread to lymph nodes. Poor histological grade is helpful, but a firm marker of the ability to metastasise would enable the surgeon to act conservatively where possible. This would also be helpful in cases in which the surgeon believes he or she has removed a malignant polyp and there are adverse pathological features which indicate an aggressive tumour. Markers which help with the above parameters, such as prognosis and response to therapy, might also be useful in the context of the management of malignant polyps and the small rectal cancer which might be removed locally. Most valuable in this situation would be knowledge as to whether the patient's tumour has metastasised. In colorectal cancer, *nm23*, a putative marker of metastasis has not been confirmed as valuable and at present no accurate molecular marker is available.

Synchronous and Metachronous Cancer

Improved knowledge of the risk of synchronous cancer or of developing a subsequent metachronous carcinoma would be of value. If this risk was high, then a total colectomy could be performed at the definitive operation. For patients with a strong family history of HNPCC, it has been standard treatment to perform a total colectomy if a cancer is diagnosed; however, the question of how a patient under 40 years or with a single first-degree relative with colorectal cancer should be managed is still open. Molecular markers may be of use in determining patients who are at increased risk of further colorectal tumours. In a preliminary study we found that there was a significant association between microsatellite instability and increased risk of synchronous and/or metachronous colorectal cancers [64].

When Should the Rectum and Colon Be Removed
due to the Risk of Neoplasia in Ulcerative Colitis?

The current indications for colorectal resection for neoplasia in ulcerative colitis are biopsy-proven high-grade dysplasia verified by two pathologists or a diagnosis of adenocarcinoma. Difficulties can sometimes arise with the diagnosis of high-grade dysplasia owing to inter- or intra-observer variation, which can be substantial, and molecular markers for this stage would be of value.

Conclusions

Over the past few years, molecular biology has proved to be a very useful tool in the study of colorectal cancer. With the discovery of the genes which cause FAP and HNPCC, assays using molecular biological techniques can now be used to screen for these diseases. The search for genes involved in sporadic colorectal cancer continues, but several tumour suppressor genes and oncogenes have already been identified and these are undergoing rigorous examination. Molecular biology also has potential uses in pre- and peri-operative evaluation of colorectal cancer patients, and there are several avenues, as discussed in this chapter, which hold promise for the future.

Acknowledgements. Our research on colorectal cancer is supported by the Yorkshire Cancer Research Campaign. We are also indebted to the Special Trustees of the General Infirmary at Leeds, who purchased our DNA sequencer.

References

1. Groden J, Thliveris A, Samowitz W, Carlson M, Gelbert L, Albertsen H, Joslyn G, Stevens J, Spirio L, Robertson M, Sargeant L, Krapcho K, Wolff E, Burt R, Hughes JP, Warrington J, McPherson J, Wasmuth J, Le Paslier D, Abderrahim H, Cohen D, Leppert M, White R (1991) Identification and characterization of the familial adenomatous polyposis coli gene. Cell 66:589–600
2. Joslyn G, Carlson M, Thliveris A, Albertsen H, Gelbert L, Samowitz W, Groden J, Stevens J, Spirio L, Robertson M, Sargeant L, Krapcho K, Wolff E, Burt R, Hughes JP, Warrington J, McPherson J, Wasmuth J, LePaslier D, Abderrahim H, Cohen D, Leppert M, White R (1991) Identification of deletion mutations and three new genes at the familial polyposis locus. Cell 66:601–613
3. Kinzler KW, Nilbert MC, Su L, Vogelstein B, Bryan T, Levy DB, Smith KJ, Preisinger AC, Hamilton SR, Hedge P, Markham A, Carlson M, Joslyn G, Groden J, White R, Miki Y, Miyoshi Y, Nishisho I, Nakamura Y (1991) Identification of FAP locus genes from chromosome 5q21. Science 253:661–665
4. Nishisho I, Nakamura Y, Miyoshi Y, Miki Y, Ando H, Horii A, Koyama K, Utsunomiya J, Baba S, Hedge P, Markham A, Krush AJ, Petersen G, Hamilton SR, Nilbert MC, Levy DB, Bryan TM, Preisinger AC, Smith KJ, Su L-K, Kinzler KW, Vogelstein B (1991) Mutations of chromosome 5q21 genes in FAP and colorectal cancer patients. Science 253:665–669
5. Fishel R, Lescoe MK, Rao MRS, Copeland NG, Jenkins NA, Garber J, Kane M, Kolodner R (1993) The human mutator gene homolog MSH2 and its association with hereditary nonpolyposis colon cancer. Cell 75:1027–1038
6. Leach FS, Nicolaides NC, Papadopoulos N, Liu B, Jen J, Parsons R, Peltomäki P, Sistonen P, Aaltonen LA, Nyström-Lahti M, Guan X-Y, Zhang J, Meltzer PS, Yu J-W, Kao F-T, Chen DJ, Cerosaletti KM, Fournier REK, Todd S, Lewis T, Leach RJ, Naylor SL, Weissenbach J, Mecklin J-P, Järvinen H, Petersen GM, Hamilton SR, Green J, Jass J, Watson P, Lynch HT, Trent JM, de la Chapelle A, Kinzler KW, Vogelstein B (1993) Mutations of a mutS homolog in hereditary nonpolyposis colorectal cancer. Cell 75:1215–1225
7. Bronner CE, Baker SM, Morrison PT, Warren G, Smith LG, Lescoe MK, Kane M, Earabino C, Lipford J, Lindblom A, Tannergård P, Bollag RJ, Godwin AR, Ward DC, Nordenskjöld, Fishel R, Kolodner R, Liskay RM (1994) Mutation in the DNA mismatch repair gene homologue hMLH1 is associated with hereditary non-polyposis colon cancer. Nature 368:258–261
8. Papadopoulos N, Nicolaides NC, Wei Y-F, Ruben SM, Carter KC, Rosen CA, Haseltine WA, Fleischmann RD, Fraser CM, Adams MD, Venter JC, Hamilton SR, Petersen GM, Watson P, Lynch HT, Peltomäki P, Mecklin J-P, de la Chapelle A, Kinzler KW, Vogelstein B (1994) Mutation of a mutL homolog in hereditary colon cancer. Science 263:1625–1629
9. Nicolaides NC, Papadopoulos N, Liu B, Wei Y-F, Carter KC, Ruben SM, Rosen CA, Haseltine WA, Fleischmann RD, Fraser CM, Adams MD, Venter JC, Dunlop MG, Hamilton SR, Petersen GM, de la Chapelle A, Vogelstein B, Kinzler KW (1994) Mutations of two PMS homologues in hereditary nonpolposis colon cancer. Nature 371:75–80
10. Drummond JT, Li G-M, Longley MJ, Modrich P (1995) Isolation of an hMSH2-p160 heterodimer that restores DNA mismatch repair to tumor cells. Science 268:1909–1912
11. Palombo F, Gallinari P, Iaccarino I, Lettieri T, Hughes M, D'Arrigo A, Truong O, Hsuan JJ, Jiricny J (1995) GTBP, a 160-kilodalton protein essential for mismatch-binding activity in human cells. Science 268:1912–1914
12. Papadopoulos N, Nicolaides NC, Liu B, Parsons R, Lengauer C, Palombo F, D'Arrigo A, Markowitz S, Willson JKV, Kinzler KW, Jiricny J, Vogelstein B (1995) Mutations of GTBP in genetically unstable cells. Science 268:1915–1917
13. Knudson AG (1987) A two-mutation model for human cancer. Adv Viral Oncol 7:1–17
14. Ponder B (1988) Gene losses in human tumours. Nature 335:400–402
15. Weber JL, May PE (1989) Abundant class of human DNA polymorphisms which can be typed using the polymerase chain reaction. Am J Hum Genet 44:388–396
16. Aaltonen LA, Peltomäki P, Leach FS, Sistonen P, Pylkkänen L, Mecklin J-P, Järvinen H, Powell SM, Jen J, Hamilton SR, Petersen GM, Kinzler KW, Vogelstein B, de la Chapelle A (1993) Clues to the pathogenesis of familial colorectal cancer. Science 260:812–816

17. Markowitz S, Wang J, Myeroff L, Parsons R, Sun L, Lutterbaugh J, Fan RS, Zborowska E, Kinzler KW, Vogelstein B, Brattain M, Willson JKV (1995) Inactivation of the type 2 TGF-beta receptor in colon cancer cells with microsatellite instability. Science 268:1336–1338
18. Bodmer W, Bishop T, Karran P (1994) Genetic steps in colorectal cancer. Nat Genet 6:217–219
19. Hockenbery D, Nunez G, Milliman C, Schreiber RD, Korsmeyer SJ (1990) Bcl-2 is an inner mitochondrial membrane protein that blocks programmed cell death. Nature 348:334–336
20. Kerr JFR, Winterford CM, Harmon BV (1994) Apoptosis. Its significance in cancer and cancer therapy. Cancer 73:2013–2026
21. Martin SJ, Green DR (1995) Apoptosis and cancer: the failure of controls on cell death and cell survival. Crit Rev Oncol Hematol 18:137–153
22. Steeg PS, Bevilacqua G, Kopper L, Thorgeirsson UP, Talmadge JE, Liotta LA, Sobel ME (1988) Evidence for a novel gene associated with low tumor metastatic potential. J Natl Cancer Inst 80:200–204
23. Arch R, Wirth K, Hofmann M, Ponta H, Matzku S, Herrlich P, Zoller M (1992) Participation in normal immune responses of a metastasis-inducing splice variant of CD44. Science 257:682–687
24. Powell SM, Zilz N, Beazer-Barclay Y, Bryan TM, Hamilton SR, Thibodeau SN, Vogelstein B, Kinzler KW (1992) APC mutations occur early during colorectal tumorigenesis. Nature 359:235–237
25. Smith AJ, Stern HS, Penner M, Hay K, Mitri A, Bapat BV, Gallinger S (1994) Somatic APC and K-ras codon 12 mutations in aberrant crypt foci from human colons. Cancer Res 54:5527–5530
26. Rubinfeld B, Souza B, Albert I, Muller O, Chamberlain SH, Masiarz FR, Munemitsu S, Polakis P (1993) Association of the APC gene product with B-catenin. Science 262:1731–1734
27. Su L-K, Vogelstein B, Kinzler KW (1993) Association of the APC tumor suppressor protein with catenins. Science 262:1734–1737
28. Yamashita N, Minamoto T, Ochiai A, Onda M, Esumi H (1995) Frequent and characteristic K-ras activation and absence of p53 protein accumulation in aberrant crypt foci of the colon. Gastroenterology 108:434–440
29. Jen J, Powell SM, Papadopoulos N, Smith KJ, Hamilton SR, Vogelstein B, Hamilton SR (1994) Molecular determinants of dysplasia in colorectal lesions. Cancer Res 54:5523–5526
30. Barbacid M (1987) Ras genes. Annu Rev Biochem 56:779–827
31. Burmer GC, Loeb LA (1989) Mutations in the KRAS2 oncogene during progressive stages of human colon carcinoma. Proc Natl Acad Sci USA 86:2403–2407
32. Scott N, Martin I, Jack AS, Dixon MF, Quirke P (1996) Genes mediating programmed cell death: an immunohistochemical study of bcl-2, c-myc and p53 expression in colorectal cancer. J Clin Pathol: Mol Pathol 49:M1–M8
33. Vogelstein B, Fearon ER, Hamilton SR, Scott EK, Reisinger AC, Leppart M, Nakamura Y, White R, Alida MM, Smits BS, Bos JL (1988) Genetic alterations during colorectal tumour development. N Engl J Med 319:525–532
34. Fearon ER, Cho KR, Nigro JM, Kern SE, Simons JW, Ruppert JM, Hamilton SR, Preisinger AC, Thomas G, Kinzler KW, Vogelstein B (1990) Identification of a chromosome 18q gene that is altered in colorectal cancers. Science 247:49–56
35. Fearon ER, Jones PA (1992) Progressing toward a molecular description of colorectal cancer development. FASEB J 6:2783–2790
36. Baker SJ, Fearon ER, Nigro JM, Hamilton SR, Preisinger AC, Milburn Jessup J, vanTuinen P, Ledbetter DH, Barker DF, Nakamura Y, White R, Vogelstein B (1989) Chromosome 17 deletions and p53 gene mutations in colorectal carcinomas. Science 244:217–221
37. Baker SJ, Preisinger AC, Jessup, Paraskeva C, Markowitz S, Willson JKV, Hamilton S, Vogelstein B (1990) p53 gene mutations occur in combination with 17p allelic deletions as late events in colorectal tumorigenesis. Cancer Res 50:7717–1722
38. Scott N, Sagar P, Stewart J, Blair GE, Dixon MF, Quirke P (1991) p53 in colorectal cancer: clinicopathological correlation and prognostic significance. Br J Cancer 63:317–319
39. Forrester K, Almoguera C, Han K, Grizzle WF, Perucho M (1987) Detection of high incidence of K-ras oncogenes during human colon tumorigenesis. Nature 327:298–303

40. Aaltonen LA, Peltomäki P, Mecklin J-P, Järvinen H, Jass JR, Green JS, Lynch HT, Watson P, Tallqvist G, Juhola M, Sistonen P, Hamilton SR, Kinzler KW, Vogelstein B, de la Chapelle A (1994) Replication errors in benign and malignant tumors from hereditary nonpolyposis colorectal cancer patients. Cancer Res 54:1645–1648
41. Leister I, Weith A, Bruderlein S, Cziepluch C, Kangwanpong D, Schlag P, Schwab M (1990) Human colorectal cancer: high frequency of deletions at chromosome 1p35. Cancer Res 50:7232–7235
42. Laurent-Puig P, Olschwang S, Delattre O, Remvikos Y, Asselain B, Melot T, Validire P, Muleris M, Giridet J, Salmon RJ, Thomas G (1992) Survival and acquired genetic alterations in colorectal cancer. Gastroenterology 102:1136–1141
43. Yaremko ML, Wasylyshyn ML, Paulus KL, Michelassi F, Westbrook CA (1994) Deletion mapping reveals two regions of chromosome 8 allele loss in colorectal carcinomas. Genes Chromosomes Cancer 10:1–6
44. Fujiwara Y, Ohata H, Emi M, Okui K, Koyama K, Tsuchiya E, Nakajima T, Monden M, Mori T, Kurimasa A, Oshimura M, Nakamura Y (1994) A 3-Mb physical map of the chromosome region 8p21.3-p22, including a 600-kb region commonly deleted in human hepatocellular carcinoma, colorectal cancer, and non-small cell lung cancer. Genes Chromosomes Cancer 10:7–14
45. Keldysh PL, Dragani TA, Fleischman EW, Konstantinova LN, Perevoschikov AG, Pierotti MA, Della Porta G, Kopnin BP (1993) 11q deletions in human colorectal carcinomas: cytogenetics and restriction fragment length polymorphism analysis. Genes Chromosomes Cancer 6:45–50
46. Young J, Leggett B, Ward M, Thomas L, Buttenshaw R, Searle J, Chenevix-Trench G (1993) Frequent loss of heterozygosity on chromosome 14 occurs in advanced colorectal carcinomas. Oncogene 8:671–675
47. Cohn KH, Wang F, DeSoto-LaPaix F, Solomon WB, Patterson LG, Arnold MR, Weimar J, Feldman JG, Levy AT, Leone A, Steeg PS (1991) Association of nm23-H1 allelic deletions with distant metastases in colorectal carcinoma. Lancet 338:722–724
48. Tanabe KT, Ellis LM, Saya H (1993) Expression of CD44R1 adhesion molecule in colon carcinomas and metastases. Lancet 341:725–726
49. Greenwald BD, Harpaz N, Yin J, Huang Y, Tong Y, Brown VL, McDaniel T, Newkirk C, Resau JH, Meltzer SJ (1992) Loss of heterozygosity affecting the p53, Rb, and MCC/APC tumor suppressor gene loci in dysplastic and cancerous ulcerative colitis. Cancer Res 52:741–745
50. Kern SE, Redston M, Seymour AB, Caldas C, Powell SM, Kornacki S, Kinzler KW (1994) Molecular genetic profiles of colitis-associated neoplasms. Gastroenterology 107:420–428
51. Suzuki H, Harpaz N, Tarmin L, Yin J, Jiang H-Y, Bell JD, Hontanosas M, Groisman GM, Abraham JM, Meltzer SJ (1994) Microsatellite instability in ulcerative colitis-associated colorectal dysplasias and cancers. Cancer Res 54:4841–4844
52. Bell SM, Kelly SA, Hoyle JA, Lewis FA, Taylor GR, Thompson H, Dixon MF, Quirke P (1991) c-Ki-ras gene mutations in dysplasia and carcinomas complicating ulcerative colitis. Br J Cancer 64:174–178
53. Yin J, Harpaz N, Tong Y, Huang Y, Laurin J, Greenwald BD, Hontanosas M, Newkirk C, Meltzer SJ (1993) p53 point mutations in dysplastic and cancerous ulcerative colitis lesions. Gastroenterology 104:1633–1639
54. Sidransky D, Tokino T, Hamilton SR, Kinzler KW, Levin B, Frost P, Vogelstein B (1992) Identification of ras oncogene mutations in the stool of patients with curable colorectal tumours. Science 256:102–105
55. Thomas GDH, Dixon MF, Smeeton NC, Williams NS (1983) Observer variation in the histological grading of rectal carcinoma. J Clin Pathol 36:385–391
56. Grossman PD, Bloch W, Brinson E, Chang CC, Eggerding FA, Fung S, Iovannisci DA, Woo S, Winn-Dean ES (1994) High-density multiplex detection of nucleic acid sequences: oligonucleotide ligation assay and sequence-coded separation. Nucleic Acids Res 22:4527–4534
57. Ellis LA, Taylor GR, Banks R, Baumberg S (1994) MutS binding protects heteroduplex DNA from exonuclease digestion in vitro: a simple method for detecting mutations. Nucleic Acids Res 22:2710–2711

58. Moerkerk P, Arends JW, van Driel M, de Bruïne A, de Goeij A, ten Kate J (1994) Type and number of Ki-ras point mutations relate to stage of human colorectal cancer. Cancer Res 54:3376–3378
59. Cawkwell L, Bell SM, Lewis FA, Dixon MF, Taylor GR, Quirke P (1993) Rapid detection of allele loss in colorectal tumours using microsatellites and fluorescent DNA technology. Br J Cancer 67:1262–1267
60. Cawkwell L, Lewis FA, Quirke P (1994) Frequency of allele loss of DCC, p53, RB1, WT1, NF1, NM23 & APC/MCC in colorectal cancer assayed by fluorescent multiplex polymerase chain reaction. Br J Cancer 70:813–818
61. Bell SM, Scott N, Cross D, Sagar P, Lewis FA, Blair GE, Taylor GR, Dixon MF, Quirke P (1993) Prognostic value of p53 overexpression and c-Ki-ras gene mutations in colorectal cancer. Gastroenterology 104:57–64
62. Dix BR, Robbins P, Soong R, Jenner D, House AK, Iacopetta BJ et al (1994) The common molecular genetic alterations in Dukes' B and C colorectal carcinomas are not short-term prognostic indicators of survival. Int J Cancer 59:747–751
63. Jen J, Kim H, Piantadosi S, Liu Z-F, Levitt RC, Sistonen P, Kinzler KW, Vogelstein B, Hamilton SR (1994) Allelic loss of chromosome 18q and prognosis in colorectal cancer. N Engl J Med 331:213–221
64. Cawkwell L, Li D, Lewis FA, Martin I, Dixon MF, Quirke P (1995) Microsatellite instability in colorectal cancer: improved assessment using fluorescent polymerase chain reaction. Gastroenterology 109:465–471
65. Hayashi N, Hirofumi A, Hiroki N, Akio Y, Yo K, Hirotoshi O, Sadamu T, Michio O, Yusuke N (1994) Genetic diagnosis identifies occult lymph node metastases undetectable by the histopathological method. Cancer Res 54:3853–3856
66. Johnston PG, Lenz HJ, Leichman CG, Danenberg KD, Allegra CJ, Danenberg PV, Leichman L (1995) Thymidylate synthase gene and protein expression correlate and are associated with response to 5-fluorouracil in human colorectal and gastric tumors. Cancer Res 55:1407–1412

The Anatomical Basis for Rectal Cancer Surgery

CHAPTER 8

Rectal and Pelvic Anatomy with Emphasis on Anatomical Layers

Johan N. Wiig and Robert J. Heald

Introduction

Two of the major problems experienced after rectal cancer surgery are the high number of local recurrences and frequent bladder and sexual dysfunction [6]. Traditional technical teaching in this kind of surgery has emphasised a blunt dissection of the rectum with its mesorectal fat from the sacrum, division of the so-called lateral ligaments between forceps and a 2- to 5-cm free distal margin on the resected bowel.

Numerous sophisticated anatomical illustrations show the pelvic autonomic nerves located directly on the rectal wall. From there, the nerves run to the genital organs. If these illustrations were correct, a rectal resection should inevitably lead to nerve damage and malfunction of the urinary and sexual organs. Enker has shown that by applying the total mesorectal excision (TME) technique, the neurological consequences can be drastically reduced [2]. Thus it seems that our anatomical maps are not in line with the surgical terrain. It is also a fact that the autonomic nerves are hardly mentioned in even the most highly esteemed surgical textbooks.

In this chapter, we will demonstrate how a thorough knowledge of the anatomical layers in the pelvis may be of help when performing radical surgery for rectal cancer.

Fasciae

Heald [5] and later Enker [3] have drawn attention to and taken advantage of the fact that the major part of rectum lies within a sheath of areolar tissue. This perirectal fat, i.e. mesorectum, is a separate compartment covered by a thin visceral fascia, the fascia propria of rectum or the mesorectal fascia. The pelvic wall is covered by a similar parietal fascia. This pre-sacral fascia is thin in the mid-line and tough over the piriformis, internal obturator and levator ani muscles. It also covers the pelvic arteries and somatic nerves to the lower extremities. These fasciae are continuations of the abdominal fasciae. The mesorectal fascia is the extension of the visceral fascia covering the dorsal aspect of the descending and ascending colon. The pre-sacral fascia is continuous with the parietal fascia on the retroperitoneal vessels and ureters. Thus, by staying in the plane between the mesorectal and pre-sacral fasciae, damage to the ureter or pre-sacral veins is avoided.

On the dorsal aspect of the pelvis over the sacrum, the mesorectal and pre-sacral fasciae are separated by loose connective tissue. In some places, there may be minor fibrous adhesions between the fasciae. These adhesions are important, as they may give rise to tears in the mesorectum during blunt dissection. Only a few tiny vessels and nerves cross the pre-sacral space. The mesorectal and pre-sacral fasciae therefore represent a flexible interface between the mesorectum and the pelvic wall, allowing movement of one structure upon the other. The discontinuation of tissues also represents a physical barrier. Rectal cancer fairly seldom seems to penetrate this barrier [7, 8].

In the pelvis at the S4–S5 level, the pre-sacral fascia toughens in the mid-line to become the rectosacral fascia, which strenghtens the pelvic floor. This is clearly identified as a tough membrane from below during the perineal part of an abdominoperineal resection. The name "Waldeyer's fascia" has been applied to the entire pelvic parietal fascia. However, it should probably only be applied to the rectosacral fascia.

Laterally, the pre-sacral fascia thins and merges with the mesorectal fascia where the so-called lateral ligament is found. The fascia is not easily seen in vivo at this location. During dissection of fresh cadavers, the fat of the pelvic wall and the mesorectum is hardened. A space can then be partly opened between the parietal and visceral fascia, showing that the two fasciae have not actually merged into one (J.N. Wiig, unpublished data).

In front, the Denonvilliers fascia is interposed between the urogenital organs and the rectum. It is a shiny, smooth anterior surface to the pre-rectal component of the mesorectum. It separates easily from the seminal vesicles, but is adherent to the mesorectal fat. In males, it fuses distally with the posterior prostatic capsule. This is the point at which it must be cut through to separate the distal rectum from the back of the prostate. The comparable fascia in the female between the rectum and vagina is less distinct, and the pre-rectal component of the mesorectum much thinner.

Pelvic Autonomic Nerves

Figure 1 is a schematic illustration of the pelvic autonomic nerves. To show the relation between the nerves and the urogenital organs, the bladder, seminal vesicles and prostate have been lifted up from behind the symphysis. The mesorectum has been reduced in size to afford a better view of the pelvic floor and walls.

In the context of rectal cancer surgery, the autonomic nerves start outside the pelvis around the inferior mesenteric artery. Here, filaments of sympathetic

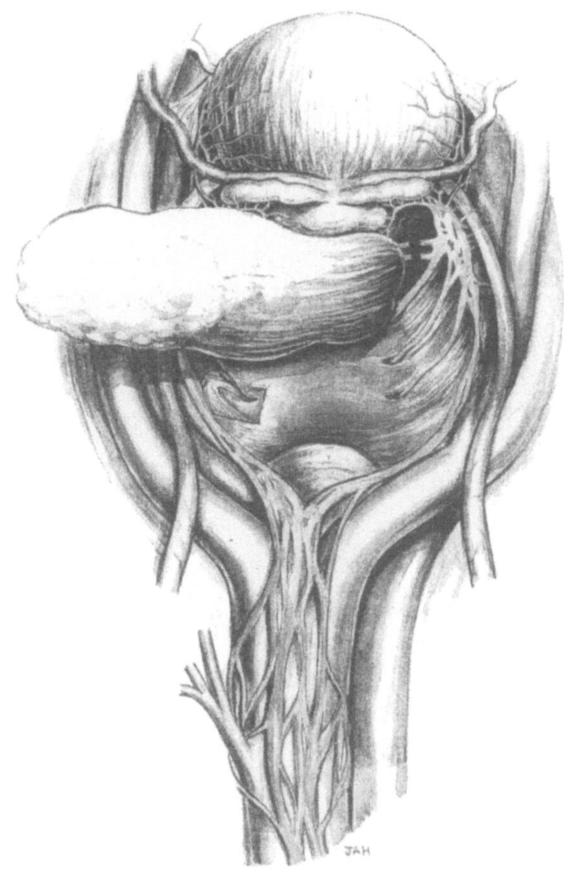

Fig. 1. Pelvis after total mesorectal excision (TME). The rectum is drawn on a smaller scale, and the bladder, prostate and seminal vesicles are lifted up to allow a better view of the autonomic nerves. The hypogastric plexus is on the aortic bifurcation; the pre-sacral nerves run along the pelvic wall dorsal to the ureter towards the pelvic autonomic plexus. From there, nerves enter the lateral ligament to the rectum, and urogenital nerves run along the dorsal and caudal aspect of the vesicles to the bladder, prostate and penis. On the *left*, a window is cut in the pelvic fascia to show some somatic nerves heading for the lower extremity

nerves join in the hypogastric or superior hypogastric plexus. From the plexus, the hypogastric or pre-sacral nerves emerge sagittally near the mid-line within the aortic bifurcation. They diverge below the promontory as "the wishbone", and each passes along the pelvic wall 2–3 cm dorsal to the ureter towards the fundus of the seminal vesicles. The relation to the fasciae is discussed below. On the side wall lateral to the lateral ligaments, the nerves join the para-sympathetic nerves originating from the sacrum. The hypogastric nerves vary in gross anatomy. Sometimes they consist of fine filaments spreading out over a width of about 1 cm, and sometimes they are distinct flat nerves 5–8 mm wide. These nerves can nearly always be easily identified. They are accompanied by small vessels which may bleed during dissection.

The parasympathetic nerves arise from the S2–S3 and S4 roots, the S3 lying in the most curved part of the sacrum. These nerves are known as the pelvic splanchnic nerves or the errigent nerves. From each root one or two nerves 1–3 mm in diameter pass anteriorly and caudally for 2–3 cm. Either S3 or S4 may be the largest. In cadaveric dissections, the nerves can nearly always be seen. During operations, this may be somewhat difficult, mostly due to slight oozing of blood. These nerves join with the hypogastric nerves in the pelvic splanchnic or inferior hypogastric plexus (Fig. 1). The plexus is about 5–6 cm long and passes forward to the lateral end of the seminal vesicles. Some of the filaments in the plexus are so thin that the plexus may hardly be visible during operation except as a flat "plate" on the pelvic side wall. Branches of the pelvic plexus nerves enter the rectum, giving rise to the structure often referred to as the lateral ligament [9].

From the lateral end of the seminal vesicles, the nerves to the urogenital organs pass along the back and lower border of the vesicles towards and along the lateral border of the prostate.

The location of the sympathetic nerves is from a practical point on the surface of the parietal fascia connected to the fascia by loose connective tissue. On the aorta this is clearly seen. Surgically, it is demonstrated when traction is applied to the upper rectum. The hypogastric nerves are then pulled forward with the mesorectum. This opens a space between the nerves and the sacrum. However, if the nerves have been carefully dissected off the mesorectum at the level of the promontory, forward traction on the rectum will leave the nerves safely on the sacrum. The nerves can then be separated from the mesorectum without damaging the mesorectal fascia.

The proper plane at the promontory is best approached from the abdomen. From the left side, it is entered by incising the fusion between the parietal and the visceral peritoneum lateral to the left colon, the so-called white line and entering the areolar tissue layer between the visceral and parietal tissue layers between the mesosigmoid and the ureter and gonadal vessels. From the right side, the approach to the plane in front of the nerves can be identified by incising the peritoneum and lifting the caecum and terminal ileum forward and upwards. As the nerves lie on the aorta at the origin of the inferior mesenteric artery, they may be damaged if the artery is divided flush on the aorta.

The parasympathetic nerves penetrate the pre-sacral fascia laterally and follow the surface of this to the pelvic splanchnic plexus. The nerves to the urogenital organs are located in front and laterally close to Denonvilliers fascia, where they are surrounded by numerous veins which may bleed during dissection. During surgery for rectal cancer, they can be protected by dissecting the plane behind them; during surgery for prostatic cancer, they can be dissected in front, showing that also at this location the nerves are not firmly bound to the surrounding organs.

Lateral Ligaments

The lateral ligaments are the main fixing points that prevent surgeons from lifting up the rectum during attempts at low anterior resection. They are defined by Goligher as the fibrous tissue between the pelvic wall, the rectum and the peritoneum [4], forming a pyramid with the base on the pelvic wall. This definition is not very precise. In contrast, both Enker and Heald suggest that what surgeons call the lateral ligament is often formed by surgeons during the operation by coning into the mesorectum [3]. This is partly in line with our cadaveric dissection studies, suggesting that most of the ligament is due to adhesions between the mesorectal and pelvic fasciae.

There are, however, structures in the so-called ligaments located at an angle of about 60° on either side of the symphysis which keep the rectum down in the pelvis. When these tethering structures are cut, the rectum can often be lifted up several centimetres (see below). These tethering structures are thus the stronger anchoring points between closely approximated stuctures. They are not ligaments in the sense that they can be developed for a certain length.

Several authors have studied ligaments in cadavers, and the results differ considerably. A middle rectal artery was found in 12%–35% of examined corpses [1, 9]. If present at all, it appeared unilaterally in less than half of the cadavers. It appeared on the pelvic wall within the autonomic pelvic splanchnic plexus, and one to five branches were found. These studies conclude that its importance for the rectal blood supply is limited. In fact, a major middle rectal artery is a rarity. If present and cut, it will not usually cause significant bleeding. The so-called inconsistent sacral artery [1] is only identified if the dissection reaches the mesorectum in the mid-line at the base of the rectosacral fascia near the anorectal junction.

The autonomic nerves to the rectum pass through the lateral ligament. In meticulous studies, Sato has shown numerous fine filaments in the ligaments which are nerves and lymphatic vessels. Heald has suggested that the major autonomic nerves leave the pelvic splanchnic plexus at a T junction, which he suggests is part of the tethering points of the rectum. Preliminary studies seem to support this. As the "lateral ligaments" do not have any length and the pelvic splanchnic plexus is located on the surface of the pelvic fascia, the nerves of the plexus are at quite a high risk of being damaged during division of the "ligaments".

Thus it seems that the rectum is kept in place in the pelvis due to minor, strong "anchoring" points consisting of nerves and vessels, by adhesions between the pelvic fasciae and, to some extent, by minor tethering neurovascular structures.

Conclusion

Knowledge of the pelvic planes enhances the possibility of a complete removal of the mesorectum and allows a more anatomical and radical operation to be performed. Identification of nervous structures diminishes the risk of impairing sexual and bladder function due to damage of the urogenital nerves or other surrounding structures. The principal and most constant component of the lateral ligaments is the autonomic nerve supply to the rectum rather than a structural and or "supportive" ligament.

References

1. Ayoub S (1978) Arterial supply to the human rectum. Acta Anat 100:317–327
2. Enker WE (1992) Potency, cure and local control in the operative treatment of rectal cancer. Arch Surg 127:1396–1402
3. Enker WE, Thaler HT, Cranor ML, Polyak T (1995) Total mesorectal excision in the operative treatment of carcinoma of the rectum. J Am Coll Surg 181:335–346
4. Goligher JC (1980) Surgery of the anus, rectum and colon, 4th edition. Ballière Tindall, London, p 539
5. Heald RJ, Husband EM, Ryall RDH (1982) The mesorectum in rectal cancer surgery – the clue to pelvic recurrence? Br J Surg 69:613–616
6. McCall JL, Cox MR, Wattchow DA (1995) Analysis of local recurrence rates after surgery alone for rectal cancer. Int J Colorect Dis 10:126–132
7. Ng IOL, Luk ICS, Yuen ST, Lau PWK, Pritchett CJ, Ng M, Poon GP, Ho J (1993) Surgical lateral clearance in resected rectal carcinoma. Cancer 71:1972–1976
8. Quirke P, Dixon MF, Durdey P (1986) Local recurence of adenocarcinoma due to inadequate surgical resection: histopathological study of lateral tumour spread and surgical excision. Lancet II:996–998
9. Sato K, Sato T (1991) The vascular and neuronal composition of the lateral ligament of the rectum and rectosacral fascia. Surg Radiol Anat 13:17–22

Regional Anatomy of the Male Pelvic Nerve Plexus: Composition, Divisions and Relationship to the Lymphatics

Tatsuo Sato and Kenji Sato

Introduction

In function-preserving operations of rectal cancer, a detailed and precise understanding is crucial not only of the rectal blood supply but also of the regional anatomy of the autonomic nerves and lymphatics. Complete comprehension of the pelvic plexus (inferior hypogastric plexus) and the related lymphatic pathways facilitates the development of function-preserving surgical procedures. As the field of dissection is very limited in this region, the structural relationships are difficult to assess during surgery.

In this chapter, we present data and photographs obtained during minute dissection of the pelvis. We have used the lateral approach after removal of the hip bones, enabling precise demonstration of the composition and detailed divisions of the pelvic nerve plexus in addition to their relationships to blood vessels and lymphatics.

Basic Anatomy

The nomenclature of this region is very complicated and sometimes misunderstood. Here we adopt the English terminology of *Nomina Anatomica* (5th and 6th edn.) [1–3, 10–12] and define the terms in a simplified diagram (Fig. 1) [4].

The pelvic or inferior hypogastric plexus supplies numerous autonomic nerve branches to the intrapelvic organs as well as to the left hemicolon. The plexus forms a thin quadrangular meshwork, the dimensions of which are about 25–30 mm in height and about 40 mm in length (Fig. 2) [4]. In men, the plexus lies lateral to the rectum, prostate, seminal vesicle and the posterior part

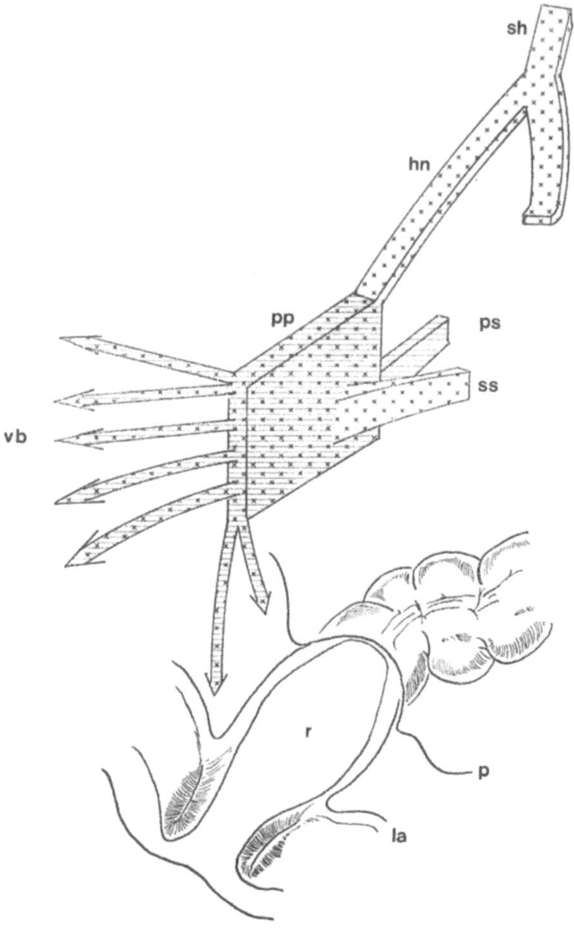

Fig. 1. Composition and divisions of the pelvic plexus (inferior hypogastric plexus). Reproduced with permission from [4] (*hn*, hypogastric nerve; *la*, levator ani; *p*, peritoneum; *pp*, pelvic plexus; *ps*, pelvic splanchnic nerves; *r*, rectum; *sh*, superior hypogastric plexus; *ss*, sacral splanchnic nerves; *vb*, visceral branches) (reproduced by permission)

of the bladder. In women, the uterine cervix and vaginal fornix take the place of the prostate and seminal vesicle. The plexus lies medial to the internal iliac vessels: in other words, it intervenes between these vessels and the intrapelvic organs. Due to its anatomical position, the visceral branches of the internal iliac vessels and their accompanying lymphatics are intimately related to the plexus. Therefore, precise knowledge of the pelvic nerve plexus is crucial in rectal cancer surgery.

The major sympathetic components are the continuation of the hypogastric nerve from the bifurcation of the superior hypogastric plexus, and these are supplemented by the sacral splanchnic nerves from the sacral sympathetic

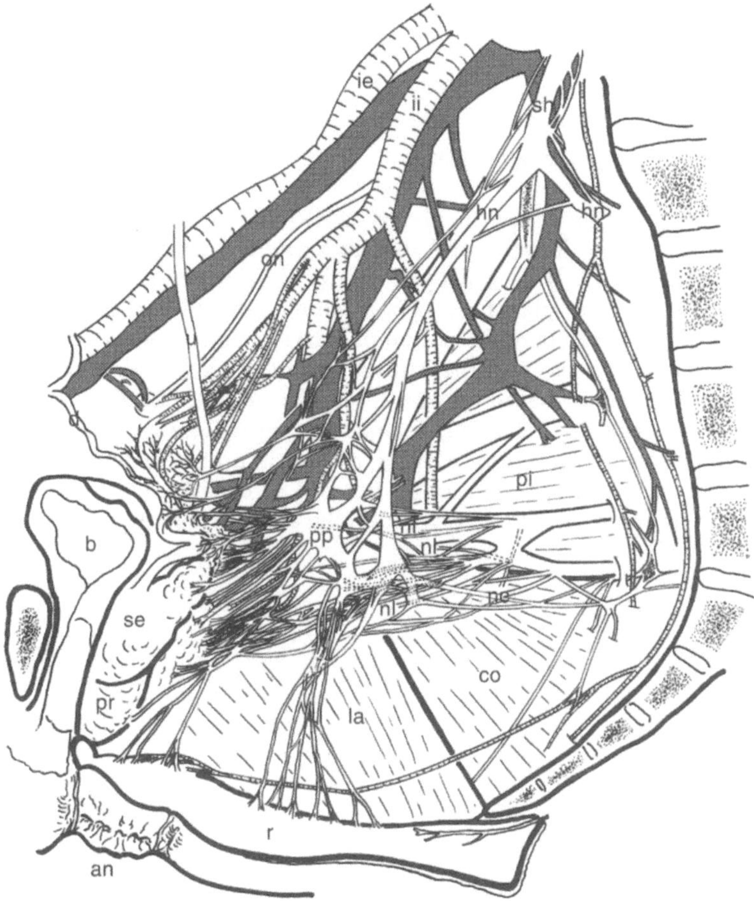

Fig. 2. Right male pelvic plexus of a midsagittally sectioned pelvis. The rectum has been pulled medially and posteriorly. Reproduced with permission from [4] (*an*, anus; *b*, urinary bladder; *cn*, cavernous nerve; *d*, ductus deferens; *hn*, hypogastric nerve; *ie*, external iliac artery/vein; *ii*, internal iliac artery/vein; *la*, levator ani; *nl*, nerve to levatory ani; *pp*, pelvic plexus (inferior hypogastric plexus); *pr*, prostate; *on*, obturator nerve; *r*, rectum; *se*, seminal vesicle; *sh*, superior hypogastric plexus; *u*, ureter)

trunk. The parasympathetic components, the pelvic splanchnic nerves, arise from the sacral plexus. These autonomic nerve components and the middle rectal vessels together with the surrounding connective tissue form the lateral ligament of the rectum (for details refer to [7]).

Composition of the Pelvic Nerve Plexus

As the sympathetic superior hypogastric plexus and the parasympathetic pelvic splanchnic nerves are important nerve structures, we will give a brief description for orientation and clarity before discussing the intricate relationships between these nerve components based on detailed dissections of the pelvis.

Superior Hypogastric Nerve Plexus

The superior hypogastric plexus (SHP) has generally been regarded as the downward continuation of the abdominal aortic nerve plexus. The chief component of SHP is, however, not the descending aortic plexus but the right and left lumbar splanchnic nerves which generally arise from the roots of L2 and L3 [5]. The site of formation of SHP (the union of the right and left lumbar splanchnic nerves) and the bifurcation of the aorta were on average situated only 5 mm apart based on our dissection of 84 cadavers [5] (Fig. 3). The SHP may be regarded as being formed at approximately the same level as the bifurcation of the aorta. SHP, a ribbon-like bundle which is approximately 5 mm wide and 42.4 mm long (mean of 84 cadavers), bifurcates into the right and left hypogastric nerves generally at the level of the intervertebral disc

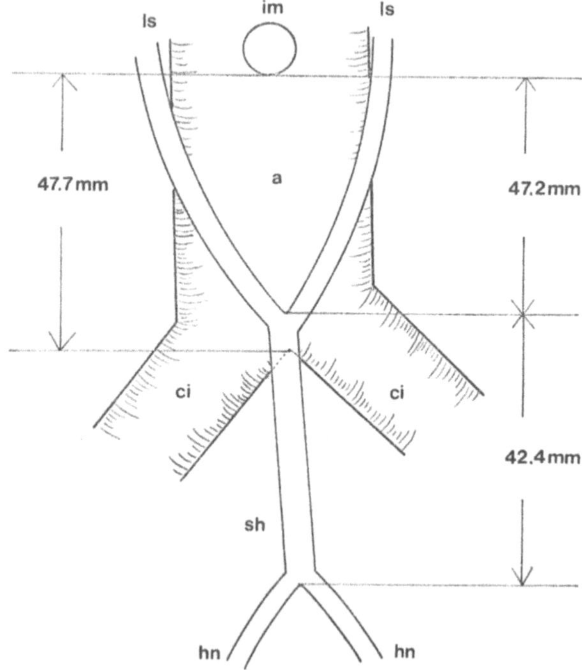

Fig. 3. Diagramatic scheme showing the topographical relationship of the superior hypogastric plexus and the bifurcation of the abdominal aorta. The numerals represent the mean length of 84 Japanese adult specimens. Reproduced with permission from [5] (*a*, abdominal aorta; *ci*, common iliac artery/vein; *hn*, hypogastric nerve; *im*, inferior mesenteric artery; *ls*, lumbar splanchnic nerve)

between L5 and S1 [5]. The SHP can therefore be found at the level between the bifurcation of the aorta and S1 during function-preserving operations.

Due to the numerous communicating branches of the inferior mesenteric and superior rectal nerve plexuses, SHP is not in direct contact with the lumbosacral vertebral column, but tends to be slightly displaced.

Pelvic Splanchnic Nerves

Textbooks commonly describe the pelvic splanchnic nerves as being formed from the roots of S2–S4 [1, 11]. In the Japanese, the main components of these nerves are typically lower and originate from the roots of S3 and S4 [4].

Dissection of the Pelvic Plexus

After removal of the right hip bone (Fig. 4a), the upper lateral edge of the levator ani (two white pins in the figure) becomes clear. The levator ani muscle serves as a septum; the pudendal nerve runs inferior to the muscle, while the pelvic plexus and levator ani supplying nerve lie superior to the muscle. The fascial structures have been removed above and medial to the levator ani (Fig. 4b).

A rich venous plexus intervenes between the fascial structures and the pelvic plexus. In the specimen on which this figure is based an "accessory pudendal artery" (accessory pudic artery as termed by Quain [9] is observed which runs obliquely inside the levator ani and reaches the dorsum of the penis. In Fig. 4c the venous plexus has been removed. The sympathetic hypogastric nerve and parasympathetic pelvic splanchnic nerves unite to form the pelvic plexus lateral to the rectum. Numerous vesical and prostatic branches of the pelvic plexus traverse to reach the urinary bladder and prostate with the lowermost prostatic branches reaching the area near the pudendal nerve.

In another specimen (Fig. 5), the lowermost branch of the pelvic plexus runs between the rectum and prostate; it then passes through the gap between the symphysis pubis and the anterior margin of the levator ani to join the dorsal nerve of the penis.

Dissection of the Lateral Lymphatics

The two major lateral pathways of the rectal lymphatics via major intermediary lymph node groups are illustrated in Fig. 6 [8]. One pathway ascends along the inner margin of the internal and common iliac arteries to reach the nodes of the aortic bifurcation (A). The other and more dominant pathway crosses the internal iliac artery and reaches the node group in the angle between the internal and external iliac arteries (B). Both pathways ascend along the common iliac artery and finally reach the para-aortic nodes.

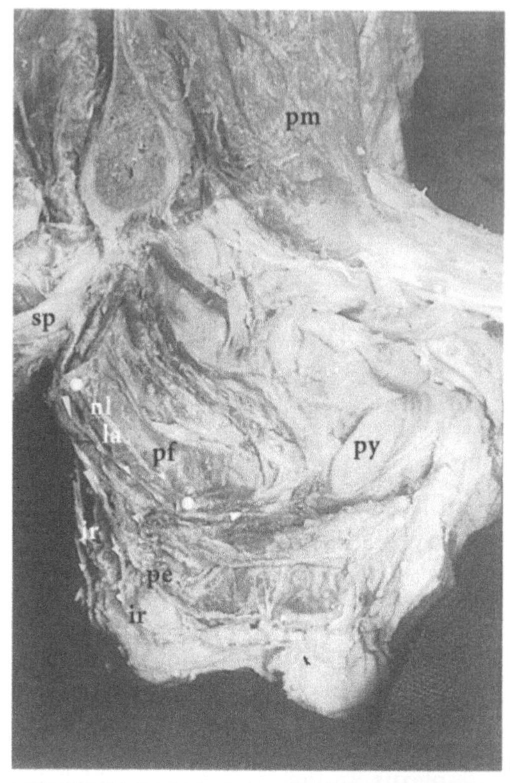

Fig. 4a–c. Serial dissections of a right male pelvic plexus as viewed from the right after removal of the hip bone (specimen 1). [*ap*, accessory pudendal artery; *b*, urinary bladder; *dp*, dorsal nerve of the penis; *ir*, inferior rectal nerves; *la*, levator ani; *nl*, nerve to the levator ani; *pe*, perineal nerves; *pf*, superior fascia of the pelvic diaphragm; *pm*, psoas major; *pp*, pelvic plexus (inferior hypogastric plexus); *pr*, prostate; *ps*, pelvic splanchnic nerves; *pu*, pudendal nerve; *py*, pubic symphysis; *r*, rectum; *sp*, sacral plexus; *sv*, superior vesical artery; *u*, ureter; *ul*, medial umbilical ligament; *vp*, vesical venous plexus]

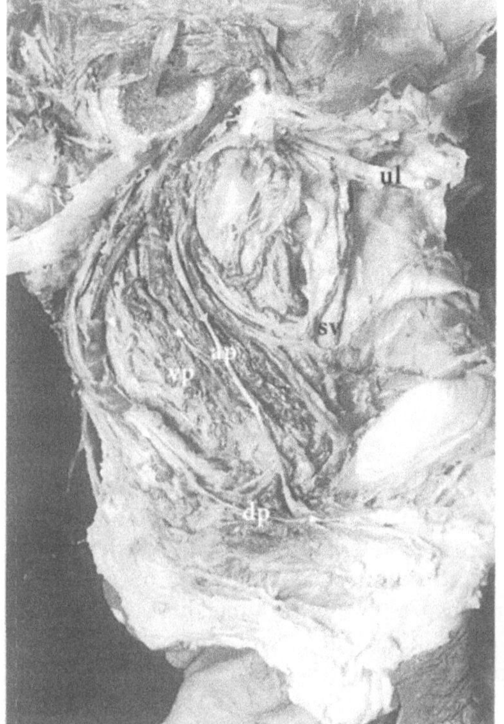

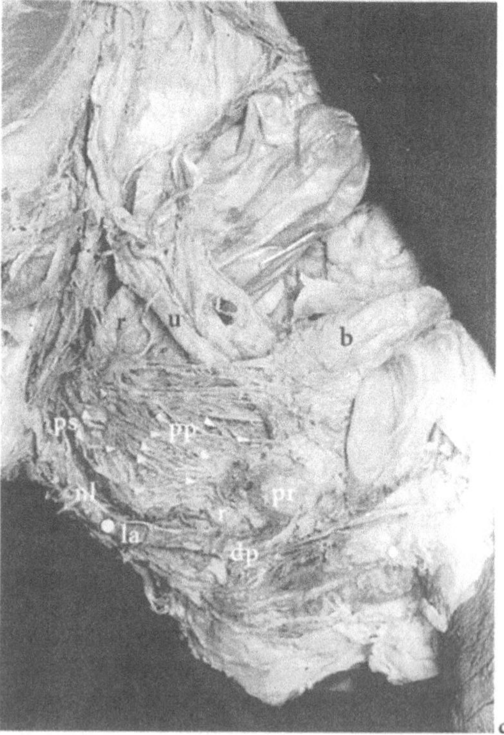

Fig. 5. Male right pelvic plexus dissection showing the course of the lowermost branch (small inlaid black papers) which joins the pudendal nerve (long inlaid black paper) (specimen 2). (*cn*, cavernous nerve; *b*, urinary bladder; *dp*, dorsal nerve of the penis; *p*, penis; *pp*, pelvic plexus; pr, prostate; *pt*, promontorium; *pu*, pudendal nerve; *r*, rectum; *se*, seminal vesicle; *sh*, superior hypogastric plexus; *sp*, sacral plexus)

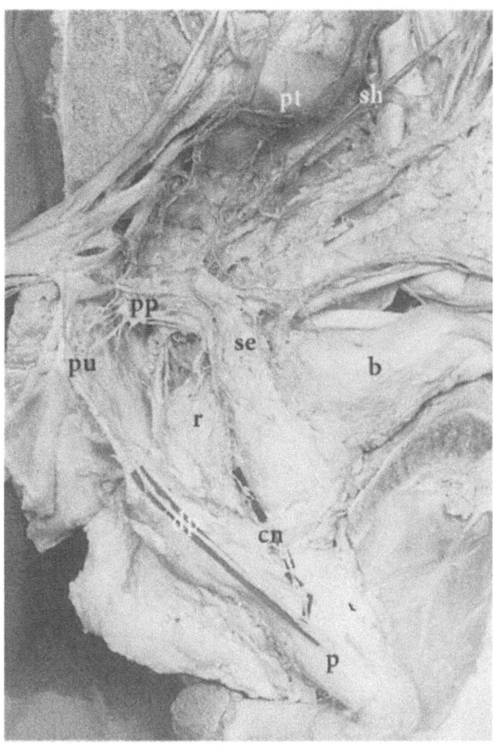

In Fig. 7a the right common, external, and internal arteries are seen and the lymphatics along and around these vessels are dissected.

After the ureteric and testicular vessels have been removed (Fig. 7b), the two lateral chains are clearly visible; one ascends along the medial margin of the internal iliac artery, while the other crosses this artery and the obturator nerve to reach the interiliac area.

After removal of the internal iliac and external iliac vessels (Fig. 7c), lymphatics which pass behind the blood vessels are seen. Due to their critical position, these lymphatics should be considered in cancer dissection procedures.

In Fig. 7d the lower portions of the abdominal aorta and inferior vena cava have been exposed, revealing the inferior mesenteric artery and the superior hypogastric plexus. The lymphatics reach the aorta and inferior vena cava and there intertwine with the autonomic nerves. It is important to note the transverse communications (tc) between SHP and the inferior mesenteric and/ or the superior rectal plexus.

Dissection of Denonvilliers' Fascia

The rectovesical septum, the so-called Denonvilliers' fascia, separates the rectum from the urogenital organs. The upper end of this fascia is connected to

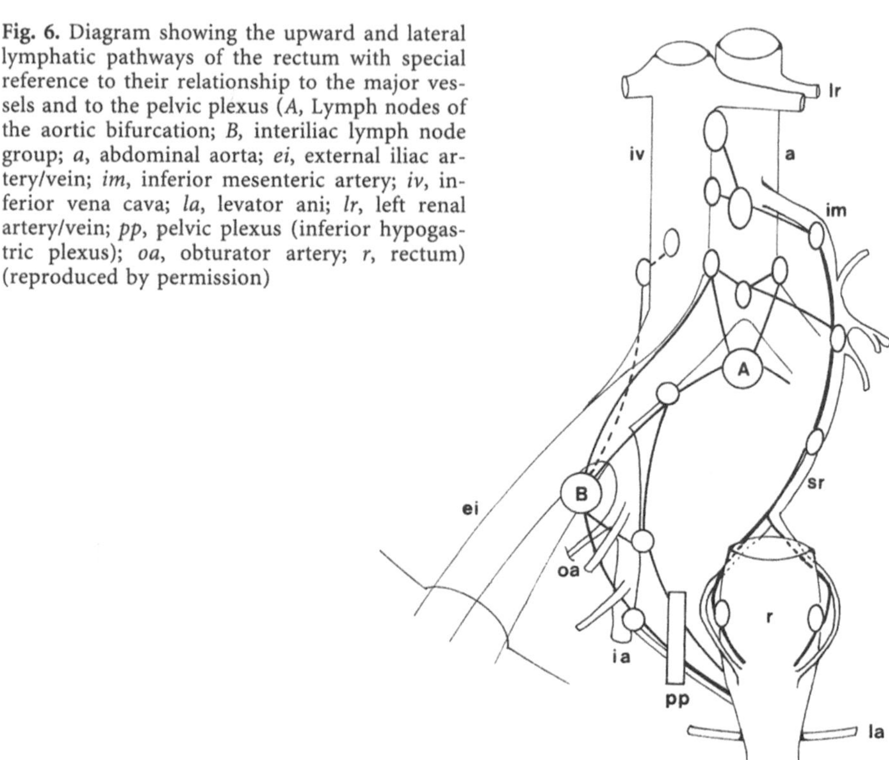

Fig. 6. Diagram showing the upward and lateral lymphatic pathways of the rectum with special reference to their relationship to the major vessels and to the pelvic plexus (*A*, Lymph nodes of the aortic bifurcation; *B*, interiliac lymph node group; *a*, abdominal aorta; *ei*, external iliac artery/vein; *im*, inferior mesenteric artery; *iv*, inferior vena cava; *la*, levator ani; *lr*, left renal artery/vein; *pp*, pelvic plexus (inferior hypogastric plexus); *oa*, obturator artery; *r*, rectum) (reproduced by permission)

the lowermost portion of the peritoneal reflection. Inferiorly this fascia is attached to the prostate and to the perineal body. In a median-sectioned specimen (Fig. 8) [6], the peritoneal reflection is seized by two forceps, revealing two transverse grooves indicative of the firm connection to Denonvilliers' fascia. With Denonvilliers' fascia removed, the inside view of the pelvic plexus is clear between the rectum and urinary bladder (Fig. 9) [6]. It becomes evident that this critical fascia divides not only these two organs but also the branches of the plexus to these organs.

Fig. 7a–d. Serial dissection of the lateral lymphatic pathways in the male right pelvis (specimen 3). [*a*, abdominal aorta; *b*, urinary bladder; *ci*, common iliac artery/vein; *d*, ductus deferens; *ei*, external iliac artery/vein; *hn*, hypogastric nerve; *ii*, internal iliac artery/vein; *iv*, inferior vena cava; *oa*, obturator artery; *on*, obturator nerve; *pp*, pelvic plexus (inferior hypogastric plexus); *pt*, promontorium; *r*, rectum; *sh*, superior hypogastric plexus; *sp*, sacral plexus; *sr*, superior rectal artery/plexus; *tc*, transverse connection between the superior hypogastric and superior rectal plexuses; *te*, testicular artery/vein; *u*, ureter]

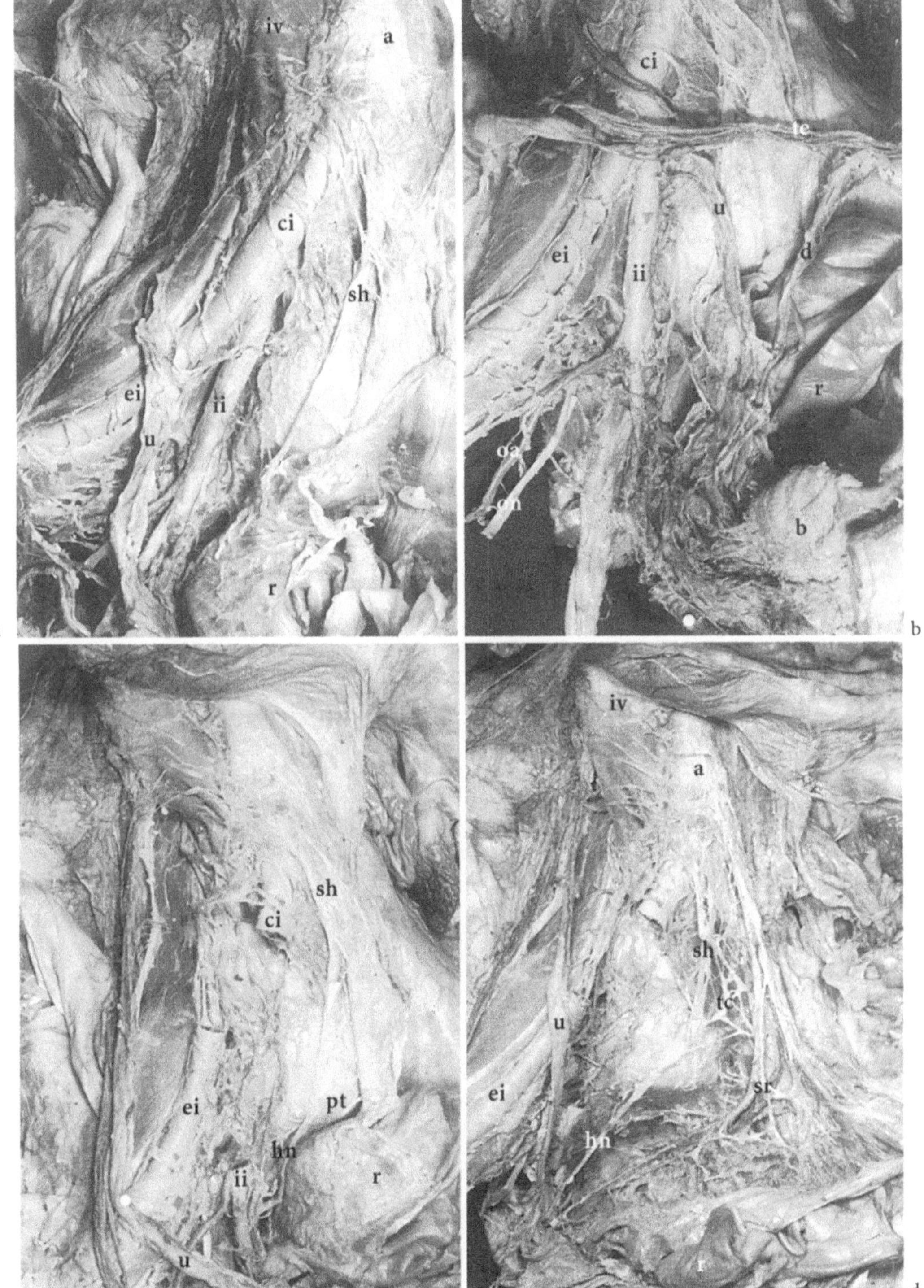

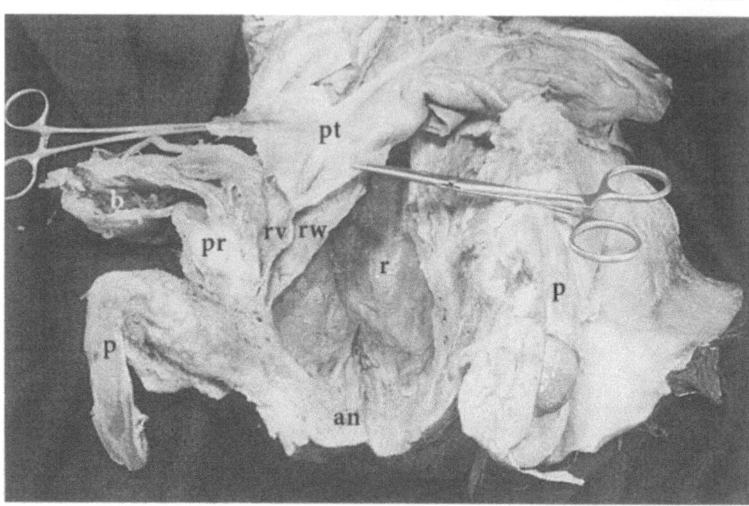

Fig. 8. Male median section dissection showing Denonvilliers' fascia with the posterior rectal wall intact (specimen 4, right side). Reproduced with permission from [6] (*an*, anus; *b*, urinary bladder; *p*, penis; *pr*, prostate; *pt*, peritoneum; *r*, rectum; *rv*, rectovesical septum (Denonvilliers' fascia); *rw*, rectal wall)

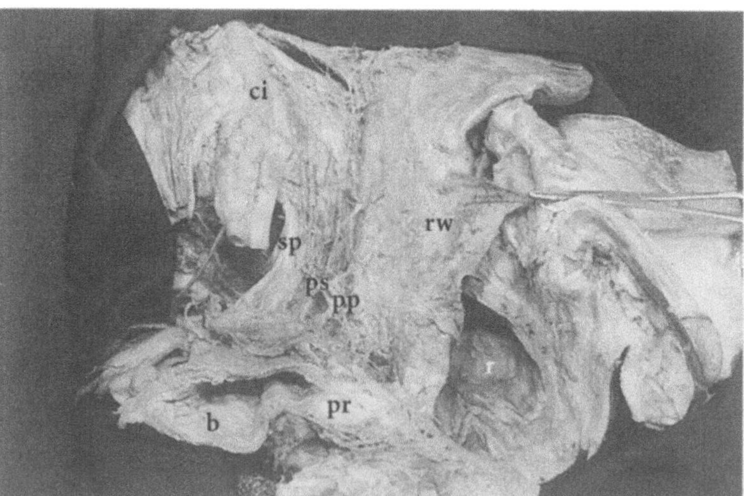

Fig. 9. With Denonvilliers' fascia removed, the pelvic plexus between the bladder, prostate and rectum is viewed from the medial side (specimen 4, right side). Reproduced with permission from [6] (*b*, urinary bladder; *ci*, common iliac artery/vein; *pp*, pelvic plexus (inferior hypogastric plexus); *pr*, prostate; *ps*, pelvic splanchnic nerves; *r*, rectum; *rw*, rectal wall; *sp*, sacral plexus)

References

1. Clemente CD (1985) Gray's anatomy of the human body, 30th edn. Lea and Febiger, Philadelphia, pp 1250-1251
2. International Anatomical Nomenclature Committee (1983) Nomina anatomica, 5th edn. Williams and Wilkins, Baltimore, pp A78-A79
3. International Anatomical Nomenclature Committee (1989) Nomina anatomica, 6th edn. Churchill Livingstone, Edinburgh, pp A84-A85
4. Sato K, Sato T (1981) Composition and distribution of the pudendal and pelvic plexuses. J Jpn Soc Coloproctol 34:515-529 (in Japanese with English abstract)
5. Sato K, Sato T (1989) Topographical relationship of the lymph nodes surrounding the abdominal aorta, the inferior mesenteric artery, and the superior hypogastric plexus. J Jpn Soc Coloproctol 42:1178-1192 (in Japanese with English abstract)
6. Sato T, Sato K (1989) Regional anatomy for urological surgery. (part 13), Intrapelvic fascia. Jpn J Clin Urol 43:576-584 (in Japanese)
7. Sato K, Sato T (1991) The vascular and neuronal composition of the lateral ligament of the rectum and the rectosacral fascia. Surg Radiol Anat 13:17-22
8. Sato K, Sato T (1993) Regional anatomy for rectal cancer surgery with special reference to the lymphatics. Geka (Surgery, Tokyo) 55:400-408 (in Japanese)
9. Schäffer EA, Thane GD (1894) Quain's elements of anatomy. 10th edn (vol 12/part 2). Longmans Green, London, pp 477-480
10. Thorek P (1985) Anatomy in surgery. 3rd edn. Springer, Berlin Heidelberg New York, p 628
11. Williams PL et al. (eds) (1995) Gray's anatomy, 38th edn. Churchill Livingstone, Edinburgh, pp 1297-1309
12. Woodburne RT, Burkel WE (1988) Essentials of human anatomy. 8th edn. Oxford University Press, Oxford, pp 549-553

Anatomical Basis of Total Mesorectal Excision and Preservation of the Pelvic Autonomic Nerves in the Treatment of Rectal Cancer

Klaas Havenga, Warren E. Enker, Marco C. DeRuiter, and Kees Welvaart

Introduction

The rectum can be defined as the final 15 cm of the large intestine. Despite its name, it is curved within the sagittal and coronal planes. Sagittally, the rectum curves anteriorly along the sacrum and makes a sharp posterior curve when the rectum penetrates the levator ani and reaches the anal canal. In the coronal plane the rectum is S-shaped.

The rectum is surrounded by an integral layer of fatty tissue: the mesorectum. Most of the arterial blood supply and the venous and lymphatic drainage of the rectum passes through the mesorectum. The proximal third of the mesorectum is covered with peritoneum on the anterior and partly on the lateral sides. The middle third of the mesorectum may be covered with peritoneum but only on its anterior side, while the distal third of the mesorectum is not covered with peritoneum at all. All of these structures are contained within the visceral pelvic fascia.

Visceral Pelvic Fascia

The posterior and lateral surfaces of the mesorectum are covered with a thin fascial leaf; the visceral fascia (Figs. 1, 2). The caudal border of the visceral fascia is at the internal anal spincter, where it joins with the parietal pelvic fascia. Laterally, the visceral fascia ends on the internal iliac arteries where it forms dense fibrous connections with the parietal pelvic fascia. Superiorly, the visceral fascia ends gradually as it meets the sigmoid mesocolon close to the sacral promontorium. The visceral fascia resembles a hammock, suspending the mesorectum between the left and right internal iliac arteries.

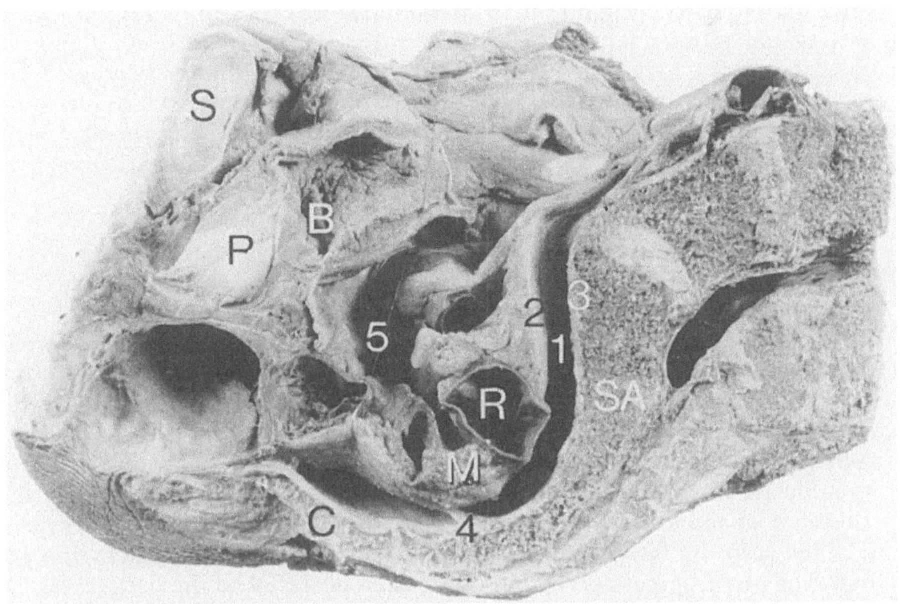

Fig. 1. Midsagittal hemisection of a male pelvis in supine position. *1*, Retrorectal space; *2*, visceral fascia; *3*, parietal fascia; *4*, rectosacral fascia; *5*, peritoneal cavity; *R*, rectum; *M*, mesorectum; *B*, bladder; *P*, prostate; *S*, symphysis pubis; *SA*, sacrum; *C*, coccyx

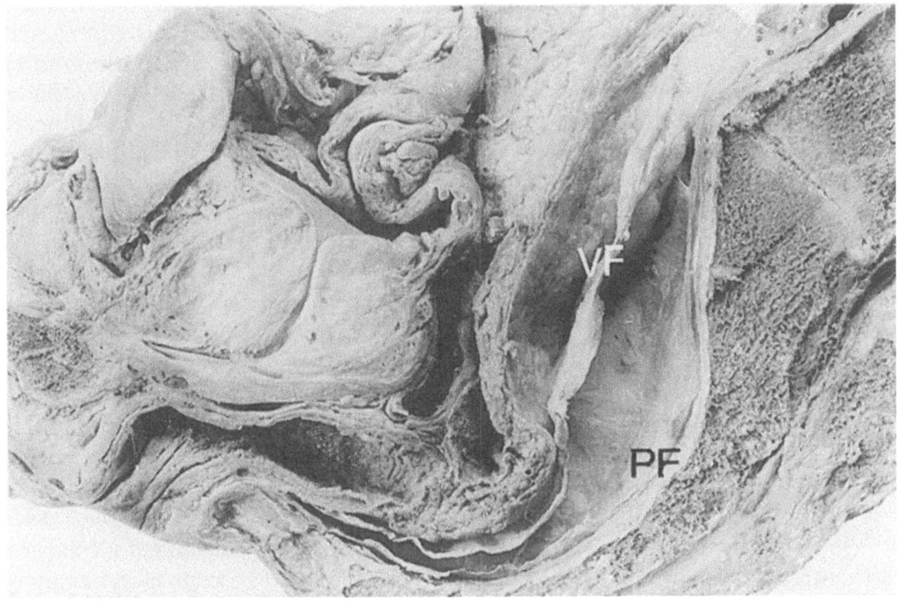

Fig. 2. Midsagittal hemisection of a male pelvis in supine position. Visceral fascia (*VF*) and parietal fascia (*PF*) are demonstrated

The embryological origin of the visceral fascia was studied by Fritsch [3]. In a 9-week-old human fetus, a rectal adventitia can be found, consisting of condensed mesenchyme. In 18- to 20-week-old fetuses, this mesenchyme develops into fibrous connective tissue. Later in the development, fat tissue starts to grow within this adventitia, separating the adventitia into lamellae. The outermost lamella forms a dense sheath which envelops all of the other visceral layers and can be regarded as the visceral fascia.

Parietal Pelvic Fascia

The parietal pelvic fascia pertains, as its name implies, to the pelvic walls (Fig. 2). On the posterior aspect of the pelvis, the parietal fasica covers the muscles of the pelvic side walls (piriformis, coccygeal, and levator ani muscles) and the anterior surface of the sacrum and coccyx.

The parietal fascia is continuous with the fasciae of the pelvic muscles and can easily be demonstrated in these areas. The parietal fascia covering the periosteum of the sacrum and coccyx is very thin. Posterior to the parietal fascia, between the fascia and the sacrum, the presacral artery and veins are found. The sacral spinal nerves are also located posterior to the parietal fascia.

Retrorectal Space and Rectosacral Ligament

Between the visceral and parietal fascia a layer of loose connective tissue is found. This layer can easily be divided so that a space is opened: the retrorectal space (Fig. 1). The borders of this retrorectal space are identical to the borders of the visceral fascia: inferiorly, the internal anal sphincter; laterally, the internal iliac artery; and, cranially, a vague border as the visceral fascia thins out in the sigmoid mesocolon. Some small branches of the internal iliac veins and the presacral venous plexus cross the retrorectal space. The loose connection of the visceral fascia to the parietal fascia allows the rectum some functional mobility, so that the rectum can straighten out during defecation as the pelvic floor lowers.

Anterior to the fourth sacral vertebra, the parietal and visceral fascia are more strongly connected by a dense band of fibers: the rectosacral ligament or rectosacral fascia (Figs. 1, 3). This ligament runs in a craniocaudal direction from the parietal fascia to the visceral fascia. The middle 3–4 cm of this ligament is a strong fibrous structure. As the rectosacral ligament extends laterally to the lateral border of the retrorectal space it becomes thinner and sometimes transparent. A small branch of the middle rectal artery or vein may be found within the rectosacral ligament.

Distal from the rectosacral ligament, the visceral fascia is a bilayered structure, with an anterior and posterior leaf (Fig. 4). The rectosacral ligament is continuous with the posterior leaf of the visceral fascia. Although the rectosacral fascia is sometimes referred to as Waldeyer's fascia, this is, in fact, incorrect as the rectosacral fascia is the only fascia not described by Waldeyer

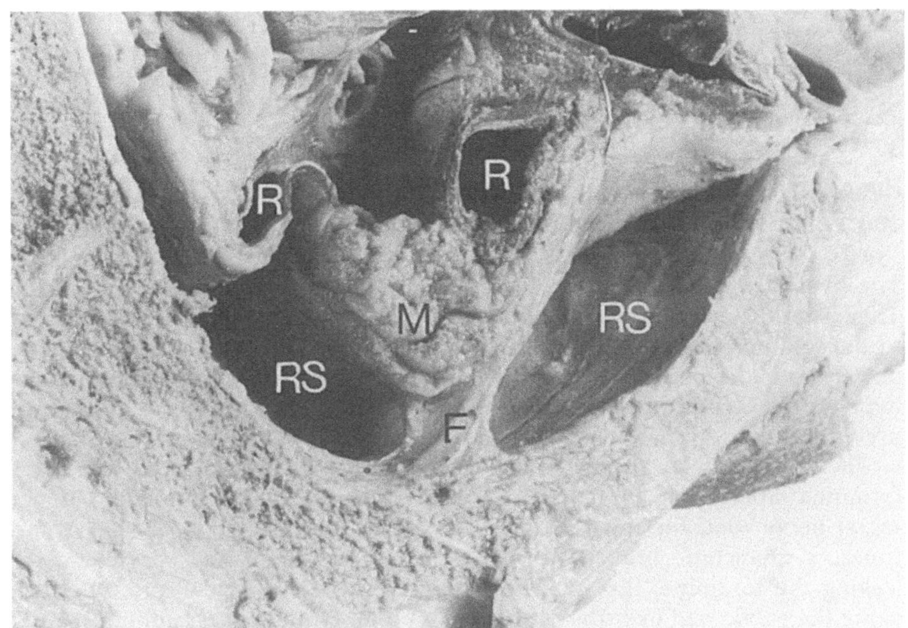

Fig. 3. Midsagittal hemisection of a male pelvis in supine position. Detail of rectosacral fascia. *RS*, retrorectal space; *F*, rectosacral fascia; *R*, rectum; *M*, mesorectum

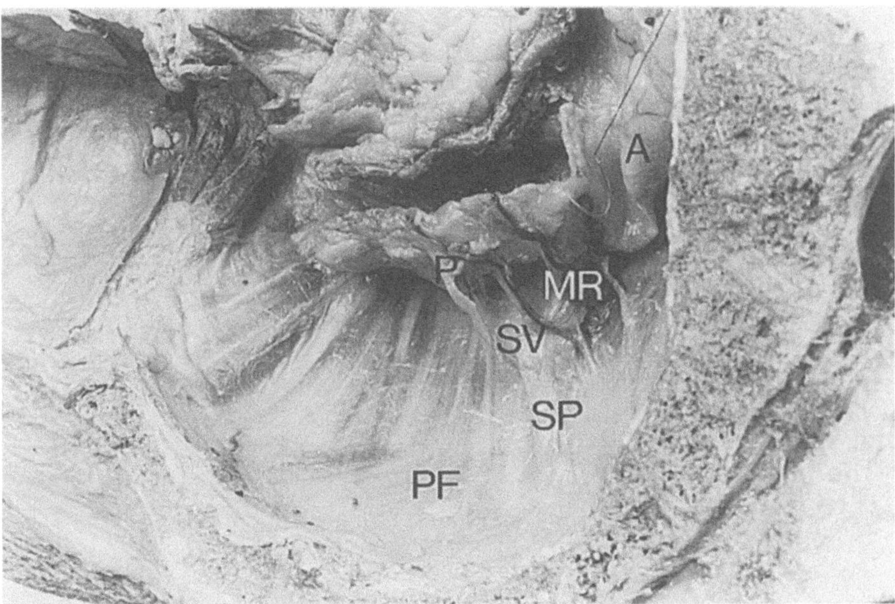

Fig. 4. Detail of the pelvic side wall. *A*, anterior leaf of visceral fascia; *P*, posterior leaf of visceral fascia; *PF*, parietal fascia, *SP*, sacral splanchnic nerve covered by parietal fascia; *SV*, sacral splanchnic nerve covered by visceral fascia; *MR*, branches of middle rectal artery and vein

[l, 7]. A functional role for the rectosacral ligament may be the anchorage of the rectum to the sacrum, preventing prolapse.

Hypogastric Nerves, Sacral Splanchnic Nerves, and Pelvic Autonomic Nerve Plexus

The hypogastric nerves are formed from the pre-aortic sympathetic plexus. They enter the pelvis at the sacral promontorium, approximately one cm lateral to the midline and two cm medial to the ureters. The hypogastric nerves lie posterior to the peritoneum and directly anterior to the visceral fascia. The hypogastric nerve continues caudal and laterally, following the course of the ureter and the internal iliac artery along the pelvic wall (Figs. 2, 5–8).

The splanchnic branches of the sacral nerves originate from the sacral foramina. Splanchnic branches are usually formed by the third and fourth sacral nerve root, the third root usually being the major contributor. Sometimes, a splanchnic branch from the second sacral nerve is present. After leaving the foramina, the splanchnic nerves run laterocaudal and anteriorly along the pelvic wall over the piriformis muscle. From the sacral foramina to a point approximately 3 cm more lateral, the splanchnic nerves are covered by the parietal fascia. To enter the visceral compartment the nerves then pierce the parietal fascia, cross the retrorectal space, and continue anteriorly to the

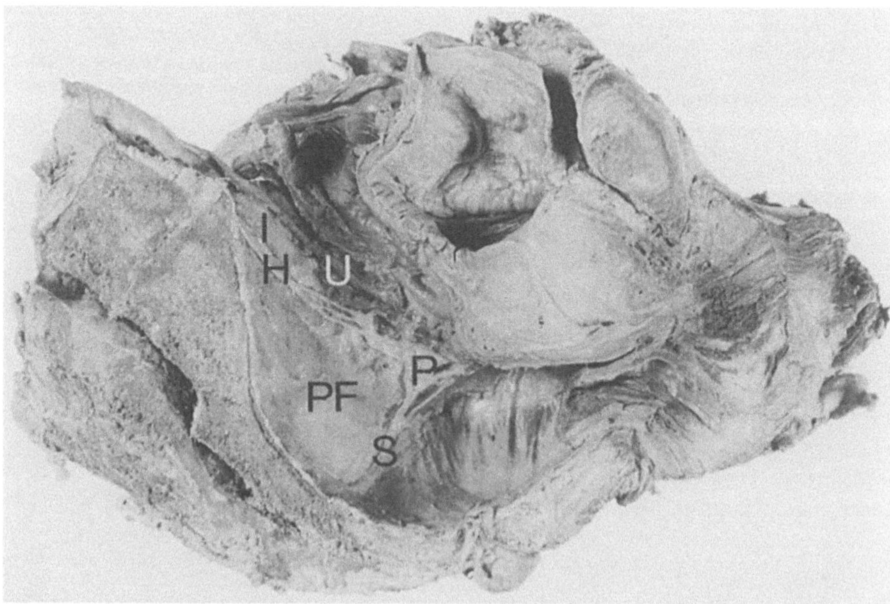

Fig. 5. Midsagittal hemisection of a male pelvis in supine position after removal of the rectum and mesorectum. *H*, hypogastric nerve; *S*, sacral splanchnic nerves; *P*, pelvic autonomic nerve plexus; *PF*, parietal fascia; *I*, internal iliac artery; *U*, ureter

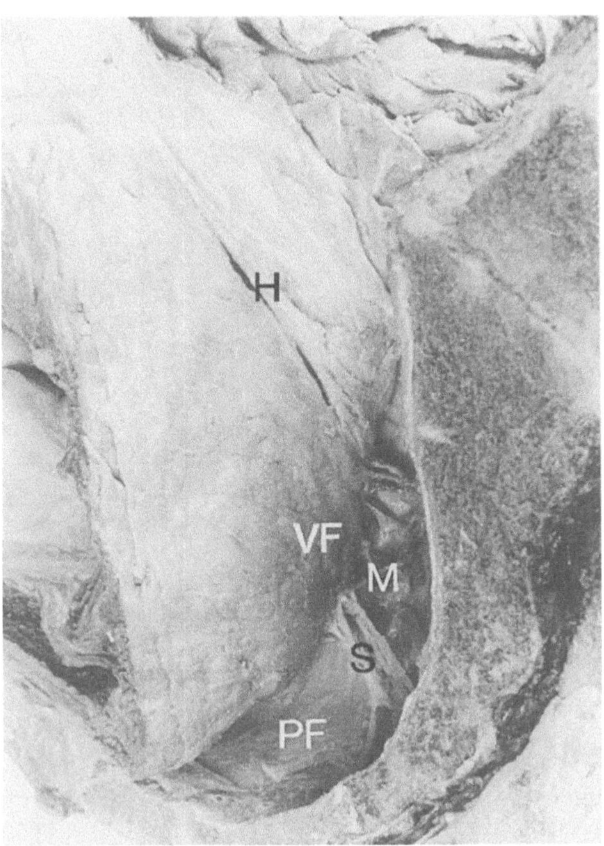

Fig. 6. Midsagittal hemisection of a male pelvis in supine position. *H*, hypogastric nerve, *S*, sacral splanchnic nerves, *M*, middle rectal vein, *VF*, visceral fascia, *PF*, parietal fascia

parietal fascia between the posterior and anterior leaves of the visceral fascia caudal to the rectosacral fascia. During the crossing of the splanchnic nerve from the parietal to the visceral compartment, the splanchnic nerves are always ensheathed by fascia. As the splanchnic nerves enter the visceral compartment, small branches from the splanchnic nerves can be identified running medially, entering the mesorectum. These branches constitute the specific parasympathetic nerve supply of the rectum. However, most fibers of the splanchnic nerve continue forward to the anterior visceral compartment, i.e., the genitourinary organs (Figs. 4, 5, 9, 10).

The hypogastric nerve and the sacral splanchnic nerves come together on the lateral pelvic wall to form the pelvic autonomic nerve plexus (Fig. 5). This plexus is a rhomboid-shaped plaque of nervous tissue. From this plexus the nerves to the genitourinary organs originate as do branches to the rectum. Just cranial from the pelvic autonomic nerve plexus branches of the middle rectal artery and vein can be identified.

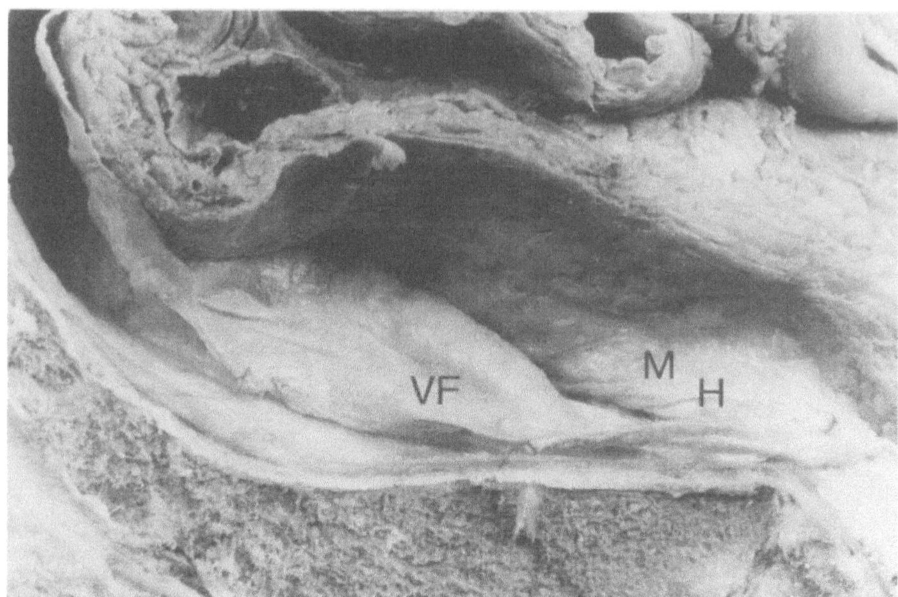

Fig. 7. Midsagittal hemisection of a male pelvis in supine position. Demonstration of the position of the hypogastric nerve (*H*) between the visceral fascia (*VF*) and the mesorectal fat (*M*)

The middle rectal artery invariably crosses the third sacral splanchnic nerve cranially. The autonomic nerves to the rectum, along with the middle rectal vessels, are embedded in fat and fibrous tissue. When the mesorectum is pulled medially, this complex of vessels and nerves forms a "ligament," extending from the pelvic wall to the mesorectum. This structure has been described as the "lateral ligament" by surgeons [2, 4, 5]. It is important to realize that the lateral ligament is merely an artifact created by surgical dissection and traction and not an anatomical structure.

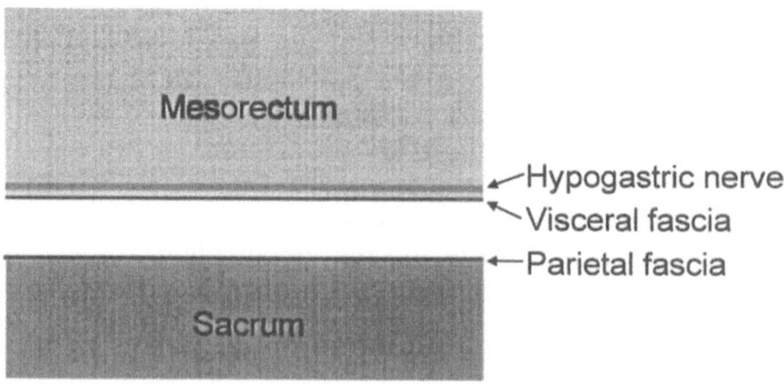

Fig. 8. The relation of the hypogastric nerve to the visceral, parietal fascia, and mesorectum

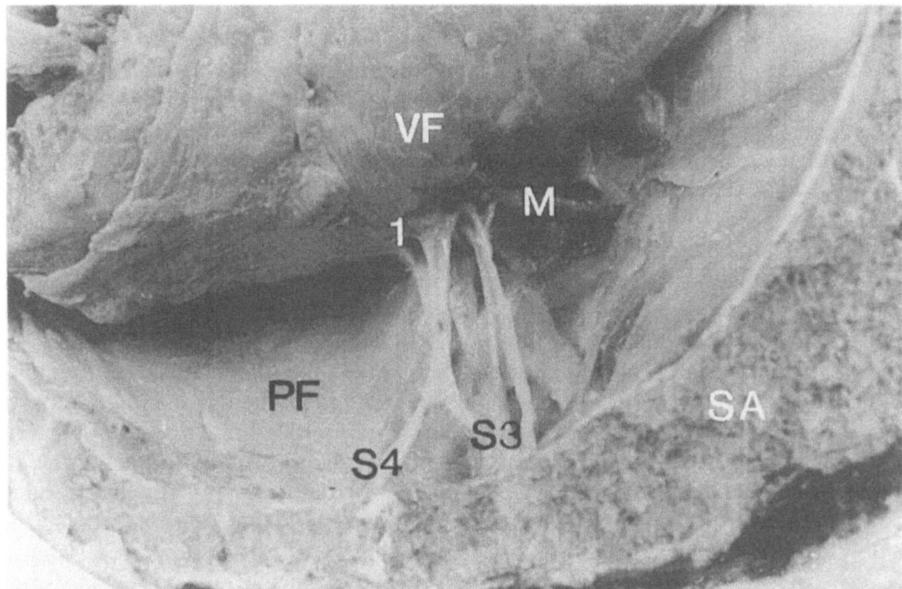

Fig. 9. Detail of the sacral splanchnic nerve, dissected from the parietal fascia. *S3*, third sacral splanchnic nerve; *S4*, fourth sacral splanchnic nerve; *1*, medial splanchnic branches (to rectum); *M*, middle rectal vein; *VF*, visceral fascia; *PF*, parietal fascia; *SA*, sacrum

Surgical Relevance

Total mesorectal excision in the surgical treatment of rectal cancer consists of removal of the intact mesorectum, the mesentery of the hindgut (see Chap. 15). Important to this operation is a bloodless, sharp dissection in the presacral plane under direct vision (see Chaps. 15, 16). Slight differences in surgical technique exist. Some choose their presacral plane between the parietal and

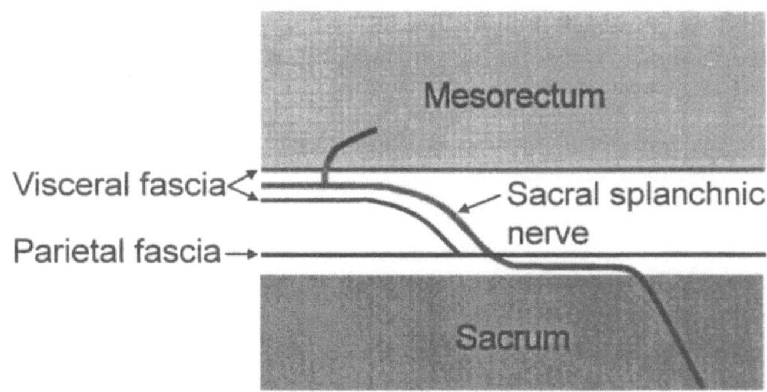

Fig. 10. The relation of the sacral splanchnic nerve to the visceral, parietal fascia and mesorectum

visceral fascia, leaving the visceral fascia on the specimen. The visceral fascia can easily be demonstrated on their specimens (see Chaps. 16, 17). Alternatively, the plane of dissection can be between the mesorectal fat and the visceral fascia, leaving the thin visceral fascia on the pelvic wall (see Chap. 15).

When the level of dissection between the visceral and parietal fascia is chosen, a step in level is neccessary when the hypogastric nerves are encountered. Medially to the hypogastric nerves, the visceral fascia will be on the specimen. Laterally to the hypogastric nerves the visceral fascia along with the hypogastric nerves will be on the pelvic wall.

The rectosacral ligament may play an important role in the outcome of surgery for rectal cancer. During conventional surgery, which is associated with blunt dissection, the rectum is traditionally mobilized by entering the hand in the presacral space. During this procedure, the rectosacral ligament will be encountered. If the rectosacral ligament is pushed bluntly, avulsion of the ligament from the sacrum may occur, causing bleeding from the presacral venous plexus. To avoid this possibility, most surgeons instinctively deviate anteriorly, unaware that the rectosacral ligament guides the dissecting hand into the mesorectum, leaving portions of the mesorectum behind, attached to the pelvic wall (Fig. 3). Quirke has shown that locally recurrent rectal cancer can be directly predicted by positive circumferential margins of the specimen [6] and the defects in the mesorectum which are associated with blunt versus sharp dissection. There is a drastic reduction in the rates of local recurrence when the mesorectum is removed completely (5%–8%) (see Chaps. 15, 16) as compared to conventional surgery (see Chap. 14).

References

1. Crapp AR, Cuthbertson AM (1974) William Waldeyer and the rectosacral fascia. Surg Gynecol Obstet 138:252–256
2. Enker WE (1992) Potency, cure, and local control in the operative treatment of rectal cancer. Arch Surg 127:1396–1402
3. Fritsch H (1990) Entwicklung der Fascia recti. Anat Anz 170:273–280
4. Goligher J (1984) Surgery of the anus, rectum and colon, 5th edn. Baillière Tindall, London
5. Huber A, von Hochstetter AH, Allgöwer M (1984) Transsphincteric surgery of the rectum. Topographical anatomy and operation technique. Springer, Berlin Heidelberg New York
6. Quirke P, Durdey P, Dixon MF, Williams NS (1986) Local recurrence of rectal adenocarcinoma due to inadequate surgical resection. Histopathological study of lateral tumour spread and surgical excision. Lancet ii:996–998
7. Waldeyer W (1899) Das Becken. Friedrich Cohen, Bonn

Tumour Spread As a Basis for Rectal Cancer Surgery

CHAPTER 11

Spread of Rectal Carcinomas

Tor J. Eide

Introduction

The sequences of spread from rectal carcinoma are determined by the biology of the tumour and the resistance of the tissue components to invasion by neoplastic cells. Rectal carcinomas show a diverse spectrum of malignant aggressiveness: from slow-growing tumour with poor ability to invade lymphatic channels or blood vessels to a disease with rapid growth and early metastasis.

The malignant potential of a tumour cannot be measured directly by any method, but the combination of gross examination and microscopy of selected histologic slides are the most reliable methods of determining the extent of local growth and estimating the risk of distant spread and prognosis. This presentation focuses on histologic features which can be identified as statistical variables and which may express the risk of spread of the tumour and thus have independent prognostic significance. This is of importance for the evaluation of new treatment modalities, whether surgery or adjuvant therapy. New molecular markers and indirect imaging techniques have recently been introduced, but meticulous morphologic evaluation is still superior to other methods in evaluating the malignant potential and extent of spread of rectal carcinomas.

Spread of Carcinoma

Continuous Spread

Rectal adenocarcinoma is first diagnosed when dysplastic glandular tissue invades the submucosal layer of the large bowel [13]. When the lesion is limited to the mucosal membrane, the proliferation of dysplastic glands is designated as an adenoma (tubular, tubulovillous, or villous) with different grades of dysplasia. We do not recommend using the term "intramucosal carcinoma" in describing large bowel neoplasms so as to reduce the risk of surgical resection of tumours at this stage, since this is generally not required. The risk of metastasis from a tumour confined to the mucosal membrane, even with severe dysplasia, is close to zero if the tumour is small (< 1 cm) and pedunculated. More care should be taken if the adenomas are large and sessile and have severe dysplasia. Multiple sections of a locally resected broad-based tumour confined to the mucosa of the rectum, including the resection margins at the base of the lesion, should be performed before the diagnosis of an adenocarcinoma can be excluded.

By the formation of highly, moderately, or poorly differentiated glands, the tumour invades through the muscularis mucosa to the submucosal layer (T1) and muscularis propria (T2) and to the mesorectal tissue (T3) [8]. A tumour is defined as being limited to the bowel wall if it extends no further than the outer edge of the muscularis propria. Untreated, the tumour will invade the serosa, the pelvic wall, and other neighbouring organs (bladder, vagina, cervix uteri) (T4).

The continuous spread is followed by a variable desmoplastic reaction of fibrous tissue which is generally first observed when the tumour infiltrates the submucosal layer. Such a reaction is rarely observed in adenomas, even with severe dysplasia. Desmoplastic fibrosis may have diagnostic importance for the confirmation of the malignant nature when the level of tumour invasion into the bowel wall cannot be properly ascertained in small biopsies of a rectal neoplasm.

Longitudinal Spread. Ulcerating carcinomas usually undermine the lateral intact mucosa by longitudinal spread, but there is generally no neoplastic tissue beyond 1–2 cm from the macroscopic tumour margins [1]. Exceptions do exist, most commonly for the very rare occurrence of signet-ring-cell carcinomas. This allow the surgeon to resect the rectum very close to the macroscopic distal edge of a rectal carcinoma ("close shave") [7]. Only with resection margins of less than 3 cm is it recommended to take a histologic section to ascertain free margins.

Invasive Margins. The invasive margin is where the tumour penetrates the bowel wall and perirectal tissue has been claimed to be of diagnostic importance [11]. Carcinomas are called "expanding" when the invasive margin is pushing or circumscribed and "infiltrating" if the tumour invades in a diffuse manner with widespread penetration of normal tissue. The diffusely infiltrating pattern is the most unfavourable feature, whereas patients with expanding tumours seem to have a better prognosis [5]. Jass [11] found that about 25% of rectal carcinomas invaded in a diffuse manner, whereas Harrison et al. [6] found a proportion of 80%. Such differences indicate severe difficulties in diagnosing the two histologic types of invasion margin, which is probably related to poor interobserver reproducibility.

Lymphatic Spread

It has been emphasized that the diagnosis of a rectal carcinoma should only be considered if the tumour infiltrates the submucosal layer [13]. One argument is related to the assumption that the lamina propria of the mucosal membrane do not contain lymphatic vessels [14] and that, biologically, a tumour confined to the mucosa cannot spread to local or regional lymph nodes. In addition, metastases from rectal tumours confined to the mucosal membrane or even infiltrating the submucosal layer are exceedingly rare [13], according to empirical observation. Dukes [3], in his original study of rectal carcinomas, did not record any tumour with lymph node metastasis if the tumours were confined to the bowel wall. However, lymphatic vessels, particularly at the lower third of the mucosal membrane, do exist and can frequently be identified by light microscopy in biopsy material in inflammatory bowel disease. Series of rectal carcinomas have demonstrated that the frequency of lymph node metastases is around 5% when the tumour invades the submucosal layer [13].

The dissection of lymph nodes is a key element for pathologists in the proper evaluation of tumour spread. The presence or abscence of lymph node involvement determine the stage of the disease and is one of the most important variables for estimating prognosis [11]. Hida and coworkers [9] found an average of 21.2 lymph nodes in the mesorectal tissue in patients with carcinoma of the rectum examined by a conventional manual method. This increased to 73.7 lymph nodes when a "clearing method" was used. The TNM staging system requires that a minimum of 12 lymph nodes be examined in a resection specimen from the colon or rectum. The necessity of detecting a high number of lymph nodes is based on the fact that a strong statistical association between the number of dissected perirectal lymph nodes and the detection rate of lymph node metastasis exists [8]. The number of positive lymph nodes with metastatic tissue is also of importance. A significant drop in survival rate between patients with 1–3 (N1) and those with more than four positive lymph nodes (N2) has repeatedly been demonstrated in several series and is thus included in the TNM staging system.

However, there is individual variation in the number of detected lymph nodes, which may be related to the patient's constitution, but also to other factors such as T stage of the tumour and preoperative radiation. In Dukes' stage A carcinomas the number of lymph nodes may be few and they may be small in size [11] and thus difficult to identify using a conventional dissection technique even in mesorectal tissue adjacent to the tumour. Such identification problems also exist in patients who have had preoperative irradiation [8]. In Dukes' stage B and C carcinomas the lymph nodes frequently display reactive hyperplasia in addition to metastatic tissue and are thus easier to find during preparation of the specimen.

Lymphatic tissue may be detected microscopically in the mesorectal tissue without any discernible lymph node structure. The capsule and the internal sinusoidal system are lacking in such lymphatic tissue. However, metastasis to these lymphatic elements may frequently occur and give rise to tumour islands in the mesorectal tissue at a distance from the main tumour margins (Fig. 1).

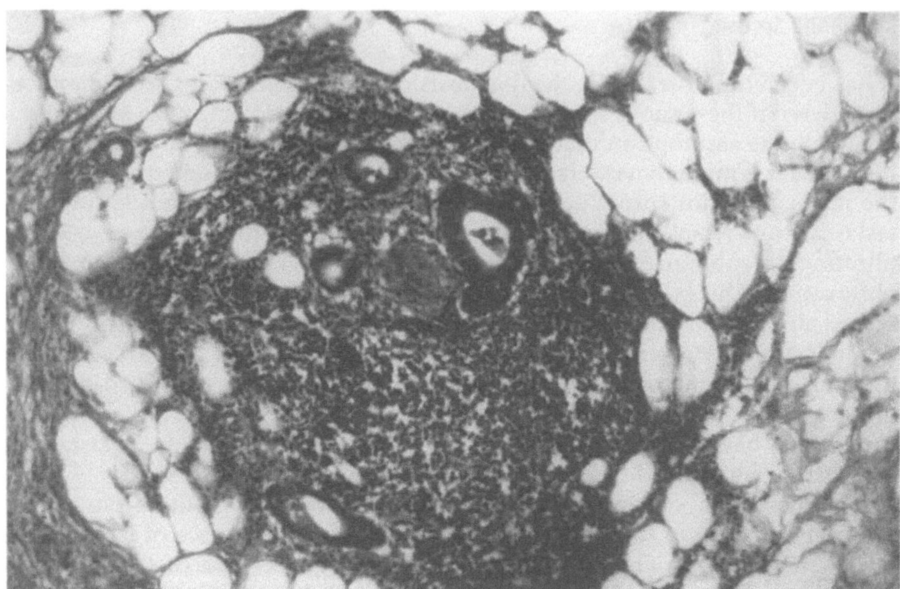

Fig. 1. "Discontinuous growth" with clusters of metastatic glands to lymphatic tissue with no lymph node structure located in the mesorectum remote from the main tumour. (H&E, 800)

These tumour satellites are defined as "discontinous growth" if they are less than 3 mm in diameter and if no lymph node structure can be identified [8]. Tumour satellites larger than 3 mm without any remnants of lymph node structure are, for practical reasons, defined as a lymph node metastases.

Apart from the presence or absence of metastasis to lymph nodes and the total number of lymph nodes involved, it may be of importance to know where the involved lymph nodes are located (adjacent or remote from the tumour). The "apical node" (N3) – the lymph node most remote from the tumour at the proximal end of the resected specimen along the vascular channel – should always be examined [11]. In addition, we prefer to devide lymph nodes into "adjacent," i.e., nodes in the mesorectal tissue within 3 cm distal and proximal from the tumour margins, and "remote" lymph nodes, which include all nodes more than 3 cm from the tumour margins. This gives the opportunity to evaluate the metastatic tumour burden at different longitudinal levels from the tumour in the mesorectal tissue.

Vascular Spread

Rectal carcinomas may infiltrate blood vessels in the bowel wall or in the mesorectal tissue. Intramural vascular infiltration, especially of thin-walled vessels in the submucosa and muscular layer may be difficult to diagnose in a tumour penetrating the bowel wall. The prognostic implication of vascular

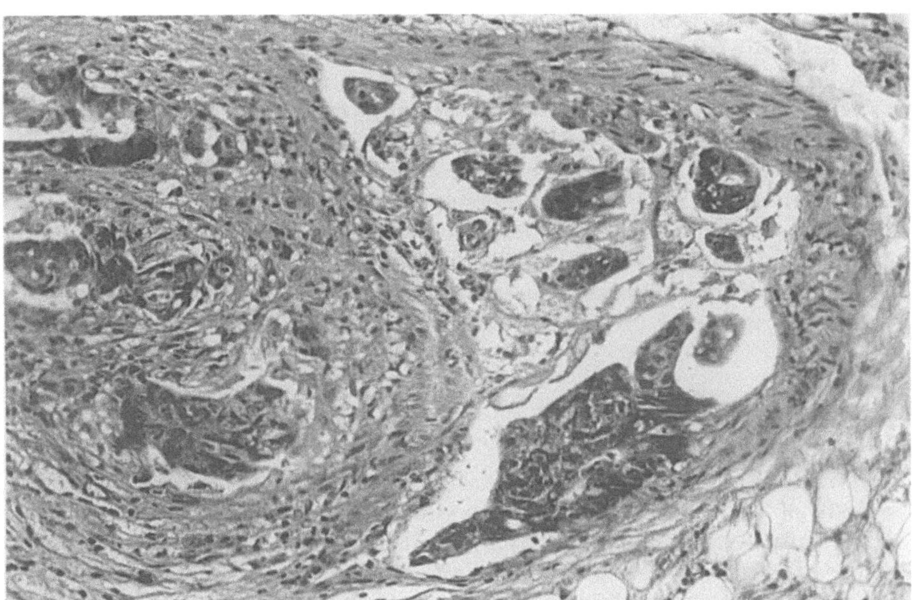

Fig. 2. A thick-walled vein with cluster of tumour cells invading the wall and also present in the vessel lumina. (H&E, 800)

infiltration in the bowel wall is not properly documented. Of more importance is infiltration of extramural vessels (Fig. 2). The presence of extramural venous invasion can be demonstrated in 10%–22% of all carcinomas of the large bowel (Table 1) and has been shown to have independent prognostic significance in

Table 1. Influence of venous invasion on survival among patients with colorectal cancer and rectal cancer

Author	Tumour localization	No of patients	Frequency of venous invasion	Statistical significance on survival	
				Univariate analyses	Multivariate analyses
Deans et al. [2]	Colon and rectum	312	10%	$p=0.02$	p=0.17
T. Eide (unpublished)	Colon and rectum	152	18%	$p < 0.001$	p < 0.01
Horn et al. [10]	Rectum	128	22%	$p < 0.0001$	p < 0.002
Harrison et al. [6]	Rectum	348	20%	$p < 0.001$	p < 0.001
Newland et al. [16]	Colon and rectum	579	19%	$p < 0.001$	p < 0.001
Shirouzu et al. [18]	Colon and rectum	376	–	$p < 0.005$	–

multivariate statistical analyses. The presence of this histologic feature correlates well with the risk of hepatic metastases. Shirouzu et al. [18] found metachronous liver metastases in about 30% of all patients with venous invasion. Efforts have been made to classify different histologic types of venous invasion and to grade the extent of the vessel infiltration [15]. It is probable that the interobserver reproducibility may be poor by the inclusion of different features of venous invasion. We therefore recommend that only the presence or absence of neoplastic cells within thick-walled veins in rectal carcinomas be reported. If doubt exists as to true venous infiltration, an elastin stain, or factor VIII immunohistochemical examination or both should be performed to confirm the nature of the luminal structure.

Perineural Spread

Tumour infiltration of the mesorectal tissue may involve nerves. Univariate analysis of perineural infiltration has shown that such a feature correlates significantly with tumour recurrence [10]. However, the typical histologic feature of perineural infiltration observed in adenoid cystic carcinomas of the salivary glands is generally not present in rectal carcinomas. The observation of clusters of tumour cells adjacent to nerves in the bowel wall and the mesorectum may be a coincidence in most of the cases and not reflect a specific biological behaviour of the tumour. Multivariate analyses have not shown perineural infiltration to be a statistically strong factor predicting survival, but may to some extent predict an increased risk of local recurrence [10, 19].

Crohn's-Like Lymphoid Reaction

Lymphocytic infiltration adjacent to the tumour margins has long been considered to be a marker of a more favourable prognosis of malignant tumours than in those cases in which no such reaction can be observed. This is also so for colorectal carcinomas. The interobserver reproducibility of the presence of lymphocytic infiltration is, however, weak [6], since there always are some lymphocytes in the bowel wall, especially if ulceration and secondary infection are present. Graham and Appelman [4] introduced the term "Crohn's like lymphocytic reaction" and this feature has been shown to have a higher degree of reproducibility [6]. The typical nodular arrangement of lymphoid tissue, often with germinal centres in the vicinity of the tumour margins, especially at the interface between the mesorectal tissue and muscularis propria (Fig. 3), could indicate a host reaction against the tumour and seems to have independent prognostic importance [6].

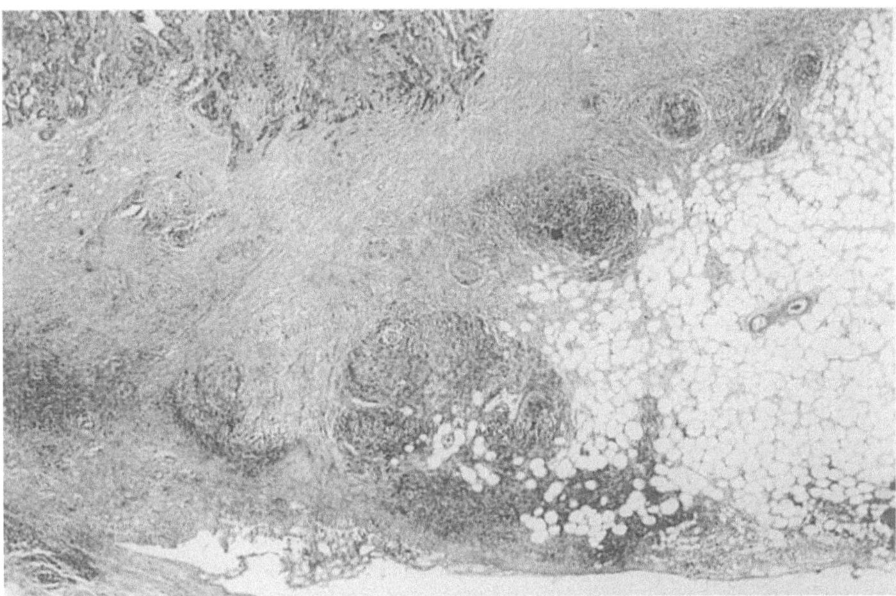

Fig. 3. Crohn's like lymphocytic reaction with lymphoid nodules in the interface between the mesorectal adipose tissue and bowel wall invaded by adenocarcinoma (*upper left corner*). (H&E, 100)

Conclusion

The gross appearance of local spread of rectal carcinomas through the bowel wall into the mesorectal tissue corresponds fairly well with the subsequent histologic evaluation in most of the cases. Therefore, a meticulous macroscopic examination of 5-mm-thick sections of the tumour with a subsequent selection of section for histologic confirmation is the method of choice for evaluating the extent of local spread of rectal carcinomas. It is particularly important to describe the spread related to the excision margin of the mesorectum [17]. The final description should always be based on histologic confirmation.

Further, it is decisive that the mesorectal tissue is meticulously dissected in order to identify an appropriate number of lymph nodes. For a standard rectal resection this should be at least 12 nodes, particularly for Dukes' stage B and C tumours. All lymph nodes adjacent to the tumour within 3 cm proximal and distal to the tumour margins should be included. Lymph nodes remote from the tumour (more than 3 cm) and the apical node should be examined separately to confirm the presence or absence of distant lymph node involvement.

Infiltration of extramural, thick-walled veins should be recorded when present and the lymphocytic infiltration close to the tumour with the appearance of Crohn's like reaction should also be included in the pathology report.

References

1. Cross SS, Bull AD, Smith JHF (1989) Is there any justification for the routine examination of bowel resection margins in colorectal adenocarcinomas? J Clin Pathol 42:1040–1042
2. Deans GT, Patterson CC, Parks TG, Spence RA, Heatley M, Moorhead RJ, Rowlands BJ (1994) Colorectal carcinoma: importance of clinical and pathological factors in survival. Ann R Coll Surg (Engl) 76:59–64
3. Dukes CE (1932) The classification of cancer of the rectum. J Pathol 35:323–332
4. Graham DM, Appelman HD (1990) Crohn's like lymphoid reaction and colorectal carcinoma: a potential histologic prognosticator. Mod Pathol 3:332–335
5. Halvorsen TB, Seim E (1989) Association between invasiveness, inflammatory reaction, desmoplasia and survival in colorectal cancer. J Clin Pathol 42:162–166
6. Harrison JC, Dean PJ, El-Zeky F, Zwaag RV (1994) From Dukes through Jass: pathological prognostic indicators in rectal cancer. Hum Pathol 25:498–505
7. Heald RJ, Karanjia ND (1992) Results of radical surgery for rectal cancer. World J Surg 16:848–857
8. Hermanek P, Henson DE, Hutter RUP, Sobin LH (1993) TNM supplement 1993. A commentary on uniform use (International Union Against Cancer). Springer, Berlin Heidelberg New York
9. Hida J, Mori N, Kubo R, Matsuda T, Morikawa E, Kitaoka M, Sindoh K, Yasutomi M (1994) Metastases from carcinoma of the colon and rectum detected in small lymph nodes by the clearing method. J Am Coll Surg 178:223–228
10. Horn A, Dahl O, Morild I (1991) Venous and neural invasion as predictors of recurrence in rectal adenocarcinoma. Dis Colon Rectum 43:798–804
11. Jass JR (1990) Prognostic factors in colorectal cancer. In: Williams GT (ed). Gastrointestinal pathology. Springer, Berlin Heidelberg New York, pp 295–322 (Current topics in pathology, vol 81)
12. Jass JR, Love SB, Northover JMA (1987) A new prognostic classification of rectal cancer. Lancet I:1303–1306
13. Jass JR, Sobin LH, In collaboration with pathologists in 9 countries (1989) Histological typing of intestinal tumors (WHO), 2nd edn. Springer, Berlin Heidelberg New York
14. Kaye GJ, Fenoglio CM, Pascal RR, Lane N (1973) Comparative electronmicroscopic features of normal, hyperplastic and adenomatous human colonic epithelium. Gastroenterology 64:926–945
15. Krasma MJ, Flancbaum L, Cody RP, Shneibaum S, Ari GB (1988) Vascular and neural invasion in colorectal carcinoma: incidence and prognostic significance. Cancer 61:1018–1023
16. Newland RC, Dent OF, Lyttle MNB, Chapuis PH, Bokey EL (1994) Pathologic determinants of survival associated with colorectal cancer with lymph node metastases. Cancer 73:2076–2082
17. Quirke P, Scott N (1992) The pathologist's role in the assessment of local recurrence in rectal carcinomas. Surg Oncol Clin North Am 1:1–17
18. Shirouzu K, Isomoto H, Kakegawa T, Morimatsu M (1991) A prospective clinicopathologic study of venous invasion in colorectal cancer. Am J Surg 162:216–222
19. Shirouzu K, Isomoto H, Kakegawa T (1993) Prognostic evaluation of perineural invasion in rectal cancer. Am J Surg 165:233–237

CHAPTER 12

Importance of Lymphatic Spread

Yoshihiro Moriya

Introduction

Spread of rectal cancer occurs via lymphatics and blood stream, by direct invasion into adjacent organs and by peritoneal seeding. The goal of surgical treatment is en bloc resection of both the primary growth and lymphatic metastasis. A comprehensive understanding of both intrapelvic lymphatics and lymph node status in patients with rectal cancer is therefore required in order to offer the patient an optimal surgical procedure.

Extramural Lymphatics of the Rectum and Anal Canal

Extramural lymphatics in the mesorectum mainly follow the blood vessels, especially the arterial system supplying the rectum and anal canal. The lymphatic distribution can be divided into three categories: (1) upward or mesenteric, (2) lateral or extramesenteric, and (3) downward (Fig. 1).

Upward Lymphatics

Upward lymphatics are the main stream in any part of the rectum and anal canal. They follow the superior rectal vessels and join the lymphatics from both

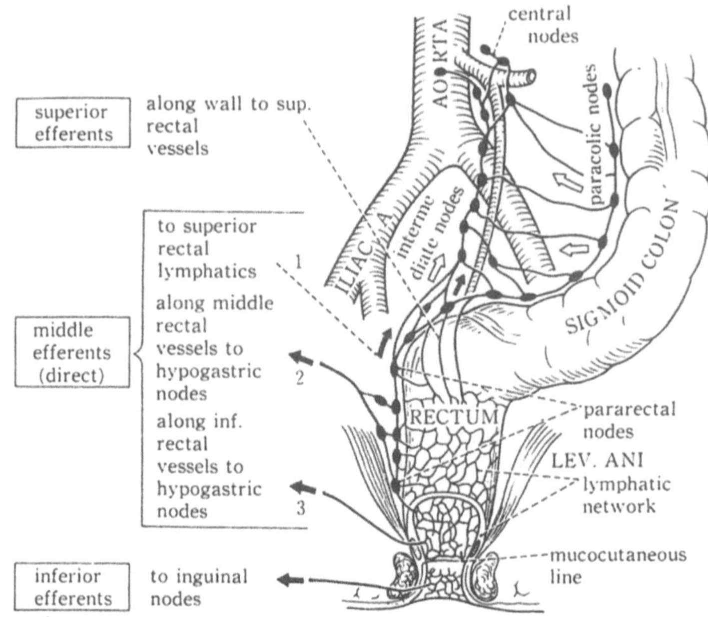

Fig. 1. Rectal lymphatic channels as outlined by Blair and coworkers [1]

the sigmoid and descending colon to drain into the inferior mesenteric nodes and then into the lumbar para-aortic lymphatic chain. Upward lymphatics also form anastomoses with the lateral and downward lymphatic vessels, as well with the lymphatics of other pelvic organs such the bladder and the genital organs.

Lateral Lymphatics

Lateral lymphatics are found along the middle rectal arteries, where they meet lymphatics along the internal iliac vessels. Together they join the lymphatics from the external iliac vessels at the bifurcation of the common iliac vessels. As absence of middle rectal arteries was observed in more than 50% of the studied cadavers [6], it is not clear that the lateral lymphatics always follow the middle rectal arteries.

It is well known that the lymphatic drainage pattern is related to the level of rectum. In other words, lymphatics from the upper or intraperitoneal rectum drain exclusively in an upward direction, while lymphatic flow from rectum at or below the peritoneal reflection can occur either laterally or in an upward direction. Lateral lymphatics in the pelvis consist of channels from pelvic organs such as the bladder, genital organs and rectum. Generally speaking, lymphatics from organs located more anteriorly in the pelvis tend to drain into a more proximal part of the internal iliac vessels. As the rectum is located in the most posterior part of the pelvic space, lateral lymphatics of the rectum drain into the distal part of the internal iliac vessels near the root of internal pudendal artery. Lymphatic vessels from the rectum extending laterally are relatively small compared with lymphatic channels from other pelvic organs such as the bladder and genital organs. The relative density of lymphatics, however, does not reduce their importance in the lymphatic spread of rectal cancer.

The history of research in lateral pelvic lymphatics may provide important information. In 1895, Gerota described the presence of lateral lymphatics for the first time. In 1925, the French researcher Villemin described the detailed lymphatic pathways in the pelvis, using the dye injection technique [7]. At that time, surgery of rectal cancer was dominated by the influence of Ernest Miles and his description of abdominoperineal resection (APR) [3]. Miles, however, had a misconception concerning the intrapelvic lymphatics (clearly demonstrated in Fig. 34 of his 1908 paper), which he believed to pass through the levator ani muscle to the bifurcation of the iliac artery. This misconception prevailed until 1950, when Blair [1] documented the three directions of lymphatic drainage from the rectum precisely in the way we describe them here.

Downward Lymphatics

Downward lymphatics drain directly into inguinal nodes. In the case of rectal adenocarcinoma, inguinal lymph node metastasis occurs when the primary lesion grows down to the anal cancer. Downward metastasis appears to be fairly infrequent in anal canal cancer and/or peri-anal skin cancer.

Concept of Lymphadenectomy

Generally speaking, primary rectal cancer is characterized by the fact that it is localized for a long time and is slow growing compared with other gastrointestinal malignancies. This localized and slow tumour growth is also quite often observed not only in lymph node metastases, but also in metastases to the liver and lung. The concept of extended lymphadenectomy is based upon such biological behaviour.

Lymph node metastasis first occurs along the lymphatic channels and follows a well-known pattern. Figure 2 shows a schematic presentation of such spread. It starts at the pararectal nodes (curve N1) and finally reaches the para-aortic nodes (curve N4). In the case of N2 metastasis, lymph node dissection performed along the limited surgical line would result in only a temporary curative resection, and the patient will most likely develop local recurrence about 1 year later. In patients with T3 rectal cancer, it is therefore our well-founded opinion that lymph node dissection should be carried out along the standard or extended line illustrated in Fig. 2.

The upward lymphatics are in the perirectal mesenteric lymphatic complex and are enclosed within the proper rectal fascia. This fascia is a strong

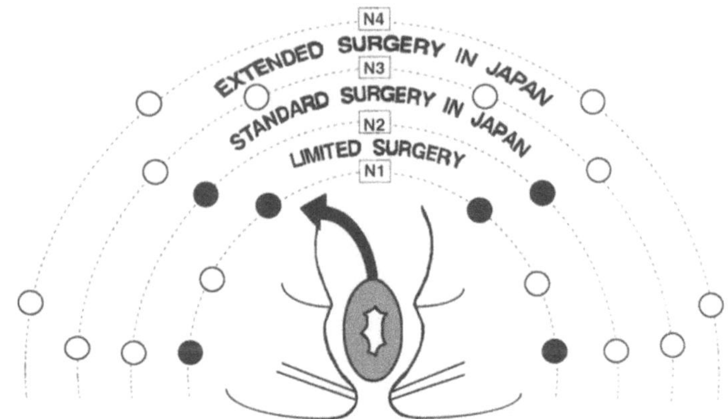

Fig. 2. Concept of lymph node dissection. *Black circles*, metastasis; *white circles*, no metastasis

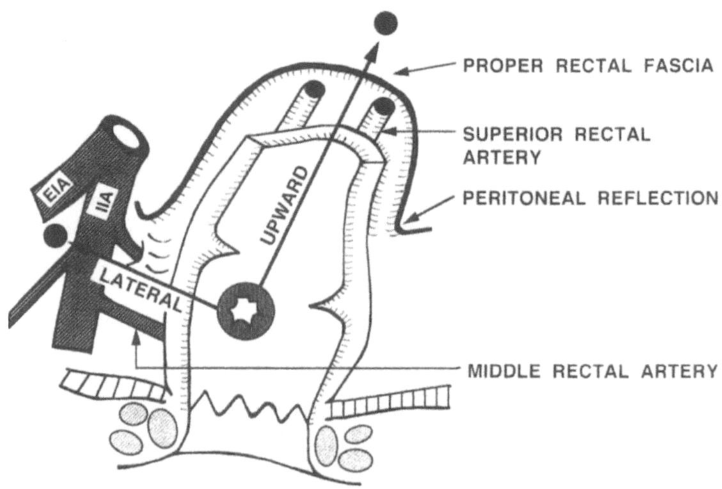

Fig. 3. Relation between upward and lateral lymphatic channels

membrane and may play a role as a barrier against cancer spread directly into extramesenteric lymphatics, such as to the internal iliac nodes. However, there is no strong membrane along the lateral lymphatic channels similar to the proper rectal fascia. Due to the surgical anatomy (Fig. 3) and the lack of a well-defined fascial covering of either the pelvic nerve plexus or the internal iliac vessels, it is more difficult to dissect lateral lymph nodes compared with upward or mesenteric lymph nodes.

Incidence of Lymph Node Metastasis According to Site and Depth of Invasion

According to the Japanese guidelines for colorectal cancer [2] (Fig. 4), regional lymph nodes for colon and rectum are identified by numbers. For example, pararectal nodes are given the number 51. This numbering is similar to that used for gastric cancer. The extent of lymphatic spread according to Japanese guidelines is classified into pararectal and/or paracolic nodes (N1 nodes), intermediate node (N2) and main node (N3) and is identical for both cancer forms. This N classification is therefore different from the N category in the TNM system; the latter combines both the number of lymph node metastases and the level of lymphatic spread (see Chap. 4).

Description of lymphatic site involvement is as follows: *upward* spread consists of pararectal (51), superior rectal (52), and inferior mesenteric lymph node (53) metastases, and *lateral spread* consists of middle rectal (62), obturator (82), internal iliac (72) and common iliac lymph node (73) metastases.

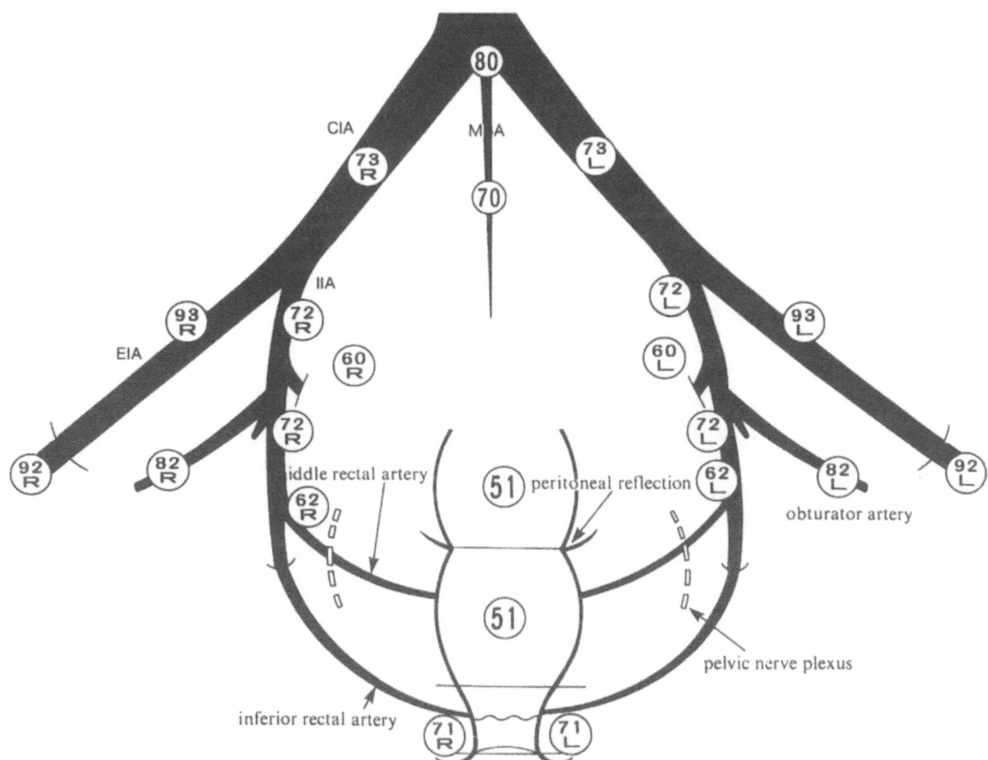

Fig. 4. Grouping map of extramesenteric or lateral lymphatics for rectal cancer, modified from guidelines for treatment of large bowel cancer in Japan [2]

Table 1. Lymph node (LN) spread in 149 patients with Dukes' C tumour and node mapping according to Japanese guidelines

Direction of LN spread	Patients	
	(*n*)	(%)
Upward alone	91	61
Upward and lateral	44	30
Lateral alone	12	8
Downward and upward	2	1
Total lateral node metastasis	56	38
Unilateral	43	29
Bilateral	13	9
Lymph node site		
Inferior mesenteric artery (site 53)	3	2
Superior rectal artery (site 52)	32	21
Pararectal (site 51)	102	67
Common iliac artery (site 73)	3	2
Internal iliac artery (site 72)	18	12
Middle rectal artery (site 62)	38	26
Obturator artery (site 82)	25	17
External iliac (site 93)	0	0

Also see Fig. 4.

The incidence of lymph node metastasis in 149 patients with Dukes' C tumour at or below the peritoneal reflection showed upward spread in 61%, and upward plus lateral spread in 30%. Lateral spread alone was seen in only 6% of patients with Dukes' C tumour at or below the peritoneal reflection. Needless to say, the most commonly affected site in upward direction were the pararectal lymph nodes (lymph node site 51; 67%), followed by the superior rectal lymph nodes (lymph node site 52; 21%).

To simplify the matter, there were two distinct categories: the incidence of upward spread was 91%, and lateral spread 38%. Frequently affected lateral lymph node sites were the middle rectal (lymph node site 62; 26%) and obturator nodes (lymph node site 82; 17%). The incidence of common iliac and external iliac node metastases, however, was low in patients operated on with curative intent (Table 1).

A further analysis was undertaken to elucidate the relation between depth of wall invasion and the incidence of lateral spread. The incidence of lateral metastasis was nearly 15% in patients with lower rectal cancer. In those with cancer invasion of the proper muscle layer, the overall rate of lateral spread was 12%, increasing to 37% in patients with Dukes' C cancer invading the proper muscle layer (Table 2). On the basis of these node findings, we recommend that a wide intrapelvic lymphadenectomy should be added, in contrast to the practice of a more limited node dissection and more localized excision often seen in Western hospitals.

Retrograde lymphatic spread is reported, and in patients with massive lymphatic infiltration, retrograde spread is a real possibility. However, retro-

Table 2. Rate of lateral lymph node (LN) metastasis according to depth of invasion

Depth	Total patient population			Patients with Dukes' C tumour		
	Total	Lateral LN spread		Total	Lateral LN spread	
	(n)	(n)	(%)	(n)	(n)	(%)
Proper muscle	59	7	12	19	7	37
Beyond muscle layer	80	7	9	36	7	19
Through rectal wall	134	35	26	80	35	43
Invasion into neighbouring organ	24	7	29	14	7	50
Total	297	56	19	149	56	38

grade lymphatic spread in patients undergoing resection with curative intent is quite rare, and in these patients a distal surgical margin of 2 or 3 cm will suffice.

A case history will demonstrate the importance of lateral dissection. A 44-year-old woman was admitted with a 2-month history of difficulties in defaecation. A rectal carcinoma was found in the lower rectum down to the anal canal. A vaginal examination revealed a recto-vaginal fistula in the posterior wall of the vagina. Preoperative computed tomography (CT) and magnetic resonance imaging (MRI) demonstrated a circular rectal cancer with enlarged lymph nodes in the obturator space (Fig. 5). Endorectal ultrasonography showed multiple nodes in the mesorectum. On the basis of these findings at imaging, a Miles-type resection (APR) was performed combined with resection of the internal female genitalia. An extended lateral lymph node dissection on the right side and partial preservation of the pelvic nerves on the left side were also performed. The patient received no adjuvant therapy after surgery. Histologically, the lesion was a signet-ring cell carcinoma. Nodal metastasis was

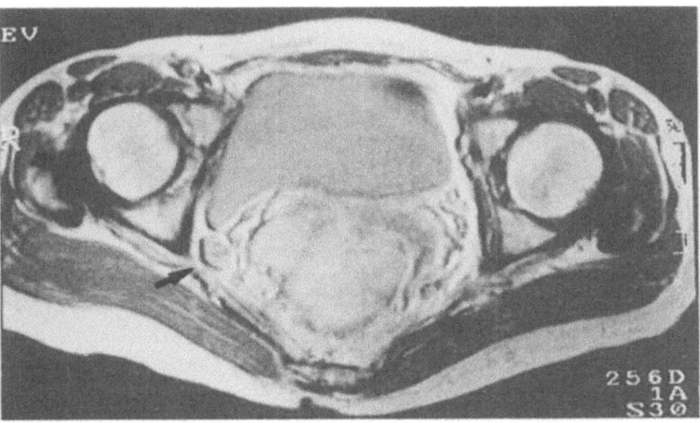

Fig. 5. Magnetic resonance imaging (MRI) of a patient with rectal cancer. The *black arrow* points to lymph node metastasis in the right obturator space

diagnosed in four out of 64 nodes, with one positive node in the right obturator space (Fig. 6). The patient has regained her health and is still alive after 5 years without recurrence.

Indication for Lymph Node Dissection
Based on the Extent of Primary Growth

As there is a close correlation between the extent of lymphadenectomy and the risk of denervation of the autonomic nervous system, the surgical procedures undertaken can be classified into four types [5]:

1. Limited surgery with total autonomic nerve preservation
2. Standard surgery with complete preservation of pelvic nerves
3. Extended surgery with partial preservation of pelvic nerves and lateral dissection
4. Extended surgery without autonomic nerve preservation

Based on our extensive experience and documentation, procedure 1 should be used in patients with Dukes' A tumour, procedure 2 in patients with Dukes' B lesion, procedure 3 in patients with Dukes' C tumour and procedure 4 in patients with suspected or definite metastasis in the lateral lymphatic nodes. The final selection of operative approach should be based on combined findings obtained from endorectal ultrasonography, CT scan, MRI and intra-operative palpation of the mesorectum. Owing to the progress of pelvic imaging, especially using endorectal ultrasonography, the extent of the primary growth (depth of invasion and lymph node metastasis in the mesorectum) can be ascertained with an accuracy up to 83% and 74%, respectively. In diagnosing lateral lymph node metastasis prospectively, however, there are still unsolved problems, particularly in how to detect nodes less than 1 cm in size.

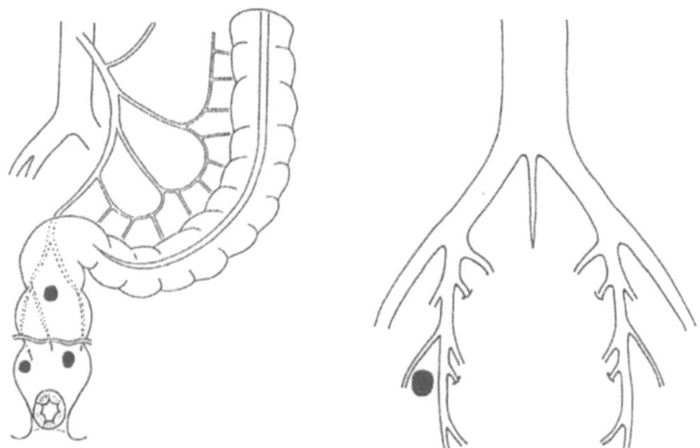

Fig. 6. Sites of four lymph node metastases (see text for details)

Technique of Lymphadenectomy Emphasizing Lateral Dissection

Upward Dissection

In procedures 2–4, para-aortic and paracaval lymphatic tissues from the level of the left renal vein to their bifurcation are completely removed along the adventitial layers of the inferior vena cava and abdominal aorta (Fig. 7). In procedure 1, in which sympathetic nerves are preserved, upward dissection is carried up to the root of the inferior mesenteric artery (Fig. 8).

Lateral Dissection

After the anterior and posterior aspects of the rectum have been mobilized from the adjacent organs, dissection along the internal iliac artery and vein are carried out in procedures 2 and 3. First of all, the internal iliac vessels are exposed and dissected from the common iliac vessels to uncover, if possible, the root of the middle rectal artery and the middle rectal vein. A meticulously sharp cut of the fascia on the piriform muscle can expose not only the recto-sacral fascia posterior to the internal iliac vein, but also the roots of the S3 and S4 pelvic nerves close to these structures. The middle rectal vessels are ligated and divided at their root. After complete mobilization of the lateral aspect of the rectum, the lateral vesical and obturator spaces are opened between the internal iliac vessels and the pelvic side wall, and clearance of lateral lymphatic tissue in these spaces is carried out while preserving the obturator nerve and

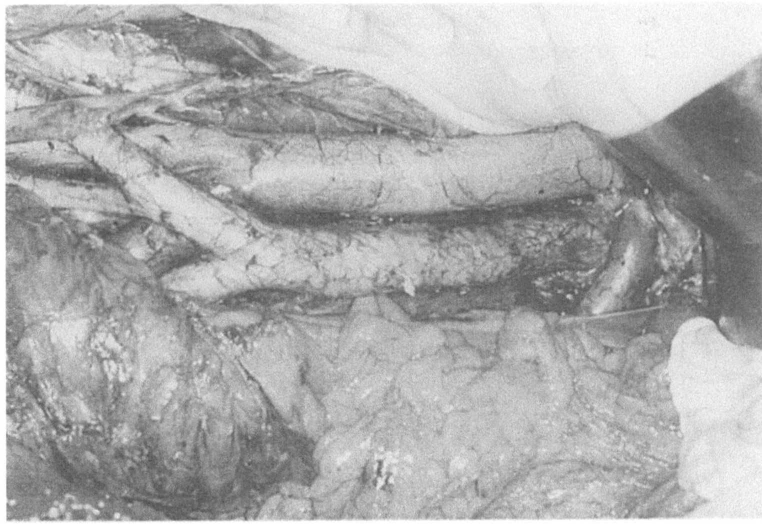

Fig. 7. Upward dissection in procedure 2–4 (see text). Sympathetic nerve fibers are completely resected

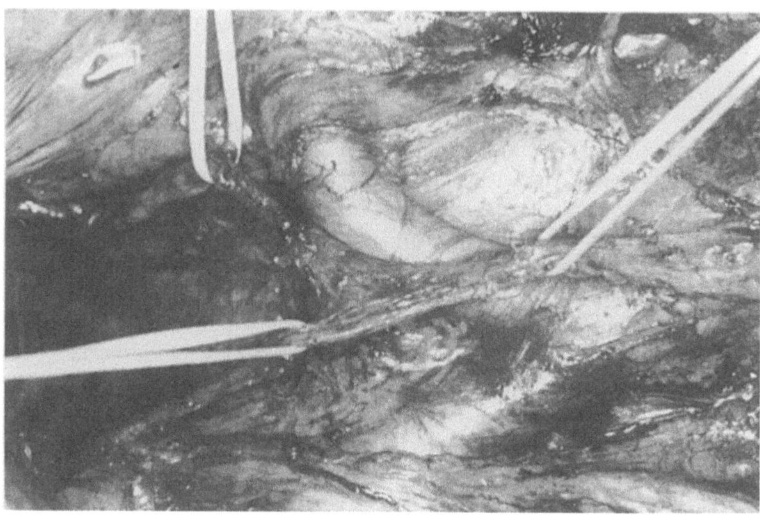

Fig. 8. Upward dissection in procedure 1. The superior sympathetic plexus and paired hypogastric nerves are preserved and demonstrated

vessels and the visceral and parietal branches of the internal iliac vessels, such as the superior gluteal and the pudendal vessels (Fig. 9). In cases where there are metastatic nodes or if metastases are suspected along the internal iliac vessels, in particular around the middle rectal artery (lymph node site 62) and in the obturator spaces (lymph node site 82), en bloc excision of the internal iliac vessels (both artery and vein) must be performed, preserving the superior

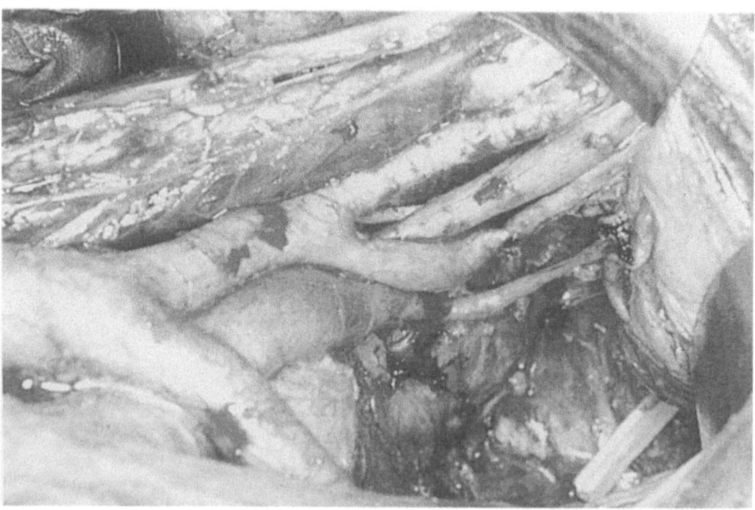

Fig. 9. Completed lateral node dissection without preservation of autonomic nerves

vesical artery and obturator nerve. This type of dissection is called extended lateral dissection [4].

Perineal Phase

After the rectum has been completely mobilized, it is attached to the pelvic wall only by the levator ani muscles and the anal canal. In patients with distal rectal cancer, the problem is whether to perform an APR or a sphincter-saving procedure. The final decision is made in the light of tumour site, histological type and node status. During a Miles-type APR, the perineal procedure consists of wide peri-anal skin resection and clearance of ischio-rectal adipose tissues and levator ani muscles from their attachment to the pelvic wall.

Survival After Extended Lymphadenectomy

The disease-free 5-year survival rate was analysed in 147 patients with Dukes' C tumour who had undergone lateral lymph node dissection for low rectal cancer according to direction of spread (Fig. 10). The 5-year survival rate was 54% in patients who had only upward lymph node spread. A similar survival rate (58%) was obtained in patients with only lateral lymph node spread. However, the disease-free survival rate was relatively poor in patients with spread in two directions (upward plus lateral). Consequently, two-directional spread offers important prognostic information.

Furthermore, survival rates were analysed according to the mode of lateral spread (uni- versus bilateral; Fig. 11). The overall survival rate was 41% in patients who had lateral node metastasis (including any combination of di-

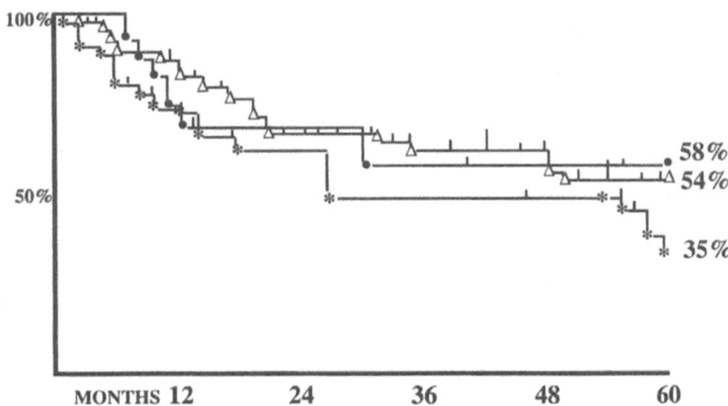

Fig. 10. Disease-free survival rate in 147 patients with Dukes' C tumour according to direction of spread. *Black circles*, lateral alone (*n*=12); *triangles*, upward alone (*n*=91); *asterisks*, upward and lateral (*n*=44)

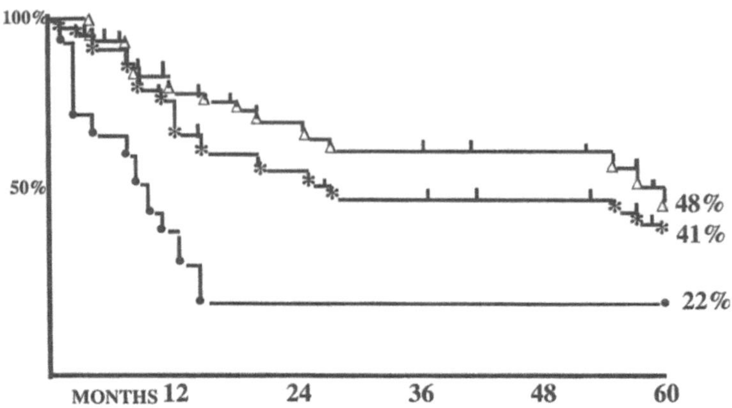

Fig. 11. Disease-free survival rate in patients with lateral node metastasis. *Triangles*, unilateral (*n*=43); *asterisks*, overall lateral (*n*=56); *black circles*, bilateral (*n*=13). *p*<0.01

rection spread). The disease-free 5-year survival rate was significantly better in patients with unilateral than in those with bilateral lateral node metastases (48% versus 22%, respectively).

Extended lymphadenectomy offers the potential to improve survival rates in patients with rectal cancer and lymph node metastasis. However, survival rates in patients with two-directional spread or bilateral lateral node metastases are still poor. Consequently, adjuvant chemo-radiotherapy should be offered to patients with local extension of primary growth.

References

1. Blair JB, Holyoke DA, Best RR (1950) A note on the lymphatics of the middle and lower rectum and anus. Anat Rec 108:635–644
2. Jinnai D (1983) General rules for clinical and pathological studies on cancer of the colon, rectum and anus. Jpn J Surg 13:557–598
3. Miles E (1908) A method of performing abdominoperineal excision for carcinoma of the rectum and of the terminal portion of the pelvic colon. Lancet II:1812–1813
4. Moriya Y, Hojo K, Sawada T, Koyama Y (1989) Significance of lateral node dissection for advanced rectal carcinoma at or below the peritoneal reflection. Dis Colon Rectum 32:307–315
5. Moriya Y, Sugihara K, Akasu T, Fujita S (1995) Nerve-sparing surgery with lateral node dissection for advanced lower rectal cancer. Eur J Cancer 31A:1229–1232
6. Sato K, Sato T (1991) The vascular and neuronal composition of the lateral ligament of the rectum and the rectosacral fascia. Surg Radiol Anat 13:17–22
7. Villemin F, Huard P, Montagne M (1925) Recherches anatomiques sur les lymphatiques du rectum et de l'anus. Rev Chir 63:39–80

The Lymphatic Spread of Rectal Cancer and the Effect of Dissection: Japanese Contribution and Experience

Takashi Takahashi, Masashi Ueno, Kaoru Azekura, and Hirotoshi Ota

Introduction

The History of Rectal Cancer Surgery

The history of modern rectal cancer surgery, which started with Kraske in 1885, can be divided into four periods, each initiated by an epoch-making proposal of a specific surgical procedure addressing a particular clinical issue. Kraske and Quenu argued for sacral or perineal approach to the primary tumor, but how to approach a higher located rectal tumor was still discussed and was undergoing research.

In 1908, Miles [1] described the abdominoperineal resection (APR) as a radical procedure for rectal cancer. He suggested furthermore that lymph node dissection played an important role in curing cancer. Discussion centered now on the extent to which lymph node dissection should be carried out.

Just as consensus formed that there were no other radical operations for rectal cancer apart from APR, Dixon [2] proposed the alternative of anterior resection which not only cured cancer, but also preserved the anal sphincter. Later, several sphincter-preserving procedures were designed and used.

The fourth period started in the early 1980s, when we in Japan started devising an autonomic nerve-preserving procedure with the intention of preserving intrapelvic organ functions.

Rectal Cancer Surgery in Japan

The history of rectal cancer surgery in Japan goes back to Dr. Yoshikiyo Senba, a Japanese surgeon and anatomist, who investigated lymphatic drainage of the rectum in 200 fetuses. He published his findings and conclusions in 1927 making special reference to their clinical importance [3] (Fig. 1). In 1940, Dr. Masaru Kuru reported his results on the clinical use of Senba's research and stressed the importance of lateral lymph node dissection and high ligation of the inferior mesenteric artery in radical surgery [4]. His successor, Dr. Tamaki Kajitani, clarified the well-defined dissecting planes around the rectum in accordance with the anatomy of lymphatics [5]. Currently, the nerve-preserving procedure is the preferred treatment option for rectal cancer surgery nationwide in Japan.

As outlined above, the development of surgical procedures in Japan has followed a different route from that taken in the West. The history of rectal cancer surgery in Japan also started with the sacral excision. Soon after, abdominoperineal amputation became the standard operative procedure. As a consequence of Senba's and Kuru's investigations, lateral dissection (clearance of lymph nodes around the internal iliac artery and in the obturator space) and high ligation of the vascular pedicle were added to rectal amputation.

Even after sphincter-preserving procedures became standard in radical surgery, the latter two technical steps were considered to be necessary if cure of a rectal cancer should be the goal of treatment. Then, autonomic nerve pre-

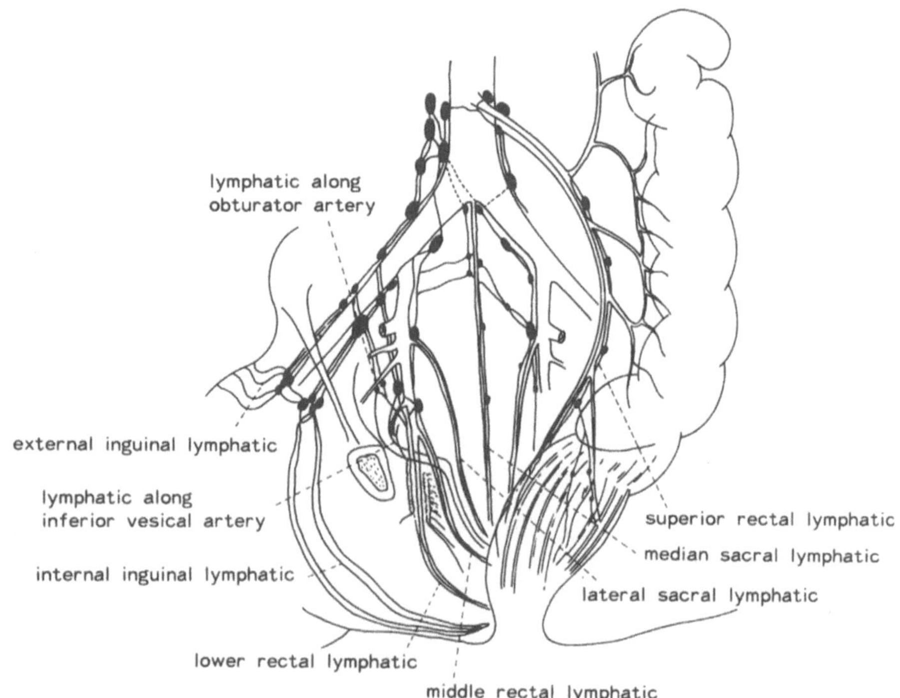

Fig. 1. Lymphatic pathway of the rectum. Original drawing by Yoshikiyo Senba (1927) with modifications

servation (ANP) was introduced as another possible option for rectal cancer surgery in around 1980 (Fig. 2).

Determining Factors for Improvements

Four factors led to improvements in rectal cancer surgery in Japan:

- There has always been a tendency toward extending the areas of dissection;
- The primary objective of surgery is to develop a procedure which can cure 100% of all patients;
- There has been little consideration given to operative morbidity and quality of life after surgery; and
- Neither time nor money is spared to achieve cure.

The only important issue was the balance between the proposed largest extent of dissection and the mortality rate. Morbidity, quality of life, and cost benefit were not seen as particularly relevant. Such considerations are based on two concepts in the Japanese way of thinking:

- People exist for the community, usually for their family, not for themselves. They are not afraid of losing nonessential body functions;
- Recovering from illness is the deepest concern in people's lives; not only for themselves but also for their family or relatives. They easily give up all money, assets, and time for that goal.

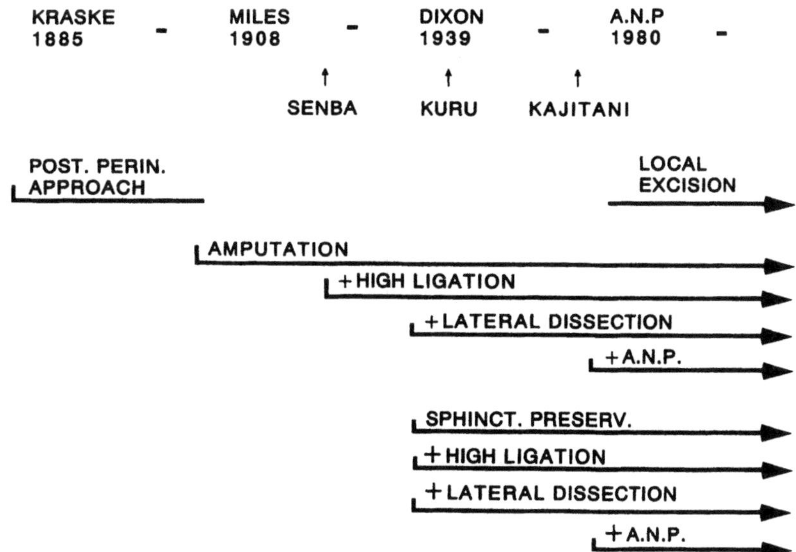

Fig. 2. Historical milestones in the development of surgery for rectal cancer (*ANP*, autonomic nerve preservation)

It can be said that the trend toward larger dissections in cancer surgery in Japan reflects a trend in clinical experimentation as a whole. Larger dissections give us the benefit of analyzing:

- Spread of rectal cancer, i.e., the main risk factor affecting the patient's outcome after a surgical procedure;
- Types of morbidity, commonly postoperative dysfunctions of intrapelvic organs with reference to clinical anatomy.

These analyses can be done on the basis of data from patients operated on in a uniform and standardized way with the maximum amount of dissection. Consequently, we can discuss and set up precise indications for several types of dissection.

Personal Experience

Lymphatic spread of rectal cancer was analyzed retrospectively on the basis of data from 1136 curative rectal resections in the period 1950–1989 at the Cancer Institute Hospital, Tokyo. The modes of upward and lateral lymphatic flow are analyzed separately, and a correlation between the two is made with special reference to the incidence of metastases and the effect of nodal dissection. Then, dissecting planes around the rectum are discussed related to the lymph node dissection procedure, as is the rationale for attending to a particular dissecting plane. Finally, results after surgery are given in two groups of patients, those treated before and after the introduction of ANP. This has been done to document the appropriateness of dissecting in defined tissue planes and the efficacy of ANP by analyzing 5-year survival rates for each type of dissection, the sites and rates of tumor recurrence after surgery, and sexual dysfunction after surgery in male patients.

Lymphatic Spread of Rectal Cancer

General State

From the rectum, the lymphatics drain in three directions; upward along the inferior mesenteric artery to the origin from the aorta; laterally along the internal iliac artery and inside the obturator space; and downward to the inguinal nodes. The direction of the lymphatic flow is related to the level in the rectum. Therefore tumor location (defined as level of the lower tumor margin) is categorized as Rs (rectosigmoid; 12–15 cm above dentate line, DL), Ra (upper rectum; 6–12 cm above DL), Rb (lower rectum; 1–6 cm above DL), and P (anal canal; less than 1 cm from DL). Each location has almost the same incidence of nodal involvement in the three directions of lymphatic flow (Table 1). The rate of nodal metastases in upward dissection was independent of level of tumor. We can therefore conclude that upward lymphatic flow has an uniform collecting basin in the entire rectum. For lateral flow, the Rb and

Table 1. Lymphatic spread of rectal cancer related to tumor location

Lower margin of tumor	Number of patients	Cases of node +ve		Upward node +ve[a]		Lateral node +ve[b]		Downward node +ve	
		n	%	n	%	n	%	n	%
Rs	26	11	42.3	11	42.3				
Ra	355	148	41.6	148	41.6	11	3.1		
Rb	561	257	45.8	251	44.7	70	12.5		
p	194	97	50	93	47.9	44	22.6	20	10.3
All	1136	513	45.1	503	44.2	125	11	20	0.7

Data based on findings in 1136 patients undergoing a curative rectal resection in the period 1950–1988.
Rs, location at 12–15 cm from dentate line; Ra, 6–12 cm from dentate line; Rb, 1–6 cm from dentate line; P, anal canal < 1 cm from dentate line.
[a]Pararectal, intermediate and main node(s).
[b]Internal iliac and obturator node(s).

the P groups have a high incidence of involvement in contrast with very low, almost negligible rates for tumors at Ra and Rs. Lateral lymphatic flow therefore has its collecting area exclusively in the lower rectum and anal canal. The data also suggest that the lower the level of the tumor, the more important the lateral flow.

Upward Spread

In the Japanese staging system of lymph node metastases, there are three grades of upward lymphatic spread determined by the anatomic site of the lymph nodes involved. These are N1 (lymph nodes along the superior rectal artery or anorectal nodes of Gerota; pararectal), N2 (lymph nodes along the main trunk of the inferior mesenteric artery; intermediate), and N3 (lymph nodes around the origin of the inferior mesenteric artery; main).

The incidence of involvement for each N stage and the crude 5-year survival rates for patients with nodal involvement are shown in Table 2. N1-positive patients have a high survival rate of 54.6%, and N2-positive patients also have a high survival rate of 41.7%. Even for N3 positive patients, we can expect that 13.6% of the patients will survive for more than 5 years.

Lateral Spread

There are also three stages of lateral lymphatic spread, namely, N1 (lymph nodes along the superior rectal artery; same as for upward spread); N2 (lymph nodes along the internal iliac artery); and N3 (lymph nodes inside the obturator space).

The incidence of and crude 5-year survival rates for N1-positive lateral spread are quite the same as for N1-positive upward spread as the N1 stage

Table 2. Lymphatic spread of rectal cancer: upward spread

	Anatomic site		
	Pararectal (anorectal)	Intermediate	Main
Japanese lymph node stage (N stage)	N1	N2	N3
Incidence of node +ve (%; n)	22.8 (260/1136)	17.5 (199/1136)	3.8 (44/1136)
5-Year survival rate of node +ve patients (%; n)	54.6 (142/260)	41.7 (83/199)	13.6 (6/44)

Data based on findings in 1136 patients undergoing a curative rectal resection in the period 1950–1988.

designates the same lymph nodes. The incidence of N2-positive and N3-positive involvement is almost the same. On the other hand, the 5-year survival rate for N2-positive patients is significantly higher than that for N3-positive patients (Table 3).

Relation Between Upward and Lateral Spread

The combination of lateral with upward spread was analyzed in 755 patients with Rb and P level cancer. As already discussed, these cancers tend to spread laterally to the iliac and obturator nodes as well as upwards along the inferior mesenteric artery.

N1 nodes are common in both directions of spread, showing a 25.5% node-positive rate and a 52.3% 5-year survival rate in these patients. The incidence of N2-positive lateral nodes is lower than that of N2-positive upward nodes, although the 5-year survival rate for N2-positive patients is quite similar (Fig. 3). For N3 nodes, the incidence of lymph node involvement and 5-year

Table 3. Lymphatic spread of rectal cancer: lateral spread

	Anatomic site		
	Pararectal (anorectal)	Internal iliac	Obturator space
Japanese lymph node stage (N stage)	N1	N2	N3
Incidence of node +ve (%; n)	22.8 (260/1136)	5.7 (65/1136)	5.2 (60/1136)
5-Year survival rate of node +ve patients (%; n)	54.6% (142/260)	41.5 (27/65)	18.3 (11/60)

Data based on findings in 1136 patients undergoing a curative rectal resection in the period 1950–1988.

survival rate of involved patients are almost equal. On the basis of these figures, we can make two conclusions related to the clinical importance of lymph node dissection for rectal cancer:

- The lateral and upward spread of Rb and P rectal cancers are equally prevalent.
- The staging system is reasonable and corresponds for both directions.

Analysis of Lateral Node Involvement

In order to analyze the mode of lateral spread further, the incidence of positive nodes was calculated for relevant tumor variables. First, tumors were categorized by the depth of invasion (Table 4). The deeper the tumor invades, the higher the incidence of lateral node involvement. For tumors with penetration of the bowel wall (A1 or A2 invasion), lateral node metastases rate was 17.4%. Ten out of 114 patients (8.8%) in this series showed metastatic nodes limited to the lateral flow only.

Next, the patients were analyzed by level of the lower margin of tumor. The incidence of lateral node involvement increases the lower the tumor is located. For tumors located less than 3 cm above the dentate line, the rate of positive lateral nodes is 13.8% or more (Table 5).

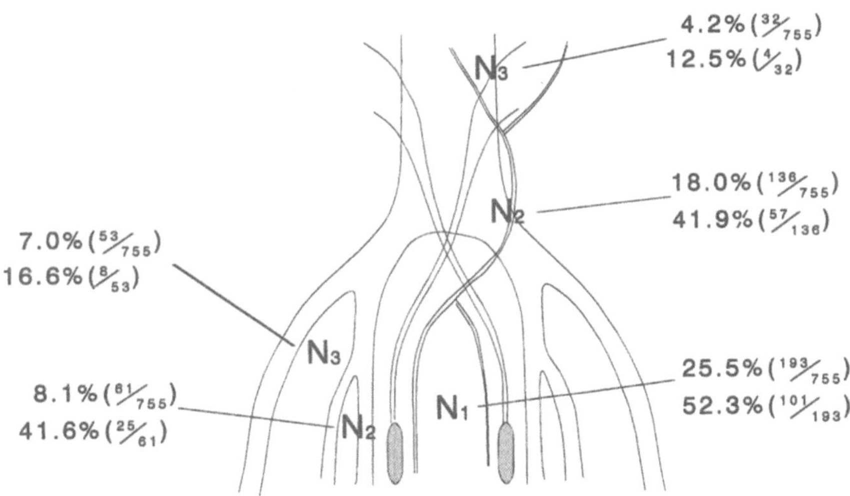

Fig. 3. Lymphatic spread of rectal cancer. Comparison between upward and lateral spread in 755 patients with lower margin of tumor at Rb (1–6 cm above dentate line) or P (< 1 cm from dentate line). First figure gives incidence of node positive patients, second figure 5-year survival rate

Table 4. Analysis of lateral spread: depth of tumor invasion

Depth of invasion	Number of patients	Number of node +ve patients	
		n	%
SM	41	1	2.4
MP	185	14	7.5
A1	222	36	16.2
A2	255	46	18
Ai	52	17	32.6
All	755	114	15

Incidence of involved iliac and/or obturator nodes according to the depth of invasion of the tumor in 755 patients with lower margin of tumor at Rb (1–6 cm from dentate line) or P (anal canal < 1 cm from dentate line). SM, Submucosa; MP, muscularis propria; A1, reached adventitia; A2, exposed on adventitia; A3, invasion of organ.

Table 5. Analysis of lateral spread: level of lower tumor margin

Level of lower margin (distance from dentate line)	Number of patients	Node +ve	
		n	%
5.1–6.0	122	10	8.1
4.1–5.0	132	13	9.8
3.1–4.0	123	17	13.8
2.1–3.0	88	14	15.9
1.1–2.0	96	16	16.6
0–1.0	194	44	22.6
All	755	114	15

Incidence of involved iliac and/or obturator nodes according to level of lower tumor margin in 755 patients with lower margin of tumor at Rb (1–6 cm from dentate line) or P (anal canal < 1 cm from dentate line).

Dissection Strategy

Dissecting Planes Around the Rectum and Extent of Nodal Dissection

The correct dissecting plane around the tumor is carefully attended to during the operation, not only to obtain a safe margin around the tumor but also to carry out appropriate lymph node dissection. The dissecting plane is, therefore, clearly linked to the extent of lymph node dissection. The dissecting plane followed for an operation will automatically define the grade of lymph node dissection for that operation.

Figure 4 is a transectional schematic drawing of the pelvis at the level of midrectum. The rectum is located in the center and is surrounded by three "ellipses", with three natural, anatomic spaces between them. There are two anatomic landmarks in the border of the spaces, namely, the pelvic nerve

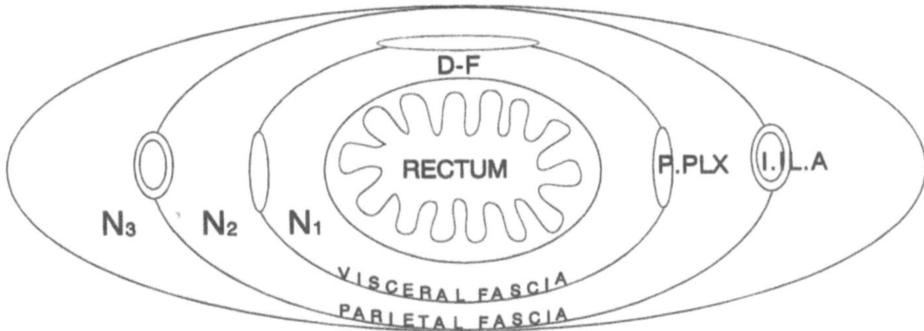

Fig. 4. Schematic transection of the midrectum. *P. PLX*, pelvic nerve plexus; *I. IL. A*, internal iliac artery; *D-F*, Denonvilliers' fascia

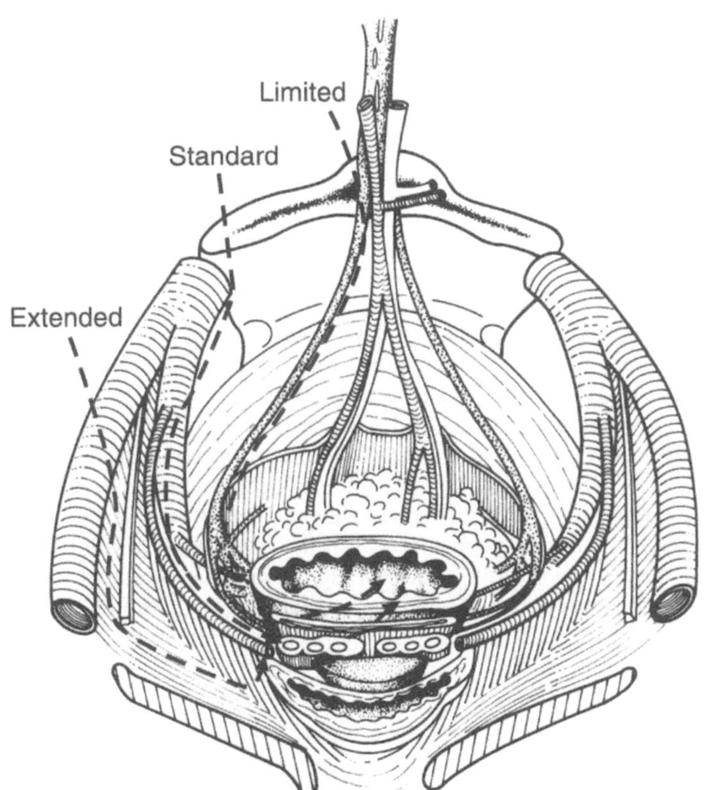

Fig. 5. Schematic presentation of three dissecting planes

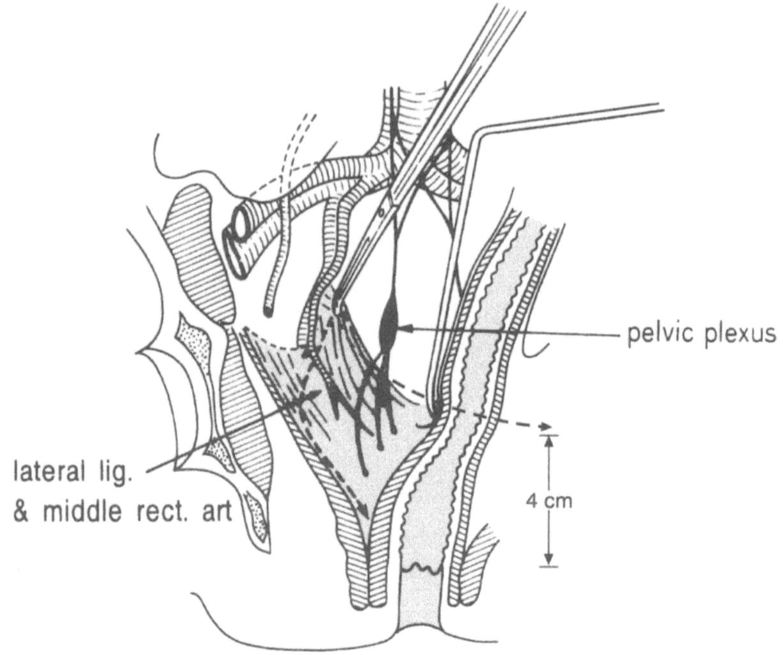

Fig. 6. Location of the pelvic nerve plexus

plexus on the border between the innermost and middle compartment, and the internal iliac artery between the middle and outer compartment. Each compartment has a group of lymph nodes staged as N1, N2, and N3 in that order from the inner to the outer compartment.

On a technical note, and with reference to Chaps. 8–10 in this volume, it is important to realize that the visceral endopelvic fascia is the border between N1 and N2 and that the parietal endopelvic fascia divides N2 from N3.

Figure 5 gives a different view of the three dissecting planes around the rectum. If the surgeon dissects in the innermost plane (the limited dissection), N1 nodes are removed by clearing tissue inside the proper rectal fascia, i.e., the visceral endopelvic fascia, from all elements of the autonomic nerve system of the pelvis and anteriorly from the Denonvilliers' fascia.

Table 6. Indication for type of dissection

	Upward node dissection	Lateral dissection	Indicated for
Limited dissection	N1,N2	N1	Early stage cancer
Standard dissection	N1,N2,N3	N1,N2	Advanced cancer upper rectum
Extended dissection	N1,N2,N3	N1,N2,N3	Advanced cancer lower rectum

In the middle plane (standard plane in Fig. 6), a clearing process is carried out along the parietal pelvic fascia posteriorly and the internal iliac artery laterally. The Denonvilliers' fascia is also excised anteriorly. Attending to the middle plane results in a complete excision of N2 lymph nodes and nerve system. The middle plane is called the standard dissecting plane in Japan.

The outer plane or extended dissecting plane is an addition to the standard dissection. In this plane, the excision of tissue inside the obturator space, which is located between the iliac artery and true pelvic side wall, is carried out. It is, therefore, apparent that the extended dissecting plane is designed for complete clearance of lateral lymph nodes (N3 nodes).

In summary (Table 6), dissection in the limited plane removes only lateral N1 nodes and N1 and N2 upward nodes. Such operation is indicated for an early stage cancer. By dissection in the middle plane, the surgeon excises N2 lateral nodes and N2 and N3 upward nodes, and is chosen for an advanced cancer located in the upper rectum. Staying in the extended plane, both lateral and upward N3 nodes are removed. Such operation is indicated for advanced cancer of the lower rectum.

Results Related to Surgical Strategy

Five-Year Survival Rates in Patients Operated on from 1974 to 1983 (Series I)

During the 10-year period from 1974, 341 patients underwent operation for rectal cancer with a curative intent along one of the three dissecting planes discussed above. Most of the "limited operations" were for Dukes' A stage cancers. The 5-year survival rate in these patients was 97.4% (Table 7).

Cancer in the upper rectum (located above the peritoneal reflection) were operated on within the "standard" dissecting plane. The 5-year survival rates were 90.9% for Dukes' A patients, 84.0% for Dukes' B and 64.7% for Dukes' C patients.

Lower rectal cancers were removed using the "extended" dissecting plane. The survival rates of 97.8% (Dukes' A), and 80.6% (Dukes' B) were as high as that for standard dissection for upper rectal cancer. Even Dukes' C cancer in the lower rectum had a 5-year survival rate of 51.1%, which was almost as high as that for standard dissection for upper rectal cancer.

These figures contrast with the general consensus that lower rectal cancer usually has a worse prognosis than upper rectal cancer. A survival rate for

Table 7. 5-Year survival rates of series I (1974–1983)

	Patients		Dukes' A		Dukes' B		Dukes' C	
	%	n	%	n	%	n	%	n
Limited dissection	97.4	(38/39)	97.4	(38/39)	–	–	–	–
Standard dissection	75.4	(80/106)	90.9	(10/11)	84.1	(37/44)	64.7	(33/51)
Extended dissection	71.4	(140/196)	97.8	(45/46)	80.6	(50/62)	51.1	(45/88)

lower rectal cancer as high as that for upper rectal cancer is considered to be a reflection of an effective clearance of the lymphatic spread of the lower cancer.

Sexual Dysfunction in Male Patients Operated on from 1974 to 1983 (Series I)

Significant pelvic dysfunction was seen after radical surgery with standard and extended dissection. One and 2 years after surgery, 155 male patients were surveyed for sexual dysfunction, i.e., loss of erection and ejaculation. Radical surgery with limited dissection did not damage any element of the pelvic autonomic nerve system. There were no patients who lost erection or ejaculation following this operation (Table 8).

As discussed above, standard dissection was used for cancer in the upper rectum and all cancers were excised by anterior resection of the rectum. Therefore, the operations using standard dissection comprise two groups, one with "high" anastomosis (more than 4 cm above dentate line) and the other with "low" anastomosis (less than 4 cm above dentate line). Almost none of the patients in the "high" anastomosis group lost the ability of erection. On the contrary, the "low" anastomosis group did not regain this function after surgery. All patients in both groups lost the ability to ejaculate.

These results are a clear reflection of the anatomic location of the hypogastric nerve fibers and the pelvic nerve plexus. The hypogastric nerves, which control ejaculation, are included in the tissue to be excised in a standard N2 lymph node dissection. In patients with "high" anastomosis, the dissection does not reach the level of the pelvic nerve plexus located 4 cm above the dentate line, which plays a role in promoting erection. In patients with "low" anastomosis, both the hypogastric nerves and the pelvic nerve plexus are completely excised (Fig. 6) which results in loss of erection and ejaculation in nearly all patients.

Patients with low rectal cancer operated on with extended dissection, and with either coloanal anastomosis or rectal amputation, and patients with low anastomosis following a standard dissection complained of loss of erection and

Table 8. Sexual dysfunction in 155 men 1 and 2 years after surgery, results of series I (1974–1983)

	Loss of erection at				Loss of ejaculation at			
	1 year		2 year		1 year		2 year	
	n	%	n	%	n	%	n	%
Limited dissection (n=16)	0	0	0	0	1	6	1	6
Standard dissection[a]								
High anastomosis (n=28)	2	7	1	4	26	93	24	86
Low anastomosis (n=31)	30	96	30	96	31	100	31	100
Extended dissection (n=80)	78	97	78	97	80	100	80	100

[a] Higher or lower than 4 cm from dentate line

ejaculation. All elements of the autonomic nerve system are sacrificed in an extended dissection and in a standard dissection with low anastomosis.

Tumor Recurrence in Patients Operated on from 1974 to 1983 (Series I)

In 75 out of 341 patients in Series I, tumor recurrence was diagnosed clinically, and verified by imaging (X-rays, computed tomography, CT, scans, or ultrasonography). No recurrence was found in patients undergoing limited dissection (Table 9).

For "standard" and "extended" dissection, the modes of recurrence were investigated. Hematogenous metastases was the most frequent type of recurrence for both groups, with an incidence of approximately 15%. The rate of local recurrence after "standard" and "extended" dissection was low (6%). This indicates that the complex lymphatic spread of low rectal cancer is eradicated by means of extended dissection.

Five-Year Survival Rates in Patients Operated on from 1984 to 1988 (Series II)

During the 5 years from 1984, 197 patients were operated on with curative intent. In this group, an ANP, either partial or complete preservation, was added to a "standard" or "extended" dissection. The operative details of ANP are as follows: As an initial step, a limited dissection is carried out, leaving every element of the autonomic nerve system intact. Then, a "peeling process" of tissue lateral to the nerve system is started from the hypogastric nerve plexus down to the pelvic plexus if required. Finally, a "standard" or an "extended" dissection is performed so precisely that the hypogastric nerve plexus and fibers, and pelvic nerve plexus and fibers on both sides can be isolated.

Partial nerve preservation means that one or more parts of the autonomic nerve system, like a unilateral side of the system or a part of the pelvic plexus, are preserved. Complete preservation indicates that the entire system of the

Table 9. Recurrences in series I (1974–1983)

| | Number of patients | Patients with recurrence | | Tumor recurrence | | | | | | | |
| | | | | Hematogenous | | Local | | Lymphatic | | Peritoneal | |
		n	%	n	%	n	%	n	%	n	%
Limited dissection	39	0	0	0	0	0	0	0	0	0	0
Standard dissection	106	27	25.4	19	17.9	7	6.6	4	3.7	7	6.6
Extended dissection	196	48	24.4	31	15.8	12	6.1	7	3.5	1	0.5
All	341	75	21.9	50	14.6	19	5.5	11	3.2	8	2.3

autonomic nerves, from the lumbal splanchnic nerves cranially to the neuro-vascular bundle of the urinary bladder on the anal side, is completely preserved on both sides.

Five-year survival rates in this series are almost the same as for patients operated on in the period 1974–1983 (Series I). Even for Dukes' B and Dukes' C tumors treated with "extended" dissection, 5-year survival rates are fairly similar to those of the group operated on before 1983 (Table 10). This shows that the modification of ANP in radical rectal cancer surgery does not reduce curability.

Sexual Dysfunction of Male Patients Operated on with ANP from 1984 to 1988 (Series II)

The 58 men in Series II were surveyed for the ability of erection and ejaculation 1 and 2 years after surgery (Table 11). After "standard" dissection with ANP and with high anastomosis, 75% of the men could regain the ability of ejaculation 2 years after surgery. This contrasts with the fact that all patients lost ejaculation function after an identical operation without ANP. Around 75% of

Table 10. 5-year survival rates of series II (1984–1988 after introduction of autonomic nerve preservation)

	Patients		Dukes' A		Dukes' B		Dukes' C	
	%	n	%	n	%	n	%	n
Limited dissection	96.2	26/27	100	26/26			0	0/1
Standard dissection	83.6	51/61	100	12/12	100	15/15	70.5	24/34
Extended dissection	70.6	77/109	86.3	19/22	87.0	27/31	55.3	31/56

Table 11. Sexual dysfunction in 58 men 1 and 2 years after surgery, results of series II (1984–1988)

	Loss of erection at				Loss of ejaculation at			
	1 year		2 year		1 year		2 year	
	n	%	n	%	n	%	n	%
Limited dissection (n=8)	0	0	0	0	0	0	0	0
Standard dissection[a]								
High anastomosis (n=12)	2	16	1	8	3	25	3	25
Low anastomosis (n=10)	3	30	2	20	4	40	3	30
Extended dissection (n=28)	7	25	5	17	14	50	9	33

[a]Higher or lower than 4 cm from the dentate line

patients with low anastomosis or "extended" dissection could also resume erection and ejaculation after surgery modified by ANP. Sexual function tended also to improve as time passed after surgery.

Tumor Recurrence in Patients Operated on from 1984 to 1988 (Series II)

Out of 197 patients, 38 (19.3%) had recurrence of the tumor within 5 years after surgery (Table 12). This is almost the same rate of proven recurrence as in the former group (Series I). Hematogenous metastases were the most prevalent mode of recurrence. As for local recurrence, rates of 4.9% and 6.4% for "standard" and "extended" dissection, respectively, were about the same as for the former group. This is highly suggestive of the notion that ANP as used in Japan does not adversely affect the radicality of rectal cancer.

Conclusion

A retrospective analysis of a large series of patients operated on for rectal cancer using a technique of extended dissection demonstrated the modes of lymphatic spread of rectal cancer. The importance of lateral lymphatic spread as well as upward spread for the outcome of the patients with low-lying rectal cancer was emphasized, and it was conclusively shown that "standard" dissection should be used for cancer of the upper rectum and "extended" dissection with lateral clearance for cancer of the lower rectum.

"Standard" and "extended" dissection decrease the patient's postoperative quality of life, with sexual dysfunction seen in male patients. ANP, however, could preserve sexual function in most without reducing survival.

Table 12. Recurrence in series II (1983–1988 after introduction of autonomic nerve preservation)

	Number of patients	Patients with recurrence		Tumor recurrence							
				Hematogenous		Local		Lymphatic		Peritoneal	
		n	%	n	%	n	%	n	%	n	%
Limited dissection	27	1	3.7	1	3.7	–	–	–	–	–	–
Standard dissection	61	13	21.3	8	13.1	3	4.9	1	1.6	1	1.6
Extended dissection	109	24	22	15	13.7	7	6.4	2	1.8	0	0
All	197	38	19.3	24	14.6	10	5.0	3	1.5	1	0.5

References

1. Miles WE (1908) A method of performing abdomino-perineal excision for carcinoma of the rectum and the terminal portion of the pelvic colon. Lancet II:1812–1813
2. Dixon CF (1939) Surgical removal of lesions occurring in the sigmoid and rectosigmoid. Am J Surg 46:12–17
3. Senba Y (1927) An anatomical study of lymphatic system of the rectum (in Japanese). J Hukuoka Med Coll 20:1213–1268
4. Kuru M (1940) Cancer of the rectum (in Japanese). J Jpn Surg Soc 41:832–877
5. Takahashi T, Kajitani K (1986) Considerations on recent improvements in five-year survival rate of colon and rectal cancer. In: Inokuchi K, Murphy GP, Sugano H, Sugimura T, Veronesi U (eds) Digestive tract tumors. Japan Scientific Press, Tokyo, pp 177–184 (GANN Monograph on Cancer Research vol. 31)

Surgical Technique – Options

CHAPTER 14

Surgical Options in Rectal Cancer

Carlo W. Taat, C. Paul Maas, Willem-Hans Steup,
and Cornelis J.H. van de Velde

Introduction

Despite advances made in diagnostic, anaesthetic and operative technology
over the past five decades, results after curative surgery for rectal cancer have
not improved, reflected by a reported local failure rate varying from 4% to over
30%, and an overall survival of less than 50% [1]. Although figures on recurrence rate may be partially dependent on the length of follow-up, and the
diagnostic tools and the diagnostic criteria employed, such variation is unique
in cancer surgery [18].

Recurrence is mainly found within the pelvis, and in contrast to colonic
cancer, often unaccompanied by distant metastatic disease [102]. Obviously the
traditional surgical approach is not optimal and readjustment must be considered.

The basic surgical principles in the treatment of colorectal cancer was for-
mulated by Lord Moynihan in 1908 [89]. Early in this century the local recurrence rate following surgery for rectal cancer was nearly 100%. Miles
developed a combined radical abdominal and perineal approach (APR) to
remove the pelvic mesocolon and the "zone of upward spread" to solve this
problem [81]. The procedure carried a 42% mortality rate in his first 12 patients reported on in 1908. In 1923 he reported a postoperative mortality rate of
9.5% and a local recurrence rate of 29.5% in 65 patients, which indicated that
APR could cure rectal cancer [82]. However, recurrence rates remained around
50% up to the 1950s with survival rates varying from 16.6% to 37.5% [44].

The Initial Standard Operation

Mr. Miles' operation was for a long time the "gold standard" for treatment of rectal cancer, even for tumours above 15 cm from the anal verge. This is somewhat surprising in view of its mutilating nature and its impact on urinary and sexual function. Indeed, "one had not done a proper cancer operation if the man was not impotent thereafter" was a frequently heard comment.

The standard dissection in rectal cancer surgery is a blunt dissection of the rectum along the presacral pelvic fascia, as is even illustrated in a recently edited textbook on colorectal surgery [21]. Little attention is paid to the mesorectal integrity and the urogenital nerves. In order to prevent nerve damage, a "cone-wise" dissection of the mesorectum is often carried out, which results in incomplete removal of lymphatic tissue. This increases the risk for tumour regrowth [63].

The choice between low anterior resection (LAR) or APR for distal rectal cancer is still a controversial issue. Even in major institutions, APR is performed in more than half of the patients [58, 66, 95]. A general trend towards sphincter-saving procedures is, however, evident (Table 1). Today APR can be limited to 15% of the total rectal cancer population.

LAR Versus APR

Sphincter-preservation techniques were introduced early in this century and were popularised in the late 1940s [12, 68]. This initiated the still ongoing controversy as to which method gives the lowest risk of local recurrence. Analysis of the Large Bowel Cancer Project in UK demonstrated that LAR for rectal and rectosigmoidal carcinoma was followed by a 18% local recurrence

Table 1. Decreasing role of APR in rectal cancer surgery

Author	Year	Country	Reference	Patients (n)	APR (proportion)
Mettlin	1981	USA	77	4610	61%
Jones	1982	UK	62	269	65%
Phillips	1984	UK	98	848	56%
Enker	1986	USA	26	412	62%
Neville	1987	USA	91	373	52%
Carlsson	1987	Sweden	102	319	41%
Gerard	1988	Europe	36	341	81%
Horn	1990	Norway	58	309	60%
Treurniet	1991	Netherlands	113	174	48%
Amato	1991	Italy	3	147	47%
Dixon	1991	UK	23	211	33%
Fändrich	1994	Germany	29	353	39%
Goldberg	1994	UK	38	468	24%
Cedermark	1995	Sweden	20	849	61%
Enker	1995	USA	28	246	28%
Heald	1995	UK	47	303	14%

Table 2. Incidence of local recurrence after APR and LAR for rectal cancer

Author	Year	Reference	APR		LAR		
			n	%	n	%	
Jones	1982	62	15/917	8.5	12/92	13.0	NS
Williams	1984	118	7/83	8.0	8/71	11.0	NS
Phillips	1984	98	57/478	12.0	67/370	18.0	NS
Neville	1987	91	36/192	19.0	36/181	20.0	NS
Amato	1991	3	7/69	11.0	9/78	12.0	NS
Dixon	1991	23	3/61	5.0	6/150	4.0	NS
Fändrich	1994	29	13/137	9.5	24/216	11.0	NS
Isenberg	1995	61	3/53	5.7	11/89	12.5	NS

NS; not significant

rate compared with 12% after APR [74]. In a group of patients with tumours located 7–10 cm from the anal verge the local recurrence rate in stapled anastomosis was 32% versus 13% for APR [91]. Similar results have been found in a recent German study, although the difference between the two methods was not significant [61].

Fändrich could not demonstrate a significant influence of the type of operation on long-term results, although a higher local recurrence rate was seen after LAR for low T4 tumours [29]. They concluded that patients with large tumours of the lower rectum seemed to benefit from APR. Others have demonstrated a 74% 5-year survival rate after sphincter-saving procedures and 62% after APR, but this difference was not statistically significant [118]. The general consensus is now that there are no differences in recurrence rates between APR and LAR (Table 2).

One explanation for the observed poor local tumour control following sphincter-saving procedures could be the so-called "coning effect" [4, 103]. The plane of dissection during a LAR will potentially be closer to the rectal wall than during APR. However, excellent local control after LAR can be achieved if careful sharp dissection under direct vision in well-defined anatomic planes is carried out [45].

All patients should therefore be considered for a sphincter-saving procedure provided that the tumour does not involve the anal sphincter and that pre-operative evaluation does not indicate irresectability [117]. APR remains the procedure of choice for patients with large cancers in the lower third of the rectum while some still advocate APR in patients with tumours of the mid-rectum [61].

We conclude that any difference in outcome between the two operations is likely to be related to the skill and experience of the surgeons.

No Touch Isolation Technique

Turnbull introduced the technique of lymphovascular isolation and ligation prior to mobilization of the tumour-bearing colonic segment, ligation of the bowel lumen, and retroperitoneal lymph node dissection in 1967 [114]. This concept was based on the observation that tumour cells often appeared in venous blood after surgical manipulation [32]. An increase in (uncorrected) 5-year survival of 16% in favour of this technique was demonstrated in Turnbull's original non-randomized study. In Dukes' C patients, the survival benefit increased to 30%. Others demonstrated that venous invasion was associated with worse prognosis, although no correlation could be demonstrated between the presence of circulating tumour cells and survival [40].

A prospective randomized multicentre study evaluating the effect of the "no touch" concept failed, however, to demonstrate a benefit with respect to overall survival. Subgroup analysis revealed a significant benefit if microscopic vascular invasion was present in the tumour [116]. This phenomenom was particularly evident in tumours of the rectum [80].

Although the concept on which this "no touch" technique is based may be correct, its impact will be greatly restricted by wide variations in lymphatic and vascular anatomy and numerous bypass routes through retroperitoneal communications between the caval and portal system.

High Ligation of the Inferior Mesenteric Artery

En bloc resection of lymph nodes at the origin of the inferior mesenteric artery (IMA) from the aorta, often called "high ligation", was assumed in the 1960s to give a survival benefit compared with "low" ligation, which allows selective preservation of the left colic artery. Such benefit was demonstrated for cancer of both the left colon and the rectum [6].

Two more recent comparative studies have failed, however, to show a survival benefit for "high" ligation irrespective of Dukes' stage [96, 110]. Unfortunately no information has been given as to the indication for "high" or "low" ligation. This raises the possibility that selection bias may affect outcome. Lymphatic drainage may not only be along the primary route following the inferior mesenteric artery, but may occur along alternative routes following the portal vein [109].

The number of involved lymph nodes is a significant factor determining survival. Hojo and Koyama [55] demonstrated in a retrospective study that life expectancy decreased with increasing number of affected nodes, with the IMA nodes only rarely being involved. In a prospective study, Moran showed prognosis to be poor if more than four nodes were involved [84]. The number of involved nodes is often underestimated, as nearly 75% will be found in nodes smaller than 5 mm by special node-clearing techniques [54]. It might be argued that once tumour has spread to the "high" nodes the disease is generalized and surgery for cure cannot be achieved.

In our opinion, the level of IMA ligation does not influence recurrence and survival rates significantly. As yet, no conclusive data on the merits of "high" IMA ligation have been published.

Resection Margins

Intramural Spread

The length of the distal bowel resection margin has been repeatedly discussed in the literature, particularly after the introduction of the circular stapling device. A much cited study reporting distal intramural spread up to 4 cm distal to the rectal cancer was used as an argument for wide distal resection margins. This finding was also responsible for the adoption of the "5 cm rule" [42]. This was allowed to happen although it had already been shown in 1949 that only in less than 1% of resection specimens was tumour extension found more than 2 cm away from the primary lesion [12].

Pollet and Nicholls [100] attempted later to define safe margins based on recorded length of the distal resection margin. A total of 334 patients were divided into three groups, namely those with a resection margin of less than 2 cm; those with a margin of between 2 and 5 cm; and those with a margin of more than 5 cm. No difference in crude 5-year survival, cancer-specific death and recurrence rates were demonstrated.

In another well-performed study, the importance of distal intramural spread in resection specimens was examined. Patients with distant spread beyond 1 cm were found to have a poorly differentiated Dukes' C carcinoma. All patients were dead within 3 years of the operation [119]. The authors concluded that extensive retrograde intramural spread signifies aggressive disease with unfavourable prognosis. Such findings should, therefore, not constitute the basis for distal margin guidelines. We will argue that routine application of the 5 cm rule is against the patient's best interest, unnecessarily sacrificing the anal sphincter in many patients. The palpable lower edge of a rectal carcinoma is nearly always also its microscopic lower edge [119].

Extramural, Mesorectal Spread

The problem of extramural distal spread has been addressed by Heald and his group [51]. He described five patients in whom minute foci of adenocarcinoma were present in the mesorectum several centimetres distal to the apparently lower edge of the tumour. Based on their findings, Heald and coworkers argued that distal mesorectal deposit(s) could not be detected before or during surgery, or even suspected after routine histological examination. Therefore mesorectal spread was presumably more dangerous than distal intramural spread and led to the recommendation that complete excision of the mesorectum should be performed routinely [51].

They also demonstrated that the distal bowel resection margin could be safely reduced to less than 1 cm. No difference in local recurrence rates were found between a group of 42 patients with distal resection margin of up to 1 cm and a group of 110 with distal margins of more than 1 cm following a curative TME [63]. Although the more than 1 cm margin group had significantly less Dukes' A tumours and selection criteria were not given, these results are impressive. Admittedly, however, no formal consensus on distal margins exists among surgeons [120].

Pelvic Lymph Node Dissection

The orderly pattern of lymphatic spread from perirectal to inferior mesenteric lymph nodes has been noted by several authors in the past [33, 41]. Lateral lymphatic spread was infrequently found [41].

The presence of lymphatic tissue draining laterally was demonstrated in vivo by injecting dye in the rectal mucosa [106]. It was argued that such findings could explain the high local failure rate. Failure was also related to the site of the tumour, i.e. the lower the tumour in the rectum, the higher the frequency of local recurrence, ranging from 30% for the lowest lesions to 6.3% for the upper third of the rectum [7]. This justified the plea for a more radical pelvic lymph node dissection (PLND) [106].

Data on survival in 80 patients who underwent radical abdominopelvic lymph node dissection failed to demonstrate a significant survival benefit in rectal and distal left colonic cancers [8]. Later Stearns and Deddish [108] reported on 122 patients with cancer within 20 cm from the anal verge. Lymph node dissection was performed along the aorta and caval vein, between the ureters from the duodenum to the levator ani muscles, including presacral external and internal iliac and obturator spaces.

In 91% of Dukes' C patients lymph node metastases were found in dissected tissues beyond the standard excision area. The 5-year survival rate for all patients was 54%, comparable to the results demonstrated in an earlier series. Though Dukes' C patients undergoing extensive node clearance fared better than patients who underwent conventional operations, the procedure-related complications and the long recovery time led the authors to conclude that radical abdominopelvic lymph node dissection should not be used routinely.

Radical lymph node dissection in colorectal cancer has also been addressed by other authors from different centres [25, 89, 37]. Enker and co-workers [25] reported on patients treated between 1966 and 1970; 5-year survival was 45.5% in 48 patients with rectal cancer. The local recurrence after resection of Astler Coller C2 stage tumours was 27.9%. C2 patients, who had a hypogastric lymph node dissection added, experienced a local recurrence rate of 18.2% [24, 25].

A report in 1986 from the same group [26] gave the results in 192 patients with rectal cancer. The aortoiliac pelvic lymphadenectomy included removal of nodes caudad to the aortocaval bifurcation, along the common iliac arteries and veins and the internal iliac and middle haemorrhoidal branches. The results were compared with those of 220 patients who underwent a conventional rectal cancer resection. Superior 5-year survival rate was observed in Dukes' C patients after LAR plus en bloc pelvic lymphadenectomy (57.6% versus 32.1% after conventional resections). Following APR, the 5-year survival was 37.0% in the extended group and 20.8% for the Dukes' C patients operated on conservatively.

The overall pelvic recurrence rate after LAR or APR with or without extended node dissection was 27.8% and 28.6%, respectively. The extent of the procedure did not have an impact on the pelvic recurrence rate [26]. It was concluded that only patients with tumours penetrating the bowel wall should be selected for this operation as the incidence of nodal metastases in such patients exceeded 50%.

In another American series of 154 rectal cancer patients, 64 had extended pelvic node dissection. Although the local recurrence rate in these patients was 9.4% versus 16.4% in the patients who underwent conventional operations, this difference did not reach statistically significance [78].

McCall and coworkers [75] reviewed 51 papers published between January 1982 and December 1992 reporting on 10 465 rectal cancer patients operated on for cure, without adjuvant therapy. The median local recurrence rate was 18.5%, and for Dukes' C tumours 28.6%. In 476 patients, collected from four papers, who underwent extended pelvic lymphadenectomy, the local recurrence rate was 12.4%. Patients in this group tended to have slightly more advanced disease (based on Dukes' stage) than 1033 patients, collected from eight papers, who underwent TME. These patients were reported to have a local recurrence rate of 7.1%.

At the National Cancer Center Hospital in Tokyo, Japan, experience with PLND for rectal cancer has been accumulated over a long period. In the past, patients with rectal cancer below the peritoneal reflection were found to have metastases to the lateral pelvic nodes in 23% [55]. Metastases to such sites indicated a 5-year survival below 10%. Extended lateral PLND was, therefore, added, the rationale being to reduce failure rates.

Their 'conventional' operation included dissection along the adventitia of the major abdominal and pelvic vessels removing para-aortic and para-caval lymphatic tissue, and resecting the aortic sympathetic plexus from the level of the left renal vein. The IMA was divided flush with the aorta. The pelvic iliac nodes were removed, and the obturator fossa was cleared of all lymphatic tissue. If metastatic involvement in the lymphatics around the internal iliac artery and vein was suspected, extended lateral dissection was added. The internal iliac vessels were sacrified to the branching of the superior gluteal vessels, preserving only the superior vesical artery and obturator nerve. No long-term sequelae of the procedure were reported.

The first report on 163 patients in whom such an extensive lateral PLND was added showed statistically increased 5-year survival rates in Dukes' B and C staged patients (83.2% and 52.5% versus 62.7% and 30.8%, respectively compared with patients who underwent conventional dissection). The frequency of pelvic recurrence was 24.5% for Dukes' C patients with extended lateral dissection versus 44.3% in patients who underwent conventional dissection [65].

Later Moriya and associates reported on lateral dissection in 232 patients with advanced rectal cancer at or below the peritoneal reflection [86]. After 'conventional' dissection, disease-free 5-year survival was 67.4%, while after 'extended' lateral dissection, survival increased to 75.8%. The survival benefit was, however, not statistically significant. In Dukes' C patients, the disease-free survival appeared better in the 'extended' group (68.0% versus 43.7%), but even this difference did not reach statistical significance. The local pelvic recurrence rate was 12% in the 'extended' group versus 19% in patients operated on "conventionally". Again no statistically significant difference could be demonstrated. Involvement of lateral nodes only was observed in 6% of patients. Postoperative neurogenic bladder and sexual dysfunction developed in virtually all of 232 patients and intermittent self-catheterisation was required in 10% of patients. Some 90% regained their ability to void after 1 year, while sexual function rarely improved.

Critics of PLND focus on the increased operation time and blood loss, and particularly the high rate of urinary and sexual dysfunction. To limit the frequency of such comorbidity which follow PLND, the concept of pelvic autonomic nerve preservation (ANP) gradually emerged [27, 87]. The principle was based on the surgical anatomy of the pelvic nerves so well described for benign disease by Lee and associates in 1973 [67].

Enker presented in 1992 a series of 42 men who underwent a curative ANP side wall dissection in conjunction with a sphincter-preserving procedure for rectal cancer below 11 cm [27]. This procedure is less extensive than the Japanese pelvic dissection as no clearance of lateral pelvic nodes was performed. Out of 38 patients, 33 remained potent, and 29 of these had normal ejaculation. Only one local recurrence was seen (2.4%) after a follow up of 20 months.

In a small series Michelassi and Block [79] reported on 91 patients who underwent wide pelvic lymphadenectomy, a more extensive dissection than that described by Enker. Three patients needed self-catheterisation postoperatively, but not for more than 8 months. Only two out of seven sexually active males regained postoperative sexual potency.

Recently Moriya reported results of his autonomic nerve sparing technique in 185 patients with rectal cancer at or below the peritoneal reflection [87]. Depending on the stage of the disease, the surgical approach allowed for different types of ANP, varying from selective unilateral or a bilateral sacrifice of the inferior hypogastric nerves or presacral nerves to a combination of these. In 81 patients, the autonomic nerves in the pelvis and preaortic region were preserved. When evaluated 30 days after operation, 91% of patients could void spontaneously. None of them was incapable of erection, but 30% experienced difficulties with ejaculation.

In the remaining patients who had either partial or near complete sacrifice of the autonomic nerves, all had severely impaired erection and none of them had normal ejaculation. Pelvic recurrence rate in this series was 4%, which is a surprisingly low figure given the 24.5% local recurrence rate in Koyama' series [65] following the more extended en bloc lateral pelvic lymphadenectomy. One may wonder whether this remarkable difference was caused either by operating on patients with less advanced tumours or by accomplishing a more complete excision of the mesorectal structures, and not due to the pre-aortic and lateral PLND.

Others have reviewed the long-standing controversy on the questionable comparability of Western and Japanese patients and emphasised the absence of prospective randomized trials required to determine the true value of radical pelvic node dissection [107].

In a comment to a much cited paper by Hojo and coworkers [56], it was concluded that lateral lymph node metastases were demonstrated in only 3% of patients, and that the corresponding 5-year survival even after extended lymphadenectomy was only 6% [46]. Support comes from Moreira et al. who compared retrospectively 95 Japanese patients who had undergone extended lateral PLND with 83 patients who had conventional dissection [85]. Recurrence and survival rates correlated more with intrinsic tumour factors, i.e. venous and neural invasion and tumour spread, than with the extent of nodal dissection.

Most studies on PLND are retrospective and lack proper control groups, and some even lack information on the effect of radical lymphadenectomy in patients whose excised nodes contained metastases [1]. An additional confusing aspect is the lack of uniformity in surgical technique, in the extent of the procedures, and in the anatomical nomenclature.

Total Mesorectal Excision

In 1982 Heald and coworkers pointed out that spread of rectal cancer occurred not only upwards, but also distally within the mesorectum. He (and others) also stated that extensive downward intramural spread is an infrequent occurrence [42, 51, 52]. The distal spread is restricted to only a few millimetres [52].

The pathology data and the experience that division of the mesorectum itself was bloody and non-anatomical led Heald to suggest a different surgical approach, dissecting in the avascular plane surrounding the mesorectum (Chap. 15). This resulted in complete removal of the mesorectum, sparing the anal sphincter and leaving a small rectal remnant to be anastomosed with the colon. The autonomic nerves were unharmed. Complete excision of the mesorectum and the mesentery containing the inferior mesenteric artery and vein gives, according to Heald, a "perfect tumour and pedicle package".

This "package" is the block of tissue in which rectal tumour spread commonly occurs [47]. In general rectal cancer will not spread beyond the borders of the mesorectum, embryologically defined by the plane between the visceral and parietal fascia. This forms the basis of the "total mesorectal excision hypothesis" [45, 47]. TME should theoretically decrease the incidence of local recurrence following surgery for cancer of the mid and low rectum. Furthermore, TME comprises a meticulous sharp dissection under direct vision along the delicately defined fascial layers, to prevent tearing into the mesorectum and opening up tumour "areas" and disrupting lymphatic channels, thereby reducing potential contamination of the operative field with tumour cells [93].

Since April 1978, 333 patients have been operated on with 261 "curative" resections at the Colorectal Research Unit of the North Hampshire Hospital. The local recurrence rate is 4% [47]. This contradicts the expectations of his critics that, with time, the local recurrence rate will undoubtedly increase. In a previous publication [50] reporting on 115 curative anterior resections, a cumulative risk of local recurrence at 5 years was 3.7% and the overall survival at 5 year 87.5% (tumour free survival 81.7%). All operations were performed or closely supervised by Mr. Heald. No patient received adjuvant therapy.

However, many investigators have questioned these findings and have pointed to the possibility of patient 'case mix' and analytical techniques [60], vague selection processes [90], and incorrect use of definitions [72] as explanations for such results.

MacFarlane and associates [70], revised independently the Basingstoke data and compared them to results from the much cited North Central Cancer Treatment Group (NCCTG) adjuvant trial [66]. In 'high-risk' patients (Dukes' B and C), only five out of 126 (3.8%) developed local recurrence after LAR in the Basingstoke series. Two of nine (22%) patients developed local recurrence after APR. The overall local-plus-distant recurrence rate was 18%. These results were clearly superior to those reported after conventional surgery and adjuvant radiotherapy in the NCCTG study (5% local recurrence at 5 years in Basingstoke compared with 25% in the NCCTG study). In the latter study, conventional surgery followed by radiotherapy and chemotherapy gave a 13.5% local recurrence rate.

A point of concern is the anastomotic leakage rate associated with the TME procedure. Out of 219 patients who underwent TME at Basingstoke symptomatic anastomotic leakage was found in 24 of them (11.0%); in 14 patients (6.4%) a minor leak was detected by contrast enema [64]. Three patients with major leaks died.

The relatively high incidence of anastomotic leakage might be caused by devascularization of the anorectal stump during dissection of the distal 'tail' of the mesorectum in TME, presumably due to the vascular anatomy of the posterior lower part of the rectum [5, 115]. In that area there is no anastomosing vascular bed between the superior and inferior rectal artery. Such vascular anastomosis is present ventrally. Furthermore the middle rectal artery is only present in 50% of cases, and in 50% of these only found unilaterally. Dissection may further compromise the already poorly vascularised dorsal aspect, subsequently impairing anastomotic healing. The problem with postoperative anastomotic dehiscence led Heald to recommend a temporary colostomy in patients with low anastomosis (less than 6 cm from the anal verge) [64].

Dixon has reported on 202 patients with cancer of the distal sigmoid and rectum in whom TME was performed by one single surgeon. In 150 patients undergoing a curative anterior resection, only six developed local recurrence. The 5-year survival was 64% after anterior resection [23]. McCall reported a pooled (eight papers) local recurrence rate of 7.3% in 1033 patients who underwent TME [75].

Major support for the impact of precise excision of the mesorectum on local recurrence rate has come from pathologists. Quirke and associates [101] demonstrated that an involved circumferential margin carried more than 80% risk for local recurrence. Quirke suggested that lateral spread of tumour at the lateral circumferential margin of the specimen might well have been encompassed by total removal of the mesorectum. Others have failed to confirm the correlation between lateral margin involvement and local recurrence [19].

A prospective study on 190 patients by Quirke's group [2] demonstrated that involvement of the circumferential margin affected independently both local recurrence rate and survival. The status of the lateral margins and the distance between tumour and the lateral margin are now accepted as independent prognostic factors [120].

A regional project in The Netherlands has demonstrated that these results are reproducible in a multicentre setting [43]. The lateral resection margins of 253 patients operated on for rectal cancer were examined according to Quirke's method. A positive resection margin was in this study an independent prognostic factor for both local recurrence and distant metastases.

Enker actually performs the same procedure as Heald. This was documented and video-taped during a joint effort in Basingstoke where each of these two surgeons performed one side of the dissection in a patient with a lower third rectal cancer [47].

One should bear in mind that Heald's results are a personal series of which the epidemiological characteristics have not been studied in detail. The Basingstoke study is challenging and provocative but otherwise inconclusive [31]. The benefit of this technique for instance on a national level can only be demonstrated through evaluation of large-scale multicentre studies, whether these are randomized or "benchmark" studies.

Local Excision

Local excision has been used to treat low rectal cancer to reduce morbidity, such as male impotence and bladder and sexual dysfunction, and to avoid permanent colostomy. Such local approaches should be considered in low-lying tumours otherwise needing APR, or when APR or LAR is not justified.

Local excision may be performed by transsphincteric, transsacral or transanal routes [69, 73]. In view of the risk for postoperative complications affecting anal continence [11], transanal local excision is the preferred route. This has met with success, results in early cancers being comparable with that of radical procedures [34, 57]. Graham et al. [39] reported on published series and found a cancer specific 5-year survival of 89% in mainly T1 (submucosal invasion only) and T2 (muscularis propria invaded) tumours, within 6 cm of the anal verge, and without enlarged lymph nodes. The local recurrence rate was 19%.

The tumour should be excised in toto to allow histological examination with assessment of resection margins, depth of penetration of the bowel wall, tumour grade, and other tumour-related prognostic features. Such an approach will not clarify the nodal status, and recommendations as to adjuvant therapy or surgery will often be difficult. Accurate assessment of lymph node status is difficult and reliable in only 80% of patients [13, 22].

Criteria used for selection are: tumours should be no more than 3 cm in diameter, mobile at palpation, within 10 cm of the anal verge, not within the range of the vaginal wall, and histologically moderately or well differentiated. Tumours should be confined to the rectal wall (T1 or T2), without evidence of lymph node metastases, as established by preoperative intraluminal ultrasound. An extension of the transanal local excision technique is transanal endoscopic microsurgery with special instruments [16, 88].

The risk for locoregional failure is high in all local excision techniques. One should realise that patients who undergo a salvage APR or LAR for subsequent local recurrence have a significantly worse prognosis than those who undergo a primary radical procedure for adverse pathologic features found in the initial local excision specimen [9, 88]. The impact of adjuvant radiotherapy has been the subject of other studies [71, 83]. Future randomized studies are required to evaluate the merits of adjuvant radiotherapy following local excision of rectal cancer.

Results After Rectal Cancer Surgery

Local recurrence is the most important outcome variable when reporting on results of rectal cancer surgery. A note of caution should be given when comparing and interpreting published data. There is no uniformity as to the applied nomenclature of either "rectal cancer" or "local recurrence". Some authors include in their series tumours that are localised in the rectum or rectosigmoid, others include only patients with tumours at or below the peritoneal reflection [2, 86, 87, 94, 105, 121]. In general, rectal cancer is defined on the basis of the distance from the anal verge to the distal tumour margin as measured by a rigid sigmoidoscope. Unfortunately this distance varies to a great extent. Thus different 'rectal cancer' series may well represent a wide variety of tumours, with different growth and spreading patterns (Table 3).

The distance from the tumour to the anal verge depends on the type of endoscope used. With a rigid scope, the distances are smaller than if a flexible endoscope is used in the same patients. Several papers lack accurate in-

Table 3. Definitions of rectal cancer

Author	Year	Reference	Distance tumour–anal verge
Enker	1979	25	< 12 cm
Phillips	1984	97	< 18 cm
McDermott	1985	76	< 18 cm
GITSG	1985	35	< 12 cm
Neville	1986	91	< 15 cm
Heald	1986	50	< 15 cm
Krook	1991	66	< 12 cm or below the sacral promontory
Amato	1991	3	< 15 cm far below promontory at laparotomy
Michelassi	1992	80	< 14 cm
Enker	1992	27	< 11 cm
MacFarlane	1993	70	< 12 cm
Moriya	1993	87	at or below the peritoneal reflection
Fändrich	1994	29	< 15 cm

formation on how the height of the tumour has been assessed [29, 45, 99]. There is an urgent need for an internationally accepted, standardized definition of "rectal cancer" to be used in communications and publications.

The site of the tumour is of prognostic importance. Tumours at or above 12 cm carry a significantly lower risk for local recurrence than more distally located lesions [99]. Anteriorly located tumours in the middle and lower third of the male rectum are said to carry a higher risk for local recurrence than posteriorly located tumours, but no reliable data are found in literature concerning this aspect.

The risk of tumour recurrence is also stage related; patients with Dukes' B or C lesions within 10 cm from the anal verge have a two- to fourfold increased risk for locoregional recurrence compared with patients with a tumour above that level [10, 61]. McCall, Cox and Watchow found in their survey a local recurrence rate of 8.5% for Dukes' A tumours, 16.3% for Dukes' B, and 28.6% for Dukes' C [75].

Recurrent disease is either local, distant or a combination of the two. It is called "local recurrence" if found adjacent to the primary tumour site or in the lesser pelvis [1]. The incidence of local recurrence after curative resection varies widely and Table 4 gives an overview of reported results.

The term "local recurrence" covers a wide range of definitions, each having an impact on reported results. In a recently published series on 284 patients, it was demonstrated that the local recurrence rate could vary from 4% to 43.3% by in- or excluding patients according to the definition of "local recurrence" [72]. Local recurrence after operation for rectal carcinoma should therefore be defined as: "any detectable local disease at follow-up, occurring either alone or

Table 4. Local recurrence after 'curative' surgery

Author	Year	Reference	Patients	Type of tumour recurrence					
				Local		Local + distant		Total local	
			(n)	n	%	n	%	n	%
Rich	1983	105	142	24	16.9	19	13.3	43	30.2
Phillips	1984	99	848	124	14.6	–		–	
Pilipshen	1984	97	382	87	14.4	50	13.1	105	27.5
McDermott	1985	76	934	107	11.0	84	9.0	193	20.0
Carlsson	1987	19	231	16	7.0	56	24.2	72	31.1
Zirngibl	1990	121	1153	265	23.0	–		–	
Amato	1991	3	147	16	10.9	–		–	
Dixon	1991	23	224	9	4.0	–		–	
Moriya	1993	87	185	8	4.3	–		–	
Norstein	1993	94	275	69	25.1	12	4.4	81	29.5
Adam	1994	2	141	32	23.0	–		–	
Fändrich	1994	29	371	42	11.3	10	2.7	52	14.0
Bognel	1995	14	339	53	15.9	10	3.0	63	18.6
SAKK	1995	111	185	47	25.4	–		–	
Isenberg	1995	61	142	14	9.9	–		–	
McCall	1995	75	10465	167	18.8	167	2.7	2183	21.5
Heald	1995	48	261	–		7	3.0	7	3.0

in conjunction with distant recurrence, in patients who underwent resection of rectal cancer". Furthermore, it is common practice to report only isolated local recurrence after 'curative' surgery, although local recurrence in combination with distant disease none the less constitutes treatment failure. Evaluation of rectal cancer surgery should include all failure areas [1, 72].

There are also problems related to the term 'curative' surgery, which generally means that all visible tumour is removed. Such a statement is based on the surgeon's judgement, and inclusion of only 'curative' patients may well introduce bias. This could partially be overcome if only postsurgical "curative resection" cases were included, where "curative" is defined as a histologically complete excision of the tumour and free resection margins (including circumferential margin).

Another confounding factor in the analysis of local recurrence rates is the potential impact of follow-up. The methods used for detecting local failure differ in accuracy, and the incidence of local recurrence increases with time [18]. Autopsy in all patients with a history of cancer surgery who die is probably not routine anywhere, but may affect recurrence rates [18, 112]. The reported incidence of local recurrence might be an underestimation of reality in many studies [1]. Authors should clearly define the outcome variables to avoid confusion and to facilitate interstudy comparison or evaluation of future novel therapies.

The individual surgeon seems also to be a prognostic factor. Among 20 consultant surgeons who reported on more than 30 patients in The Large Bowel Cancer Project in UK [74], local recurrence rates ranged from below 5% to more than 20%. The "surgeon factor" persisted after correction for other prognostic tumour characteristics. This surgeon-related phenomenon, first reported by Phillips et al. [97] in 1984, has been confirmed by McArdle and coworkers [74]. With recurrence rates ranging from nil to 21% among 13 surgeons, we may assume that some of the differences in outcome reflect differences in patient characteristics, but even after adjusting for known risk factors substantial differences remained.

Recently Hermanek reported on local recurrence rates from surgical departments entering patients into the German Colorectal Cancer Study [53]. Local failure rate ranged from 1% to 18% for TNM stage II patients, and from 9%–38% for stage III patients. The local recurrence rates related to individual surgeons ranged from 5% to more than 50%. The subsequent 5-year survival ranged from 80% to 40% and was inversely correlated to local failure rates. This shows that optimal local control does have an impact on survival [49]. The failure rate in the German study did not show any relation with the total number of rectal operations performed by each surgeon. The operating surgeon appears to be an independent prognostic factor even after stratification for tumour-related factors, a finding confirmed by others [30].

The best results in Table 4 come from personal series where surgeons nearly always have adopted the principle of TME. Despite possible confounders, as discussed above, the unprecedented good results do suggest that the TME technique will contribute significantly to the future outcome of rectal cancer surgery. Others report less favourable outcomes (Table 4). It is apparent that conventional resection technique for rectal cancer does not meet the standards set by "TME surgeons".

The presented data support the contention that surgery for rectal cancer should be performed by surgeons with a special interest and skill in colorectal surgery. This is supported by a recent investigation on the effect of the surgeon's specialty interest on the type of resection performed [104]. Surgeons with experience and interest in colorectal cancer did wider resections in left-sided colonic and rectal cancers than surgeons with other interests.

The surgeon as a prognostic factor has also impact on the interpretation of results of adjuvant studies. The Gastro-Intestinal Tumour Study Group (GITSG) and the NCCTG demonstrated the efficacy of postoperative adjuvant radio- and chemotherapy in rectal cancer, treatments leading to significantly reduced recurrence rates and improved survival [35, 66, 95]. Local recurrence rate in the 'surgery alone' control group in the GITSG study [35] was 25%, and 5-year local recurrence rate in the NCCTG study [66] after surgery plus radiotherapy was 24%. The local recurrence rate following adjuvant treatment was 13% [95], a figure regularly encountered in European publications following surgery alone. Notably, only in the NCCTG study were the operative records reviewed by a surgical board to ascertain that minimal surgical criteria had been met. Quality control of surgery should be an essential item in future studies.

On the basis of the GITSG and NCCTG studies, the NIH Consensus Development Conference (1990) recommended that combined surgical and adjuvant therapy was the optimal management for rectal cancer patients with a poor prognosis (TNM stage II and III) [92]. Given the impact of the operating surgeon on patient outcome, the results from any trial addressing the question of adjuvant therapy needs to be interpreted with caution [2].

The system of specially trained surgeons has been validated in the previously conducted Dutch Gastric Cancer Trial comparing Japanese style D2 lymph node dissection to routine dissection [15]. Surgical quality control turned out to be crucial in testing the hypothesis [17]. In addition to quality control within the operating theatre, the role of the pathologist, which has been discussed before, is emphasized [2, 19, 101]. For rectal cancer trials, the method of examination of the specimen as described by Quirke (Chap. 5) should be introduced as the "gold standard". Through accurate feedback from the pathologist, the surgeon can evaluate the completeness of his rectal excision.

A more careful attention to surgical details should be followed by improved results. The impact on patient outcome might be greater than that of any of the adjuvant therapies currently under study [53]. Hermanek predicted that optimal surgery would increase 5-year survival from 45% to around 80%, a 75% improvement, whereas the contribution of adjuvant modalities is commonly not greater than 10%–20%.

References

1. Abulafi AM, Williams NS (1994) Local recurrence of colorectal cancer: the problem, mechanisms, management and adjuvant therapy. Br J Surg 81:7–19
2. Adam IJ, Mohamdee MO, Martin IG et al. (1994) Role of circumferential margin involvement in the local recurrence of rectal cancer. Lancet 334:707–711
3. Amato A, Pescatori M, Butti A (1991) Local recurrence following abdominoperineal excision and anterior resection for rectal carcinoma. Dis Colon Rectum 34:317–322
4. Anderberg B, Enblad P, Sjödahl R, Wetterfors J (1983) The EEA stapling device in anterior resection for carcinoma of the rectum. Acta Chir Scand 149:99–103
5. Ayoub SF (1978) Arterial blood supply of the human rectum. Acta Anat 100:317–327
6. Bacon HE, Khubchandani IT (1964) The rationale of aortoiliopelvic lymphadenectomy and high ligation of the inferior mesenteric artery for carcinoma of the left half of the colon and rectum. Surg Gynecol Obstet 119:503–508
7. Bacon HE, Sauer I (1950) Surgical treatment of cancer of the lower bowel. Cancer 3:773–778
8. Bacon H, Dirbas F, Myers T, Ponce de Leon F (1958) Extensive lymphadenectomy and high ligation of the inferior mesenteric artery for carcinoma of the left colon and rectum. Dis Colon Rectum 1:457–465
9. Baron PL, Enker WE, Zakowski MF, Urmacher C (1995) Immediate vs salvage resection after local treatment for early rectal cancer. Dis Colon Rectum 38:177–181
10. Bentzen SM, Balslev I, Pedersen M et al. (1992) Time to loco-regional recurrence after resection of Dukes' B and C colorectal cancer with and without adjuvant postoperative radiotherapy. A multivariate regression analysis. Br J Canc 65:102–107
11. Bergman L, Solhaug JH (1986) Posterior trans-sphincteric resection for small tumours of the lower rectum. Acta Chir Scand 152:313–316
12. Best RR, Blair JB (1949) Sphincter preserving operations for rectal carcinoma as related to the anatomy of the lymphatics. Ann Surg 130:538–576
13. Beynon J, Mortensen NJ, Foy DM et al. (1989) Preoperative assessment of mesorectal lymph node involvement in rectal cancer. Br J Surg 76:276–279
14. Bognel C, Rekacewicz C, Mankarios H et al. (1995) Prognostic value of neural invasion in rectal carcinoma: a multivariate analysis on 339 patients with curative resection. Eur J Cancer 31A:894–898
15. Bonenkamp JJ, Songun I, Hermans J et al. (1995) Randomized comparison of morbidity after D1 and D2 dissection for gastric cancer in 996 Dutch patients. Lancet 345:745–748
16. Buess G, Kipfmüller K, Ibald R, Heintz A et al. (1989) Transanale endoskopische Mikrochirurgie beim Rectumcarcinom. Chirurg 60:901–904
17. Bunt AMG, Hermans J, Smit VTHBM et al. (1995) Surgical/pathological-stage migration confounds comparisons of gastric cancer survival rates between Japan and Western countries. J Clin Oncol 13:19–25
18. Carlsson U, Larson A, Ekelund G (1987) Recurrence rates after curative surgery for rectal cancer with special reference to their accuracy. Dis Colon Rectum 30:431–436
19. Cawthorn SJ, Parums DV, Gibbs NM et al. (1990) Extent of mesorectal spread and involvement of lateral margin as a prognostic factor after surgery for rectal cancer. Lancet 335:1087
20. Cedermark B, Johansson H, Rutqvist LE et al. for the Stockholm Colorectal Cancer Study Group (1995) The Stockholm I trial of preoperative short-term radiotherapy in operable rectal carcinoma. Cancer 75:2269–2275
21. Cohen AM, Winawer SJ (eds) (1995) Cancer of the colon, rectum and anus. McGraw-Hill, New York, p 583
22. Derksen EJ (1992) New aspects in diagnoses and treatment of rectal cancer. Academic Thesis, Free University, Amsterdam
23. Dixon AR, Maxwell WA, Thornton Holmes J (1991) Carcinoma of the rectum: a 10-year experience. Br J Surg 78:301–311
24. Enker WE (1978) Surgical treatment of large bowel cancer. In: Enker WE (ed) Carcinoma of the colon and rectum. Yearbook Medical, Chicago, pp 97–100

25. Enker WE (1992) Potency, cure, and local control in the operative treatment of rectal cancer. Arch Surg 127:1396–1402
26. Enker WE, Laffer UT, Block GE (1979) Enhanced survival of patients with colon and rectal cancer is based upon wide anatomic resection. Ann Surg 190:350–360
27. Enker WE, Pilipshen SJ, Heilweil ML et al. (1986) En bloc pelvic lymphadenectomy and sphincter preservation in the surgical management of rectal cancer. Ann Surg 203:426–433
28. Enker WE, Thaler HT, Cranor ML, Polyak T (1995) Total mesorectal excision in the operative treatment of carcinoma of the rectum. J Am Coll Surg 181:335–346
29. Fändrich F, Schröder DW, Saliveros E (1994) Long term survival after curative resection for adenocarcinoma of the rectum. J Am Coll Surg 178:271–276
30. Fielding LP (1988) Surgeon-related variability in the outcome of cancer surgery. J Clin Gastroenterol 10:130–132
31. Fielding LP (1993) Colorectal carcinoma: mesorectal excision for rectal cancer (letter). Lancet 341:471–472
32. Fisher ER, Turnbull RB (1987) The cytologic demonstration and significance of tumour cells in the mesenteric venous blood in patients with colorectal carcinoma. Surg Gynecol Obstet 100:102–108
33. Gabriel W, Dukes C, Bussey H (1935) Lymphatic spread in cancer of the rectum. Br J Surg 23:395–413
34. Gall FP, Hermanek P (1988) Cancer of the rectum – local excision. Surg Clin N Am 68:1353–1365
35. Gastrointestinal Tumor Study Group (1985) Prolongation of the disease-free interval in surgically treated rectal carcinoma. N Engl J Med 312:1465–1472
36. Gerard A, Buyse M, Nordlinger B et al. (1988) Preoperative radiotherapy as adjuvant treatment in rectal cancer. Ann Surg 208:606–614
37 Glass R, Ritchie J, Thyompson H, Mann C (1985) The results of surgical treatment of cancer of the rectum by radical resection and extended abdominoiliac lymphadenectomy. Br J Surg 72:599–601
38. Goldberg PA, Nicholls RJ, Porter NH et al. (1994) Long-term results of a randomized trial of short-course low-dose adjuvant preoperative radiotherapy for rectal cancer. Reduction in local treatment failure. Eur J Cancer 30A:1602–1606
39. Graham RA, Garnsey L, Jessup JM (1990) Local excision of rectal carcinoma. Am J Surg 160:306–312
40. Griffiths JD, McKinna JA, Rowbotham HD (1973) Carcinoma of the colon and rectum: circulating malignant cells and 5 year survival. Cancer 31:226
41. Grinnell RS (1942) The lymphatic and venous spread of carcinoma of the rectum. Ann Surg 116:200–216
42. Grinnell RS (1954) Distal intramural spread of carcinoma of the rectum and rectosigmoid. Surg Gynecol Obstet 99:421–430
43. Haas-Kock de D, Baeten C, Jager J et al. (1995) The prognostic significance of the lateral resection margin in rectal cancer. Presented at IKA 15th Anniversary International Congress Colorectal Cancer: From Gene to Cure, 9–11 February 1995, Academic Medical Center, Amsterdam
44. Harnsberger JR, Vernava AM, Longo WE (1994) Radical abdominopelvic: lymphadenectomy historic perspective and current role in the surgical management of rectal cancer. Dis Colon Rectum 37:73–87
45. Heald RJ (1988) The "Holy Plane" of rectal surgery. J Royal Soc Med 81:503–509
46. Heald RJ (1991) Function preserving rectal surgery (letter). Dis Colon Rectum 34:627–628
47. Heald RJ (1995) Invited lecture: rectal cancer: the surgical options Presented at IKA 15th Anniversary International Congress "Colorectal Cancer: From Gene to Cure", February 9–11, 1995, Academic Medical Center, Amsterdam, The Netherlands
48. Heald RJ (1995) Rectal cancer: the surgical options. Eur J Cancer 31A:1189–1192
49. Heald RJ, Karanjia ND (1992) Results of radical surgery for rectal cancer. World J Surg 16:848–857

50. Heald RJ, Ryall RDH (1986) Recurrence and survival after mesorectal excision for rectal cancer. Lancet I:1479–1482
51. Heald RJ, Husband EM, Ryall RDH (1982) The mesorectum in rectal cancer surgery – the clue to pelvic recurrence? Br J Surg 69:613–616
52. Hermanek P (1982) Evolution and pathology of rectal cancer. World J Surg 6:502–509
53. Hermanek P (1994) Local control and long-term prognosis. Results of the German Multicenter Study on Colorectal Cancer. Presentation to the European Society of Surgical Oncology. Joint Meeting of ESSO, BASO and CAO. Heidelberg, June 10, 1994
54. Herrera L, Villarreal JR (1992) Incidence of metastases from rectal adenicarcinoma in small lymph nodes detected by a clearing technique. Dis Colon Rectum 35:783–788
55. Hojo K, Koyama Y (1982) Lymphatic spread and its value in rectal cancer. Am J Surg 144:350–354
56. Hojo K, Sawada T, Moriya Y (1989) An analysis of survival and voiding, sexual function after wide iliopelvic lymphadenectomy in patients with adenocarcinoma of the rectum, compared with conventional lymphadenectomy. Dis Colon Rectum 32:128–133
57. Horn A, Halvorsen JF, Morild I (1989) Transanal extirpation for early rectal cancer. Dis Colon Rectum 32:769–772
58. Horn A, Halvorsen JF, Dahl O (1990) Preoperative radiotherapy in operable rectal cancer. Dis Colon Rectum 33:823–828
59. Houbiers J, Brand A, van de Watering LMG et al. (1994) Randomized controlled trial comparing transfusion of leucocyte-depleted or buffy-coat-depleted blood in surgery for colorectal cancer. Lancet 334:573–578
60. Isbister WH (1990) Basingstoke revisited. Aust NZ J Surg 60:243–246
61. Isenberg J, Keller HW, Pichlmaier H (1995) Middle and lower third rectum carcinoma: sphincter saving or abdominoperineal resection? Eur J Surg Oncol 21:265–268
62. Jones PF, Thomson HJ (1982) Long term results of a consistent policy of sphincter preservation in the treatment of carcinoma of the rectum. Br J Surg 67:564–568
63. Karanjia ND, Schach DJ, North WRS, Heald RJ (1990) "Close shave" in anterior resection. Br J Surg 77:510–512
64. Karanjia ND, Corder AP, Bearn P, Heald RJ (1994) Leakage from stapled low anastomosis after total mesorectal excision for carcinoma of the rectum. Br J Surg 81:1224- 1226
65. Koyama Y, Moriya Y, Hojo K (1984) Effects of systematic lymphadenectomy for adenocarcinoma of the rectum. Jpn J Clin Oncol 14:623–632
66. Krook JE, Moertel Ch, Gunderson LL et al. (1991) Effective surgical adjuvant therapy for high-risk rectal carcinoma. N Engl J Med 324:709–715
67. Lee JF, Mauer VM, Block GE (1973) Anatomic relations of pelvic autonomic nerves to pelvic operations. Arch Surg 107:324–328
68. Lloyd-Davies OV (1948) Radical excision of carcinoma of the rectum with conservation of the sphincters. Proc R Soc Med 41:822–826
69. Localio SA, Eng K, Coppa GF (1983) Abdominosacral resection for midrectal cancer. Ann Surg 198:320–324
70. MacFarlane JK, Ryall RDH, Heald RJ (1993) Mesorectal excision for rectal cancer. Lancet 341:457–460
71. Marks G, Mohiuddin MM, Masoni L, Pecchioli L (1990) High dose radiation and full-thickness local excision. Dis Colon Rectum 33:735–759
72. Marsh PJ, James RD, Schofield PF (1995) Definition of local recurrence after surgery for rectal carcinoma. Br J Surg 82:465–468
73. Mason AY (1977) Trans-sphincteric approach to rectal lesions. Surg Ann 9:171–194
74. McArdle CS, Hole D (1991) Impact of variability among surgeons on postoperative morbidity and mortality and ultimate survival. Br Med J 302:1501–1505
75. McCall JL, Cox MR, Wattchow DA (1995) Analysis of local recurrence rates after surgery alone for rectal cancer. Int J Colorect Dis 10:126–132
76. McDermott FT, Hughes ERS, Pihl E et al. (1985) Local recurrence after potentially curative resection for rectal cancer in a series of 1008 patients. Br J Surg 72:34–37
77. Mettlin C, Mittelman A, Natarajan N et al. (1981) Trends in the United States for the management of adenocarcinoma of the rectum. Surg Gynecol Obstet 153:701–706

78. Michelassi F, Block GE, Vannuci L, Montag A, Chappell R (1988) A 5-to 21-year follow-up and analysis of 250 patients with rectal adenocarcinoma. Ann Surg 208:379–380
79. Michelassi F, Block GE (1992) Morbidity and mortality of wide pelvic lymphadenectomy for rectal adenocarcinoma. Dis Colon Rectum 35:1143–1147
80. Michelassi F, Vannuci L, Alaya JA, Chappel R, Goldberg R, Block GE (1990) Local recurrence after curative resection of colorectal carcinoma. Surgery 108:787–793
81. Miles WE (1908) A method of performing abdomino-perineal resection for carcinoma of the rectum and of the terminal portion of the pelvic colon. Lancet II:1812–1813
82. Miles WE (1923) Cancer of the rectum. Lettsomiam Lectures. Harrison and Sons, London, p 63
83. Minsky BD, Cohen AM, Enker WE, Mies C (1991) Sphincter preservation in rectal cancer by local excision and postoperative radiation therapy. Cancer 67:908–914
84. Moran MR, James EC, Rothenberger DA, Goldberg SM (1992) Prognostic value of positive lymph nodes in rectal cancer. Dis Colon Rectum 35:579–581
85. Moreira LF, Hizuta A, Iwagaki H et al. (1994) Lateral lymph node dissection for rectal carcinoma below the peritoneal reflection. Br J Surg 81:293–296
86. Moriya Y, Hojo K, Sawada T, Koyama Y (1989) Significance of lateral node dissection for advanced rectal carcinoma at or below the peritoneal reflection. Dis Colon Rectum 32:307–315
87. Moriya Y (1993) Pelvic node dissection with autonomic nerve sparing for invasive lower rectal cancer: Japanese experience. In: Wanebo HJ (ed) Colorectal cancer. Mosby, St. Louis, p 274
88. Morson BC, Bussey HJR, Samoorian S (1977) Policy of local excision for early rectal carcinoma of the colorectum. Gut 18:1045–1050
89. Moynihan BGA (1908) The surgical treatment of cancer of the sigmoid flexure and rectum: with special attention to the principles observed. Surg Gynecol Obstet 6:463–466
90. Nelson H, Beart RW Jr (1993) Surgical management: optimal procedures and overall results. In: Wanebo HJ (ed) Colorectal cancer. Mosby, St. Louis, p 199
91. Neville R, Fielding LP, Amendola C (1987) Local tumor recurrence after curative resection for rectal cancer: a ten hospital review. Dis Colon Rectum 30:12–17
92. NIH Consensus Conference (1990) Adjuvant therapy for patients with colorectal cancer. JAMA 264:1444–1450
93. Norgren J, Svensson JO (1985) Anal implantation metastasis from carcinoma of the sigmoid colon and rectuma risk when performing anterior resection with the EEA-stapler? Br J Surg 72:602
94. Norstein J, Bergan A, Langmark F (1993) Risk factors for local recurrence after radical surgery for rectal carcinoma: a prospective multicentre study. Br J Surg 80 [Suppl]:S22
95. O'Connell MJ, Martenson JA, Wieand HS et al. (1994) Improving adjuvant therapy for rectal cancer by combining protracted infusion fluorouracil with radiation therapy after curative surgery. N Engl J Med 331:502–507
96. Pezim ME, Nicholls RJ (1984) Survival after high or low ligation of the inferior mesenteric artery during curative surgery for rectal cancer. Ann Surg 200:729–733
97. Phillips RK, Hittinger R, Blesovsky L, Fry JS, Fielding P (1984) Local recurrence following "curative" surgery for large bowel cancer: I. The overall picture. Br J Surg 71:12–16
98. Phillips RKS, Hittinger R, Bleskovsky L et al. (1984) Local recurrence following "curative" surgery for large bowel cancer: II. The rectum and rectosigmoid. Br J Surg 71:17–20
99. Pilipshen SJ, Heilweil M, Quan SHQ et al. (1984) Patterns of pelvic recurrence following definitive resections of rectal cancer. Cancer 53:1354–1362
100. Pollett WG, Nicholls RJ (1982) The relationship between the extent of distal clearance and survival and local recurrence rates after curative anterior resection for adenocarcinoma of the rectum. Ann Surg 198:159–163
101. Quirke P, Dixon MF, Durdey P, Williams NS (1986) Local recurrence of rectal cancer due to inadequate surgical resection. Lancet II:996–999
102. Rao AR, Kagan AR, Chan PM, Gilbert HA, Nussbaum H, Hintz BL (1981) Patterns of recurrence following curative resection alone for adenocarcinoma of the rectum and sigmoid colon. Cancer 48:1492–1495

103. Reid JD, Robins RE, Atkinson KG (1984) Pelvic recurrence after anterior resection and EEA stapling anastomosis for potentially curable carcinoma of the rectum. Am J Surg 147:629–632
104. Reinbach DH, McGregor JR, Murray GD et al. (1994) Effect of the surgeon's specialty interest on the type of resection performed for colorectal cancer. Dis Colon Rectum 37:1020–1023
105. Rich T, Gunderson LL, Lew R et al. (1983) Patterns of recurrence of rectal cancer after potentially curative surgery. Cancer 52:1317–1329
106. Sauer I, Bacon H (1951) Influence of lateral spread of cancer of the rectum on radicality of operation and prognosis. Am J Surg 81:111–120
107. Scholefield HJ, Northover JMA (1995) Surgical management of rectal cancer (for debate). Br J Surg 82:745–748
108. Stearns MW, Deddish MR (1959) Five-year results of abdominopelvic lymphnode dissection for carcinoma of the rectum. Dis Colon Rectum 3:169–172
109. Sugarbaker PH, Corlew S (1982) Influence of surgical techniques on survival in patients with colorectal carcinoma. Dis Colon Rectum 25:545–557
110. Surtees P, Ritchie JK, Phillips RKS (1990) High versus low ligation of the inferior mesenteric artery in rectal cancer. Br J Surg 77:618–621
111. Swiss Group for Clinical Cancer Research (SAKK) (1995) Long-term results of single course of adjuvant intraportal chemotherapy for colorectal cancer. Lancet 345:349–353
112. Tornquist A, Ekelund J, Leandoer L (1982) The value of intensive follow-up after curative resection for colorectal carcinoma. Br J Surg 69:725–728
113. Treurniet-Donker AD, Putten WLJ van, Wereldsma JCJ (1991) Postoperative radiation therapy for rectal cancer. Cancer 67:2042–2048
114. Turnbull RB, Kyle K, Watson FR et al. (1967) Cancer of the colon; the influence of the no-touch technique on survival rates. Ann Surg 166:420–427
115. Vogel P, Klosterhafen B (1988) Die chirurgische Anatomie der Rectum- und Analgefäße. Langenb Arch Chir 373:264–269
116. Wiggers T, Jeekel J, Arends JW et al. (1985) The no-touch isolation technique in colon cancer: a prospective controlled multicentre trial. Br J Surg 72 (Suppl):S135
117. Williams NS (1993) Surgical treatment of rectal cancer. In: Keighly MRB, Williams NS (eds) Surgery of the anus, rectum and colon. Saunders, London, p 393
118. Williams NS, Johnston D (1984) Survival and recurrence after sphincter saving resection and abdominoperineal resection for carcinoma of the middle third of the rectum. Br J Surg 71:278–282
119. Williams NS, Dixon MF, Johnston D (1983) Reappraisal of the 5 centimetre rule of distal excision for carcinoma of the rectum: a study of distal intramural spread and of patients' survival. Br J Surg 70:150–154
120. Wolff BG (1992) Lateral margins of resection in adenocarcinoma of the rectum. World J Surg 16:467–469
121. Zirngibl H, Husemann B, Hermanek P (1990) Intraoperative spillage of tumor cells in surgery for rectal cancer. Dis Colon Rectum 33:610–614

CHAPTER 15

Total Mesorectal Excision:
History and Anatomy of an Operation

Richard J. Heald

Introduction

Surgery has never been a science. Most of the "standard" operations that are regularly performed were established, like the boundaries of the countries in which we live, as accidents of history. Most of the surgical papers with pretensions to real scientific method are about the trappings of surgery rather than the actual craft which is the essence of its daily practise. Chemotherapy, anaesthetic and antibiotic agents, and sometimes the consequences and outcomes of surgery are often well reported and are the subject of controlled prospective trials, but the actual building blocks themselves remain poorly defined.

Perhaps this is the reason why the assumption is widely made in the medical profession by those concerned with colorectal cancer that the only major improvements to be achieved are in respect of adjuvant therapies. Indeed, from the management of this, the commonest of all curable major cancers, a worldwide chemotherapy health care revolution is daily reaching the headlines and the corridors of power, while major changes in the daily practise of surgery are regarded as being largely matters of technical detail.

In Great Britain, for example, plans are afoot to reorganise cancer services on the basis of the availability of medical oncology services with scant regard for the background realities. It is surgeons, radiologists and radiotherapists, backed by the skills of histopathologists, who currently manage and, for practical purposes, are the only sources of permanent cure of any of the major epithelial neoplasms.

The standard operation for rectal cancer in most of the Western world throughout the whole of this century has been the abdominoperineal resection (APE), as advocated by Miles in 1908 [13]. As recently as 1993, Murray and Veidenheimer described it as the "gold standard by which all other operations must be judged, not only for carcinomas of the distal third of the rectum but for all bulky tumours of the middle third as well" [14].

There can be few more dramatic examples of the limitations of historically based "standard operations". Miles had scarcely published his procedure before it had become standard practice, and relatively few references appear in the literature apart from the written proceedings of the Medical Society of London, where he gave three Lettsomian lectures on the subject many years after it had become widely practised.

In the English-speaking world, the more thoughtful and scholarly contributions of Henri Hartmann [7, 8] have been largely disregarded, and a huge block of tissue including the levator ani muscle, the anal sphincter and the contents of the ischio-rectal fossa have been offered up by the surgical profession on a daily basis as a "ritual sacrifice". In my opinion, the sacrifice of these tissues is a "standard" for which no scientific evidence can in fact be adduced at all.

A history of restorative excision would not be appropriate here, but its arrival in the 1940s and 1950s did seem on a common sense basis to threaten the apparent "radicality" of Miles' original operation as illustrated in his own diagram from the Lettsomian Lecture (Fig. 1a). The cluster of lymph nodes in the ischio-rectal fossa on his diagram have not once occurred in the last 407 cases referred to me. Their existence was largely a figment of Miles' imagination based on the frequency with which he saw recurrences after APE.

Some early reports of anterior resection (AR) raised doubts in many minds about whether the local control and cure rates would be unacceptably increased by this challenge to orthodoxy [11]. Famous surgeons such as Gabriel at St. Mark's intoned against the evils of such irresponsible challenges to established practice. Those who were determined to persevere produced a further orthodox "standard" for which no scientific evidence whatever was forthcoming, i.e. the "5 cm rule" [2, 3, 6]. All subsequent data have demonstrated quite clearly that the palpable lower edge of the tumour is indeed the microscopic lower edge in all but a very tiny percentage of cases [16]. The arbitrary choice of the 5 cm rule for the muscle wall of distal clearance has cost millions of people their anal canals!

The battles of the 1940s and 1950s were to be fought again in the 1970s and early 1980s after the introduction of circular stapling devices. These instruments, which were developed and improved rapidly by American technological know-how, made it easier for surgeons to go lower with their anastomoses than they had felt happy and safe to do with manual anastomoses. Early reports gathered in profusion to suggest that this new wave of liberties was being paid for by both anastomotic leakage and, more seriously, by locally recurrent disease [11].

Fig. 1. a Ernest Miles' original diagram demonstrating his concept of a "cylindrical" field of spread justifying abdominoperineal excision. **b** Our opinion on lymphatic spread within the mesorectum

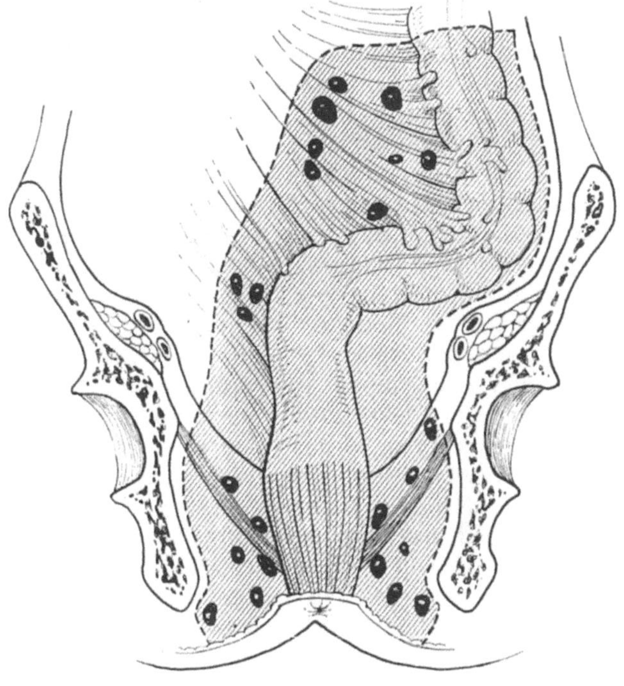

a

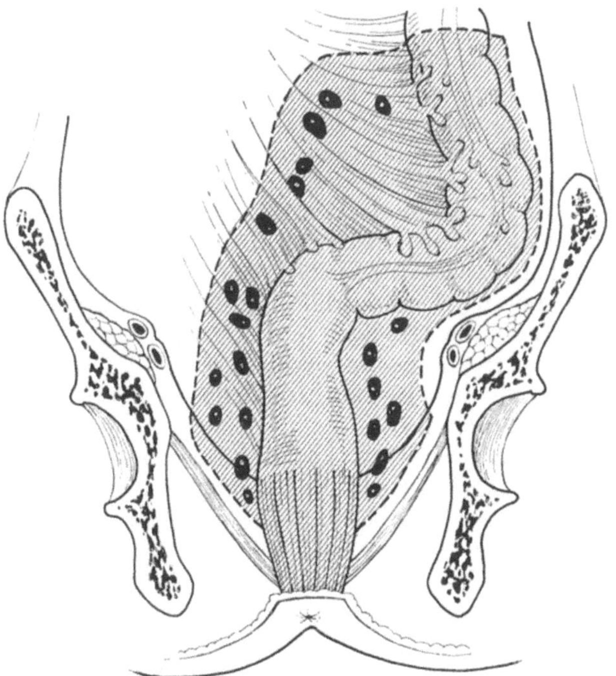

b

Concept of the Mesorectum

The word "mesorectum" appears in no anatomical textbooks, and a Medline search of the surgical literature conducted in June 1995 shows no references to the structure prior to 1980. I believe that I can claim responsibility for writing about it first, although its existence was alluded to by Dukes and pointed out to me by one of my chiefs at Guy's Hospital, Rex Lawrie [9]. It commanded attention then because its division during anterior resection as performed in the 1960s constituted a tiresome and haemorrhagic phase of the operation. A later mentor in my surgical upbringing, Professor John Goligher, elaborated on the word mesorectum by clarifying my own concept of an "integral visceral mesentery of the hind gut" – precise words with a precise meaning. He did so to explain to others what he believed I meant by the word and in doing so gives us a perfect definition for standardising a block of tissue which it is rational for us to excise in a rectal cancer operation.

At the beginning of this century, Moynihan, that hero of British surgical history, very beautifully described cancer surgery as being "the applied anatomy of the lymphatic system". This is most particularly true of colorectal cancer, which has been frequently shown to have lymphatic involvement in more than one half of all cases; modern "best" results confirm that this is often the only spread, i.e. it is present without distant metastases which would preclude cure. The very fact that an avascular plane could be developed around the mesorectum and that it is embryologically distinct from the surrounding parietal structures led me to argue the inherent probability that this lymphatic spread would be confined within it (Fig. 1b). This may be the first example of the practical reality that the field of spread of cancer may remain for a considerable time within a specific embryological entity – and that optimal surgery requires removal of this entity intact.

The concept of the mesorectum, however, does not appear in the anatomy books because it does not readily come from the dissection of the cadaver – a fact which has been brought home to us in recent months when we have tried to establish anatomical prosection workshops at the Royal College of Surgeons in London. This anatomical concept comes instead from surgeons dissecting human tissues in their live state. The areolar planes between tissues of embryologically distinct origins are the essential stock in trade of every abdominal surgeon. They are much more clearly apparent in the live patient, where they provide the means of movement of one tissue upon another, and the means of access for the surgeon to a relatively bloodless separation zone between one organ and another.

Surgeons in the first half of this century were more than a little restricted by the inaccessibility and the bleeding which tended to occur when they strayed into the lower reaches of the pelvis. Thus when most of today's surgeons were taught about anterior resection and about APE, there was more than a hint of "sleight of hand" and "mystery" to the delivery from the depths of a tattered and sometimes torn tube of rectum with an irregular and patchy covering of fat. Most of us "trainees" could not really see how this block of tissue had been created, and very few of our chiefs explained it to us. Miles considered that the procedure was easy enough and stated that it should be accomplished in less than 45 min.

As has been recently emphasised by Enker and others [5], the practice of inserting one's hand into the loose areolar tissue between the mesorectum and the sacral promontory was fraught with hazard because of the condensation that occurs lower down, rather firmly binding the back of the mesorectum to the front of the middle part of the sacrum. This condensation has been called the recto-sacral ligament and, as Enker emphasises [5], the hand thrust down in this way will be directed by the ligament straight into the mesorectum and thus across the commonest field of spread of the typical mid-rectal carcinoma. It must be particularly borne in mind in this regard that the superior rectal artery and vein with their surrounding lymph nodes are very close to the posterior margin of the mesorectum, so that respect for its covering areolar tissue is crucial to the whole practice of total mesorectal excision: involved nodes may be only 1–2 mm away from the plane of excision.

Operative Technique

Total mesorectal excision and stapled reconstruction were therefore an attempt at a spoken and written description of what I felt in the early 1980s to be a sensible way to improve this "snatch and run" approach. The mesorectum was a rational monobloc to remove to optimise rectal cancer cure and to preserve as many anal canals as possible [9]. Criticism and attention had been drawn to the dangers of going still lower with AR after the arrival of the circular stapling devices in the late 1970s [11]. It was therefore determined in Basingstoke at that time that fastidious efforts would be directed towards the complete excision of the mesorectum by careful pursuit of the innermost proper areolar plane around the integral visceral mesentery of the hind gut.

The upper limit was determined as the origin of the inferior mesenteric artery from the aorta, but preserving 1 cm so as to safeguard the divisions of the sympathetic nerves around its origin. On occasions where it was deemed desirable, several more centimetres of the artery would be stripped distally of their mesenteric surround so that the ascending left colic artery could be preserved. Subsequent studies showed this to be of rather little practical value, and it is certainly of little oncological importance in defining the upper limit of the mesorectal package [4].

Following the posterior plane downwards towards the aortic bifurcation, the "pedicle package" is carefully dissected from the sympathetic nerves on the front of the aorta and its bifurcation and the top of the mesorectum identified within the "wishbone" bifurcation of the pre-sacral nerves. This is carefully preserved, and there is good clinical evidence that its sacrifice leads to retrograde ejaculation.

In the mid-line posteriorly, the plane between mesorectum and pre-sacral tissues is developed downwards and the condensation called the rectosacral ligament cut through under direct vision in such a way as to preserve the coverings of the mesorectum. This provides access to the depths of the pelvis, where the bi-lobed mesorectum can be painstakingly dissected out from the levator gutters.

Laterally, the plane is developed between the hypogastric nerves (pre-sacral nerves) and the lateral surface of the mesorectum. As this plane is developed, it becomes apparent that the tethering points of the mesorectum are in reality points of adherence between the mesorectum and the flattened confluence of sympathetic and parasympathetic nerves, which is called the inferior hypogastric plexus. The principal parasympathetic contributor to this plexus comes forward from the anterior aspects of the third and fourth sacral nerve roots and comprises the principal pelvic splanchnic parasympathetic outflow. In the experience of the author, the largest of these is to be found just distal to the piriformis muscle under the sacral fascia, sometimes a prominent pillar running from back to front adherent to the mesorectum and sometimes covered with fascia and somewhat overshadowed by piriform muscle itself. Thus in conventional surgery it is presumably protected in some people, though it is often damaged or removed. This flattened nerve plexus curves slightly medially behind the vas deferens to become the neurovascular bundle, which has been so well described and demonstrated by Walsh lower down in his descriptions of the operation of radical prostatectomy [12]. Where they most obviously abut on to the rectal surgeons "tumour package", they are running along the lateral edge of Denonvillier's fascia behind the lateral extremities of the seminal vesicles. Lower still, they run along the postero-lateral aspect of the prostate, where only a little areolar tissue separates them from the anterior aspect of the muscle of the anorectum. Damage to them at this point is rather common if the surgeon feels motivated to remove a "sliver" of prostate in his attempt to clear an anteriorly situated cancer below 5 cm in a male patient.

The definition of the anterior plane of the rectal cancer specimen deserves special attention in male patients; if the seminal vesicles are approached anterior to the peritoneal reflection by division of the peritoneum a perfect plane can be entered anterior to Denonvillier's fascia. This distinct fascia is well developed in men as a shiny anterior surface of a complete circumferential surrounding mesentery, i.e. the mesorectum. Thus the pathologist can readily identify the front of the specimen because it is the site of the peritoneal reflection and, below it, of the shiny Denonvillier's fascia. Lower down, this fascia becomes adherent to the tissues at the back of the lower part of the seminal vesicles and the top of the prostate, so that the lowest part of the anterior wall of the rectum has little intervening tissue between muscle and the posterior wall of the prostate, i.e. at this level the mesorectum is virtually absent.

Lower down at the back, however, the mesorectum is generously provided as a bilateral globular expansion of the mesentery out into the lower recesses of the pelvis, distal to the pillars of the autonomic nerves at the sides. This is clearly the basis for the damage which so often occurred in the past to the parasympathetic nerves with consequent loss of sexual potency and the ability to achieve an erection. It is said that many of the great names in British surgery used to teach that "if you had not made the patients impotent you would not have cured them of cancer". A second site for possible damage, as already described, is behind the prostate, where the lowest anterior rectal cancers pose the greatest technical difficulties of all.

The middle rectal arteries are usually absent or negligible in size, and the so-called lateral ligaments have been confirmed in six out of six biopsy examinations to be what I believe they are, i.e. the parasympathetic and sympathetic nerve supply of the rectum itself. The secret of not making the patient impotent is the division only of the horizontal limb of the "stub" of nerve entering the mesorectum, i.e. of not removing the whole T junction.

Standardisation of Rectal Cancer Surgery

The first requirement for standardisation of rectal cancer surgery is to define the package of tissue to be removed. In surgical terms, this is as described as above. In terms of conventional anatomy, the relations of the block of tissue can readily be described.

Anteriorly within the pelvis in males, the upper third of the rectum is covered with peritoneum and related therefore to intraperitoneal structures such as ileum. Below the peritoneal reflection Denonvillier's fascia, its anterior surface, is related to the back of the seminal vesicles, while below this again the lower third is related to the back of the prostate.

Posteriorly, the mesorectum is related to the aorta and its bifurcation with its covering nerve plexuses. Lower in the pelvis lie the pre-sacral fat pad and the sacrum, coccyx and ano-coccygeal raphe, which give the mesorectum its bi-lobed appearance posteriorly. Hence my rule of thumb that if you have not seen the bi-lobed lipoma you have not done a proper TME.

On each side, the nerve plexuses and fasciae lie on the surface of the piriformis muscle and, beyond this, the pelvic floor and levator ani muscles. At its extreme caudal end, the rectum joins the internal sphincter of the anus with an acute posterior curve. At this point, the anorectal junction is within the sling of the puborectal muscle, which is important in the maintenance of continence – particularly in guarding against faecal and flatal stress incontinence.

In females, these relations are altered anteriorly, where both the middle and the lower third of the rectum lie behind the posterior vaginal wall. Denonvillier's fascia and anterior mesorectum between it and the anterior rectal wall are often rudimentary in females. However, it is common, even in anteriorly placed cancers, for there to be a satisfactory mobile plane due to the areolar tissue which lies between the vagina and the anterior aspect of the rectum.

"On table" vaginal examination is a key precursor to TME, as this mobility determines whether excision of the posterior vaginal wall is necessary. This is important because surgical orthodoxy used to dictate that the posterior vaginal wall must be sacrificed – most particularly in all anteriorly placed rectal carcinomas. It is inherent in the hypothesis of TME that cure and local control depend upon the liberation of the embryologically determined specimen *only* along such planes. I would suggest that sacrifice of the posterior vaginal wall is rarely necessary, except when it is tethered to or involved by the primary tumour.

In addition to the basic definition of the mesorectum given above, there are two major practical objectives for the operating surgeon. The first relates to the avoidance of tearing of the specimen – a TME may conceivably be "total" but not "curative" if it is torn close to the edge of the primary tumour. The second of these "dynamic" objectives for the surgeon is the avoidance of implantation of exfoliated cells. This, like so many other aspects of cancer surgery, remains unproven as a significant hazard. Nevertheless, it is my view that steps should be taken to guard against it. Therefore it is necessary that the lower edge of the specimen along the muscle tube should be defined and either clamped or stapled. This staple line may be called the pathologist's staple line and is an alternative to the clamp. It is essential that the distal segment is thoroughly washed below this seal. Either a manual purse string or a second staple line (the patient's staple line) will be needed prior to the use of a circular stapling device to join the colon or a short colon pouch to the anal canal.

The actual technique for stapling has undergone steady development during the last 17 years and has been the crucial facilitator in improving the quality of deep pelvic dissection. The original Russian SPTU gun of the late 1970s has been replaced by successively improved circular and linear staplers. The mid-1990s "state of the art" combination for low pelvic reconstruction would involve a U.S. Surgical Corporation (USSC) GIA (or equivalent) for creating an ultra-short colon pouch (2×5 cm) and two PI30 linear staple cartridges (or equivalent), one to seal the specimen and another in place of a "purse string". These set the scene for a stapled low colorectal or coloanal anastomosis with a flip-top Premium EE 31 or 34 circular stapler (or equivalent). This is a lot of staplers, and it is expensive. However, it represents one of the most worthwhile examples of higher initial costs saving money in the end – colostomy bags for life and a higher risk of local recurrence are the two largest "real" costs of rectal carcinoma, and they can both be avoided by better technique. The cost of the staplers is readily recouped in under 6 months in terms of colostomy bags alone. In national terms (e.g. for the UK) this could save £ 10 million in one year – a figure which would be cumulative with each year of survival.

Personal Results

The application of these principles has been tested in Basingstoke on 407 consecutive patients referred with rectal cancer. Figure 2 shows the distribution of operations, reflecting a profound distaste on my part for the performance of APE. A total of 86% of patients had AR of the rectum and only 7% had APE, both incorporating TME. Only for the very highest rectal tumours between 12 and 15 cm where 5 cm of mesorectum distal to the tumour could readily be excised without tapering inwards closer than 5 cm was the low pelvic dissection avoided and mesorectal transection and anastomosis around 8–10 cm undertaken.

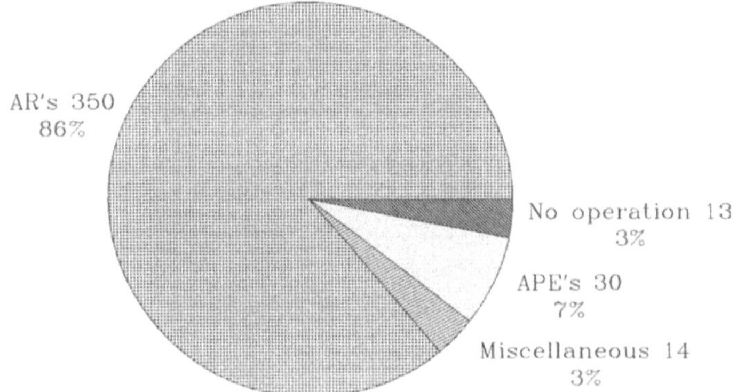

Fig. 2. Choice of operation in 407 consecutive referrals. *AR*, anterior resection; *APE*, abdominoperineal excision

Thirteen patients in a 17-year period were excluded because they failed to reach the operating theatre (97% operability). Thus over 90% of those undergoing radical surgery had AR and 85% of these TME.

Survival analysis by the lifetable method in 359 patients with sufficient data for inclusion on 1 June 1994 is given in Fig. 3a. In the two minority survival curves at the top and bottom of the lifetable, it will be seen that local excision was used very rarely and so far without adverse consequence in terms of local failure. It will also be seen that the small number of patients undergoing palliative Hartmann surgery or colostomy only died very rapidly indeed.

A number of critics of this series have alluded that undue selectivity has been applied to the referrals. We will refute the assertion that any significant differences that may exist between this series and other published series can be attributed to the exclusion of unfavourable cases. We agree with Hermanek's observation that the general rule is that, provided prospective and consecutive data collection has been used, those units with the best results are usually those with the least exclusions [10]. This is important because the view that good results reflect selection bias is very widely held and has significantly slowed the acceptance of TME. The failure to identify clearly in the past every single exclusion, even those 13 who died before reaching the operating room, has perhaps contributed to this delay.

The survival data are based on an unusually comprehensive regime of intensive follow-up; 3-monthly for 2 years, 6-monthly for 3 years and annually thereafter. Senior consultant staff have examined the patients on virtually every visit, carcino-embryonic antigen (CEA) tests have been undertaken routinely, and endoscopies, ultrasound and computed tomography (CT) scans as clinically indicated, and no patient has been lost to follow-up. Figures 4–6 refer to both local recurrence and overall recurrence including local recurrence; only deaths proven to be from other causes with proven freedom from recurrent disease are censored at the point on the lifetable where the relevant death occurred. Figure 4 shows the expectation of cure in all patients considered to

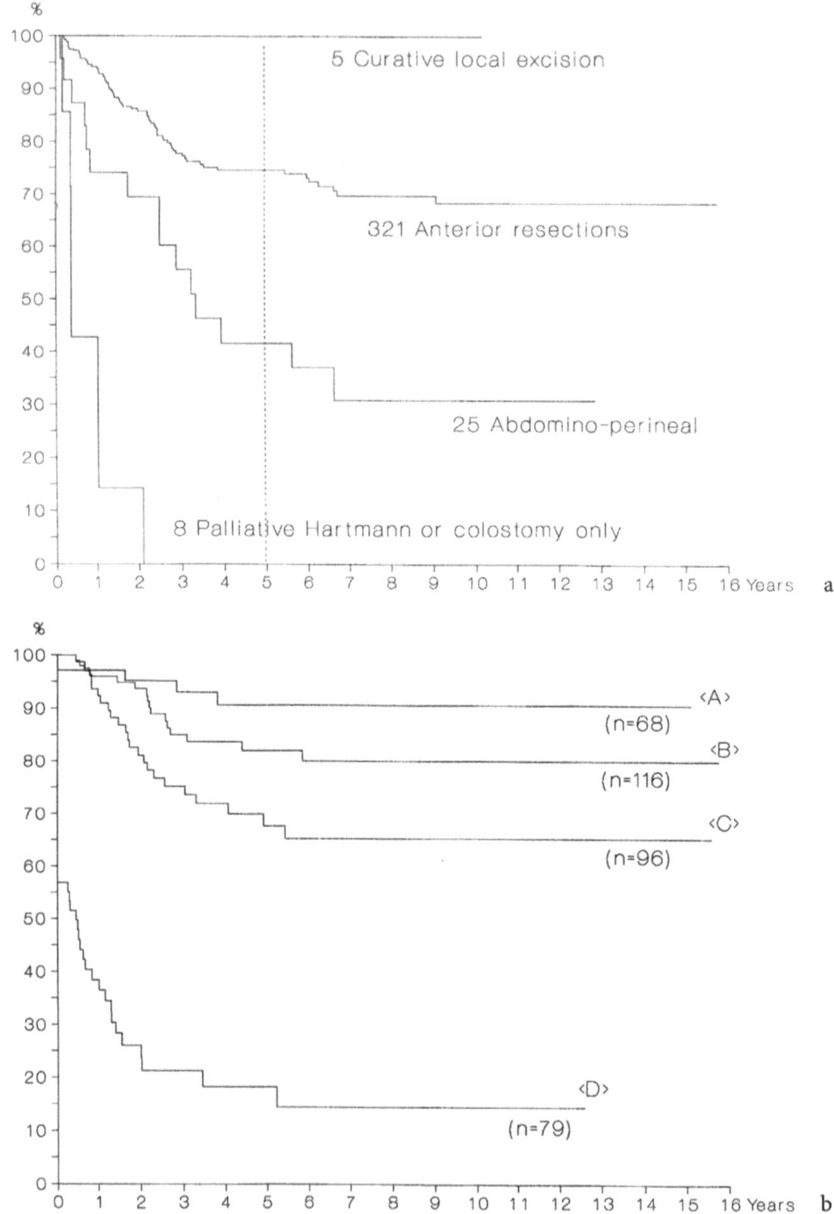

Fig. 3. a Survival analysis (by lifetable method). Event is death with recurrence of any kind. Only deaths proven to be from other causes in patients free of tumour are censored. **b** Survival until recurrence by Dukes' stage at operation

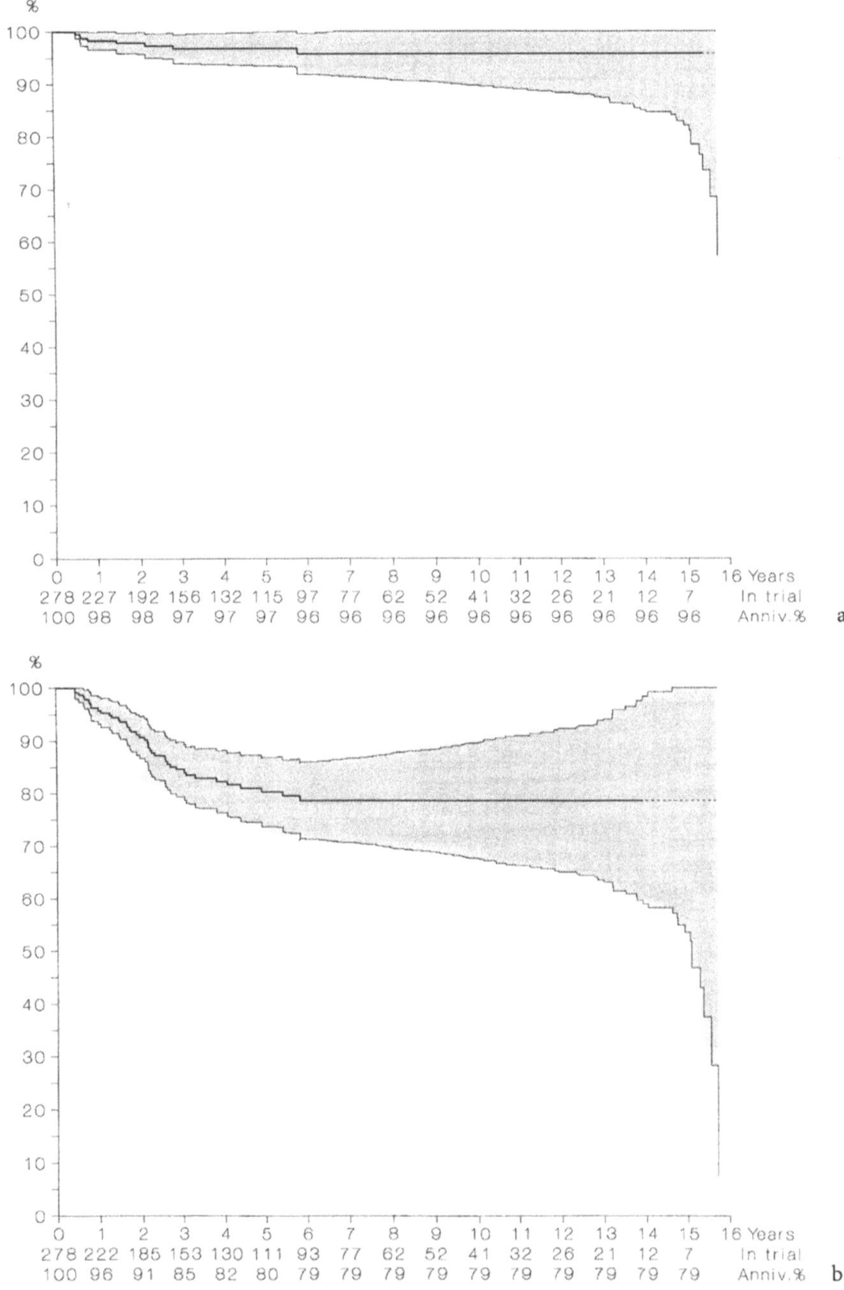

Fig. 4. a Local recurrence. Lifetable analysis until recurrence with or without metastatic disease in "curative" operations. The local recurrence rate is 3% at 5 years (95% confidence interval, CI, 0%–7%), and 4% at 10 years. **b** Lifetable analysis until recurrence of any kind in "curative" operations. The recurrence rate is 20% at 5 years (95% CI, 13%–26%), and 21% at 10 years

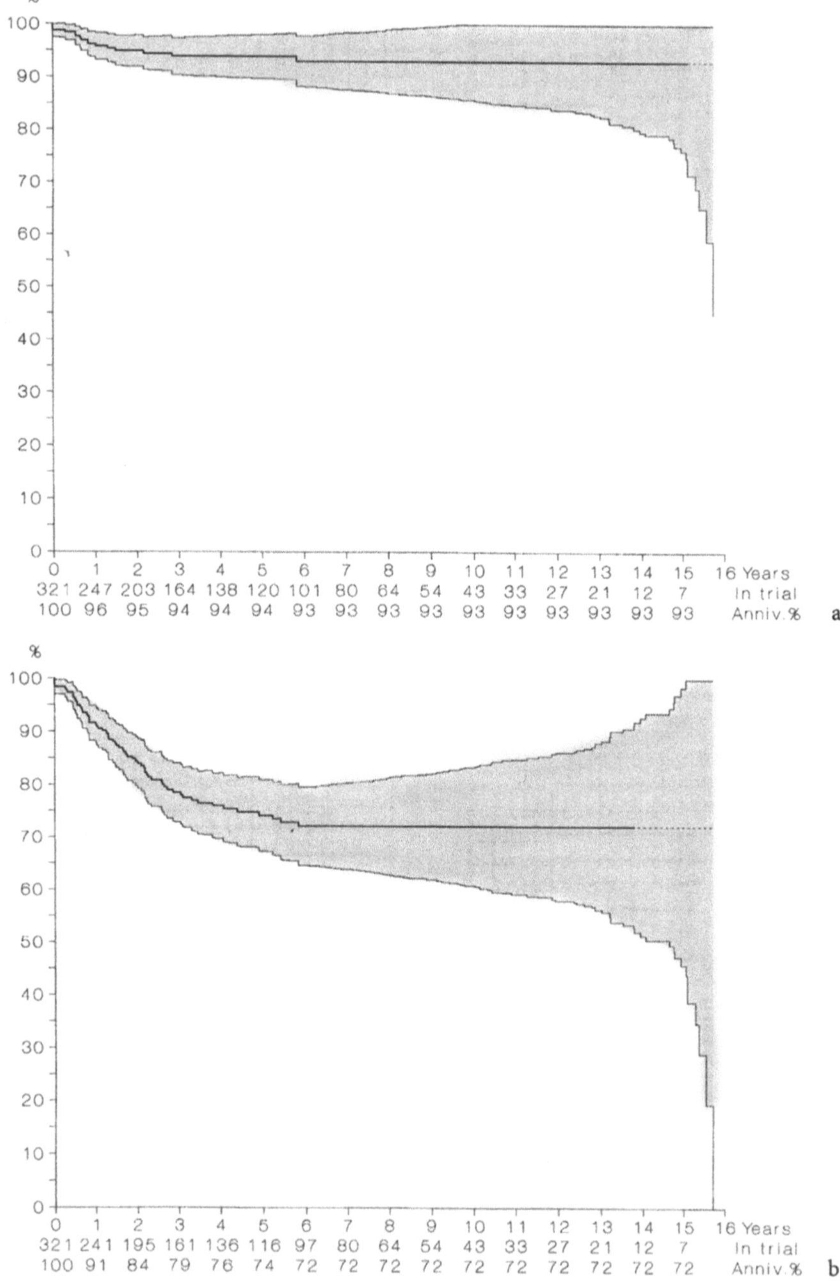

Fig. 5. a Survival analysis until local recurrence of all rectal cancer operations excluding only those with distant metastases, i.e. no exclusion for local residual disease. The local recurrence rate is 6% at 5 years (95% confidence interval, CI, 2%–10%), and 7% at 10 years. **b** Survival until recurrence of any kind of all rectal cancer operations, excluding only those with distant metastases, i.e. no exclusion for local residual disease. The recurrence rate is 26% at 5 years (95% CI, 19%–32%), and 28% at 10 years

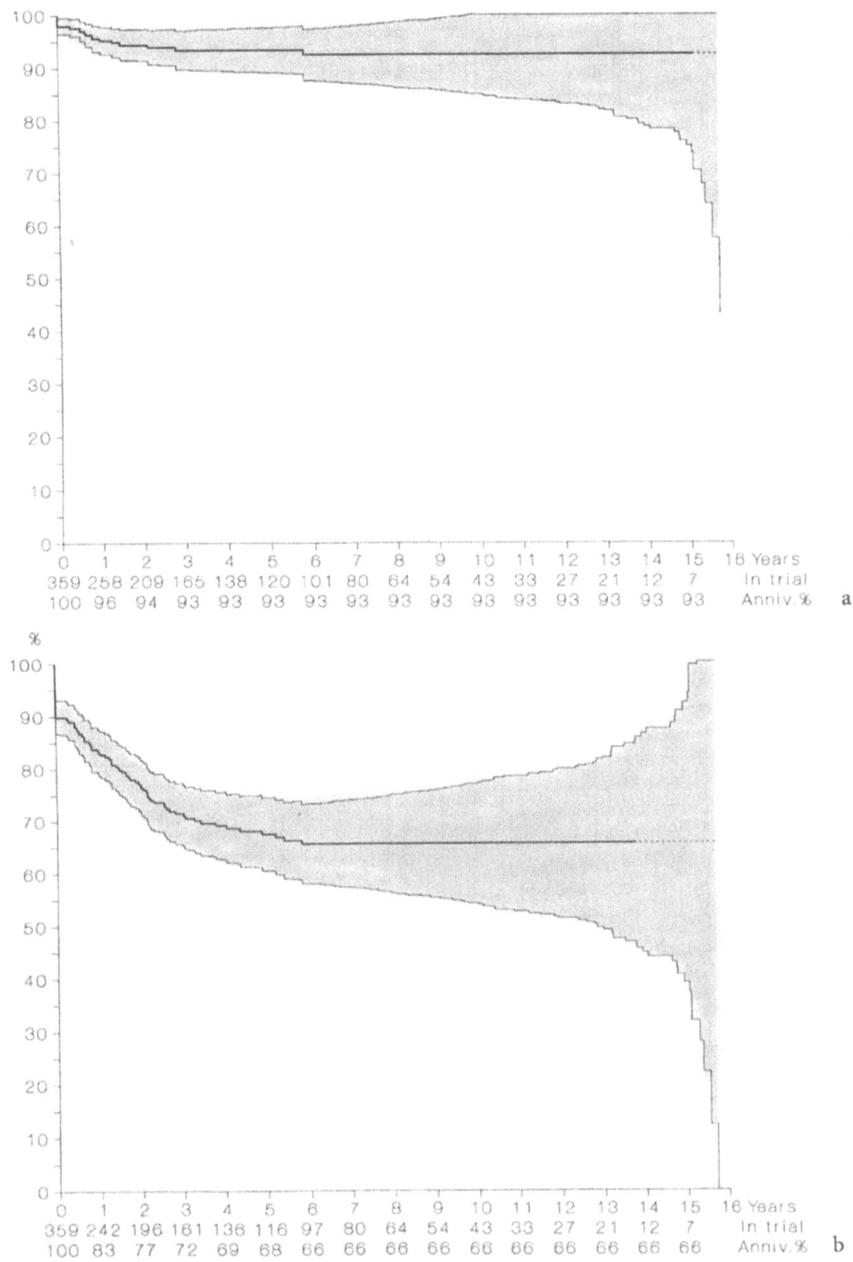

Fig. 6. a Survival until local recurrence for all rectal cancers including locally incurable and those with metastases. Local recurrence is defined as any recurrence detectable within the pelvis by any means. Actual local recurrence was 7% (95% confidence interval, CI, 3%–11%), and 7% at 10 years. **b** Survival until recurrence for all rectal cancers, including locally incurable and those with metastases. 32% overall recurrence at 5 years (95% CI, 25%–38%), and 34% at 10 years

have had a curative operation, Fig. 5 in all those who had an operation without metastases with no exclusion for adjudged local failure and Fig. 6 the results for all patients whether presenting with metastatic disease or not.

Conclusion

The figures presented raise the possibility that specialisation in and concentration on the detailed technique of TME can virtually eliminate locally recurrent disease as a problem in patients with rectal carcinoma. This is potentially one of the most exciting developments in cancer treatment at this time. It does, however, pose enormous problems in both the organisation of surgical services and the need for the establishment of specialised surgical training facilities.

In the organisation of hospital operating lists, it entails a fundamental change in the attitude to one of the common branches of surgery. Rectal carcinoma ceases to be a 2-h operation which can be performed by any general surgeon and becomes instead the ultimate endeavour of a specialist taking anything from 3 to 5 h. Two committed specialist surgeons are necessary to achieve the best results. Demand on blood transfusion and support services is increased, and the markedly increased risk of anastomotic leakage means that short-term morbidity rates are likely to be increased unless the profession can accept the need for routine temporary defunctioning.

It is necessary to take the longer view on behalf of the patient before the major benefits and cost saving become apparent. The disadvantages for surgeons are substantial both in time and in terms of acceptance that the responsibility for local failure rests with them.

I have spent most of my surgical lifetime steeped in the performance of this one operation and yet I still consider it to be the most difficult operation which I ever perform. Once the defined objectives have been accepted, the rough compromise of former times must be abandoned and the rigorous demands of a lengthy, precise, deep dissection accepted and incorporated in the working week.

Specialisation itself poses huge organisational problems. Most hospitals in most countries still embrace rectal carcinoma as a part of general surgery. In the United Kingdom, most of the six to ten trained surgeons that might be at work in a District General Hospital would regard themselves as qualified to undertake rectal carcinoma operations. If we accept that standardisation is desirable and that it brings substantial benefits to patients, then the number of surgeons in each unit performing such surgery must be reduced to one or two. The educational institutions will need to provide a new kind of surgical training facility which enables people actually to see in the depths of the pelvis.

Happily in the aftermath of the widespread introduction of laparoscopic surgery, much of the basic infrastructure necessary for television teaching of surgery is coming into existence in most Western countries. In the Royal College of Surgeons in England, for example, a new skills workshop (the Hill Skills Centre) has been established largely on the back of the urgent demands posed on surgical training by the introduction of laparoscopy. In Elancourt, South of Paris, the U.S. Surgical Corporation has opened a truly magnificent teaching facility which could similarly be harnessed to this enterprise. My visits to Scandinavia have combined with developments at the Royal College and with a background interest in audiovisual matters to give me some insight into the requirements of an audiovisual teaching programme for TME.

The first need is for a high-quality image. The impact of video in surgical training has probably been minimal in the past for the simple reason that the quality of readily accessible formats such as VHS and of readily affordable cameras was inadequate. Only the highest-quality images can command the attention of surgeons for the time necessary to acquire the expertise. High-definition television would be ideal, but it is formidably expensive and it seems likely that broadcast-quality conventional television, 625 lines in Europe and 525 lines in the United States, will prove to be the most effective compromise. Standard broadcast cameras are too bulky for the operating theatre, and most operating room gantries are unsatisfactory for one reason or another. Even cameras mounted on operating lights are not ideal because of the tendency of surgeons to get their head in the way of the camera. Thus for the Scandinavian Workshops and for the first live transmission to the Royal College of Surgeons "Masterclass", a special Sony camera was used which has a broadcast-quality lens and camera head block mounted on a mobile counterbalanced arm which can be moved by the surgeon with a sterile handle similar to those used for operating room lights. The rest of the camera electronics are mounted on a trolley some way from the patient, while all the modalities of lens control and adjustment are in the hands of a cameraman with a monitor. The scene for a typical workshop is completed by two-way sound communication and a suitable intermediary expert in the room with the workshop participants. In theory, such a workshop could be transmitted to, or involve, very large audiences, but at the present time attempts to increase the size of the audience have been rather unsuccessful. Small participating groups taking turns to scrub and to be involved in the viewing room alternately seem to have been the most effective, as the sense of participation and involvement appears to be a crucial ingredient. The new digital formats will probably bring virtually broadcast-quality images within ready reach of hospital departments using less bulky equipment at lower cost.

At the time of going to press this teaching programme has expanded to more than 80 TV demonstration operations in over forty cities in 11 countries. Nothing of this kind has ever occurred in the history of surgery. Problems remain in the collection of data to facilitate measurement of the impact of all of this work. It is possible to prescribe standards for TME, and it is possible to provide practical training workshops to describe the operation. It is more difficult to define the number of surgeons who are genuinely convinced that the extra effort is worthwhile so that they embark on the painstaking performance of the operation in their future practice. Thus identification of "TME surgeons" that may be tagged in the cancer registries is clearly a practical problem. Fortunately, the efforts of Quirke in the correlation of outcomes with the involvement of circumferential margins on careful histopathological assessment provide a way of auditing the specimens produced by any surgeon [1]. Histopathological workshops to demonstrate detailed audit and to correlate details of surgical technique with success or failure of tumour clearance at the margins seem a rational and constructive way forward. In January 1994, one such workshop at the Rikshospital in Oslo, Norway, attracted pathologists from 28 hospitals, and there is evidence of improved histopathology reporting in Norway as a consequence. It appears probable that really convincing data will first emerge from Norway and Sweden where major changes are already in place.

Certain key issues emerge from this broad spectrum of endeavour. The starting point is the identification of enormous variations in cancer cure rates between surgeons, first by Fielding in the United Kingdom [15] and most recently by Hermanek in Germany [10]. The latter study suggests that the "best" surgeon offers his or her patient five times the prospect of local control and doubles the prospect of permanent cure. No such differences exist in any other major cancer; they spell out clearly the need for a standard operation producing a specimen that can be accurately audited. Teaching methods need to overcome the fundamental difficulties of seeing and understanding the details of deep pelvic dissection. Broadcast-quality audiovisual technology is necessary, together with special experience by surgeons, who must commit their efforts to their surgical audience as well as to the patient. It is probably true to say that the rewards for successful training in pelvic surgery are potentially greater than in any other area of surgical development or of cancer management.

Acknowledgements. Mr. Heald's department wishes to record its special gratitude to the Wessex Cancer Trust and to the patients of southern England who have supported it. The International TME Project is supported by U.S. Surgical Corporation (Auto Suture).

References

1. Adam IJ, Mohamdee MD, Martin IG, Scott N, Finan PJ, Johnston D, Dixon MF, Quirke P (1994) Role of circumferential margin involvement in the local recurrence of rectal cancer. Lancet 344:707–710
2. Cole PP (1913) The intramural spread of rectal carcinoma. Br Med J 1:431–433
3. Connell JF Jr, Rottmo A (1949) Retrograde spread of carcinoma in the rectum and rectosigmoid. Arch Surg 59:807–813
4. Corder AP, Karanjia ND, Williams JD, Heald RJ (1992) Flush aortic tie versus selective preservation of the ascending left colic artery in low anterior resection for rectal carcinoma. Br J Surg 79:680–682
5. Enker WE, Thaber HT, Cranos ML, Polyak T (1995) Total mesorectal excision in the operative treatment of carcinoma of the rectum. J Am Coll Surg 181:335–346
6. Handley WS (1910) The surgery of the lymphatic system. Br Med J 1:922–928
7. Hartmann H (1923) Ablation abdominale des cancers rectosigmoidienne. 30th Congres francais de chirurgie, Strasbourg, p 411
8. Hartmann H (1923) Procède nouveau d'extirpation des cancers de la partie terminale du Colon. Bull et mem de la Societe de Chirurgie Paris, p 1474
9. Heald RJ, Husband EM, Ryall RDH (1982) The mesorectum in rectal cancer surgery – the clue to pelvic recurrence? Br J Surg 69:613–616

10. Hermanek P, Wiebelt H, Staimmer D, Riedl S (1995) Prognostic factors of rectum carcinoma – experience of the German Multi-Centre Study SGCRC. Tumori Suppl 81:60–64
11. Hurst PA, Prout WG, Kelly JM, Bannister JJ, Walker RT (1982) Local recurrence after low anterior resection using the staple gun. Br J Surg 69:275–276
12. Lepor H, Gregerman M, Crosby R, Mostofi FK, Walsh PC (1985) Precise localization of autonomic nerves from pelvic plexus to corpora cavernosa: detailed anatomical study of adult male pelvis. J Urol 133:207–212
13. Miles E (1923) Cancer of the rectum. Harrison, London
14. Murray JJ, Veidenheimer MC (1993) Abdomino-perineal excision of the rectum. In: Fielding LP, Goldberg SM (eds) Rob and Smith's operative surgery, 5th edn. Chapman and Hall, London, p 472
15. Phillips RKS, Hittinger R, Blesovsky L, Fry JS, Fielding LP (1983) Local recurrence after curative surgery for large bowel cancer (1). The overall picture. Br J Surg 71:12–16
16. Williams NS, Dixon MF, Johnston D (1983) Re-appraisal of the 5 cm rule of distal excision for carcinoma of the rectum: a study of distal intramural spread and of patients' survival. Br J Surg 70:150–155

Total Mesorectal Excision with Pelvic Autonomic Nerve Preservation in the Operative Treatment of Rectal Carcinoma

Warren E. Enker, Klaas Havenga, Howard T. Thaler, Alfred M. Cohen, Tatyana Polyak, Milicent Cranor, and Katherine McDermott

Introduction

Total mesorectal excision (TME) has been advocated as the appropriate operation for rectal cancer, reducing the rates of pelvic recurrence and distant spread and improving survival in comparison with conventional operations, even when accompanied by adjuvant therapy [31]. TME appropriately addresses the pathophysiology of rectal cancer, as 65%–80% of patients with rectal cancers present with regional disease limited to the mesorectum, i.e., either full-thickness penetration of the rectal wall or involvement of mesorectal lymph nodes [12]. The rectum and the potentially affected mesorectum must be regarded as a single unit of regional disease to be resected en bloc, with intact negative margins. Anatomically, this unit corresponds to the posterior visceral compartment of the pelvis, in which the rectum and the mesorectum are enveloped within the visceral pelvic fascia [7].

As an operative procedure for primary rectal cancer, TME is reported to accomplish these goals. In recent studies, MacFarlane et al. [31] and Enker et al. [14] have reported a local failure rate of only 5%–8% in over 400 Dukes' B and C patients undergoing resections utilizing the principles of TME. All patients would have been considered "high-risk" patients, meeting the conventional eligibility criteria for adjuvant radiation therapy (RT) and chemotherapy. In contrast to most studies, where metastases occur in 65% of patients, rates of distant metastases were only 23%–25% in both studies, suggesting the cure of regional disease [14, 31]. To examine the success of this approach, we have analyzed the outcome of TME in our own surgical experience.

Methods

From 1979 to 1993, all patients with primary rectal cancer (0–12 cm from the anal verge) who underwent resection for their curable primary disease were included in a personal consecutive series (WEE). Only the presence of synchronous distant disease determined incurability. If patients underwent resection of all gross disease they were considered curable. No patients were excluded from this series because of locally advanced primary rectal cancer, i.e., regional disease at risk for marginal resectability, resectable pelvic sidewall involvement, including major vascular resection (i.e., internal iliac artery), or adjacent organ involvement.

The location of the primary tumor was determined by a rigid proctoscopy in the left lateral Sims' position. Clinical, operative, and pathologic data were recorded prospectively and were included in a database, beginning in 1980.

Patients were examined quarterly to 6-monthly for 5 years or longer, depending upon their clinical circumstances. Follow-up included an updated history, a physical examination and rigid proctoscopy, colonoscopy 1 year following resection and at 1- to 3-year intervals thereafter, complete blood cell count (CBC), sequential multiple analysis (SMA; including liver function tests), and carcinoembryonic antigen (CEA) at each office visit, and annual chest X-rays. Imaging studies (i.e., computed tomography scans, CT) were performed only when clinical or laboratory evidence suggested the possibility of recurrent disease. Potentially curable solitary metastasis, i.e., liver or lung, were pursued aggressively.

Local recurrence was defined as any recurrence within the field of the resection, most commonly the true pelvis. Pelvic recurrence was defined as clinical, endoscopic, radiologic, or pathologic documentation of disease with/ without CEA elevation. Pelvic recurrence was reported in either the presence or absence of distant metastases. Distant spread was defined as metastases to the liver, lung, bone, brain, peritoneum, or other distant site.

Technique of Operation

All operations reported in this paper were performed at the Colorectal Service at the Memorial Sloan-Kettering Cancer Center and in the setting of a Surgical Oncology Fellowship Training Program. Patients underwent resection in the

Trendelenburg-lithotomy position, through a midline abdominal incision. Although not universally practiced, the majority of patients underwent high ligation of the inferior mesenteric artery (above the left colic branch). Very low anastomoses (i.e., at or below the levator ani muscle) were facilitated both by high ligation and by division of the inferior mesenteric vein at its apex.

For the most part, all operations were conducted as previously described [11]. Dissections were performed using sharp (i.e., scissors or electrocautery) technique under direct vision, along the parietal plane of the pelvic fascia, medial to the sympathetic and the pelvic parasympathetic nerves. Based upon cadaver dissections [23], some authors define this as the plane between the parietal and the visceral layers of the pelvic fascia. In contrast to the disrupted mesorectum that can be seen after some conventional resections, the meso-rectum is excised completely enveloped within the visceral pelvic fascia, pro-ducing an uninterrupted, smooth surface to the specimen. This surface feature may be photodocumented.

In rare cases, portions of a dissection were performed along the adventitia of one or the other internal iliac vessels and included a segment of the internal iliac vessels and/or other sidewall structures in order to accomplish the en bloc resection of any lateral extensions of disease or of any adjacent organ in-volvement. No routine attempt was made to perform iliac or obturator lymphadenectomy.

Over the past 7 years, a deliberate attempt has been made to identify and preserve all of the major components of the pelvic autonomic nervous system in conjunction with TME. Truncal autonomic nerve preservation (ANP) [11] is defined as preservation of the superior hypogastric nerves, the anterior nerve roots of S2, S3, and/or S4, and the pelvic autonomic nerve plexus (PANP) along the pelvic sidewall along with the deliberate sacrifice of all autonomic branches passing from these main trunks to the mesorectum and rectum. Only the direct extension of tumor to a nerve or adverse clinical circumstances (i.e., in some male patients >100 kg) have precluded the use of TME in combination with ANP [11, 24].

The pelvic dissection is begun with the division of the pelvic peritoneum, generally along the peritoneal planes which outline the entire mesorectum. The deeper dissection is performed between the parietal and visceral planes of the pelvic fascia. The parietal plane covers the presacral fascia, the piriform muscles, the internal iliac vessels, the sympathetic and parasympathetic nerves, and the pelvic autonomic plexus. The parietal plane is *not* the vascular ad-ventitia, but is a sheet of fascia located more medially and covering all of the above-named structures. The vessels and their adventitia and lymph nodes are located either within or lateral to the parietal fascia.

The dissection first separates the visceral layer of the pelvic fascia and the contained mesorectum from the adjacent hypogastric nerves. Local traction and countertraction are essential. The nerves are sharply dissected along their medial edges from the bifurcation of the nerves, overlying the sacral prom-ontory, to the pelvic sidewall, where they join the PANP. The dissection con-tinues between the parietal plane of the pelvic fascia, and the visceral plane surrounding the mesorectum, along the presacral fascia. Only minor vessels are encountered and these may be cauterized. Long instruments are required, e.g., DeBakey forceps, cautery extension, long scissors (12–14 inches). Below the level of S3 (which is invariably associated with the anterior sacral curvature), the rectosacral fascia (or ligament) is encountered [7, 22]. The rectosacral fascia, which fuses the parietal and visceral layers of the pelvic fascia in the posterior midline, is divided sharply, resulting in a wide opening of the presacral space, which is then sharply dissected to the tip of the coccyx.

At the outset of the dissection, the pelvic peritoneum is divided approximately 1 cm anterior to the pouch of Douglas. The deeper dissection continues using sharp technique anterior to Denonvillier's fascia until the prostate is reached or to the base of the rectovaginal septum.

The lateral dissection is characterized by two main features, i.e. sharp dissection of the mesorectum away from (1) the PANP and (2) the anterior parasympathetic sacral nerve roots of S3 and/or S4. The pelvic splanchnic nerves are also referred to by some as the nervi erigentes or as "the pelvic nerves."

The PANP is a dense plaque of nerve tissue situated anterolaterally along the pelvic sidewall, at the level of the seminal vesicles or the cervical vaginal junction. The PANP is the junction of the sympathetic and parasympathetic nerves. When present, the middle rectal artery penetrates the PANP heading medially towards the rectum from the lateral pelvic sidewall [59]. What is generally regarded as the "lateral ligament" is really a surgically developed structure which does not exist in the absence of medial traction. The "fixed" origin of the "ligament" is actually the fusion of the lateral mesorectum to the PANP with the middle rectal artery running through the bunched up tissues created by medial traction [59]. Meticulous sharp dissection is needed in order not to injure the plexus laterally or to penetrate the mesorectum medially.

The parasympathetic nerves, particularly S3, may be visible as they exit the sacral foramina or, more laterally, as they exit from beneath the piriform muscles. These very fine nerves course anterolaterally to meet the PANP and almost invariably run caudad to the middle rectal artery. The PANP and the nerves along and posterolateral to the lateral ligaments are the two most likely sites of nerve injury, the latter due to medial tenting of the nerves with inadvertent transection. (In blunt dissection, these nerves are commonly avulsed from the pelvic sidewall or are cut blindly, remaining entirely unrecognized.) Meticulous proactive hemostasis is important, as "chasing" a bleeding vessel into the pelvic sidewall can lead to parasympathetic nerve damage.

Once the rectosacral ligament has been divided, and the mesorectum has been dissected away from the parasympathetic nerves and the PANP, the levator ani muscles are visible. In some cases, S3 and S4 may be observed running anteriorly towards the bladder neck. The left and right paravesical tissues (or extensions of the mesorectum) must be dissected without inadvertent nerve injury.

The sharp dissection continues to the levators and the remaining dissection continues along the levator fascia to the anal hiatus. At this point, complete rectal mobilization is achieved and the rectum is straightened and elevated out of the sacral curvature. Sphincter preservation is accomplished when mobilization of the rectum produces a tumor-free rectal wall distal to the lowest palpable edge of the primary tumor. The mesorectum and the rectum are divided at the same level, at least 3–4 cm distal to the lowest palpable edge of the primary cancer. In the case of mid- to upper rectal tumors (i.e., 6–11 cm from the anal verge), no attempt is made to upwardly dissect the distal mesorectum into the specimen, a significant departure from the method of Heald. As a consequence, the level of the anastomosis varies in relation to the level of the primary and does not invariably fall within several centimeters of the levators. If any uncertainty exists as to the level of the tumor, a rectal examination may be performed prior to selecting the site for transection of the rectum. In the patient, a distal margin of normal rectal wall of 3–4 cm is generally accepted, especially in cases of lower rectal cancers being treated by coloanal anastomosis.

In the case of sphincter preservation, the anastomosis is accomplished by standard colorectal circular stapling techniques or by lower anterior resection with stapled or hand-sewn coloanal anastomosis [49]. A rectal "washout" is not routinely performed prior to transection of the rectum. Instead, the pelvis is irrigated with normal saline directly following transection of the rectum. (Clearly, this act, together with the data reported in this paper, both imply that in my opinion "seeding" plays no role in the etiology of pelvic recurrence.)

In the case of abdominoperineal resection (APR), the pelvic dissection is performed to the anal hiatus of the levator ani prior to beginning the perineal phase of the operation [10].

A temporary, defunctioning colostomy is employed in over 50% of cases, especially when the anastomosis is less than 5 cm from the anal verge. It is generally closed after 8–12 weeks.

Staging Methods

Pathologic staging was performed according to 1932 version of the Dukes' classification [9] and according to the 1987 version of the AJCC/UICC staging classification for colorectal cancer [8]. TNM stages corresponding to Dukes' stage C include all patients with lymph node involvement, i.e., T(any)N1–3M0. Nevertheless, N1 or N2 disease can encompass a wide range of Dukes' C substages, i.e., stages T1–4, as well as other adverse pathologic features. To strictly characterize our results, survival and local pelvic recurrence rates are provided for these various substages (see Tables 1–4). Adverse pathologic features, including positive margins of resection, lymphatic vascular invasion (LVI), blood vessel invasion (BVI), perineural invasion (PNI), degree of differentiation, extracapsular nodal penetration, and non-nodal mesenteric implants, were reported separately.

Adjuvant Therapy (Clinical Guidelines Determining Its Use)

Patients considered to be marginally resectable at the time of their initial presentation were offered preoperative RT under Institutional Review Board-approved protocols, which administered clinically significant doses of RT (>4500 cGy) and chemotherapy [35]. Patients with positive lymph nodes (T3N1 or T3N2), especially in the presence of adverse pathologic features, who did not receive preoperative RT were offered the option of receiving postoperative RT and/or chemotherapy in accordance with the adjuvant therapy, which ultimately became the NIH consensus guidelines [43]. Patients with T3N0 disease were routinely advised not to undergo RT. The earlier published results of TME and of my evolving experience with local control were also explained to the patient [10, 11, 31]. In view of the very low incidence of local failure associated with TME, most patients deferred postoperative adjuvant therapy. Perioperative RT (with or without chemotherapy) involving the administration of 4500 cGy or more was administered to 70 patients with Dukes' B or C stages of disease.

Statistical Methods

Survival and time to recurrence curves were estimated by the Kaplan-Meier method, which also yielded estimates of 5-year survival and recurrence percentages. Deaths due to causes unrelated to the rectal cancer were treated as censored. Statistical significance of potential prognostic factors, such as Dukes' stage (B or C) or perineural involvement (present or absent), was evaluated by the generalized Wilcoxon test. Factors were evaluated both univariately and multivariately, adjusting for other significant pathologic factors. For comparative purposes, results are reported as 5-year percentages, while significance tests are based on the full curves. All computations were done using SAS software PROC LIFETEST [58].

Results

From 1979 to 1989, a total of 246 consecutive patients with primary rectal cancers stages T3N0M0 or T(any)N1–2M0 underwent resection by one surgeon. All patients underwent resection according to the principles of TME (or TME with ANP) as outlined above, except for one female patient in whom TME was not possible because of short stature and extreme obesity, despite a gynecoid pelvis. The mean age was 61.4 years, the median age 62 years, and the range 29–90 years.

Of the 246 patients, 170 (69.1%) underwent low anterior resection (LAR), while 76 (30.9%) underwent an APR. A total of 145 patients (85.3%) with lesions between 6 and 11 cm from the anal verge underwent sphincter preservation.

The median potential follow-up time was 6 years. There were 133 men (54.1%) and 113 women (45.9%). The distal edge of the primary tumor was located between 0 and 5 cm from the anal verge in 51 patients, between 6 and 12 cm from the anal verge in 193 patients.

Stage

Of the 246 patients, there were 99 patients with Dukes' B (T3N0M0) tumors and 147 patients with Dukes C, i.e., T(any)N1–2M0 disease (of whom 105 patients with Dukes' C had T3N1–2M0 cancers). Substages of Dukes' C disease which underwent further evaluation for survival and local recurrence included stages T1–2N1–2M0, T3N1–2M0, T3N1M0, and T3N2M0, which were analyzed separately.

A separate group of patients comprising 141 patients with Dukes' A lesion (T1–2N0M0) are reported for completeness, but are not included in the significant analyses, as they are not considered "high risk" by any adjuvant therapy definitions.

Survival

Total hospital mortality (after less than and more than 30 days) was 0.8% (two out of 246 patients). Both died of cardiovascular complications ranging from the first to the 50th postoperative day. The overall 5-year survival for all patients (n=246) was 74.2% (Fig. 1). Survival by stage and by substage is listed in Table 1. The progressive worsening with increasing stage was statistically significant at each stage ($p < 0.0001$).

Survival was statistically related to nodal status ($p < 0.0003$), i.e., N0 versus N1 versus N2. Patients undergoing LAR had a 5-year survival rate of 80.7%, while patients undergoing APR had a 5-year survival rate of 60.2% ($p < 0.0003$). There were no differences in the survival attributable to sex (men, 78.1%; women, 69.5%). No differences in survival were attributable to the level of the primary tumor (0–5 cm, 74.4%; 6–11 cm, 73.4%; >11 cm, 85.1%).

Patterns of Failure

Pelvic Recurrence

A total of 246 patients had Dukes' B (n=99) or Dukes' C (n=147) rectal cancers, a group comparable to the "high-risk" groups of Krook [30] and of MacFarlane [31]. The Kaplan-Meier estimate of the overall rate of pelvic recurrence within 5 years for all stages of disease was 7.3% (18 out of 246; Fig. 2). Pelvic recurrence rates by stage are listed in Table 2. These data include all pelvic recurrences, whether in the presence or absence of distant metastatic disease.

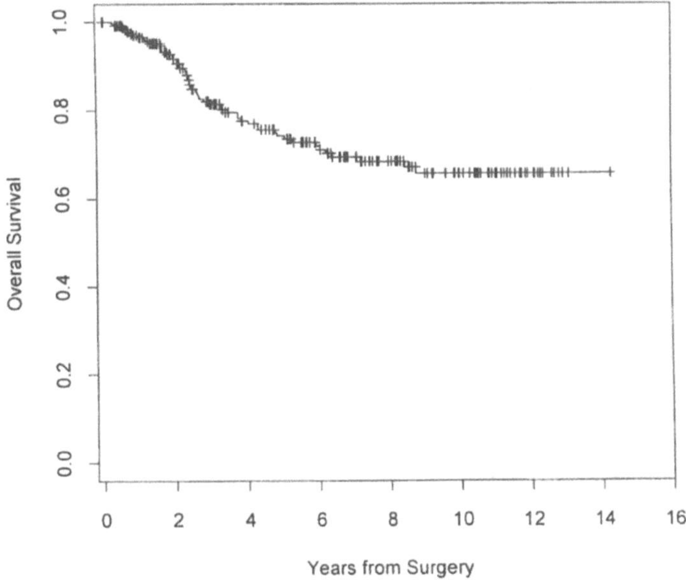

Fig. 1. Kaplan-Meier survival of 246 patients with Dukes' B and C rectal cancers

Table 1. Rectal cancer Dukes' B and C stages: Kaplan-Meier 5-year survival by stage

Dukes' stage	TNM stage	Patients (n)	Died of disease (n)	5-year survival (%)
B	T3N0M0	99	13	86.7[*]
C	T(any)N1-2M0	147	43	64[*]
	T3N1-2M0	105	29	68
	T1-3N1-2M0	141	–	67[c]
C1[a]	T3N1M0	69	–	69.9
C2[b]	T3N2M0	36	–	60

[a]One to three positive nodes.
[b]Four or more positive nodes.
[c]Excludes six patients with stage T4N1-2M0 diesease, of whom five died of disseminated disease or local failure; Kaplan-Meier 5-year survival rate, 17%.
[*]$p<0.0003$.

Pelvic recurrences were observed in 14 of 246 patients (5.7%) with stages B or C disease who did not develop evidence of distant metastases. Pelvic recurrences by stage in the absence of distant metastatic disease are listed in Table 3.

There were no differences in the overall 5-year pelvic recurrence rates by sex or by height of the tumor location. There were no pelvic recurrences observed when the primary lesion was situated more than 11 cm from the anal verge,

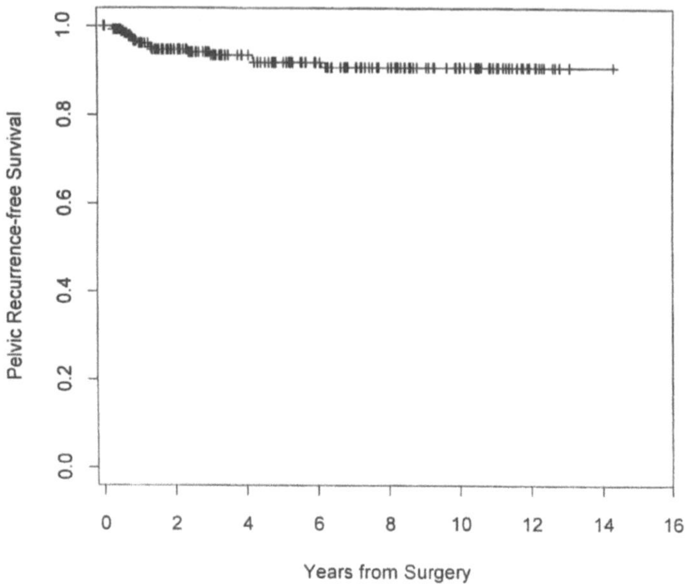

Fig. 2. Local recurrence; free survival for all "high-risk" patients

Table 2. Dukes' B and C rectal cancers: all pelvic recurrences in the presence or absence of distant metastases

Dukes' stage	TNM stage	Patients (n)	Pelvic recurrences	
			(n)	(%)[c]
B	T3N0M0	99	3	4.0
C	T(any)N1-2M0	147	15	12.0
	T1-3N1-2M0	141	13	11.0[d]
B and C	T3N0M0 and T(any)N1-2M0	246	18	7.3%[e]
C2	T3N1-2M0	105	8	8.1[f]
C1[a]	T3N1M0	69	3	4.8
C2[b]	T3N2M0	36	5	14.0

[a]One to three positive nodes.
[b]Four or more positive nodes.
[c]Kaplan-Meier estimates at 5 years.
[d]Excludes six patients with T4N1-2M0 disease, of which two had local recurrence (Kaplan-Meier local recurrence rate, 58%). Five of six patients died; 5-year survival rate, 17%.
[e]"High-risk" group of Krook (NCCTG) [30] and of MacFarlane [31].
[f]Astler-Coller Modified Dukes' Classification [3].

Table 3. Dukes' B and C stages of rectal cancer: pelvic recurrence in the absence of distant metastases

Dukes' stage	TNM stage	Patients (*n*)	Pelvic recurrences	
			(*n*)	(%)[c]
	T3N0M0	98	2	3
C	T(any)N1-2M0	147	12	10
	T1-3N1-2M0	141	8	6.8[d]
B and C	T3N0M0 and T(any)N1-2M0	245	14	5.7[e]
C2	T3N1-2M0	103	6	5.8[f]
C1[a]	T3N1M0	68	2	3.3
C2[b]	T3N2M0	35	4	11.4

[a]One to three positive nodes.
[b]Four or more positive nodes.
[c]Kaplan-Meier estimates at 5 years.
[d]Excludes six patients with stage T4N1-2M0 (see footnote d, Table 2).
[e]"High-risk" group of Krook (NCCTG) [30] and of MacFarlane [31].
[f]Astler-Coller Modified Dukes' Classification [3].

confirming our previous data that 11–12 cm seems to be a physiologically appropriate level for defining the rectum in relation to cancer [13]. The two factors which were statistically most predictive of pelvic recurrence were nodal status (N0 vs. N1 vs. N2: univariate $p=0.0002$, adjusted for perineural invasion $p=0.0043$; perineural invasion: univariate $p=0.0002$, adjusted for nodal status $p=0.0043$). Overall, no differences in local recurrence rates were observed when patients undergoing LAR were compared with patients undergoing APR. In the most advanced stage patients, i.e., those involving T4 disease, the local recurrence rate after APR was significantly higher than after LAR (Table 4).

Distant Metastases

Disseminated failure without pelvic recurrence was observed in 58 patients (23.6%). These figures are practically identical to the figures reported by MacFarlane et al. [31], who compared the results of TME with the results of conventional surgery plus adjuvant therapy, as reported by the NCCTG [40].

Radiation Therapy and Pelvic Recurrence

The influence of RT was examined in relation to the presence or absence of pelvic recurrence in group T(any)N1–2M0. Published data from the MRC Working Party indicated no differences in local control attributable to 2000 cGy of preoperative irradiation [43]. Under these circumstances, patients from the early 1980s who were included in protocols of "sandwich" radiation, receiving only 1500 cGy of preoperative irradiation, were included in the analyses as patients who have received minimal or no radiation. There were too few pelvic recurrences in Dukes' B (T3N0M0) cases (three out of 99) to analyze for significance. Of the 70 Dukes' C (T(any)N1–2M0) patients who received adjuvant perioperative RT of more than 4500 cGy, nine developed a pelvic recurrence. Of the 78 Dukes' C patients who either had minimal or no perioperative RT, six developed a pelvic recurrence. For all Dukes' C patients, there was no statistically significant difference in the incidence of local failure attributable to RT (two-tail p value=0.41).

Under specific circumstances, however, RT was marginally significant (p=0.07) in a multivariate analysis (involving multiple risk factors) of local failure after adjusting for perineural involvement and nodal status. The specific benefit of RT was observed in patients at highest risk, namely N2 nodal disease (n=70) or perineural involvement (PNI+; n=15). This group comprised 78 patients in total (seven had both factors), of whom two had missing data making them unevaluable. Among these 76 evaluable patients, full-course RT was significantly related to reduced risk of local failure (p=0.05).

Other Parameters Related to the Operation

Clinical anastomotic leaks were observed in five out of 170 patients, a leak rate of 2.9%. No patients died as a result of an anastomotic disruption. In three patients who underwent LAR, severe rectal strictures and/or fistulae led to the establishment of a permanent colostomy. All had received full-course postoperative RT.

For the most recent 100 patients undergoing LAR by means of TME with ANP, the mean patient weight was 77.8 kg (median, 79 kg; range, 41–137 kg). The average duration of the operation was 250 min (median, 4 h 10 min; range, 150–420 min). The average measured blood loss was 594 cc (range, 100–2000 cc). During this same period for APR, the mean weight was 66.6 kg (median, 71.5 kg; range, 43–91 kg). The mean operating time was 249 min (median, 4 h 9 min; range, 180–360 min), and the mean blood loss was 448 cc (median, 600 cc; range, 140–1000 cc).

Discussion

Importance of the Mesorectum in Relation to Pelvic Recurrence

In 1986, Quirke and coworkers proved that pelvic recurrence is a direct consequence of inadequate mesorectal excision, leaving regional disease in the pelvis [53]. Conventional operative technique commonly violates the circumference of the mesorectum during blunt dissection along undefined planes, leaving residual mesorectum in the pelvis. Pelvic recurrence more often than not is the clinical presentation of this persistent disease. These data and the importance of the mesorectum as the repository of regional disease have been corroborated by others [2, 42, 53, 54, 56].

Table 4. Traditional rates of pelvic recurrence in relation to conventional surgery

Author	Patients (n)	Local recurrence (%)		Adjuvant Therapy	Comments
Adam [2]	190		23	No	Positive margins, 78% Negative margins, 10% Dukes' B not a rational basis for adjuvant RT
Cass [6]	67	*B2	22	No	*Modified Dukes Classification by Astler and Coller [3]
		*C2	38		
Gilbert [20]	54	*B2	35	No	
		C2	65		
Rich [57]	142	**A	8	No	Rectum and rectosigmoid Present or absent distant metastases
		B	31		**Modified Astler-Coller staging by Gunderson and Sosin [21]
		C	50		
		B2m	17		
		B3$_g$	54		
		C1	36		
		C3	67		
Walz [64]	88	*B2	16	No	
		C2	37		
Gunderson [21]		**C1	24	No	Second look or symptomatic recurrences
		C2	70		
Patel [47]	435	A	13	No	Present or absent distant metastases
		B	17		
		C	37		
Pilipshen [51]	412	A	14	No	In some patients preoperative RT 2000 cGy; 0–11 cm 30%, >11 cm 6%
		B	30		
		C	40		
Moosa [36]	152		32	No	0–5 cm from anal verge Intraperitoneal rectum, 4%
Athlin [4]	99	*B1	27	No	
		B2	48		
		C2	55		
Williams [66]	107	APR	24	No	Cumulative LR rates at 5 years[a]
		LAR	20		

Table 4 (*Contd.*)

Author	Patients (n)	Local recurrence (%)		Adjuvant Therapy	Comments
Neville [41]	373	A	5.3	Yes	Adjuvant Rx not specified. Retrospective review
		B	14.9		
		C	36.5		
Willett [65]	261	**B2	13	≥ 4500–5040 cGy	Chemotherapy (postoperative)
		B3	17		
		C2	23		
		C3	77		
Tepper [62]		**B2	23/9	Surgery alone/	
		C1	50/20	Surgery + 5040 cGy	Postoperative RT
		C2	47/21		
		C3	67/53		
Gastro-intestinal Tumor Study Group [17]	95		17	4500 cGy+FU+MeCCNU	50% severe acute toxicity. Two (1%) treatment-related deaths
	104		16	4500cGy+escalating FU	
Fisher [15]	555	Surgery	24.5		
NSABP R-01		CRx	21.4	FU, MeCCNU, vincristine	Rectal carcinomas. Extraperitoneal Dukes' B&C. Only significant survival benefit to male patients receiving CRx
		RT	16.3 (n.s.)	4600 cGy AP-PA fields	
Påhlman [46]	209	n=26	12 (p=0.02)	4700–4900 cGy (preoperative)	*Significant difference in Dukes' B, no difference in survival
	204	n=43	21	5000–6000 cGy (postoperative)	
Stockholm	331	n=37	18 (n.s.)	2500 cGy/5–7 days	*p=0.01 (Dukes' B)
Rectal Cancer [61]	348	n=86	31	Surgery only	n.s. in Dukes C
Gerard EORTC [19]	166	n=24	15 (p=0.0003)	3450 cGy/19 days	*n.s. Survival
	175	n=49	30	Surgery only	
Krook	104		13.5 (p=0.036)	4500–5040 cGy+FU+MeCCNU	<12 cm from anal verge or at sacral promontory.

Study					
NCCTG Study Group [30]	100		25	4500–5040 cGy	Estimated 5-year recurrence. RT only 62.7% RT+CRx 41.5%
GITSG [16]	58	$n=14$	24	Surgery only	First site of
	48	$n=13$	27	FU + MeCCNU	recurrence 5-year: survival B2, 74%; C1, 52%, C2, 35%
	50	$n=10$	20	4000–4800 cGy (postoperative) RT + Crx	
	46	$n=5$	11		
MRC Working Party [40]	275		43.2	Surgery only	Actuarial rates 17 UK Centers
	277		44.6	500 cGy preoperative RT	
	272		47.1%	2000 cGy preoperative RT	
Phillips [50]	848		15	Not reported	Rectum and rectosigmoid[b]
		LAR	18		
		APR	12		
Williams [67]	154	LAR	12	Not reported	Mid-third rectum, 7.5–12 cm from the anal verge
		APR	9		
McDermott [33]	801	19–24		No	ESR Hughes series
Marsh [32]	141	36.5		Surgery	No survival difference Minimum follow-up, 4 years 0–13 cm[b]
	143	12.8 (.0001)		Surgery + 2000 cGy	
Norstein [44]	284	29			National Registry LR rate of 37% (32/86) in midrectal tumors

LAR, low anterior resection; APR, abdominoperineal resection; RT, radiation therapy; LR, local recurrence; FU, 5-fluorouracil; MeCCNU, semustine; AP-PA, anteroposterior-posteroanterior; n.s., not significant; $B2_2$, B_2 microscopic; $B3_g$, V_3 gross; R_x, therapy; CR_x, Chemotherapy.

[a]See Fig. 2.

[b]Inclusion of rectosigmoid tumors (i.e., >12 cm) favors lower rates of local recurrence. See Pilipshen [51].

In a recently reported prospective study of 190 patients, Adam and coworkers examined the circumferential margins for tumor involvement [2]. Of 141 curative cases, 35 patients (25%) had involvement of the circumferential margins by tumor, and the overall rate of local recurrence was 25%. Where the circumferential margins were positive for tumor, 78% of these patients developed pelvic recurrence, while local recurrence occurred in only 10% of those patients with no circumferential involvement. Circumferential tumor involvement significantly influenced both survival and local recurrence rates.

Quirke and coworkers have emphasized the importance of a visibly intact smooth outer surface of the dissected mesorectum, i.e., the surgical circumferential margins in the grossly examined specimen. They have also made a very compelling case for revising the standard method of examining the pathologic specimen following resection of the rectum for cancer. They suggest that serial slices through the tumor, the rectum, and the mesorectum are a more sensitive means of evaluating the pathology in relation to the prognosis than the traditional methods in current practice [52].

Defining Total Mesorectal Excision

TME is defined as the complete excision of the intact unit, i.e., rectum and its mesorectum, with negative margins of resection. TME accomplishes the removal of the mesorectum and the rectum and any potential spread, enveloped within the visceral layer of the pelvic fascia [7, 11, 31, 59]. Such spread may be represented by any number or variety of pathologic findings within the mesorectum and is not limited to lymph node involvement [2, 42, 53, 54, 56].

Virtually all regional forms of spread of disease (with the exception of pelvic sidewall attachment or adjacent organ involvement) are to be found within this anatomic unit of the rectum and the mesorectum, enveloped by the visceral layer of the pelvic fascia [7, 11].

In my opinion, TME defines the planes of pelvic down to the anal hiatus within the levator ani muscle. The bowel and the mesorectum may be transected approximately 4–5 cm distal to the lowest edge of the primary cancer. TME does not imply the dissection of the lowest parts of the mesorectum upward with every resection, particularly in the high lesions. Under such circumstances, if disease is found in the most distal mesorectum, it is a reflection of highly aggressive pathology, for which TME alone will not be curative.

Conventional Resection

Conventional operations for rectal cancer, i.e., the operations most commonly taught and practiced worldwide, are associated with blunt dissection, at best along the visceral plane of the pelvic fascia. Violation of the mesorectum, albeit inadvertent, occurs both because of the undefined planes and possibly because of resistance to blunt dissection encountered at the rectosacral fascia [23]. This structure, situated in the posterior midline in the vicinity of S3, must be incised sharply or blunt dissection deviates anteriorly into the mesorectum, precisely where regional tumor may be found.

Conventional operations are associated with a worldwide incidence of pelvic recurrence averaging 30% [2, 30, 44] (Table 4) and are also associated with a total failure rate, i.e., disseminated metastases, of 60%–65% in patients with Dukes' C disease [2, 4, 6, 20, 21, 30, 32, 33, 36, 41, 47, 50, 51, 57, 64, 66, 67]. Various trials of adjuvant RT have reduced the incidence of local failure to about 15% [17–19, 30, 40, 46, 61, 62, 65]. Nevertheless, RT alone offers no reported impact on survival. While combined modality treatment, i.e., chemotherapy and RT are reported to yield significant "reduction in risk" of recurrence [16, 17, 30, 63], the survival and local recurrence rates achieved by combined-modality adjuvant therapy following conventional resection have yet to approach the rates achieved by TME [31].

Rather than considering significant changes in the operative approach, surgeons are often influenced to consider evolving forms of combined adjuvant therapy. Often ignored in this equation is the fact that adjuvant therapies have their own significant mortality and morbidities. In the most widely referenced combined-modality adjuvant therapy trials, treatment-related mortality (two out of 46; 4.3%) exceeded any acceptable levels of operative mortality [16, 30].

Despite the survival advantage of postoperative combined-modality therapy, the incidence of grade 3+ toxicity in patients receiving RT and chemotherapy in the GITSG trial was 26% hematological and 35% nonhematological [16]. Long-term morbidity has also been encountered, with 6.7% of patients requiring reoperation for radiation-related small-bowel obstruction [30]. Long-term mortality has been attributable to methyl-CCNU (semustine)-related leukemia [5].

Recently, two institutions have reported abnormal bowel function attributable to postoperative irradiation in patients undergoing LAR or LAR with coloanal reconstruction. Statistically significant impairment of function related to both altered bowel habits and incontinence represented lifelong deleterious consequences of radiation [29, 48]. All of these factors deserve consideration in the planning of patient care. Adjuvant therapy should be examined under optimal circumstances, after the best results that surgery can offer, rather than as a compelling substitute for less than optimal surgical outcomes.

Extended Resections

Extended operations have evolved in an effort to enhance the cure of what is viewed by surgeons as a regional disease in the majority of patients with rectal cancer. The pros and cons of TME should be considered in relation to these extended operations, which include en bloc resections of the internal iliac, obturator, and paravesical lymph nodes, together with LAR or APR [26, 27].

All such potential spread is regarded as "regional" by the advocates of extended operations. Studies which initially plotted the location of excised lymph nodes from these extended operations documented an incidence of up to 7% positive lateral nodes [27]. Among patients with positive lateral nodes, fewer than 10% of patients survived 5 years, with most deaths due to disseminated disease. Subsequently, Moriya claims an incidence of positive lateral adenopathy in 14% of patients and a 5-year survival of 49% [39]. However, most Japanese surgeons do not employ radiation therapy for obturator-node positive patients, extended resections being used for cure and for local control.

Recently, Morikawa and associates [38] have reported an overall incidence of lateral lymph node spread of 8.8%. The majority of patients with lateral spread had Dukes' C primary cancers, i.e., axial mesenteric spread. Higher rates of lateral spread were only observed in low rectal cancers. Survival rates and rates of pelvic recurrence were not provided in relation to lymph node distribution.

Most recently, it has been reported that local failures and survival rates are not altered by extended operations when compared with Japanese standard operations [37]. Moreira and coworkers reported on 95 patients who underwent extended operations. Only ten patients (11%) had lateral lymph node spread, and all ten patients had Dukes' C tumors. Lymphatic invasion was present in 50%, and perineural invasion in 27%. There were no statistically significant differences in local control, distant metastases, or overall survival when compared to patients undergoing the Japanese "standard" operation, resection and internal iliac lymphadenectomy. Recurrence and metastases were related to the adverse pathologic features, and not to the extent of lymphadenectomy [37].

The survival data associated with lateral lymph node spread suggests that most "lateral" nodal spread is a form of systemic, not of "regional" disease. While dramatic individual cases of cure have been achieved, most such survival is anecdotal. The morbidity of extended operations remains high, despite attempts to preserve all sympathetic and parasympathetic fibers of the pelvic autonomic nervous system. Sexual dysfunction is observed in 75%–95% of all patients and urinary dysfunction in 40%–50%, largely due to the lateral dissection which devascularizes nerves [28, 39]. While urinary function may improve over time, sexual dysfunction remains permanent [28, 39]. In the absence of improved survival and/or local control compared with TME, the price of such significant morbidity is too high to advocate extended operations as a routine procedure. In addition, the logistics of performing extended dissections in 70- to 90-kg Western men, as opposed to 40- to 50-kg Japanese patients, virtually precludes the adoption of extended lymphadenectomy as a standard operative approach in most Western centers.

Total Mesorectal Excision Versus Extended or Conventional Operations

Total mesorectal excision solves many of the problems which are inherent in both the conventional and the extended approaches. The publications by MacFarlane [31] and Enker [14], as summarized in this report, both indicate that the local control and cure rates with TME are among the highest reported for any operative approach to rectal cancer, with or without adjuvant therapy.

In this study we confirm that local failure is observed in only 5%–10% of patients, including all "high-risk" patients, even those with locally advanced disease, without significant benefit from RT [31]. In MacFarlane's study, only a rare patient presenting with locally advanced disease received any perioperative irradiation. These results suggest that the benefits of TME are independent of RT in most patients and represent the optimal operative approach in patents with locally advanced disease which should be treated in conjunction with RT.

Regarding the reduction of morbidity, sphincter preservation was accomplished in 85% of our patients with cancers situated 6–11 cm from the anal verge. When TME is combined with truncal ANP, we have reported the preservation of sexual function in 95% of men under the age of 60 years [11] and can now report the preservation of sexual function in 85% of men and women, with no observed loss in urinary function [24]. Deterioration in sexual function following TME-ANP is observed in men over the age of 60 years and in patients undergoing APR. The results of our investigations and the possible causes associated with these changes have been reported by Havenga et al. [24].

In addition to preventing pelvic recurrence, adequate resection appears to improve survival, reducing systemic metastases from the range of 60%–65% to 23%–25% in "high-risk" patients [30, 31]. After TME, distant spread remains a far greater concern than does local recurrence, which only exceeds 10% in the presence of T4 or N2 disease. Even in N2 disease, TME reduces the local recurrence rate to 11%–14% from the 40%–67% which is commonly reported with conventional operations [55, 63].

Several studies have reported a statistically significant increase in local recurrence rates in patients undergoing APR for low rectal cancers when compared with anterior resection for midrectal cancers [1, 44, 50]. Our data indicate that local failure is not a function of sphincter preservation, so long as total regional excision of tumor is accomplished (Table 5).

Table 5. Pelvic recurrences by stage and by operation performed[a]

	LAR			APR			p Value
	Total (n)	Recurrences (n)	(%)	Total (n)	Recurrences (n)	(%)	
T3N0M0	68	1	2.6	30	0	0	n.s.
T3N1M0	48	0	0	21	1	7.7	n.s.
T3N2M0	29	2	4.5	7	0	0	n.s.
T2N1-2M0	77	2	1.5	28	1	5.3	n.s.
T1-3N1-2M0	101	4	4.5	40	4	13.7	0.018
T(any)N1-2M0	101	4	4.5	46	5	13.8	0.01
Total	167	5	3.8	76	5	7.6	n.s.

n.s., not significant.
[a]All pelvic recurrences, either in the presence or in the absence of distant metastases.

Table 6. Influence of adverse pathologic risk factors on subsequent sites of failure, i.e., patterns of recurrence

Adverse pathologic risk factor	Cases observed (n)	Total recurrences (n)	Local recurrences (n)	Distant metastases (n)
Blood vessel invasion (BVI)	34	11	0	11
BVI only[a]	24	7	0	7
Lymph vascular invasion (LVI)	16	6[b]	3[b]	4[b]
LVI only[a]	9	5	2[b]	3[b]
Perineural invasion (PNI)	9	7	2	5
PNI only[a]	6	5	2	3
Mucinous component	32	7	3[b]	5[b]
MC only[a]	23	4	2[b]	3[b]
Grade III	26	9	3[b]	7[b]
Diff only[a] (DIFF)	11	5	2[b]	4[b]
Three or more adverse pathologic features	6	2	1	1

DIFF, degree of differentiation.

[a] In the absence of any other adverse risk factors.

[b] One was both distant and local.

Adverse Pathologic Features

The role of additional risk factors is less clear. The presence of perineural invasion is a significant independent prognostic variable for local recurrence. Despite the role of PNI in local failure, the presence of any additional adverse pathologic risk factor seems to be a marker of systemic spread more than of local failure (Table 6). For each adverse pathologic feature, whether alone or in combination with other risk factors, the incidence of systemic spread considerably outweighs the incidence of local failure.

Role of Adjuvant Therapy in Relation to Total Mesorectal Excision

Our findings suggest that, after TME, the following is true:

1. Adequate resection alone offers excellent local control in stages T3N0M0 and T3N1M0 rectal cancers.
2. Risk factors for local failure are N2 disease and perineural invasion.
3. Systemic metastases outweigh local failure rates in "high-risk" patients.
4. Adverse pathologic risk factors increase the likelihood of local failure, but really suggest the stronger likelihood of systemic recurrence.

Based upon these findings, the current use of adjuvant therapy deserves serious reconsideration. Currently, it would appear that two standards of surgery exist, based upon the documented type of operation: treatment by the conventional operation or treatment by TME. In the aftermath of conventional operations, and in the absence of preoperative treatment, local failure can be expected in 30% of patients and systemic disease in 60%–65%. Under these circumstances, adjuvant therapy should be advocated consisting of combined chemotherapy and RT, as outlined by the NIH Consensus Report [43], the NCCTG [30], and by O'Connell [45].

For patients undergoing TME, adjuvant therapy should be considered under the following circumstances:

1. Preoperative combined chemotherapy and RT in patients presenting with locally advanced, i.e., marginally resectable or unresectable disease, as advocated by Minsky [34].
2. Combined postoperative chemotherapy and RT in patients with N2 disease, or perineural invasion, or with multiple adverse pathologic features in the mesorectum (even in the presence of T2 disease). Patients with T3N0M0 or T3N1M0 disease without additional risk factors need not be subjected routinely to RT [2, 10, 31]. If they are studied as part of an adjuvant therapy trial, the standard of surgery should be documented in accordance with agreed definitions.
3. For patients with T3N1M0 disease, based upon the incidence of distant spread versus local failure, systemic adjuvant chemotherapy alone should also be examined in the setting of a controlled trial, in an attempt to confirm its reported efficacy in primary rectal cancer [15]. Some compelling results of the combinations of 2500 cGy preoperatively are reviewed by Glimelius (see Chap. 28).

Surgical Oncology and Education

Recently, prospective efforts have begun involving large numbers of co-operating surgeons in Norway [44] and in the Netherlands [25], attempting to define and to alter the standards of operations for rectal cancer. The goal of these efforts is to shift the emphasis from conventional operations (together with conventional failure rates) to TME with ANP, improving cure, local control, and morbidity. Preceptorship has played a key role in these efforts.

In addition to improving cure, these efforts will influence ongoing multidisciplinary studies. The results of our study and those obtained by MacFarlane [31] suggest that future protocols in adjuvant therapy must document the standard of operation, i.e., TME or conventional resection. No matter how much improvement in local control can be accomplished by the addition of adjuvant RT and chemotherapy, the benefits of combined-modality adjuvant therapy will be best appreciated in the setting of optimal surgical results [60].

Efforts to standardize the criteria for, and to formalize the nomenclature of the various operations for rectal cancer are currently underway. There are five planes for the anatomic dissection of the pelvis in relation to rectal cancer. These are: (1) the rectum itself, (2) the visceral layer of the pelvic fascia, (3) the parietal layer of the pelvic fascia, (4) the vascular adventitia, and (5) the fascia covering the vessels, defining the spaces lateral to the true pelvis, i.e., the obturator spaces. Based upon these data, we recommend consideration of the following standards for nomenclature of operations, i.e., resections (not including any form of local excision) related to rectal cancers:

1. Operations performed along the wall of the rectum should be referred to as D0 resections. Violation of the mesorectum either by blunt dissection or by inadvertently incomplete resection of the mesorectum, lacking an intact visceral pelvic fascia as an envelope, will qualify as a D0 resection.
2. Operations performed between the parietal and the visceral planes of the pelvic fascia, producing an intact visceral layer as an envelope for the entire resected mesorectum, should be referred to as D1 resections. TME will qualify as an D1 resection. TME with ANP is a D1 resection.
3. Operations which are performed along the internal iliac, i.e., hypogastric vessels, and which include an internal iliac or hypogastric lymphadenectomy should be referred to as D2 resections.
4. Operations which dissect the lymph nodes of the obturator spaces, or which resect the internal iliac vessels and obturator nodes en bloc with the primary cancer and the mesorectum, should be referred D3 resections.
5. The en bloc resection of adjacent viscera, i.e., bladder, seminal vesicles, prostate, uterus, vagina or ovaries, small bowel or an adjacent portion of the colon, should be designated by the subscript letter A, i.e., $D1_A$.
6. Sphincter preservation or APR should not influence the D designation of the resection, although other subscript letters, i.e., $_{SP}$ or $_{AP}$ might be a useful descriptor.

Conclusions

1. TME resects the entire unit of regional spread, enveloped within the visceral fascia, achieving negative margins of resection in the vast majority of cases of rectal cancer, improving survival and reducing pelvic recurrence rates in curable patients.
2. Local recurrence rates in "high-risk" patients range from 5% to 8%, while systemic spread is observed in 23%–25% of patients.
3. As currently reported in this study, RT does not appear to reduce the local failure rate in the overall setting of TME, except for a borderline effect observed only in patients with N2 disease or with perineural invasion, conditions associated with locally advanced disease.
4. TME is compatible with ANP and with sphincter preservation, further reducing the morbidity of resections for rectal cancer.
5. In comparison with patients undergoing conventional resections, the extremely low pelvic recurrence rates in patients undergoing TME suggest that the routine use of adjuvant postoperative RT in T3N0M0 disease is not warranted and should be reevaluated in patients with T3N1M0 disease. In the setting of protocol-based treatment, preoperative RT may be of value in patients who will shortly undergo TME.
6. In view of the higher incidence of systemic spread, there is a possible role for adjuvant chemotherapy alone in high-risk rectal cancers treated by TME.
7. Efforts should be extended to teach TME to the surgical community dealing with curable primary rectal cancer.

8. Adjuvant therapy trials should document the standards of operation employed and should examine the impact of the type of surgery on rates of local recurrence and distant metastases within their trials.
9. Standard nomenclature for designating the extent of operations in rectal cancer is suggested.

Acknowledgements. This work was supported in part by the Edith and Louis Roberts Fund and the Joseph N. Bettinger Fund, Colorectal Service, Department of Surgery, Memorial Sloan-Kettering Cancer Center. The authors gratefully acknowledge the assistance of Mrs. Evelyn Santiago in the preparation of the manuscript.

References

1. Abulafi AM, Williams NS (1994) Local recurrence of colorectal cancer: the problem, mechanisms, management and adjuvant therapy. Br J Surg 81:7–19
2. Adam IJ, Mohamdee MO, Martin IG et al (1994) Role of circumferential margin involvement in the local recurrence of rectal cancer. Lancet 344:707–711
3. Astler VB, Coller FA (1954) The prognostic significance of direct extension of carcinoma of the colon and rectum. Ann Surg 139:846–851
4. Athlin L, Bengtsson NO, Stenling R (1988) Local recurrence and survival after radical resection of rectal carcinoma. Acta Chir Scand 154:225–229
5. Boice JD, Greene MH, Killen JY Jr et al (1983) Leukemia and pre-leukemia after adjuvant treatment of gastrointestinal cancer with semustine (methyl-CCNU). N Engl J Med 309:1079–1083
6. Cass AW, Million RR, Pfaff WW (1976) Patterns of recurrence following surgery alone for adenocarcinoma of the colon and rectum. Cancer 37:2861–2865
7. Church JM, Raudkivi PJ, Hill GL (1987) The surgical anatomy of the rectum – a review with particular relevance to the hazards of rectal mobilization. Int J Colorect Dis 2:158–166
8. Cohen AM, Shank B, Friedman MA (1989) Colorectal cancer. In: DeVitaV, Hellman S, Rosenberg SA (eds) Principles and practice of oncology, 3rd edn. Lippincott, Philadelphia, p 910
9. Dukes CE (1932) The classification of cancer of the rectum. J Pathol 35:323–332
10. Enker WE (1990) Cancer of the rectum. Operative management and adjuvant therapy. In: Fazio VW (ed) Current therapy in colon and rectal surgery. Decker, Toronto, pp 120–129
11. Enker WE (1992) Potency, cure, and local control in the operative treatment of rectal cancer. Arch Surg 127:1396–1402
12. Enker WE, Laffer UT, Block GE (1979) Enhanced survival of patients with colon and rectal cancer is based upon wide anatomic resection. Ann Surg 190:350–360
13. Enker WE, Pilipshen SJ (1983) Patterns of failure resulting after definitive resections for rectal and colonic cancer. Cancer Treatment Symp 2:173–180
14. Enker WE, Thaler HT, Cranor ML, Polyak T (1995) Total mesorectal excision in the operative treatment of rectal cancer. J Am Coll Surg 181:335–346
15. Fisher B, Wolmark N, Rockette H et al (1988). Postoperative adjuvant chemotherapy or radiation therapy for rectal cancer: results from NSABP Protocol R-01. J Natl Cancer Inst 80:21–29
16. Gastrointestinal Tumor Study Group (1985) Prolongation of the disease-free interval in surgically treated rectal carcinoma. N Engl J Med 312:1465–1472
17. Gastrointestinal Tumor Study Group (1992) Radiation therapy and fluorouracil with or without semustine for the treatment of patients with surgical adjuvant adenocarcinoma of the rectum. J Clin Oncol 10:549–557
18. Gerard A, Berrod JL, Pene F et al (1985) Interim analysis of a phase III study on pre-operative radiation therapy in resectable rectal carcinoma. Trial of the Gastrointestinal

Tract Cooperative Group of the European Organization for Research on Treatment of Cancer (EORTC). Cancer 55:2373–2379
19. Gerard A, Buyse M, Nordlinger et al (1988) Preoperative radiation therapy as adjuvant treatment in rectal cancer. Final results of a randomized study of the European Organization of Research and Treatment of Cancer (EORTC). Ann Surg 208:606–614
20. Gilbert SG (1978) Symptomatic local tumor failure following abdominoperineal resection. Int J Radiat Oncol Biol Phys 4:801–807
21. Gunderson LL, Sosin H (1974) Areas of failure found at reoperation (second or symptomatic look) following "curative surgery" for adenocarcinoma of the rectum. Clinicopathologic correlation and implications for adjuvant therapy. Cancer 34:1278–1292
22. Havenga K, Enker WE, De Ruiter MC et al (1996) The rectosacral ligament – an anatomic insight into the cause of local recurrence after conventional resection for rectal cancer (submitted for publication)
23. Havenga K, Enker WE, DeRuiter MC, Welvaart K (1996) Anatomical basis of autonomic nerve-preserving total mesorectal excision for rectal cancer. Br J Surg 83:384–388
24. Havenga K, Enker WE, McDermott K et al (1996) Male and female sexual and urinary function after total mesorectal excision with autonomic nerve preservation for rectal cancer. J Am Coll Surg (accepted for publication)
25. Havenga K, Huang Y, Enker WE et al (1996) Total mesorectal excision versus conventional surgery for rectal adenocarcinoma (submitted for publication)
26. Hojo K, Koyama Y (1982) The effectiveness of wide anatomical resection and radical lymphadenectomy for patients with rectal cancer. Jpn J Surg 12:111–116
27. Hojo K, Koyama Y, Moriya Y (1982) Lymphatic spread and its prognostic value in patients with rectal cancer. Am J Surg 144:350–354
28. Hojo K, Sawada T, Moriya Y (1989) An analysis of survival and voiding, sexual function after wide iliopelvic lymphadenectomy in patients with carcinoma of the rectum, compared with conventional lymphadencetomy. Dis Colon Rectum 32:128–133
29. Kollmorgen CF, Meagher AP, Wolff BG et al (1994) The long-term detrimental effect of postoperative radiation therapy for rectal carcinoma on bowel function. Proc Am Soc Colon Rect Surg 37:7
30. Krook JE, Moertel CG, Gunderson LL et al (1991) Effective surgical adjuvant therapy for high-risk rectal carcinoma. N Engl J Med 324:709–715
31. MacFarlane JK, Ryall RDH, Heald RJ (1993) Mesorectal excision for rectal cancer. Lancet 341:457–460
32. Marsh PJ, James RD, Schofield PF (1994) Adjuvant preoperative radiotherapy for locally advanced rectal carcinoma. Dis Colon Rectum 37:1205–1214
33. McDermott FT (1983) Carcinoma of the rectum. In: Hughes ESR, Cuthbertson AM, Killingback MK (eds) Colorectal surgery. Churchill Livingstone, Melbourne, pp 347–388
34. Minsky BD (1994) Preoperative combined modality treatment for rectal cancer. Oncology 8:53–61
35. Minsky BD, Kemeny N, Cohen AM et al (1991) Preoperative high-dose leucovorin/5-fluorouracil and radiation therapy for unresectable rectal cancer. Cancer 67:2859–2866
36. Moosa AR, Ree PC, Marks JE et al (1975) Factors influencing local recurrence after abdominoperineal resection for cancer of the rectum and rectosigmoid. Br J Surg 62:727–730
37. Moreira LF, Hizuta A, Iwagaki H et al (1994) Lateral lymph node dissection for rectal cancer below the peritoneal reflection. Br J Surg 81:293–296
38. Morikawa E, Yasutomi M, Shindou K et al (1994) Distribution of metastatic lymph nodes in colorectal cancer by the modified clearing method. Dis Colon Rectum 37:219–223
39. Moriya Y, Hojo K, Sawada T et al (1989) Significance of lateral node dissection for advanced rectal carcinoma at or below the peritoneal reflection. Dis Colon Rectum 32:307–315
40. MRC Working Party (1984) The evaluation of low dose preoperative x-ray therapy in the management of operable rectal cancer; results of a randomly controlled trial. Br J Surg 71:21–25
41. Neville R, Fielding LP, Amendola C (1987) Local tumor recurrence after curative resection for rectal cancer a ten-year hospital review. Dis Colon Rectum 30:12–17

42. Ng IOL, Luk IS, Yuen ST (1993) Surgical lateral clearance margins in resected rectal carcinomas: a multivariate analysis of clinicopathologic features. Cancer 71:1972–1976
43. NIH Consensus Conference (1990) Adjuvant therapy for patients with colon and rectal cancer. J Am Med Assoc 264:1444–1450
44. Norstein J, Bergan A, Langmark F (1993) Risk factors for local recurrence after radical surgery for rectal carcinoma: a prospective multicentre study. Br J Surg 80 [Suppl]:22
45. O'Connell M, Martenson J, Rich T et al (1993) Protracted venous infusion (PVI) 5-fluorouracil (5-FU) as a component of effective combined modality postoperative surgical adjuvant therapy for high-risk rectal cancer (abstract). Proc Am Soc Clin Oncol 12:193
46. Påhlman L, Glimelius B (1990) Pre or postoperative radiotherapy in rectal and rectosigmoid carcinoma. Ann Surg 211:187–195
47. Patel SC, Tovee EB, Langer B (1977) Twenty-five years of experience with radical surgical treatment of carcinoma of the extraperitoneal rectum. Surgery 82:460–465
48. Paty PB, Enker WE, Cohen AM et al (1994) Long-term functional results of coloanal anastomosis for rectal cancer. Am J Surg 167:90–95
49. Paty PB, Enker WE, Cohen AM, Lauwers GY (1994) Treatment of rectal cancer by low anterior resection with coloanal anastomosis. Ann Surg 219:365–373
50. Phillips RKS, Hittinger R, Blesovsky L et al (1984) Local recurrence following "curative" surgery for large bowel cancer of the rectum and rectosigmoid. Br J Surg 71:17–20
51. Pilipshen SJ, Heilweil M, Quan SHQ (1984) Patterns of pelvic recurrence following definitive resections of rectal cancer. Cancer 53:1354–1362
52. Quirke P (1996) Circumferential margins and pelvic recurrence in rectal cancer: pathologic evaluation. SWAP course on total mesorectal excision in rectal cancer. The Royal College of Surgeons of England, London, 27–28 April
53. Quirke P, Durdey P, Dixon MF et al (1986) Local recurrence of rectal adenocarcinoma due to inadequate surgical resection. Histopathological study of lateral tumor spread and surgical excision. Lancet I:996–999
54. Quirke P, Scott N (1992) The pathologist's role in the assessment of local recurrence in rectal carcinoma. Surg Oncol Clin North Am 1:1–17
55. Rao AR, Kagan AR, Chan PM et al (1981) Patterns of recurrence following curative resection alone for adenocarcinoma of the rectum and sigmoid colon. Cancer 48:1492–1495
56. Reynolds J (1996) The importance of the mesorectum in the operative treatment of rectal cancer (submitted for publication)
57. Rich T, Gunderson LL, Lew R et al (1983) Patterns of recurrence of rectal cancer after potentially curative surgery. Cancer 52:1317–1329
58. SAS Institute (1989) SAS/STAT User's guide, version six, vol 2, 4th edn. SAS Institute, Cary, North Carolina, pp 1027ff
59. Sato K, Sato T (1991) The vascular and neuronal composition of the lateral ligament of the rectum and the rectosacral fascia. Surg Radiol Ant 13:17–22
60. Steele GD (1994) Editorial commentary. In: Simone JV, Bosl GJ, Glatstein E, Longo DL, Ozols RF, Steele G Jr (eds) Yearbook of oncology 1994. Yearbook Medical Publishers, Chicago, pp 273–274
61. Stockholm Rectal Cancer Study Group (1990) Preoperative short-term radiation therapy in operable rectal carcinoma: a prospective randomized trial. Cancer 66:49–55
62. Tepper JE, Cohen AM, Wood WC et al (1986) Postoperative radiation therapy for rectal cancer. Int J Radiat Oncol Biol Phys 13:5–10
63. Twomey P, Burchell M, Strawn D, Guernsey J (1989) Local control in rectal cancer. Arch Surg 124:1174–1179
64. Walz BJ, Green MR, Lurstrom RE et al (1981) Anatomic prognostic factors after abdominoperineal resection. Int J Radiat Oncol Biol Phys 7:477–482
65. Willett CG, Tepper JE, Kaufman DS et al (1992) Adjuvant postoperative radiation therapy for rectal adenocarcinoma. Am J Clin Oncol 15:371–375
66. Williams NS, Durdey P, Johnston D (1985) The outcome following sphincter-saving resection and abdominoperineal resection for low rectal cancer. Br J Surg 72:595–598
67. Williams NS, Johnston D (1984) Survival and recurrence after sphincter saving resection and abdominoperineal resection for carcinoma of the middle third of the rectum. Br J Surg 71:278–282

CHAPTER 17

Nerve-Sparing Surgery:
Surgical Neuroanatomy and Techniques

Yoshihiro Moriya

Introduction

Rectal cancer is generally characterized by being relatively slow growing and localized compared with other gastrointestinal malignancies. The characteristics of localized tumour growth are also observed both in lymph node metastasis and in metastases to the liver and lung. The Japanese treatment concept of extended lymphadenectomy is based upon such biological behaviour.

However, disturbances of micturition and sexual function are frequently seen after extended rectal cancer surgery including lymphadenectomy. Such consequences imply that aggressive surgery must not only be evaluated in terms of tumour control, but also by its functional end-results. Since 1984, based on a better understanding of the anatomy of the pelvic autonomic nervous system, we have been actively undertaking autonomic nerve-sparing surgery with wide lymphadenectomy for lower rectal cancer [3, 4] in order to optimize function without compromising the concept of local and regional tumour control.

Surgical anatomy of the autonomic nervous system, patient selection and techniques for three different nerve-sparing procedures will be discussed here.

Surgical Anatomy of the Pelvis

The organs in the pelvis are supplied with both sympathetic and parasympathetic innervation. These autonomic nerves radiate and intertwine quite differently (Fig. 1) [2].

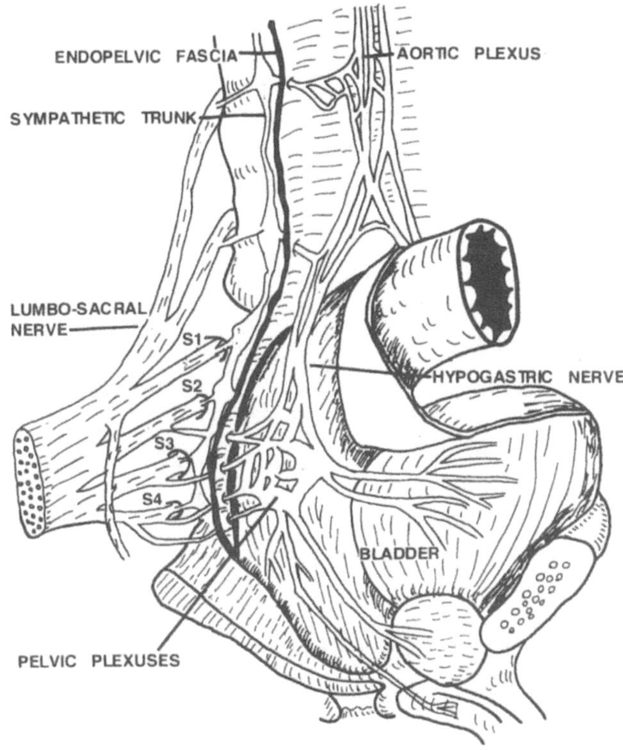

Fig. 1. Intrapelvic autonomic nervous system

The sympathetic nerve system in the pelvis arises from aortic plexuses, which represent the downward extension of the celiac plexuses on the abdominal aorta. The aortic autonomic nerve plexuses are reinforced by splanchnic branches from the bilateral lumbar sympathetic trunks located in front of the lumbar vertebrae. The fibres on the left side of the aorta are denser than those on the right and form the inferior mesenteric plexuses roughly where the inferior mesenteric artery originates from the aorta.

Fibers of the aortic plexuses extend downward in front of the abdominal aorta. At the level of the aortic bifurcation, the fibres merge to form the superior hypogastric plexus, which descends 2–3 cm and divides into the paired hypogastric nerves below the promontorium of sacrum. At this junction, the superior hypogastric plexus comes to lie in the interiliac trigon, behind the mesorectum. In order to preserve the sympathetic nervous system, an exact understanding of these anatomical details is highly important. Thus, first of all, the superior hypogastric plexuses should be identified at the interiliac trigon just behind the mesorectum after having mobilized the base of the sigmoid mesocolon. As almost all fibres forming the inferior mesenteric plexus arise from the aortic plexuses, the superior hypogastric plexus is usually displaced somewhat to the left.

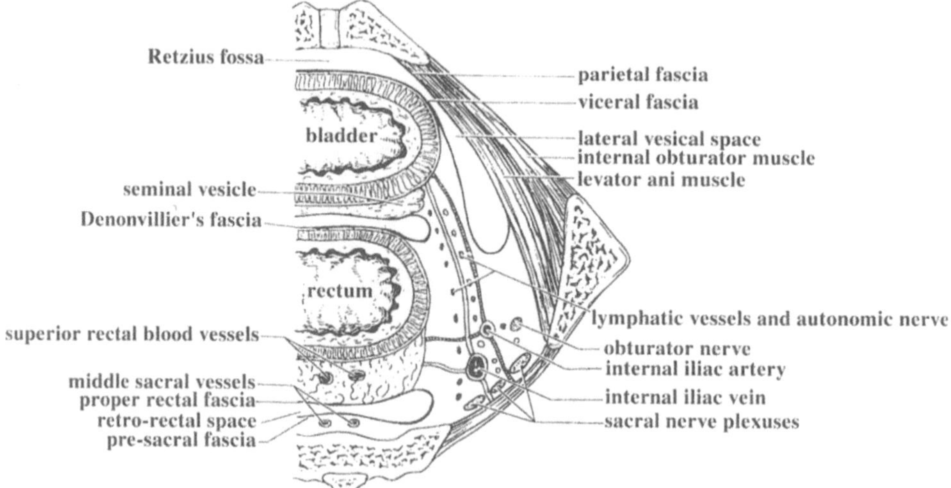

Fig. 2. Relation of intrapelvic organs, blood vessels and the pelvic nerve plexus

The superior hypogastric plexus shows several anatomical variations in its arrangement. Although progress has been made in our understanding of the anatomy and distribution of autonomic nerves, variations are not easily detected during surgery. The right and left hypogastric nerves proceed downward between the internal iliac vessels and the proper rectal fascia and finally enter the antero-superior parts of the pelvic plexuses (Fig. 2).

The paired hypogastric nerves are one of three routes of the sympathetic nervous system extending into the pelvis. The other two routes are the sacral sympathetic trunks, which extend along the anterior surface of the sacrum just medial to the internal iliac vessels, and the superior rectal plexus downward from the inferior mesenteric plexuses.

The function and anatomy of the superior rectal plexus are not important, because the plexus is included in the resected area in the case of advanced rectal cancer. Although the sacral sympathetic trunks present extremely fine connections to the pelvic plexuses, their functional importance is as yet obscure. In order to perform a nerve-sparing procedure, it is therefore important to visualize the routes of the superior hypogastric plexus in the pelvis. In the absence of visual identification in a para-aortic lymphadenectomy designed to remove upward lymphatic node spread, serious damage to the nerves may occur, adversely affecting male ejaculation.

Just below the peritoneal reflection on each side, the hypogastric nerves join at an antero-superior angle the pelvic plexus or the inferior hypogastric plexus, which lies antero-laterally close to the sidewall of rectal ampulla (Fig. 3). The pelvic plexuses are relatively narrow, flattened, plexiform bands, 3–4 cm in diameter, and are the direct continuations and extensions both of hypogastric and pelvic splanchnic nerves or nervi erigentes.

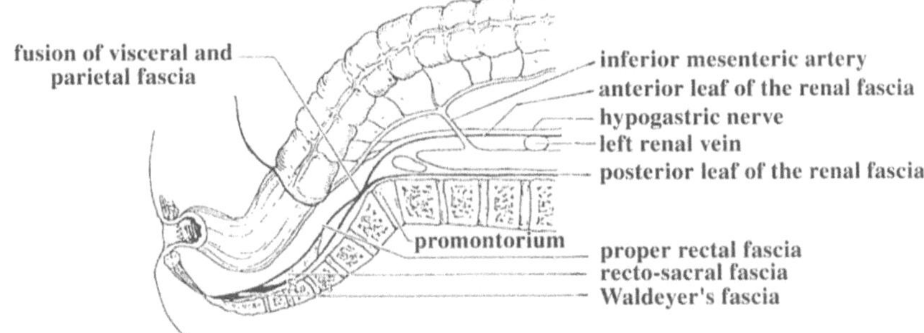

Fig. 3. Pelvic anatomy (cross-section) focusing on the fascial structures and the hypogastric nerves

The pelvic splanchnic nerves arise from the anterior surfaces of the sacral nerves located downward and laterally on the piriform muscle. In applied surgical anatomy, the largest contribution from the sacral nerve to the pelvic plexuses is from the S3 root, but with contribution also from the S2 and S4 roots. Fibres from S4 are usually larger than those from S2 [4]. The pelvic splanchnic nerves enter the postero-lateral angle of the pelvic plexuses. Intrapelvic organs receive subsidiary visceral branches from the pelvic plexuses. The main trunks of the nerves to the bladder and proximal urethra lie outside the pelvic fascia [5]. The entire left colon receives its parasympathetic supply from the pelvic plexus through the mesorectum; this parasympathetic supply reaches the inferior mesenteric plexus and finally runs along the inferior mesenteric artery.

It is of paramount importance to appreciate the anatomical relationship between the internal iliac vessels, the fascial structures and the intrapelvic autonomic nervous system, taking the following four aspects into account:

1. The entire sympathetic and parasympathetic nerves are located medial to the internal iliac vessels.
2. The endopelvic fascia covering the iliac vessels also sheathes the roots of the pelvic splanchnic nerves.
3. The parietal fascia fuses with the proper rectal fascia at or below the caval bifurcation and then gradually separates from the proper rectal fascia.
4. From the level of the third or fourth sacral segment, the rectosacral fascia are seen in the retrorectal space.

During surgery, a natural dissection layer exists between the proper rectal fascia (mesorectum) and pre-sacral fascia in the loose areolar tissue of the retrorectal space. The pelvic splanchnic nerves pierce the endopelvic fascia, which is a lateral continuation of the rectosacral fascia, in order to enter the pelvic plexuses. The importance of the rectosacral fascia when performing autonomic nerve-sparing surgery lies in the following point: a sharp dissection of the rectosacral fascia on the right and left sides brings into view the root of the pelvic splanchnic nerves, which are seen as white bundles. After dissecting the rectosacral fascia, Waldeyer's fascia appears posteriorly as a white leaf covering the sacrum and coccyx.

If urinary and sexual functions are to be preserved, a complete anatomical understanding of the nerve supply and of the musculature in the perineum is also important [6]. The main nerve in the perineum is the pudendal nerve, which is derived either from the second and third, from the second, third and fourth or from third and fourth sacral nerves. The pudendal nerves leave the pelvis below the piriform muscle and immediately enter the pudendal (Alcock's) canal, which contains three structures (artery, vein and nerve) medial to the ischial tuberosity. After branching of the inferior rectal nerves, the pudendal nerve divides into two further branches: the perineal nerves and dorsal nerve of the penis or clitoris. These branches are found along the undersurface of the ischium and pubic bone, where they innervate the striated external urethral sphincter.

The perineal muscles are more complicated than the nerve supply. The central tendon or perineal body is a fibromuscular septum intervening between the urogenital diaphragm and the anal canal. There are many aspects of coordination between urogenital and anal regions, not only neurologically but also anatomically. Therefore, in the case of abdominoperineal resection, urinary and sexual disturbances occur more frequently than after a sphincter-saving operation because of the complete resection of the levator ani muscles and impairment both of the central tendon and branches of the pudendal nerve.

Patient Selection

Based on a comprehensive understanding of the anatomy and functional consequences of denervation of the autonomic nervous system, nerve-sparing surgery can be divided into four major categories (Fig. 4).

1. *Total preservation of the autonomic nervous system.* Such an operation also include total mesorectal excision (TME). The nerve-sparing effect of this procedure has been outlined and stressed by Heald and Ryall [1].
2. *Resection of the sympathetic nervous system but complete preservation of pelvic nerves.* This ensures undisturbed micturition in both sexes and erection in males.
3. *Partial preservation of pelvic nerves.* This is designed to preserve, to some extent, undisturbed urinary function. This type of resection is commonly undertaken during lateral lymph node dissection.
4. *Extended lateral lymphadenectomy without nerve preservation.*

Based on our extensive experience and taking into account the information from TNM staging, total preservation of the autonomic nervous system (category 1 operation) is best applied in patients with T2 tumour. Complete preservation of pelvic nerves (category 2 operation) is offered to patients with T3 tumour, and partial preservation of pelvic nerves (category 3) to patients with node-positive rectal cancer. The so-called extended lymphadenectomy without

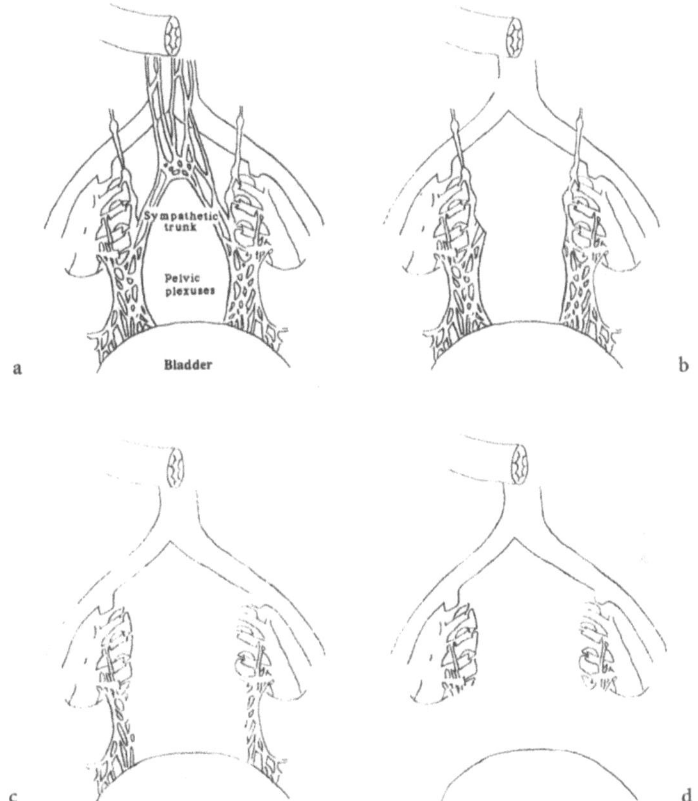

Fig. 4a–d. Types of nerve-sparing techniques. **a** Total preservation of autonomic nerve. **b** Complete preservation of pelvic nerve. **c** Partial preservation of pelvic nerve. **d** Extended lymphadenectomy without nerve preservation

nerve preservation (category 4) is carried out in patients with definite lateral node metastasis.

Such criteria of patient selection for specific procedures are based not only on the relationship between the cancer and pelvic nerves, but also on the neuroanatomical features in which the paired sympathetic hypogastric nerves after branching off from the superior hypogastric plexuses are strongly adherent to the mesorectum (Fig. 3), in particular to the proper rectal fascia.

Endorectal ultrasonography should be routinely be used to assess invasion of the rectal wall and to identify lymph node metastasis preoperatively. If further imaging is necessary, magnetic resonance imaging (MRI) and/or computed tomography (CT) scan of the pelvis should be carried out.

Surgical Technique

Proximal Dissection

The preferred approach is a long median incision extending from the pubis to a point near the level of the xiphoid process. After inserting an abdominal retractor, the loops of the entire small bowel are displaced out of the abdominal cavity using two or three large moist packs to allow better access to the inferior mesenteric artery.

While retracting the sigmoid mesocolon, an incision is made in the white tendon at the base of the sigmoid mesocolon to expose the superior hypogastric plexus in the interiliac trigon, where this plexus is easily identified between the mesorectum and a point just distal to the aortic bifurcation. After lifting the plexus with a band, fibres of the sympathetic nerves including both the aortic plexuses and the lumber splanchnic nerves are seen. They must remain untouched while the mesorectum and mesocolon are freed of sympathetic fibers up to the root of the inferior mesenteric artery.

Although such sympathetic nerve-preserving techniques were performed without technical problems for para-aortic lymph node dissection (Fig. 5) during the development of our nerve-sparing technique, the incidence of ejaculation disturbance was very high after this type of dissection owing to damage of both blood and lymphatic supply to the sympathetic nervous system. Therefore, we now recommend that the layer of separation should be more superficial to the autonomic nervous system (i.e., in front of it). Following identification of sympathetic nerves, the inferior mesenteric artery is doubly ligated and cut at its origin from the abdominal aorta. The inferior

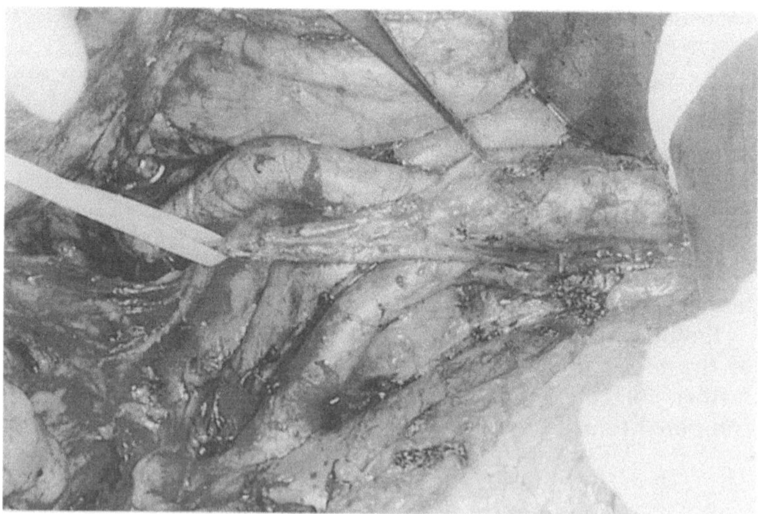

Fig. 5. Sympathetic nerve-preserving procedure with para-aortic lymph node dissection

mesenteric vein is likewise cut several centimetres cephalad to the inferior mesenteric artery at the lower border of the pancreas. The sigmoid mesocolon is fashioned to prepare the colon stump for colostomy or low anterior anastomosis.

Posterior Pelvic Dissection

Pulling the rectum antero-caudally, the retrorectal space is opened using the deep pelvic retractor or long scissors while looking for the middle sacral vessels. By sharp separation, the rectum is mobilized posteriorly down to the coccygeal bone (Fig. 6). While dissecting in the retrorectal space, three important manoeuvres have to be performed. The first is to prevent injuries to the

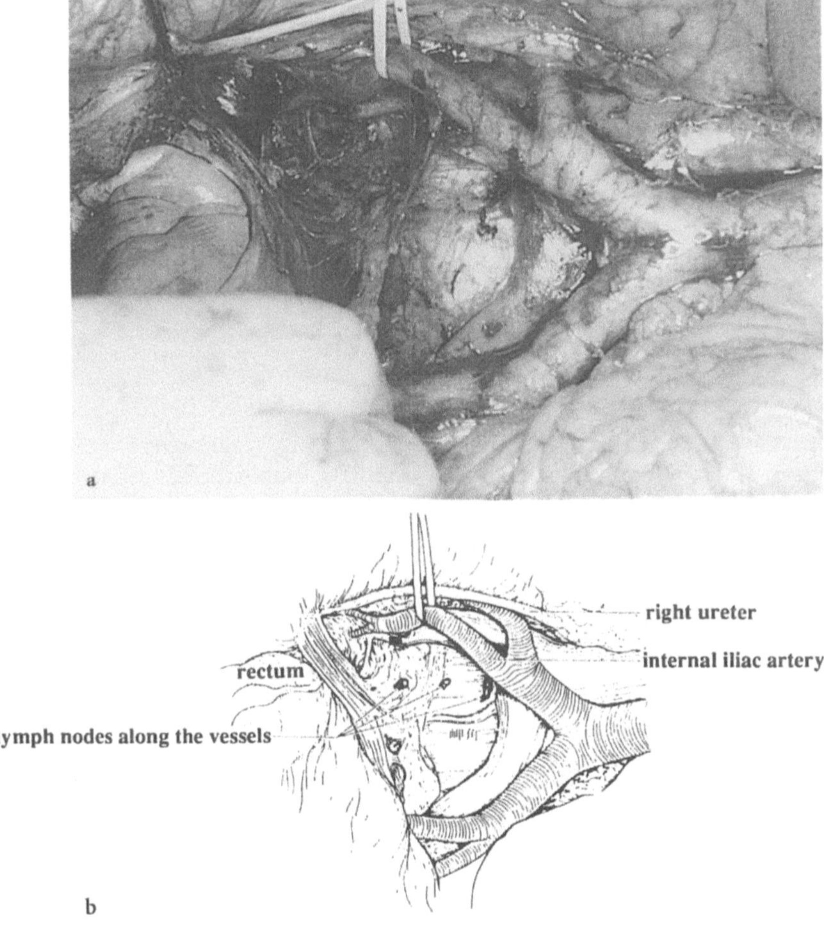

Fig. 6a,b. Dissection of the retrorectal space

hypogastric nerves, which run downward close to the proper rectal fascia along the pelvic side wall. The paired hypogastric nerves should therefore be meticulously dissected off the rectum. Secondly, the root of the pelvic splanchnic nerves arising from S3 and S4 sacral nerves should be identified. This should be an entirely bloodless process, and complete haemostasis should be achieved by diathermy coagulation if small veins between the rectum and the middle sacral veins are encountered. It is dangerous to insert the right hand (blind manipulation) to dissect the retrorectal space; bleeding into the loose areolar tissue will result in inadequate identification of the fine anatomical details that are an integral part of the nerve-sparing operation. Whenever a correct dissection of the retrorectal space is performed, the pre-sacral venous plexuses can be clearly seen. The third manoeuvre is to estimate the appearance of lymph nodes in the mesorectum by palpation.

Anterior Pelvic Dissection

The peritoneal incisions are now extended distally around the rectovesical pouch or more widely on the transverse vesical fold in patients with definite serosal invasion of the anterior wall of the rectum. While retracting the bladder toward the pubis by a long pelvic retractor, the rectum is retracted cranio-posteriorly by the surgeon's left hand, and cautious diathermy dissection is gradually deepened in the plane just behind the seminal vesicles. Denonvillier's fascia should be kept on the rectal side. The anterior dissection should proceed in this plane to the base of the prostate gland.

Lateral Dissection

In the course of the above-mentioned surgical manoeuvres, the rectum has been freed both posteriorly and anteriorly, but will still remain strongly attached on either side by the so-called lateral ligament. This "ligament" consists, however, nearly exclusively of autonomic nerves fibres. The autonomic nervous system in the pelvis is found, as previously described, between the internal iliac vessels and the rectum. Dissecting the lateral ligament is the most intense and challenging phase during a rectal excision, particularly when partial preservation of pelvic nerves is combined with lateral dissection. For this reason the nerve-sparing dissecting techniques are described in detail.

First of all, the ureter is gently lifted and retracted to prevent injury. The dissection is started along the inner side of the internal iliac vessels down to the middle rectal artery, while removing lymphatics and fatty tissue covering the vessels. While doing this, the fascia on the piriform muscle which connects with the rectosacral fascia (see Chap. 9) is identified. By meticulous sharp cuts of these fascial structures, the root of the pelvic splanchnic nerves arising from the anterior sacral foramen can be exposed (Fig. 7). It should be noted that veins from the internal pudendal venous plexuses exist in this region that

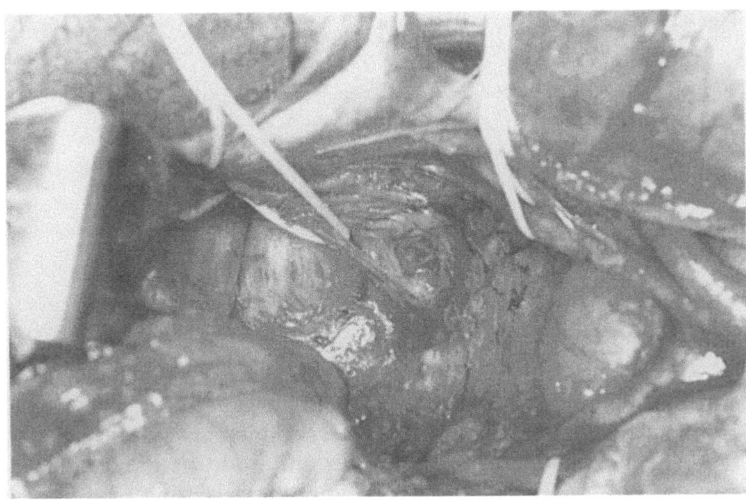

Fig. 7. Root of pelvic nerves on right side

anastomose with the internal iliac veins. To proceed successfully, bleeding in this region must be avoided at all costs.

The pelvic nerve plexuses lie closely attached to both the internal iliac vessels and the side wall of the rectal ampulla. While maintaining traction of the rectum in the antero-cephalad direction and at the same time ascertaining the position of the root of the pelvic nerve, it is essential that the pelvic plexuses are freed from the proper rectal fascia; all the branches to the rectal wall from the pelvic plexus have to be cut. After completion of nerve dissection, the deep or lower pararectal space can be opened and the superior surface of the levator ani muscle can be seen. The rectum on the right side is now completely free of any attachment to the pelvic wall. After dissection of the right lateral ligament, the opposite ligament is then dissected similarly.

Finally, the paravesical and obturator spaces are opened between the lateral border of the internal iliac vessels and the true pelvic wall, and the lateral lymphatic tissues in these spaces are cleared while preserving the obturator nerve and vessels as well as vesical and parietal branches arising from the internal iliac vessels and the sacral nerve plexuses (Fig. 8). However, when affected nodes are found or suspected in the lateral lymphatic channels around these vessels, en bloc excision of the internal iliac vessels (both arteries and veins) and re-resection of the preserved autonomic nervous system should be carried out aggressively.

Distal Dissection

After completing both rectal mobilization and lateral dissection, the rectum is attached only to the levator ani muscles and the anal canal. At this stage, the

Fig. 8. Lateral lymph node dissection

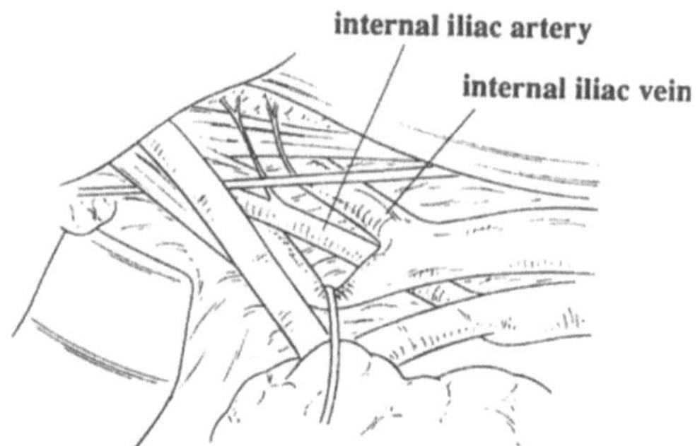

surgeon has to decide whether to perform an abdominoperineal resection or a sphincter-saving procedure. This decision is based on tumour site, histological type, local extent of primary tumour and node status. If a free distal margin of more than 2 cm can be obtained, a sphincter-saving procedure using a stapler device is the recommended alternative.

Conclusion

Our current policy focuses on individualization or case-oriented procedures. Aggressive use of various nerve-sparing operations in patients with advanced rectal cancer is the key element of the surgical procedure, taking into account the extent of cancer spread based on both preoperative imaging diagnosis and intra-operative findings.

References

1. Heald RJ, Ryall RD (1986) Recurrence and survival after total mesorectal excision for rectal cancer. Lancet II:479–482
2. Lee JF, Maurer VM, Block GE (1973) Anatomic relation of pelvic autonomic nerves to pelvic operations. Arch Surg 107:324–329
3. Moriya Y, Hojo K, Sawada T, Koyama Y (1989) Significance of lateral node dissection for advanced rectal carcinoma at or below the peritoneal reflection. Dis Colon Rectum 32:307–315
4. Moriya Y (1993) Pelvic node dissection with autonomic nerve sparing for invasive lower rectal cancer. In: Wanebo HJ (ed) Colorectal cancer. Mosby, St Louis, pp 274–289
5. Smith PH, Ballatyne B (1968) The neuroanatomical basis for denervation of the urinary bladder following major pelvic surgery. Br J Surg 55:929–933
6. Walsh PC, Schlegel PN (1988) Radical pelvic surgery with preservation of sexual function. Ann Surg 208:291–300

CHAPTER 18

Lateral Node Dissection – A Critique

John K. MacFarlane

Introduction

The stimulus to develop a wider pelvic dissection in the management of rectal cancer was initiated by the frustration of surgeons working in this area with the poor results of conventional operative approaches. Both local recurrence and death from metastatic disease seemed to be unacceptably high and it was hoped that using wider-field procedures would eliminate the last cancer cell, thus effecting a cure.

The spread of rectal cancer from the bowel wall locally into adjacent tissues, regionally into lymphatics and the draining nodes, and eventually via the blood stream to distant sites has been the subject of many classical studies dating back to Gabriel and Dukes [8]. Attempts to remove the nodes were frustrated by the location of the tumour within the bony pelvis, where the use of a wide local resection as the paradigm of management was felt to be virtually impossible.

Although the commonest pattern of spread was proximal in the mesentery, lateral spread was recognised as early as the 1950s by Stearns and Deddish [28] and Bacon [3], who reported that their more radical approach to rectal cancer nodal dissection produced better local and overall control than conventional operations.

The adoption and modification of the technique beginning in the mid-1960s by the Japanese authors Koyama [16], Moriya [22], Hojo [15], Moreira [21] and others (see Chaps. 13, 17) has stimulated considerable debate in the literature. The surgical tour de force and outstanding technical expertise of these surgeons has led to a serious look at their results in the West [7, 11, 26]. A parallel trend in the management of gastric carcinoma, again championed by the Japanese, has led to a randomised study of extended lymph node dissection in North

America and Europe. This will test the current oncological principle which views lymph nodes in general as indicators of the aggressiveness of the tumour rather than as the focus of subsequent metastatic spread.

At the same time as these reports were reaching the Western journals, Heald [13, 14], MacFarlane [18], Enker [6], Aitken [1] and others were reporting extraordinarily low local recurrence rates from an operation in which great care was taken to remove the mesorectum intact in every case of rectal cancer operated upon with the hope of cure, whether with permanent colostomy or anal preservation. Thus, although direct comparisons are not possible, the results of a less radical procedure were at least as good, if not somewhat better than those obtained with the most radical of dissections. The results of the extended operations will be reviewed and the role of this procedure assessed in the light of the total mesorectal excision (TME) experience as reported above.

Definitions of Terms

It is important to define the terms used in this paper to describe the various surgical procedures for rectal cancer treatment. The "conventional" rectal resection as performed by Western surgeons since the description of Miles [20] is a procedure to remove the pelvic mesocolon by the abdominoperineal approach comprising the "zone of upward spread", which became the gold standard for rectal cancer up to 15 cm from the anal verge. This procedure combines both sharp and blunt dissection in the pelvis and often results in residual mesorectal tissues being left in situ to provide the nidus for pelvic recurrence.

The seminal publications of Heald [13, 14] and his colleagues from Basingstoke in the early 1980s pointed out the importance of a complete dissection of the mesorectum under direct vision in a definable and relatively avascular plane. This procedure was called TME and resulted in surprisingly low local recurrence rates. TME corresponds to the category I lymph node dissection described by Japanese authors (see Chap. 17). It has subsequently been adopted by other investigators, as noted above.

Operations which extend beyond the mesorectum into the lateral pelvic tissues and remove the lymph nodes along the iliac and obturator vessels are characterised as lateral node dissection or extended pelvic lymphadenectomy (EPL). Such a procedure corresponds to category II–IV operations in the Japanese terminology (see Chap. 13). Thus the conventional resection is felt to leave perirectal lymph nodes in situ as well as tumour within the mesorectal lymphatics, whereas TME and EPL procedures remove such nodes. The extended operations incorporate pelvic lymph nodes beyond the mesorectum and are more radical and complex procedures. They result in a number of unavoidable neurological complications which are avoided by TME.

Review of Literature

Frequency of Nodal Involvement

EPL results in the retrieval of a variable number of involved lymph nodes (Table 1). Stearns and Deddish [28] reported a 9% incidence of lateral node involvement in 122 patients reported in 1959, while Moriya et al. [22] showed an overall incidence of 18.1% in 231 patients reviewed in 1989. Their results in 114 Dukes' C patients yielded 36% lateral nodal positivity. Hojo et al. [15] divided their node-positive rate into cancers above and below the peritoneal reflection and reported a 23% rate with tumours centred below the peritoneal reflection compared with only 8.8% above that point. Finally, Moreira et al. [21] reported an 11% nodal involvement in 95 patients in 1994. A detailed discussion of the current results of lateral node dissection appears in Chaps. 12, 13. The other field of putative lymph node spread is proximal along the inferior mesenteric artery and vein, and the so-called "high ligation advocates", such as Ault [2], State [27], Rosi [25] and Grinnell [10], all deserve mention in this discussion. Enthusiasm for high ligation of the inferior mesenteric and vein in an effort to clear lymphatic metastases from colorectal cancer to the para-aortic region was reported in the 1960s.

Rosi et al. [25] reported that the addition of left hemicolectomy to the Miles procedure resulted in a 6.9% improvement in the 5-year survival rate over a conventional procedure which left the left colon intact. Grinnell's report in 1965 suggested additional lymph node metastases retrieved with high ligation of the inferior mesenteric artery at the aorta. However, the results in patients with lymph node involvement at this level were discouraging, and no additional survival was felt to be achieved by this more extensive proximal dissection. The failure of high ligation to salvage patients with nodal metastases above the level of the left colic artery was attributed to the aggressiveness of the tumour with such high lymph node metastases, and the presence of microscopic metastatic disease beyond the resection margins, which became clinically relevant in follow-up, was uniformly present.

Table 1. Results of extended pelvic lymphadenectomy (EPL) – frequency of nodal involvement

Authors	Patients (n)	Frequency (%)
Stearns and Deddish [28]	122	9.0%
Moriya et al. [22]	231	18.1%
	114	36.0% (Dukes' C)
Hojo et al. [15]	389	8.8% (upper rectum)
		23.0% (lower rectum)
Moreira et al. [21]	95	11.0%
Takahashi et al. (Chap. 13)	125	11%

Table 2. Rate of pelvic recurrence

Authors	Pelvic recurrence (%)		
	Extended pelvic lymphadenectomy	Dukes' tumour stage	Conventional operation
Moriya et al. [22]	16.0	C	n.a.
Hojo et al. [15]	6.3	B	21.8*
	23.6	C	32.9*
Moreira et al. [21]	4.0	B	15.0
	12.0	C	20.0
Yasutomi et al. [29]	13.2	–	13.7
Koyama [16]	8.4	B	26.1
	24.5%	C	44.3

n.a., not applicable.
*Statistically significant difference.

Rate of Pelvic Recurrence

The results of extended pelvic dissection of lymph nodes are reported in Table 2. In each study, the pelvic recurrence rate of EPL is compared with that noted in conventional dissections. None of these studies is randomised, and significant differences are seen in the Hojo paper for Dukes' B and C lesions as well as for the overall results in the Moreira report.

The pelvic recurrence rate varies considerably from a low of 4% for the Dukes' B cases reported by Moreira [21] to a high of 24.5% for Dukes' C patients operated on by the Hojo group [15]. No comparative group is reported on by Moriya [22], and Yasutomi [29] has noted no significant difference between the EPL group and the patients subjected to conventional dissections. Additionally, he has a historical control group which does not differ substantially from the results reported in this later study. In no instance was a "conventional dissection" defined, making these comparisons somewhat difficult to interpret.

Survival

The effects on 5-year survival of EPL patients are summarised in Table 3. Each of the reported studies is non-randomised, and the results reported from conventional lymphadenectomy are either historical or contemporaneous with those reported for EPL. The Hojo report [15] and Koyama [16] claim a statistically significant difference in both the Dukes' B and C categories and additionally note a difference between Dukes' B and C both for the EPL and conventional dissection groups. Each of the other reports, although seeming to favour the EPL category, fails to reach statistical significance.

Table 3. Five-year survival (non-randomised) related to type of lymph node (LN) dissection

Authors	Survival (%)	
	Extended pelvic lymphadenectomy	Conventional operation
Stearns and Deddish [28]	54.0	46.0
Bacon [3]	54.0	49.0
Moriya et al. [22]	75.8	67.4
	68.0[a]	43.7
Hojo et al. [15]	88.0[b]	74.0[b*]
	61.0[a]	43.0[a*]
Moreira et al. [21]	76.0	72.0
Glass et al. [9]	54.0	52.0
Enker et al. [6]	48.0[a]	28.0[a]

[a]Dukes' C tumour.
[b]Dukes' B tumour.
[*]Statistically significant difference.

Complication of Pelvic Dissection

Finally, the complication rate of pelvic dissection was reported on by four authors and is presented in Table 4. Hojo [15] notes a 39.4% bladder dysfunction at 1 year following EPL and a 76% overall sexual dysfunction rate in patients under the age of 60 years with previous normal sexual function. Moriya [22] notes that 10% of his patients who underwent EPL require periodic catheterisation for bladder emptying at 1 year, and virtually no return of sexual function is noted with time following an initial experience of over 90% impotence. In contrast, Enker [5], with his autonomic nerve-preserving mesorectal excision, has an overall 4.7% bladder dysfunction with a 13.3% sexual dysfunction rate in the long-term follow-up of patients in his series.

Hojo [15] reports the morbidity rates in terms of anastomotic pelvic infection and intestinal obstruction as being the same in both groups. Overall operative mortality rates in all of the series remain acceptably low at 2% or less, and no differences are seen between patients treated with EPL when compared with the conventional surgical approach.

Table 4. Complications of pelvic dissection

Authors	Type of operation	Complications (%)	
		Bladder	Sexual
Hojo [15]	EPL	39.4	76.0
Moriya [22]	EPL	10.0 (catheter)	>90.0
Enker [5]	TME	4.7	13.3
Michelassi [19]	EPL	18.0	100.0

EPL, extended pelvic lymphadenectomy; TME, total mesorectal excision.

In North America, Fabrizio Michelassi [19] retrospectively analysed 27 patients treated at the University of Chicago Medical Centre between 1988 and 1990 as to the effect of wide pelvic lymphadenectomy on early and late complications. The study defined wide pelvic lymphadenectomy as an en bloc resection of the left colon rectosigmoid and rectum as outlined by Block [4]. The choice of lymphadenectomy was left to the discretion of the surgeon, but the more conventional approach was reserved for patients with "earlier tumours".

The morbidity and mortality associated with the two procedures was not significantly different in terms of intra-operative blood loss, length of post-operative hospital stay or mortality. The neurogenic complications of the wide pelvic lymphadenectomy produced a temporary neurogenic bladder in 18% of the patients so treated. However, sexual dysfunction was high in both groups in that only seven of the 16 males in the series were sexually active prior to their surgery and two from the conventional dissection group remained so postoperatively, whereas none of the four patients treated in the wide pelvic lymphadenectomy group were sexually active postoperatively. This suggests that the morbidity of the wider pelvic lymphadenectomy is significant in the long term and deserves serious consideration.

Attempts at autonomic nerve preservation associated with wide pelvic lymphadenectomy (for technical details see Chap. 17) are reported by Moriya and his colleagues [23, 24] and by Takahashi and co-workers (see Chap. 13). While the results reported in these recent papers are very good in terms of local recurrence and disease-free survival, specific reference to functional results indicate that 84% of male patients had "acceptable urinary function after surgery", and of 31 patients with total preservation of the autonomic nerves, ten were unable to ejaculate and only three were capable of erection. Although these recent results of a concerted effort to preserve the autonomic nerves are somewhat better than prior results, these meticulous efforts at nerve-sparing do not produce the kind of results reported by Enker [5] and others with TME alone.

Comments

The postulated mechanism for spread of cancer cells into adjacent lymphatic drainage sites is retrograde flow due to blockage of local and regional nodes in the mesorectum. Involvement of adjacent soft tissues outside the mesorectal envelope and occasional skipped metastases occur with high-grade histologies noted by Dukes in his original studies. The presence of lateral lymph node spread therefore implies a poor prognosis malignancy [17]. The rationale for extending the limits of lymph node dissection resides in the apparent lack of completeness of traditional dissection methods, the nodes themselves being a focus for both metastatic disease and local recurrence, and the hoped-for improvement in long-term survival. Further stimulus to surgical innovation in this area comes from the relative failure of adjuvant therapy strategies in rectal cancer. Early efforts in surgical innovation were championed by Stearns and

Deddish [28] as well as Bacon [3] and his co-workers. The results of their attempts at improving the 5-year survival rates using extended lymph node dissection produced a minor impact on the overall survival, ranging from 5% to 8% improvement. Subsequent studies by Glass [9] and co-workers failed to show any such improvement in results, and the concept of extended lymph node dissection was abandoned in the Western surgical world until re-introduced in the late 1960s by the Japanese. During this interval, the paradigm of lymph nodes as a focus for dissemination came under some scrutiny, especially in studies of breast, lung, melanoma and other tumours. Thus the current notion that nodal involvement is more an indicator of aggressive behaviour than a focus for dissemination has gained favour. Nonetheless, the mesorectal envelope in rectal cancer may well place the rectum in a somewhat different category, and thus the results of the Japanese experience become a focus of interest.

There is no question that the completeness of the lateral node dissection is greater than that in the traditional or mesorectal dissections. A large number of nodes is always recovered, and 8%–23% node-positivity rates have been reported. The question is to the clinical relevance of these positive nodes. The results would seem to favour their presence as a potential for local (pelvic) recurrence, although the modest improvement in survival reported suggests that the dissemination of tumour has already occurred in most of the patients in whom the nodes are found to be involved.

The best figures for local control of rectal cancer are reported with mesorectal dissection (TME). The additional of lateral node removal has failed to improve on the results reported from series where TME is practised. It is tempting, therefore, to postulate that the observed improvement in results reported from lateral pelvic dissection over conventional surgery could be attributed to the inclusion of the total mesorectum in the more radical approach and not to the removal of nodes at a distance.

It should be noted that the best 5-year survival results reported by the Japanese in the range of 76% overall do not differ significantly from the 78% 5-year actuarial survivals reported by Heald and the Basingstoke group [12] using TME without lateral lymph node removal.

The frustration that adjuvant strategies have failed to cure more patients challenges the surgeon to adopt the best surgical procedure as the operation of choice and to investigate new approaches to adjuvant treatment, including biological, genetic and targeted radiation methodologies.

Finally, the complications of lateral node pelvic dissection, which do not differ significantly from conventional approaches in terms of anastomotic leaks, pelvic infections or subsequent obstruction, do differ considerably when long-term effects on bladder and sexual function are included in the follow-up. There is no doubt that the wide dissection compromises neurological function in the pelvis and results in an unacceptably high long-term dysfunction rate in both of these categories.

Conclusions

It must be concluded, therefore, that the inclusion of lateral node dissections of any magnitude is not warranted in the management of primary operable rectal cancer. The increased long-term morbidity and the lack of significant improvement in either local control or actuarial survival of EPL over TME support this position. The challenge for the future remains in the appropriate utilisation of adjuvant therapy strategies, both conventional and investigative, in the attempt to improve on the results of mesorectal excision as the cornerstone of treatment for cancer of the rectum.

References

1. Aitken RJ (1996) Mesorectal excision for rectal cancer. Br J Surg 83:214–216
2. Ault GW, Castro AF, Smith RS (1950) Carcinoma of upper rectum and rectosigmoid; clinical report on high inferior mesenteric ligation. Postgrad Med 8:176–183
3. Bacon HE (1956) Abdomino-perineal proctosigmoidectomy with sphincter preservation: 5 year and 10 year survival after "pullthrough" operation for cancer of the rectum. JAMA 160:628–634
4. Block GE (1991) Abdominoperineal resection. In: Zydema GD (ed) Surgery of the alimentary tract, 3rd edn. Saunders, Phildelphia, pp 213–220
5. Enker WE (1992) Potency, cure and local control in the operative treatment of rectal cancer. Arch Surg 127:1396–1402
6. Enker WE, Heilweil ML, Hertz RL et al (1986) En bloc lymphadenectomy and sphincter preservation in the surgical management of rectal cancer. Ann Surg 203:426–433
7. Enker WE, Thaler HT, Cranor ML, Polyak T (1995) Total mesorectal excision in the operative treatment of rectal cancer. J Am Coll Surg 181:335–346
8. Gabriel WB, Dukes C, Bussey HJR (1935) Lymphatic spread in cancer of the rectum. Br J Surg 23:395–413
9. Glass RE, Ritchie JK, Thompson HR et al (1985) The results of surgical treatment of cancer of the rectum by radical resection and extended abdomino-iliac lymphadenectomy. Br J Surg 72:599–601
10. Grinnell RS (1965) Results of ligation of inferior mesenteric artery at the aorta in resections of carcinoma of the descending and sigmoid colon and rectum. Surg Gynecol Obstet 120:1031–1036
11. Harnsberger JR, Vernava III AM, Longo WE (1994) Radical abdominopelvic lymphadenectomy: historic perspective and current role in the surgical management of rectal cancer. Dis Colon Rectum 37:73–87
12. Heald RJ (1995) Rectal cancer: the surgical options. Eur J Cancer 31A(7–8):1189–1192
13. Heald RJ, Husband EM, Ryall RDH (1982) The mesorectum in rectal cancer surgery: the clue to pelvic recurrence? Br J Surg 69:613–616
14. Heald RJ, Ryall RDH (1986) Recurrence and survival after total mesorectal excision for rectal cancer. Lancet I:1479–1482
15. Hojo K, Sawada T, Moriya Y (1989) An analysis of survival and voiding, sexual function after wide iliopelvic lymphadenectomy in patients with carcinoma of the rectum, compared with conventional lymphadenectomy. Dis Colon Rectum 32:128–133
16. Koyama Y, Moriya Y, Hojo K (1984) Effects of extended systematic lymphadenectomy for adenocarcinoma of the rectum – significant improvement of survival rate and decrease of local recurrence. Jpn J Clin Oncol 14:623–632
17. MacFarlane JK (1996) Nodal metastases in rectal cancer. The role of surgery in outcome. Surg Oncol Clin North Am 5:191–202
18. MacFarlane JK, Ryall RHD, Heald RJ (1993) Mesorectal excision for rectal cancer. Lancet 341:457–460

19. Michelassi F, Block GE (1992) Morbidity and mortality of wide pelvic lymphadenectomy for rectal adenocarcinoma. Dis Colon Rectum 35:1143–1147
20. Miles WE (1926) Cancer of the rectum. Harrison's, London, p 63
21. Moreira LF, Hizuta A, Iwagaki H, Tanaka N, Orita K (1994) Lateral lymph node dissection for rectal carcinoma below the peritoneal reflection. Br J Surg 81:293–296
22. Moriya Y, Hojo K, Sawada T, Koyama Y (1989) Significance of lateral node dissection for advanced rectal carcinoma at or below the peritoneal reflection. Dis Colon Rectum 32:307–315
23. Moriya Y, Sugihara K, Akasu T, Fujita S (1995a) Nerve-sparing surgery with lateral node dissection for advanced lower rectal cancer. Eur J Cancer 31A:1229–1232
24. Moriya Y, Sugihara K, Akasu T, Fujita S (1995b) Patterns of recurrence after nerve-sparing surgery for rectal adenocarcinoma with special reference to loco-regional recurrence. Dis Colon Rectum 38:1162–1168
25. Rosi PA, Cahill WJ, Carey J (1962) A ten year study of hemicolectomy in the treatment of carcinoma of the left half of the colon. Surg Gynecol Obstet 114:15–24
26. Scholefield JH, Northover JM (1995) Surgical management of rectal cancer. Br J Surg 82:745–748
27. State D (1951) Combined abdominoperineal excision of the rectum. A plan for standardization of the proximal extent of the dissection. Surgery 30:349–354
28. Stearns MW Jr, Deddish MR (1959) Five year results of abdominopelvic lymph node dissection for carcinoma of the rectum. Dis Colon Rectum 2:169–172
29. Yasutomi M, Shindo K, Mori N, Matsuda T (1991) Does the pelvic node dissection for the rectal cancer patients make any contribution to end results of surgery? Gan To Kagaku Ryoho 18:541–546

CHAPTER 19

Laparoscopic Approaches to Malignant Disease

John E. Hartley, Graeme S. Duthie, and John R.T. Monson

Introduction

The recent application of laparoscopic surgical techniques to colorectal resection is controversial, and the value of this new treatment modality is, as yet,
unclear. The laparoscopic approach may confer benefit to the patient in terms
of reduced wound-related morbidity, shorter duration of ileus and decreased
hospital stay [6, 7, 12, 17, 20, 29]. However, the oncological safety of laparoscopic techniques is unproven. Histological examination of resected specimens
has provided data suggesting that the lymph node clearance and excision
margins achieved laparoscopically may be comparable to those obtained using
conventional surgical techniques [7, 8, 12, 24, 25]. However, the loco-regional
recurrence rates consequent upon the laparoscopic approach are not yet
known. There are also reports of wound recurrence following laparoscopic
surgery, some of which have occurred after "curative excision" of early cancers, and these have yet to be adequately explained [18, 28].

These issues are of particular relevance in surgery for rectal cancer. The only
hope of cure of rectal cancer lies in adequate surgery [21]. The consequence of
inadequate surgery is commonly disease recurrence within the pelvis with the
likelihood of untold misery and debilitation. Wide variations in the success of

rectal cancer surgery both between surgeons and institutions are apparent [21]. While the principal prognostic variable in rectal cancer is the tumour stage and grade, the major treatment variable is the surgeon. Routine excision of the intact mesorectum during resection of cancers of the mid- and lower rectum has resulted in the lowest results of local recurrence ever reported [14]. These standards, established by Heald and co-workers, are those against which any new technique must be evaluated.

These factors have led many surgeons to argue that, given the current state of laparoscopic technology and its uncertain efficacy, tumours of the low rectum and their corresponding mesorectum should only be excised by specialist surgeons using conventional techniques [19]. However, we have been struck by the excellence of the magnified views, deep within the pelvis, which may be obtained at laparoscopy. It is possible that this technology may permit the combination of a mesorectal excision, comparable to that advocated by Heald and co-workers, with the potential advantages of minimally invasive surgery. Unfortunately, during laparoscopic-assisted anterior resection, the pelvic dissection is often carried out during the open stage of the procedure so that real doubt exists as to the ability of the laparoscopic approach to perform an adequate, "closed", mesorectal excision.

After some preliminary comments on those factors pertinent to case selection and preoperative preparation, this chapter will present our techniques for laparoscopic-assisted anterior resection and abdominoperineal resection. The results of our preliminary experience with laparoscopic mesorectal excision during these procedures are also discussed.

Preoperative Preparation

The preoperative considerations in patients who are to undergo laparoscopic rectal surgery are broadly similar to those in patients subjected to conventional resection. There are certain areas which require particular attention, and these will be reviewed.

Clinical Assessment

Particular attention must be paid to the general fitness of the patient. Laparoscopic rectal surgery requires prolonged periods of pneumoperitoneum, often in extremes of patient position. The potentially hazardous effects of pneumoperitoneum include derangements of acid–base balance, altered pulmonary mechanics and cardiovascular impairment [4, 23]. It is unclear whether laparoscopic colorectal surgery is associated with an increased incidence of such complications, but we currently perform baseline arterial blood gas estimations as part of the ongoing investigation of the anaesthetic implications of laparoscopic colorectal surgery. At present we suggest that patients with significant cardiovascular impairment should be operated upon by conventional means, although there is little data with which to quantify the risks of pneumoperitoneum under such circumstances.

Gross obesity and the presence of multiple surgical scars constitute, in our view, only a relative contra-indication to the laparoscopic approach, provided such cases are approached with a low threshold for conversion to formal laparotomy.

Imaging

Computed tomography (CT), intrarectal ultrasound (USS) (Fig. 1) and, more recently, magnetic resonance imaging (MRI) enable delineation of local tumour spread and nodal metastasis [2]. Such imaging techniques are still under evaluation, but may provide a guide towards preoperative radiotherapy in patients with significant extrarectal spread or obvious nodal disease. These modalities may also have an important role in the decision as to whether to undertake laparoscopic or conventional surgery and might be based on factors such as tumour bulk and local invasion. The value of these techniques in this latter capacity is at present under intense investigation.

As with open surgery, the entire large intestine should be examined by either contrast radiology or colonoscopy to exclude the presence of synchronous tumours. In the presence of stenosing rectal lesions, such examination may not be possible and may then be legitimately postponed until the postoperative period. We feel that contrast radiology is particularly important, since colonoscopy may be inaccurate with regard to the anatomical position of lesions

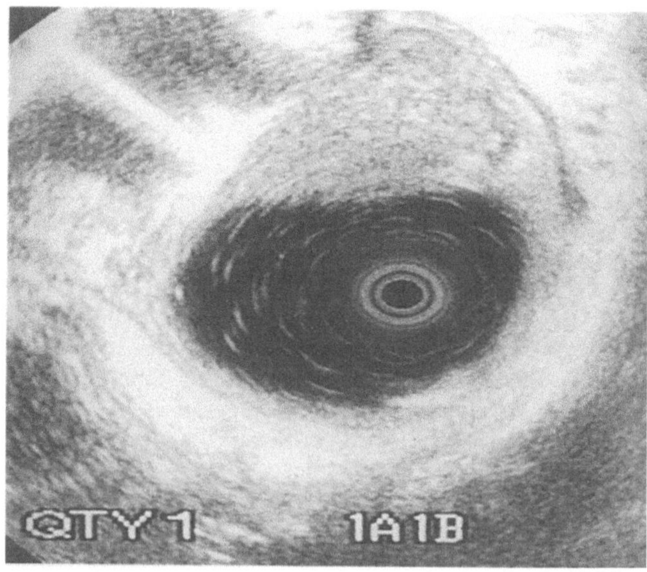

Fig. 1. Preliminary transrectal ultrasound (USS) in a patient about to undergo a laparoscopic anterior resection with full mesorectal excision (USS staging of Dukes' B was confirmed by the pathologist)

[3]. Tumours without obvious serosal involvement may be overlooked at laparoscopy, and the potential exists for removal of the wrong segment of bowel [11] or a failure to identify synchronous lesions at laparoscopy [15].

Examination Under Anaesthesia

Abdominoperineal excision must be reserved for those cancers which invade the anal sphincter complex or for tumours which are so close to the sphincter that, after full mobilisation of the rectum, a clamp cannot be placed below the palpable edge of the tumour with adequate clearance. In specialist hands, some 80%–90% of rectal cancers will be suitable for anterior resection [10]. If these strict guidelines are adhered to in patients undergoing abdominoperineal excision, the laparoscopist may not in fact visualise the tumour, which will be excised by the perineal surgeon. The whole of the rectum can be mobilised laparoscopically. However, the decision as to whether the patient is suitable for restorative resection may then require manual palpation of the tumour to assess distal clearance, which in turn necessitates an abdominal incision. Therefore, if inappropriate sphincter sacrifice is to be avoided, laparoscopic abdominoperineal excision without a facilitating abdominal incision must be reserved for patients with sphincteric involvement, where the indication for excision of the rectum is beyond doubt. This decision should be made at a preliminary examination under anaesthesia, when appropriate biopsies should also be taken.

Bowel Preparation and Other Measures

Standard regimens of bowel preparation and antibiotic prophylaxis should be utilised as for open colorectal surgery. Thrombo-embolic prophylaxis is also important. In our practice, this comprises subcutaneous heparin and graduated compression stockings commenced preoperatively and continued until the patient is mobilised. All patients should be visited by the stoma therapist and counselled as to the likelihood of requiring a stoma. For those patients undergoing abdominoperineal resection, the stoma site should be marked.

Operative Techniques

Instrumentation

Full videolaparoscopy facilities are required along with the standard range of laparoscopic instruments, including Babcock-type graspers, curved endoscopic scissors and an endoscopic linear stapling device (with vascular cartridge) which can be used to divide the bowel and mesenteric vessels. In addition, USS transducers specifically designed for laparoscopic use are now available [13] and may prove to be of value in hepatic assessment during laparoscopic colorectal surgery.

Positioning the Patient

The anaesthetised patient should be placed in a modified Lloyd-Davies position. This differs from the traditional Lloyd-Davies position in that the legs are held almost straight (if the legs are flexed at the hips, they tend to impinge upon the long-handled laparoscopic instruments). A urinary catheter and nasogastric tube should be inserted to help prevent trocar injury to the viscera. The abdomen and perineum are then prepared and draped in the usual manner. Prior to abdominoperineal excision, the anus is closed with a stout purse-string suture.

Preliminary Laparoscopy

Carbon dioxide pneumoperitoneum of 12–15 mmHg is achieved by standard insufflation techniques (either "open" or "closed", depending upon the bodily habitus of the patient and the likelihood of extensive adhesions). The pressure is thereafter maintained by an automatic insufflator. A 10-mm 0° telescope is then inserted through a subumbilical port, and preliminary laparoscopy performed. The whole of the peritoneal cavity should be systematically examined, paying particular attention to the liver, the surface of which should be inspected for the presence of metastases. We also perform a laparoscopic USS examination of the liver at this point (Fig. 2).

Subsequent trocars are inserted under direct vision to minimise the risks of visceral injury. For laparoscopic rectal surgery, we have found the most useful

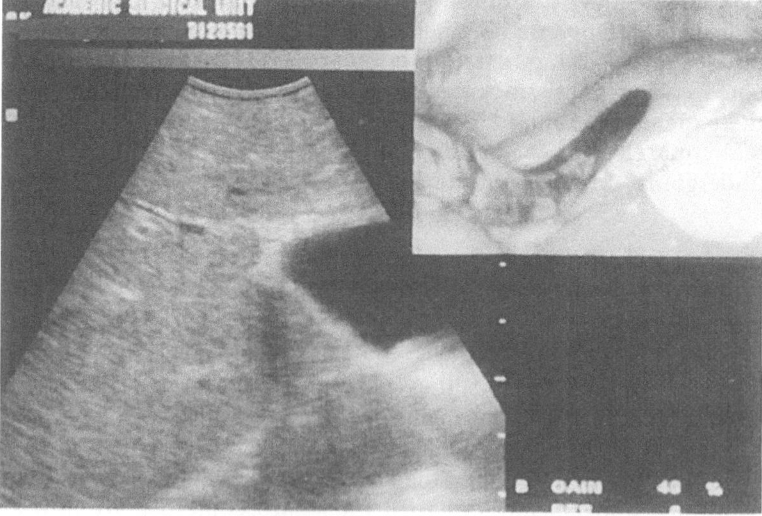

Fig. 2. Laparoscopic ultrasound (USS) examination of the liver with a flexible-tipped transducer during laparoscopic rectal surgery

configuration of the additional ports is for one to be suprapubically, with single ports in the right and left flanks. During abdominoperineal resection, the left flank port should be placed at the intended site of colostomy formation. All ports must be at least 10 mm in diameter so that instruments and camera may be interchanged.

The principle steps in laparoscopic rectal surgery are of course identical to those followed at open surgery; first the bowel is mobilised by division of its peritoneal attachments, the vascular supply to the bowel is then interrupted and the appropriate segment resected and, finally, intestinal continuity is restored or a stoma is fashioned. During laparoscopic-assisted operations, a varying proportion of the procedure can be carried out "open", through the incision required for specimen delivery. As will be evident, this leads to problems of definition and makes comparison between series difficult. Although intracorporeal left-sided anastomoses can be constructed as part of a "totally laparoscopic" approach, we remain to be convinced that the extra time required and technical difficulties are recompensed by the advantages of smaller abdominal wounds. Intracorporeal anastomosis plays no part in our current practice, so that all our procedures, with the exception of abdomino-perineal excision, are best termed laparoscopic-assisted resections.

Our techniques for anterior resection of the rectum and abdominoperineal excision will now be presented according to this schema.

Mobilisation of the Left Colon

The left colon is mobilised by a combination of medial retraction and division of the lateral peritoneal attachments. The descending colon is grasped with Babcock graspers and retracted cranially and towards the mid-line, and the sigmoid colon is retracted caudally and towards the mid-line. The left paracolic gutter is best exposed by tilting the operating table so that the patient's left shoulder is uppermost. The lateral peritoneal reflections of the colon are then divided with electrocautery scissors, commencing at the sigmoid and moving cranially towards the splenic flexure. The gonadal vessels and left ureter are at risk of injury during this stage of the procedure and must be identified and preserved.

During abdominoperineal excision, only the sigmoid colon need be mobilised. During anterior resections, we always mobilise the entire left colon and splenic flexure in order to guard against tension at the subsequent anastomosis. When taking down the splenic flexure, the patient should be placed in the reverse Trendelenburg position so that gravity is able to assist in retraction. The transverse colon is grasped at its mid-point and retracted caudally and medially, and the descending colon is grasped and retracted in the same direction. The peritoneal attachments of the flexure are then divided.

Ligation and Division of the Inferior Mesenteric Vessels

The inferior mesenteric vessels should be ligated high. During laparoscopic-assisted anterior resections, this can be performed, if desired, during the open phase of the procedure after an abdominal incision has been made for subsequent specimen delivery, but high ligation may be difficult to accomplish through the small, low, Pfannensteil-type incision normally made for specimen delivery. We always attempt to perform a high ligation of the inferior mesenteric artery close to its origin from the aorta, and of the vein close to where it disappears beneath the lower border of the pancreas. Intracorporeally, division of these vessels is accomplished with a linear stapling device with vascular cartridge (Fig. 3). In the case of laparoscopic abdominoperineal resection of the rectum, early division of the inferior mesenteric pedicle is particularly advantageous. The blood loss during the subsequent pelvic dissection is much reduced, and elevation of sigmoid and rectum during rectal mobilisation is also much facilitated.

Rectal Mobilisation

The importance of removal of the complete mesorectum as part of the optimum oncological clearance of mid- and low rectal tumours is being increasingly recognised. With care and strict attention to haemostasis, the intact mesorectum can be excised laparoscopically as follows.

Rectal mobilisation is commenced by using a Babcock forceps inserted via the left iliac fossa to elevate and retract the rectosigmoid junction cephalad and

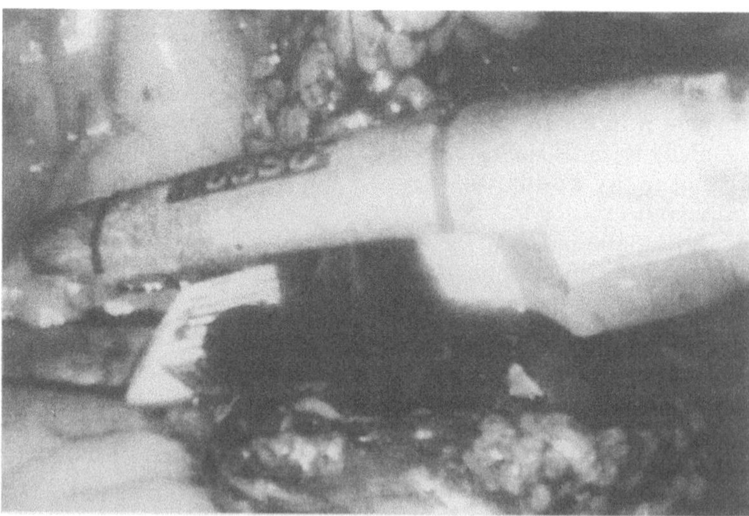

Fig. 3. High ligation of the inferior mesenteric artery with an endoscopic linear stapler during laparoscopic anterior resection

to the left. The mid-rectum is elevated by further Babcock forceps used via the suprapubic port. In this way, the peritoneal reflection to the right of the rectosigmoid junction is exposed under tension. The parietal peritoneum at this point is incised with electrocautery scissors, thus gaining access to the relatively avascular areolar tissue between the fascial capsule of the intact mesorectum anteriorly and Waldeyer's fascia posteriorly (Fig. 4) – the so-called "Holy plane" of rectal surgery [14]. This plane is developed in this way down into the pelvis by incising the peritoneum along the right pelvic side wall until the mid-line is reached in the rectovesical or rectovaginal pouch. The right ureter must be identified and preserved (Fig. 5).

The "lateral ligaments" (see Chaps. 9, 10, 15) are divided by diathermy under direct vision. Posteriorly, the pelvic nerves are readily identified thanks to the magnified views at laparoscopy and can be identified and preserved. These same magnified views permit accurate sharp dissection of the mesorectum, which can be excised intact (Fig. 6). In female patients, as this dissection proceeds towards the pelvic floor, retraction of the pouch of Douglas may be facilitated by an assistant's fingers placed in the vagina. This helps in elevation of the cervix and body of the uterus and thus dissection of the rectum from the vagina.

Most of the rectal mobilisation can be completed via this right-sided approach, in that starting on the right lateral aspect the rectum is mobilised forwards and the plane of dissection is developed posteriorly and around to the left. A small amount of dissection may remain on the left pelvic side wall, and this is best approached from the left side.

The importance of adhering to open surgical principles during laparoscopic dissection cannot be over-emphasised. On encountering difficulties in ori-

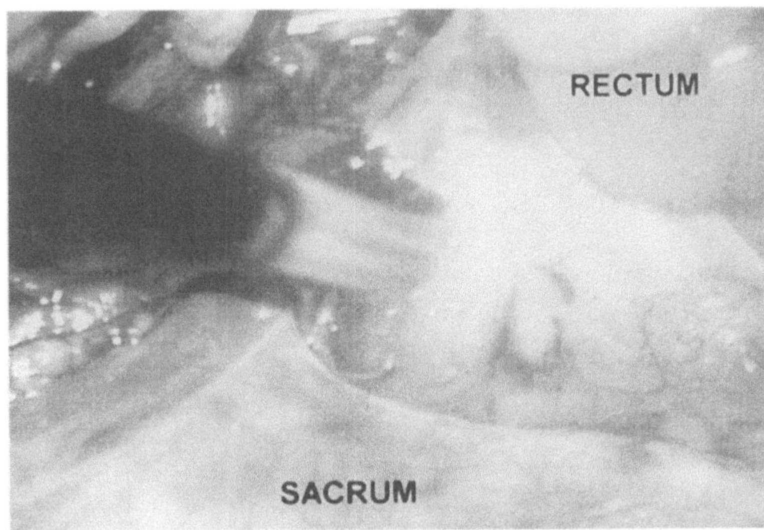

Fig. 4. The beginnings of the avascular pre-sacral plane during a laparoscopic total mesorectal excision for rectal cancer

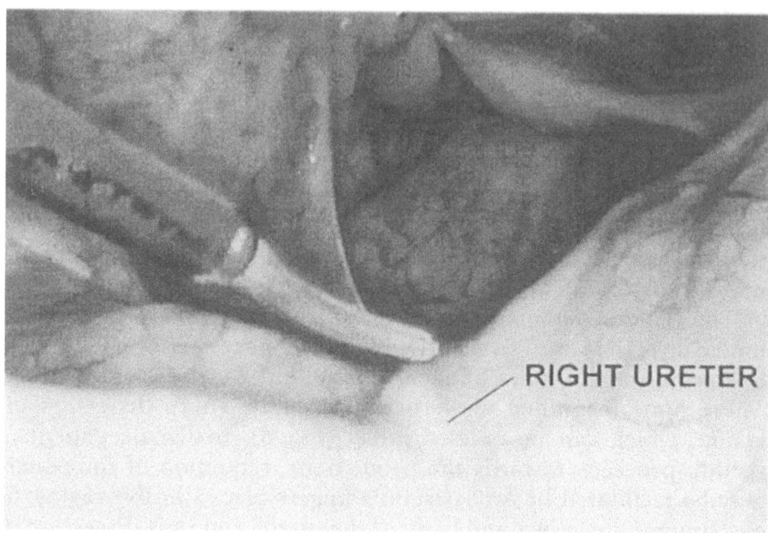

Fig. 5. Identification of the right ureter at the pelvic brim during laparoscopic rectal surgery

entation, or where there is difficulty defining the correct anatomical planes, the surgeon must not hesitate to complete the procedure through the low transverse incision that will inevitably be required for specimen delivery. It is far better to admit defeat at laparoscopy than to leave a patient with positive excision margins.

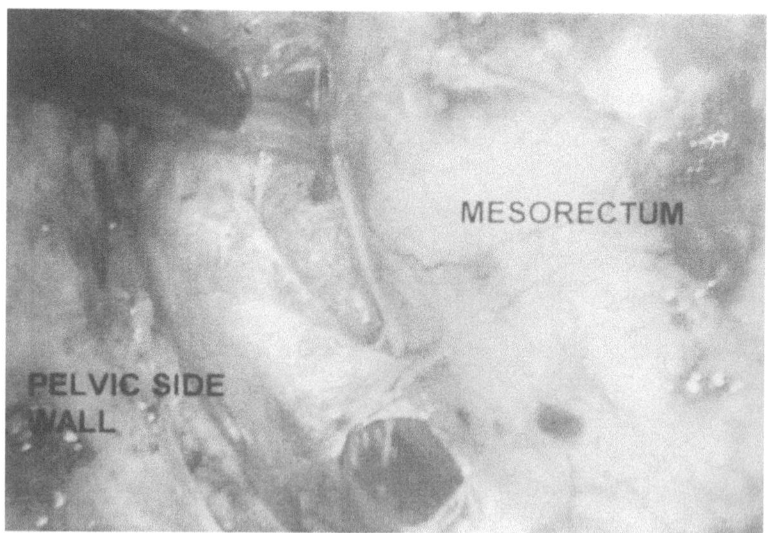

Fig. 6. The magnified views obtained deep within the pelvis at laparoscopy permit accurate accurate excision of the intact mesorectum

Resection and Anastomosis During Anterior Resection

Having completed a total rectal mobilisation, when dealing with cancers of the low or middle third of the rectum, or mobilising the rectum sufficiently to obtain an adequate distal clearance for high anterior resections, the bowel is resected. There are a number of options at this point.

The distal rectum may be transected intracorporeally using a linear stapler. The mobilised bowel is then exteriorised through a 5- to 7-cm transverse suprapubic incision, whereupon the proximal bowel is transected. A standard end-to-end anastomosis can then be completed under direct vision by placing the anvil of a circular stapling gun into the proximal bowel and then the head of the gun into the stapled rectum via the anus in the usual fashion. The "completeness" of the doughnuts is checked, and the integrity of the anastomosis is tested by air insufflation techniques.

The above approach is somewhat limited by the current generation of laparoscopic linear cutters, which are on the whole not readily capable of satisfactorily dividing the distal rectum deep within the pelvis, particularly in male patients. During laparoscopic-assisted anterior resections, we most frequently make use of the low abdominal incision in order to place a conventional linear stapler across the distal rectum under direct vision, so that the anastomosis is then constructed exactly as would be the case at open surgery.

We have adopted a policy of temporarily defunctioning all low rectal anastomoses with a loop ileostomy. A suitable loop of terminal ileum is therefore selected during the open phase of the procedure and brought out through the right iliac fossa trocar site. The stoma is then matured in the usual fashion once the abdominal wounds have been closed. These defunctioning stomas are reversed at 6 weeks after surgery, after sigmoidoscopy and a water-soluble contrast study performed down the distal limb of the loop have shown the anastomosis to be intact.

Perineal Phase of Laparoscopic Abdominoperineal Resection

As described above, the mobilisation of the rectum and mesorectal excision can, with care and strict attention to haemostasis, be continued down to the level of the pelvic floor (Fig. 7). The proximal colon must be transected with an endoscopic stapler before the perineal dissection is commenced, since this would be impossible to safely complete without an adequate pneumoperitoneum. The perineal phase is then commenced – somewhat later than is the case during open surgery. This proceeds in the conventional manner. Division of the skin and subcutaneous fat allows the laparoscopist to make a window in Waldeyer's fascia by cutting down directly onto the perineal surgeon's fingers. The seal provided by the perineal operator's fingers allows the pneumoperitoneum to be usefully maintained for some moments while the remainder of the perineal dissection is performed with laparoscopic guidance where necessary. The laparoscopist then places the proximal end of the bowel in the hand

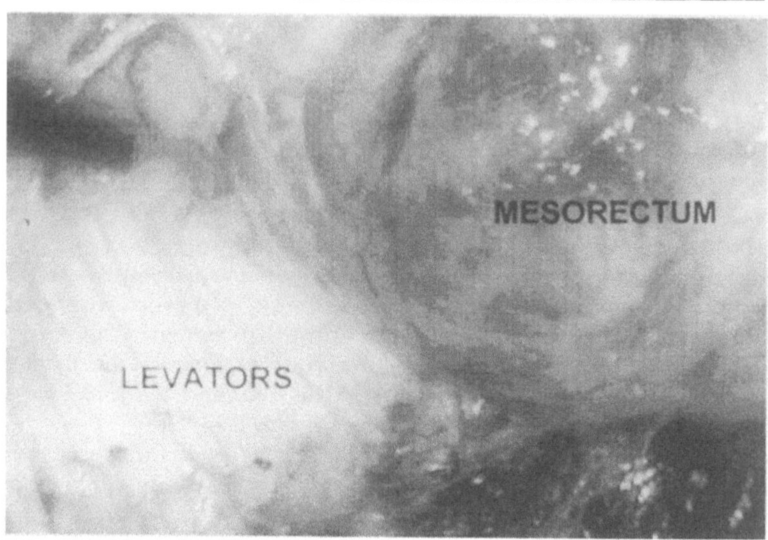

Fig. 7. Completed mobilisation of the rectum down to the level of the pelvic floor

of the perineal surgeon, who then withdraws the specimen, at which point the pneumoperitoneum is lost.

Closure

Following laparoscopic-assisted anterior resection, the abdomen is closed without drainage, the port sites are closed and the loop ileostomy matured in the usual fashion. After laparoscopic abdominoperineal excision, the port sites are closed, the colostomy matured and the perineum is closed in the usual manner, after two suction drains have first been placed into the pelvis either via the abdomen or through the perineum.

Postoperative Care

The postoperative management of patients following laparoscopic rectal surgery should be identical to that following open colorectal surgery. Antibiotic prophylaxis should be completed. The nasogastric tube is removed on the first postoperative day, and oral fluids are commenced. The oral intake is thereafter gradually increased as tolerated, and a light diet is commenced with signs of resolution of the ileus. All patients receive chest physiotherapy, and the patient is mobilised as soon as possible. Thrombo-embolic prophylaxis is continued until the patient is fully mobile. The patient is discharged when he or she is tolerating a normal diet and managing their stoma if present.

Results

Since November 1993, our unit has attempted a laparoscopic approach to elective resection in 30 consecutive patients with rectal cancer, all procedures being performed by a single surgeon (the senior author). A total of 21 of the attempted procedures were successfully completed (five laparoscopic abdominoperineal excisions and 16 laparoscopic-assisted anterior resections). Conversion to formal laparotomy was required in the remaining nine patients (giving a conversion rate of 30%), for the reasons detailed in Table 1.

Congenital absence of the left kidney was confirmed at laparotomy in the patient in whom the laparoscopic approach was terminated because the left ureter could not be identified. The patient in whom a fixed tumour was found to be lying at the rectosigmoid junction underwent a Hartmann's resection after the bladder had been opened during a trial laparoscopic dissection. On two of the three occasions on which there was definite doubt as to the resectability of the lesion at laparoscopy, irresectability was confirmed at laparotomy and the patients were simply defunctioned. The third patient underwent a Hartmann's resection. In two patients gross obesity was felt to preclude a laparoscopic approach, and an early decision was made to convert to formal laparotomy. A single patient had such dense adhesions that the tumour could not be identified at laparoscopy.

Amongst those 16 patients in whom a laparoscopic-assisted anterior resection was completed successfully, the proportion of the rectal dissection that was performed laparoscopically varied. In two patients, the open phase of the operation commenced once the left colon had been mobilised, and in a further four patients the whole of the rectal dissection was performed "open", giving a total of six patients in whom the rectal dissection was performed during the open phase of laparoscopic-assisted anterior resection.

In total, therefore, 14 patients underwent a complete laparoscopic rectal dissection with full mesorectal excision, including four patients in whom this was performed as part of an abdominoperineal excision. All but one resection was considered curative, the exception being a 55-year-old man with locally advanced disease who was felt at the time of abdominoperineal excision to have residual disease on the pelvic side wall, evidenced by microscopically and macroscopically positive resection margins.

Table 1. Reasons for conversion from laparoscopic approach to rectal cancer to formal laparotomy

Reason for conversion	Operations (n)
Fixed tumour	1
Doubtful resectability	3
Gross obesity	2
Dense adhesions	1
Ureter not identified	1
Camera failure	1
Total	9 (30%)

Table 2. Characteristics of patients undergoing curative rectal excision with total mesorectal excision

	Age (years)		Sex (n)		Dukes' stage (n)		
	Mean	Range	M	F	A	B	C
Laparoscopic approach (n=13)	66	(37–82)	10	3	3	7	3
Open surgery (n=12)	67	(53–78)	10	2	1	5	6

The total specimen length, lymph node yield, longitudinal excision margin and radial excision margins in these resection specimens were compared with the same parameters from 12 consecutive curative rectal resections, with mesorectal excision performed by a single consultant colorectal surgeon using conventional techniques. These two groups were similar in terms of age and sex distributions and in the Dukes' stage of the resected tumours (see Table 2). All resection specimens were examined according to standard techniques, as described by Quirke and co-workers [22], by a single colorectal pathologist who was blinded to the method of resection. The results of this assessment are presented in Table 3.

The operative times associated with the two surgical approaches, the duration of ileus (time to passage of flatus or first bowel motion), analgesia requirements (number of days that the patients required parenteral opiates) and length of hospital stay are presented in Table 4.

The complications which resulted from the two surgical approaches are presented in Table 5. Three of the five patients who suffered a clinical anastomotic leakage had been defunctioned at the time of surgery and were managed conservatively. The two remaining patients required a laparotomy, at which time a loop ileostomy was fashioned.

A single patient developed mechanical small-bowel obstruction after an abdominoperineal resection. This was not resolved with conservative measures, and the patient required a laparotomy and division of a band adhesion.

Table 3. Histological examination of the adequacy of surgical excision achieved using laparoscopic and conventional approaches to curative excision of rectal cancer (median values with interquartile range)

Group	Specimen length (cm)		Longitudinal margin (cm)[*]		Radial margin (cm)		Positive margins (n)	Lymph node yield	
	Median	Range	Median	Range	Median	Range		Median	Range
Laparoscopic approach (n=13)	26.0	24–30	3.75	3.13–4.5	0.65	0.33–1.25	0	7.0	4.25–9.5
Open surgery (n=12)	26.5	22.5–32.3	3.0	1.5–3.0	1.0	0.3–1.5	0	7.0	5.0–11.0

[*]$p=0.02$ (Mann-Whitney test for non-parametric data).

Table 4. Operating times and duration of ileus, analgesia requirements, and length of hospital stay associated with curative laparoscopic and conventional resections of rectal cancer, including total mesorectal excision (median values with interquartile range)

Group	Operation time (min)[*]		Duration of ileus days)		Analgesia requirements (days)		Hospital stay (days)	
	Median	Range	Median	Range	Median	Range	Median	Range
Laparoscopic approach (n=13)	180	168–218	3.0	3.0–4.0	4.0	3.0–6.0	13.5	10.25–27.0
Open surgery (n=12)	125	104–144	4.0	3.0–5.0	4.0	3.0–5.0	15.0	11.75–28.5

[*]p=0.003 (Mann-Whitney test for non-parametric data).

Table 5. Complications resulting from curative laparoscopic and open resections for rectal cancer, including complete mesorectal excision

Complication	Laparoscopic (n)	Open (n)
Wound infection	0	1
Respiratory tract infection	1	1
Wound haematoma	1	0
Clinical anastomotic leakage	4	1
Bowel obstruction	0	1
Urethral injury	1	0

A single patient sustained a partial urethral tear during the perineal phase of a laparoscopic abdominoperineal excision. This was managed conservatively with good functional results.

Comments

The application of laparoscopic techniques to colorectal surgery is in the early stages of clinical evaluation. Although these methods have yet to undergo the rigors of a randomised controlled trial, there is now sufficient experience to confirm the technical feasibility of the approach. Relatively large series of laparoscopic colorectal procedures for benign and malignant disease have been reported [6, 7, 12, 17, 20, 29]. The only study published to date which is confined to laparoscopic anterior resection did not report the radial excision margins [24]. Quirke and colleagues have established circumferential margin involvement as the key determinant of outcome after conventional surgery [1]. The single study to date which has compared radial excision margins from laparoscopic and conventional approaches to rectal cancer was confined to abdominoperineal excision [5]. Our own experience with laparoscopic resections for rectal cancer raises a number of points of discussion.

Firstly, while we would argue that total mesorectal excision can be achieved by a totally laparoscopic approach, there are inevitably patients in whom such an approach cannot be successfully pursued. Our rate of conversion to laparotomy (30%) is higher than most reported figures [12, 16, 20, 25, 29]. This may reflect our policy of offering the laparoscopic approach to all comers in the elective situation, while maintaining a low threshold for conversion. Most of our cases were converted because tumour fixity or invasion meant that there was doubt as to the resectability of the lesion. We felt it unwise to make such decisions without recourse to formal laparotomy, which on most occasions confirmed the inoperable nature of the tumour. With further experience, imaging modalities such as MRI and endorectal USS may be found to be capable of identifying those patients in whom a laparoscopic approach should not be undertaken.

Protracted operation times have been a characteristic of the laparoscopic approach in our hands, though this finding has not been confined to laparoscopic rectal surgery [9]. Disappointingly, we have demonstrated no advantage for laparoscopic rectal surgery in term of in-patient morbidity or hospital stay. These findings are at odds with most [6, 7, 12, 17, 20, 29], but not all [9, 26, 27] of the published literature. During laparoscopic-assisted anterior resections, the abdominal incision required must be of a size at least sufficient to allow insertion of a pelvic retractor and linear stapler. In practice, this means an average length of some 7–10 cm. We feel that it is questionable whether one ought to expect a major difference in clinical outcome between conventional and laparoscopic approaches under these circumstances. Indeed, to date, most of the series reporting significant differences in postoperative analgesia requirements, return of bowel function and length of stay consequent upon the laparoscopic approach have been composed largely of right- and left-sided segmental resections. At open surgery, such resections would not be considered as significant in terms of risks of morbidity and mortality as an anterior resection or abdominoperineal excision. We would speculate that such distinctions are likely to be maintained with laparoscopic surgery. This may, however, not hold true for laparoscopic abdominoperineal excision, where the requirement for a significant abdominal incision is avoided. The absence of an abdominal incision, together with the fewer cancer concerns (since the tumour is not dissected laparoscopically), may make this the ideal indication for a laparoscopic approach. Clearly, further experience is required to confirm or refute this hypothesis.

On a more negative note, the rate of anastomotic leakage among those patients who underwent laparoscopic total mesorectal excision is worryingly high. However, at open surgery, total mesorectal excision with ultra-low anastomosis is, with very few exceptions, associated with a clinical leak rate in the region of 10%–15% [10]. We feel that our own rather higher leak rate in this series of patients, while disturbing, is unlikely to be a function of the laparoscopic approach; the splenic flexure was mobilised in all cases, and the anastomosis was constructed extracorporeally in a manner identical to that used at open surgery. Our policy is now to temporarily defunction all patients in which a total mesorectal excision has been undertaken with a loop ileostomy.

Finally, it is encouraging to note the results of our histological assessment of laparoscopic resection specimens, which suggest that initial cancer clearance may at least be comparable to that which can be achieved using conventional methods. Parity in these parameters between laparoscopic and open surgery has been demonstrated by other investigators [7, 8, 12, 17, 25]; however, we are the first to report the radial excision margins achieved during laparoscopic-assisted anterior resections where the pelvic dissection is performed laparoscopically. The difference in longitudinal margins achieved using the two surgical techniques may simply be an index of the height of the lesion from the anal verge. Although reassuring, these are early data which must be viewed in the context of the long-term loco-regional recurrence rates as these become available.

In conclusion, the goals of rectal cancer treatment remain fewer stomas, low rates of local recurrence and low rates of autonomic nerve damage. Our experience confirms the technical feasibility of a laparoscopic approach to the resection of rectal cancer. However, this feasibility does not, of itself, provide justification for the approach. The short-term benefits to the patient of this form of surgery remain unproven, and the rates of recurrence and nerve damage can only be judged with larger numbers of patients and longer follow-up. The answers to these outstanding issues are likely to be provided by the properly controlled randomised studies which are underway in the United States and about to start on this side of the Atlantic.

References

1. Adam IJ, Mohamdee MO, Quirke P et al (1994) Role of circumferential margin involvement in the local recurrence of rectal cancer. Lancet 344:707–711
2. Collier BD, Foley WD (1993) Current imaging strategies for colorectal cancer. J Nucl Med 34:537–540
3. Cotton PB, Williams CB (1990) Practical gastrointestinal endoscopy. Blackwell Scientific, Oxford
4. Cunningham AJ (1994) Laparoscopic surgery – anaesthetic implications. Surg Endosc 8:1272–1284
5. Darzi A, Lewis C, Menzies-Gow N, Guillou PJ, Monson JRT (1995) Laparoscopic abdominoperineal excision of the rectum. Surg Endosc 9:414–417
6. Dean PA, Beart RW, Nelson H, Elftmann TD, Schlinkert RT (1994) Laparoscopic-assisted segmental colectomy: Early Mayo Clinic experiences. Mayo Clin Proc 69:834–840
7. Falk P, Beart R, Wexner S et al (1993) Laparoscopic colectomy: a critical appraisal. Dis Colon Rectum 36:28–34
8. Guillou P, Darzi A, Monson J (1993) Experience with laparoscopic colorectal surgery for malignant disease. Surg Oncol 2 [Suppl 1]:43–49
9. Hartley JE, Qureshi A, Duthie GS, Lee PWR, Monson JRT (1995) Laparoscopic surgery for colorectal cancer – a test of the surgeon not the equipment. Br J Surg 82:693 (abstract)
10. Heald RJ, Goligher JC (1993) Anterior resection of the rectum. In: Fielding LP, Goldberg SM (eds) Rob and Smith's operative surgery, rectum and anus. Butterworth-Heinemann, Oxford
11. Hill ADK, Banwell PB, Darzi A (1993) Laparoscopic colonic surgery: the unseen lesion. Minim Invas Ther 1:13–15
12. Hoffman G, Baker J, Fitchett C, Vansant J (1994) Laparoscopic-assisted colectomy. Initial experience. Ann Surg 219:732–743
13. Jakimowicz JJ (1993) Review: intraoperative ultrasonography during minimal access surgery. J R Coll Surg Edinb 38:231–238

14. MacFarlane J, Ryall R, Heald R (1992) Mesorectal-excision for rectal-cancer. Lancet 341:457–460
15. McDermott JP, Devereaux DA, Caushaj PF (1994) Pitfall of laparoscopic colectomy. Dis Colon Rectum 37:602–603
16. Milsom JW, Lavery IC, Church JM, Stolfi VM, Fazio VW (1994) Use of laparoscopic techniques in colorectal surgery – preliminary study. Dis Colon Rectum 37:215–217
17. Monson J, Darzi A, Carey P, Guillou P (1992) Prospective evaluation of laparoscopic-assisted colectomy in an unselected group of patients. Lancet 340:831–833
18. Nduka CC, Monson JRT, Menzies-Gow N, Darzi A (1994) Abdominal wall metastases following laparoscopy. Br J Surg 81:648–652
19. O'Rourke N, Heald R (1993) Laparoscopic surgery for colorectal cancer. Br J Surg 80:1229–1230
20. Phillips E, Franklin M, Carroll B, Fallas M, Ramos R, Rosenthal D (1992) Laparoscopic colectomy. Ann Surg 216:703–707
21. Phillips R, Hittinger R, Blesovsky L, Fry J, Fielding L (1984) Local recurrence following 'curative' surgery for large bowel cancer: I The overall picture. Br J Surg 71:12–16
22. Quirke P, Durdey P, Dixon M, Williams N (1986) Local recurrence of rectal adenocarcinoma due to inadequate surgical resection. Lancet 8514:996–999
23. Safran DB, Orlando R (1994) Physiologic effects of pneumoperitoneum. Am J Surg 167:281–286
24. Tate JJT, Kwok S, Dawson JW, Lau WY, Li AKC (1993) Prospective comparison of laparoscopic and conventional anterior-resection. Br J Surg 80:1396–1398
25. Van Ye TM, Cattey RP, Henry LG (1994) Laparoscopically assisted colon resections compare favourably with open technique. Surg Laparosc Endosc 4:25–31
26. Wexner S, Johansen O, Nogueras J, Jagelman D (1992) Laparoscopic total abdominal colectomy. A prospective trial. Dis Colon Rectum 35:651–655
27. Wexner S, Cohen S, Johansen O, Nogueras J, Jagelman D (1993) Laparoscopic colorectal surgery: a prospective assessment and current perspective. Br J Surg 80:1602–1605
28. Wexner SD, Cohen SM (1995) Port site metastases after laparoscopic colorectal surgery for cure of malignancy. Br J Surg 82:295–298
29. Zucker KA, Pitcher DE, Martin DT, Ford RS (1994) Laparoscopic-assisted colon resection. Surg Endosc 8:12–18

CHAPTER 20

Laparoscopic Resection of Rectal Cancer: Short and Long Term Results

Josep Rius Macias and Steven D. Wexner

Introduction

Surgeons have traditionally attempted to find new methods to treat their patients, methods that would concomitantly reduce injury caused by the treatment. The application of minimally invasive techniques to operations for colorectal disease follows in this tradition. The introduction of laparoscopic cholecystectomy in 1987 illustrates the potential benefits of minimally invasive approaches to gastrointestinal disease [20].

The tremendous success of laparoscopic cholecystectomy, along with the influx of new technology has stimulated application of the laparoscope in the treatment of other gastrointestinal diseases. Application of videolaparoscopic techniques to colorectal operations was initially limited by the lack of appropriate instruments [75]. Consequently, the first laparoscopic colon resections were "laparoscopic-assisted" colectomies. The introduction of laparoscopic intestinal staplers allowed intraperitoneal transection of the bowel.

The results of improved cost, less pain, shorter hospitalization and convalescence as well as other benefits obtained with laparoscopic cholecystectomy have not been universally borne out in other forms of laparoscopic surgery. Specifically, in laparoscopic colorectal surgery, these above-mentioned benefits are ill defined [2]. There are five fundamental differences between laparoscopic colorectal surgery and almost all other procedures.

Firstly, laparoscopic colorectal surgery is typically a multiquadrant procedure. Most segmental colectomies require mobilization of the colon in at least two quadrants. Therefore, it is often necessary to move personnel as well as to change position of the instruments, monitors and patient to adequately access these quadrants. These maneuvers are in marked contradistinction to laparoscopic cholecystectomy or other procedures where the target organ lies in a single quadrant.

Secondly, the colon has numerous arcades of large branching vessels that must be ligated. These vessels are often large and, at times, embedded in a thick, fatty mesentery. Either numerous clips or, more commonly, vascular staplers are used for this ligation. Although the latter method is quicker, it certainly adds to the cost of the procedure.

Thirdly, an enlarged trocar site or a formal, albeit small, incision is necessary to remove the specimen in laparoscopic colorectal surgery.

Fourthly, an anastomosis needs to be fashioned and in a tension-free, well-vascularized manner. Lastly and most importantly, a major indication for laparoscopic colorectal surgery is malignancy. All other laparoscopic procedures are performed for benign disease.

Potential Benefits of Laparoscopic Colorectal Surgery

In evaluating the benefits of laparoscopic colorectal surgery as compared to open surgery, it is important to assess postoperative length of stay, pain, cosmesis, resolution of ileus, and cost.

Length of Stay

In a collective series by Wexner et al. [93] 486 patients were compiled with a mean hospitalization of 7.1 days. This length of stay is not different from that of many standard "open" colectomies performed in the United States. Therefore, comparisons between institutions are difficult. There are some series that show a remarkably lower length of stay than 7.1 days (Table 1). However, these figures may be attributable to the fact that many patients did not undergo resectional surgery, but instead colotomy and polypectomy. We recently reviewed our experience with our initial 140 laparoscopic colectomies [95]. We found the length of hospitalization for our nonresectional procedures to be remarkably similar to that reported by Phillips et al. [60].

Pain

Several series have evaluated pain associated with laparoscopic colon surgery as compared to laparotomy. Ramos et al. [67] showed that patients who underwent standard surgery used patient-controlled analgesia for 6.2 days postoperatively versus 2.9 days if the procedure was laparoscopically performed. More recently, in a more scientifically precise manner, Pfeifer and colleagues [59] analyzed two matched groups of patients who had undergone either open or laparoscopic colorectal surgery regarding the pain associated with their procedure. There were no statistically different responses between open and

Table 1. Mean length of stay, morbidity and mortality of recent series

Author	Year	Patients (n)	Mean stay (days)	Range (days)	Morbidity (%)	Mortality (%)
Jacobs et al. [34]	1991	14/20	4	NS	15	0
Corbitt et al. [18]	1992	18	4	3–6	0	0
Monson et al. [45]	1992	40	8	NS	15	2.5
Phillips et al. [60]	1992	51	4.6	1–30	8	2
Etienne et al. [22]	1993	35	9	5–23	26	0
Franklin et al. [25]	1993	19	7.4	NS	16	0
Larach et al. [37]	1993	18	8.4	4–25	39	
Lointier et al. [40]	1993	6	10	7–16	16	0
Milsom et al. [44]	1993	9	7	5–12	0	0
Peters and Bartels et al. [58]	1993	24	4.8	NS	13	0
Quattlebaum et al. [63]	1993	20	4.4	2–12	30	0
Scoggin et al. [73]	1993	20	5	2–31	20	
Senagore et al. [74]	1993	38	7	NS	1.5	0
Wexner et al. [92]	1993	74	7	2–40	34	0
Bauer et al. [4]	1994	8	6.7	5–10	0	0
Chindasub et al. [13]	1994	10	8	NS	20	0
Musser et al. [50]	1994	24	8.5	NS	28	0
Puente et al. [62]	1994	38	4.8	3–14	24	0
Sosa et al. [77]	1994	14	6.3	4–10	14.3	
Tucker et al. [83]	1994	114	4.8	NS	7	0
Van Ye et al. [85]	1994	14	9.1	4–9	7	0
Vara-Thorbeck et al. [86]	1994	18	7.6	4–12	34	0
Zucker et al. [99]	1994	65	4.4	3–8	6	0
Total		618	7.1	1–40	18.8 (0–39)	

NS, not stated.

laparoscopic surgery when patients were asked to compare the pain associated with their respective procedures.

Cosmesis

Improved cosmesis is another proposed benefit of laparoscopic surgery. Obviously, cosmesis is a very subjective question, as shown by Pfeifer et al. [59]; patients who underwent laparoscopic and open procedures were asked to compare their incisions to those of either previous surgery or their own perceptions. There were no statistically significant differences in the responses between the open and laparoscopic groups.

Ileus

Early return of bowel function may contribute to shorter hospitalization. It has been proposed that laparoscopic surgery results in earlier recovery of bowel function (Table 2). Bohm and colleagues [9] found that, in dogs, recovery from postoperative ileus is more rapid after laparoscopic than after conventional

Table 2. Duration of ileus

Author	Year	Number of patients	Resolution of ileus
Jacobs et al. [34]	1991	20	90% oral intake day 1
Phillips et al. [60]	1992	51	100% oral intake day 2
Peters and Bartels et al. [58]	1993	24	Oral intake day 2–3 (mean)
Senagore et al. [74]	1993	38	100% oral intake day 3
Wexner et al. [92]	1993	74	Flatus on day 3 (mean)
Puente et al. [62]	1994	38	74% fluids or regular diet day 2
Tucker et al. [83]	1994	114	Liquid intake 2.4 days (mean)
Vara-Thorbeck et al. [86]	1994	18	Oral intake 3.2 days (mean)

intestinal surgery. Jacobs et al. [34], in their initial series of 20 patients, noted that 18 patients "tolerated" clear fluids on postoperative day one while similarly Peters and Bartels [58] reported that laparoscopic patients regained bowel function significantly earlier (2.7 versus 4.0 days), tolerated regular diet earlier (2.3 versus 4.6 days) and hence had a markedly shorter hospitalization (4.8 versus 8.2 days). This experience was confirmed by Senagore et al. [74], who compared 102 colectomies with 38 unmatched laparoscopic assisted colectomies. They found that bowel function resumed quicker and hospitalization was shorter in the laparoscopic-assisted group.

Scrutiny of the "Materials and Methods" sections in these articles revealed dietary advancement, despite the absence of objective return of bowel function, and passage of flatus or stool. In fact, some of the most staunch proponents even discharged their patients from hospital prior to passage of stool. Conversely, these same surgeons waited for flatus and/or bowel motions *prior to* dietary advancement after laparotomy. Thus, the data become uninterpretable as the groups are not comparable. Furthermore, Rajagopal et al. [65] have demonstrated that, without the laparoscope, postcolectomy hospitalization has decreased from 9.4 days to 6.3 days over the last 10 years. Given a 6.3 day mean length of stay after standard colectomy, it is hard to expect a significantly shorter stay after laparoscopic intervention. Early resumption of oral feeding can be safely tolerated in 89% of patients in the immediate postoperative period after open surgery, as demonstrated by Binderow et al. [7] and Reisman et al. [68] in two separate prospective randomized trials.

Cost

To address the issue of cost, Falk et al. [23] received data from four surgeons in three different institutions consisting of medical records, videotapes and hospital bills from 66 consecutive laparoscopic procedures (Table 3). Although the mean hospital stay for patients who underwent laparoscopic sigmoid or right hemicolectomies was significantly shorter, procedure and instrument costs were significantly lower in patients who underwent open surgery. The total costs were similar in both groups.

Table 3. Cost

Author	Year	Open (US $)	Laparoscopic (US $)
Falk et al. [23]	1993	14 000	13 500
Senagore et al. [74]	1993	14 449±696	12 131±612
Vayer et al. [87]	1993	22 938	26 662
Hoffman et al. [30]	1994	10 213	12 464
Musser et al. 50]	1994	11 207	9 811
Reiver et al. [72]	1994	19 384	23 294
Pfeifer et al. [59]	1995	26 903	29 626

Senagore et al. [74] reported that overall cost was lower for patients who underwent laparoscopy. They attributed the savings not only to reduction of hospital stay, but also to the use of fewer pharmaceutical agents, intravenous infusions, and intramuscular injections. When two groups (40 laparoscopic procedures and 40 open procedures) of age, sex, diagnosis and operation-matched patients from our institution were compared, there were no significant statistical differences in the total cost between the two groups [72].

Cleveland Clinic Florida Experience

At Cleveland Clinic Florida, we initiated the use of laparoscopic colon and rectal surgery after a 6-month training period (February 1991–August 1991) with animal models and laparoscopic cholecystectomy [90]. In August 1991, a prospective registry was established according to the guidelines of the American Society of Colon and Rectal Surgeons (1991). The registry included information pertaining to morbidity, mortality, duration of surgery, duration of ileus, length of hospital stay, age, sex, diagnosis, indication for surgery and surgical procedure performed.

Since the inception of the registry, over 200 laparoscopic colorectal procedures have been performed by a single surgeon. From August 1991 to January 1996, 31 cases of colorectal malignancy were performed as either laparoscopic or laparoscopic assisted operations. Indications in 14 patients were rectal adenocarcinomas (ten patients), anal carcinomas (two patients), recurrent anal leiomyosarcoma (one patient), and Kaposi's sarcoma of the rectum (one patient). The average age was 59 (range 25–79) years, with five men and nine women. The procedures performed included laparoscopic assisted low anterior resection in three cases, laparoscopic abdominoperineal resection in six cases, laparoscopic end colostomy in two cases, laparoscopic loop ileostomy in two cases, and laparoscopic liver biopsy in one case.

We experienced intraoperative complications in two cases, and an unrecognized colotomy in one case in a defunctioning Hartmann's stump. This patient developed postoperative peritonitis and required laparotomy and abscess drainage in the immediate postoperative period. The second patient had bleeding from the left external iliac artery during dissection that needed conversion to laparotomy. Another patient was converted due to confusing anatomy making dissection difficult. Fortunately, both intraoperative complications occurred within the first 12 months of performing laparoscopic surgery. No intraoperative complications have been noted in the last 4.5 years.

Only two complications were reported in the postoperative follow-up; one patient had small-bowel obstruction and another had small-bowel herniation. Five patients had a follow-up of less than 3 months; however, in the remaining nine patients, the mean follow-up was 44 (range 9–51) months. There were nine operations performed for palliation, four of these patients died in the follow-up due to their primary tumor. In the five cases performed with curative intent, two patients were lost to follow-up. In the eight patients available for long term follow-up, no local or port-site recurrences have been reported.

The mean operating time for all procedures was 176 (range 45–270) min. In procedures specifically for resection, the mean operating time increased to 213 (range 90–270) min, including the converted cases. When the cases are divided into two groups, those performed before and those after December 1993, the mean operating time decreased from 245 to 151 min, respectively ($p<$ 0.05), with all the complications and the conversions occurring in the first group. Chronologically dividing the cases demonstrates the importance of the learning curve and the impact of experience in laparoscopic colorectal surgery. In our series of all colorectal procedures, the overall complication rate was remarkably reduced from 39% in the first 28 cases, to 12% in the next 44 cases [17]. Overall complication rates in the initial series have ranged from 0% to 39% (Table 1).

For curative left-sided resections, the inferior mesenteric artery and vein were divided at their origins either with clips, endoloops, or with an endoscopic vascular stapling/cutting device (Ethicon Endosurgery Inc., Cincinnati, Ohio). During the rectal dissection, care was taken to ensure total mesorectal excision with wide lateral margins. Distal bowel transection was facilitated with the application of the 60 mm endoscopic linear stapling/cutting device (Ethicon Endosurgery Inc., Cincinnati, Ohio). Subsequently, either an incision was made or one of the ports was exchanged for the 33 mm port (Ethicon Endosurgery Inc., Cincinnati, Ohio) and the specimen was delivered. The tumor-bearing segment was then excised, and anastomosis effected with the detachable head circular stapling device.

The surgical resection margins and lymph node harvest were identical to those achieved during our routine procedures for malignancy [16]. For abdominoperineal resections, the laparoscopic procedure was the same as described above, however the left colon was intra-abdominally transected and removed through the perineal incision, with the end colostomy created in the left iliac fossa port-site position, preoperatively marked by the enterostomal therapist.

Discussion

In the absence of prospective, randomized clinical trials comparing laparoscopy with conventional surgery, most trials compare either historical controls or nonrandomized patients. Long-term follow-up studies addressing cancer recurrence and disease-free periods will not be available at least for the next few years. Some institutions have initiated these studies to establish not only differences in the immediate postoperative period relating to postoperative recovery of bowel function, pain, hospitalization, cost, and return to normal activity, but also in the long-term relative to cure of cancer. Results of these trials in relation to immediate benefit will be available in the not too distant future, although the results of cancer resections will not be available for at least 5 years.

The learning curve effect is evident in many series [69]. There are specific complications relating to the use of the laparoscopic approach, such as from insertion of the Veress needle, and damage to the major vessels and underlying structures. Specific to colorectal procedures, ureteral injury has been reported [21]. Phillips et al. [60], in his report of 51 laparoscopic colectomies, noted that the circular stapled anastomosis was incomplete in 18% of cases versus only 2%–8% during laparotomy [39].

Another potential but avoidable problem of laparoscopic colorectal surgery is the loss of sensation. Corbitt [18] reported conversion in three of 18 procedures due to the inability to identify the colonic lesions. Cohen et al. [17] in a survey of the members of the American Society of Colon and Rectal Surgeons, reported 18 instances of incorrect segment removal. Sixty-nine percent of 635 respondents advocated routine use of additional maneuvers such as intraoperative colonoscopy or preoperative lesion marking to overcome this problem. Fingerhut [24], McDermott et al. [41], and Vara-Thorbeck et al. [86] have all reported reoperating for unrecognized synchronous lesions. This embarassing problem can be avoided by the liberal use of intraoperative colonoscopy to confirm the location of the lesion(s).

At present, surgical excision of colorectal tumors remains the primary modality for the management of colorectal carcinoma [81]. The aim of surgical intervention is to maximize the chance for cure through en bloc removal of the tumor and the lymphatic nodal basin with adequate margins to ensure removal of the entire locoregional tumor burden [54]. In the excision of proximal lesions, vascular and lymphatic anatomy is fairly-well delineated [47]. In rectosigmoid and rectal lesions, however, some controversies exist in the literature. It is accepted that surgical technique closely relates to the rate of local recurrence. Incomplete surgical excision of the mesorectum and inadequate lateral margin clearance are both associated with locoregional recurrence and poor prognosis [12, 29, 42, 64].

The controversy of high ligation, however, persists even in conventional techniques [3, 49]. Miles [43] advocated ligation of the inferior mesenteric artery up to, but not including, the left colic artery in his description of the abdominoperineal resection. Morgan and Griffiths [48], however, advocated a higher level of ligation to include the left colic artery at the level of its origin from the aorta. This experience was not shared with other authors who did not glean any benefit from high ligation [27, 79].

As increasing reports of laparoscopic resections are published, the number of lymph nodes resected has been used as a denominator to compare extent and adequacy of resection. The mean number of lymph nodes excised have ranged from 4.2 to 28.4 (Table 4). The number of lymph nodes counted in a resected specimen is heavily dependent on not only the method of detecting the lymph nodes, but also the pathologist involved. Furthermore, an equal number of nodes may be harvested by a proper wedge resection or by a sleeve resection. In the former setting, paracolic, middle, and high nodes will be harvested whereas in the latter scenario, only paracolic nodes will have been retrieved. There is great variability from institution to institution in the quantification of the lymph nodes [8].

While issues such as lymph node numbers may be controversial, some current laparoscopic practices have been proven to be unacceptable. The local recurrence rate after colotomy and polypectomy is unacceptably increased [91]. The incidence of malignant change in larger sessile polyps is significant and therefore a cancer resection should be undertaken [53]. If a recurrence occurs after a laparoscopic colotomy and polypectomy, one must attribute this problem to the choice of procedure [38].

Distal resection margins are another important factor in rectal cancer surgery. It has been well accepted that adequate distal resection relates to local recurrence [98]. Although the 5 cm rule has been deemed unnecessary, the 2 cm margin is accepted [96]. The only study in which laparoscopic and standard anterior resection have been compared included 11 patients with

Table 4. Lymph node harvest in laparoscopic colectomy

Author	Year	No. of patients	No. of nodes mean (range)		Open colectomy mean (range)	
Jacobs et al. [34]	1991	4 (R. hemi)	25.5	(17–35)		
		2 (L. hemi)	8	(NS)		
Monson et al. [45]	1992	28	10	(5–21)		
Phillips et al. [60]	1992	24	14	(8–22)		
Dodson et al. [19]	1993	3	4.2	(NS)		
Franklin et al. [25]	1993	24	14	(8–22)		
Guillou et al. [28]	1993	9		(5–21)		
Larach et al. [37]	1993	13	9.8	(0–22)		
Peters and Bartels [58]	1993	NS (Sig. colect)	7.3	(NS)	4.7	(NS)
		NS (R. hemi)	9	(NS)	8.5	(NS)
Tate et al. [80]	1993	11	10	(2–14)	13	(2–18)
Wexner et al. [92]	1993	12	19	(3–84)		
Chindasub et al. [13]	1994	10	10	(8–18)		
Musser et al. [50]	1994	15	10.6	(NS)	7.9	(NS)
Puente et al. [62]	1994	22	11	(2–28)		
Van Ye et al. [85]	1994	14	10.5	(0–32)	7.6	(2–19)
Vara-Thorbeck et al. [86]	1994	17	8.5	(6–11)		
Zucker et al. [99]	1994	23 (R. hemi)	28.4	(18–35)		
		4 (Sig. colect)	8	(6–10)		
		4 (LAR)	7.3	(5–11)		

R. hemi, right hemicolectomies; L. hemi, left hemicolectomies; NS, not stated; Sig. colect., sigmoid colectomy; LAR, low anterior resection tumors located at a mean of 20 (range 7–40) cm from the dentate line in whom a laparoscopic anterior resection was undertaken. Fourteen patients with a mean tumor height of 15 (range 7–30) cm underwent laparotomy and anterior resection [80]. Despite the sigmoid location in the former group, the distal margins were as small as 5 mm, whereas the smallest margins in the open group were 20 mm. Although the authors concluded that the technique was acceptable, more critical analysis would have dictated the opposite conclusion.

The fact that remains incomprehensible is the occurrence of port-site recurrence after seemingly curative resection for carcinoma (Table 5). One might reasonably argue that these recurrences could be due to inadequate precautions, thus the routine use of specimen bags or wound protectors should prevent tumor innoculation into the wound. Surprisingly, however, port-site recurrences have not only been confined to advanced lesions as one would expect, but have appeared in Dukes' A and B lesions as well. Furthermore, Montorsi et al. [46] recently showed port site recurrence in a patient with a Dukes' B lesion in whom the specimen was placed in a plastic bag prior to extraction. A strikingly disturbing denominator in these reports is the apparent rapidity of progression of disease [24, 56, 88]. In a recent review of port site metastasis after laparoscopic colectomy, Wexner and Cohen [94] noted 33 cases. In six series, the actual incidence was reported and ranged from 1.5% to 21% with a median of 3.5% and a mean of 6.5%.

Conversely, isolated wound recurrences without carcinomatosis after laparotomy occur less in apparently 0.3% of cases [31]. The five- to tenfold increased incidence of this phenomenon in laparoscopy has led to further controversy over its role in malignancy. It has been hypothesized that elevated intra-abdominal pressure can attenuate the immune response as was hypothesized about blood transfusions [6, 98]. To refute this theory, investigators performing animal experiments have shown that host defenses are less depressed in laparoscopy than laparotomy [82].

Perhaps the advent of gasless laparoscopy will help reduce the number of early recurrences. However, Kockerling [36] failed to show any malignant cells in the aerosol, but found them in all of the dissecting instruments during diagnostic laparoscopy without resection in patients with malignancies. If the answer is to proceed then the surgeon, already capable of performing laparoscopic colectomy for benign disease, can proceed with application of these techniques in a colectomy for malignancy. If the answer is to stop, then many patients with benign disease will have already benefitted from the laparoscopic approach. Thus, it remains that until an adequate theory is proposed, caution should be exercised in laparoscopic cancer resections [94].

In the interim, laparoscopic and laparoscopic-assisted colectomies for cure of malignancies should be performed only within the confines of an Institutional Review Board-approved prospective randomized trial. Laparoscopy is a wonderful tool for the treatment of benign disease of the colon, rectum, and anus [35, 55, 70, 71, 76]. Thus, the surgeon can develop expertise and surpass the learning curve operating on benign disease. During that time, the answer to the question about malignancy will be found. This finding certainly helps explain the implantations which have occurred in cases in which no resection

Table 5. Port site recurrences

Author	Year	Dukes' stage	Interval to recurrence (months)
Alexander et al. [1]	1993	C	3
Walsh et al. [89]	1993	C	6
Fusco and Paluzzi [26]	1993	C	10
Guillou et al. [28]	1993	C	NS
O'Rourke et al. [57]	1993	B	2.5
Stitz [78]	1993	D	NS
Cirocco et al. [14]	1994	C	9
Wilson et al. [97]	1994	NS	NS
Nduka [51]	1994	C	3
Prasad et al. [61]	1994	B	6
		A	26
Berends et al. [5]	1994	B	NS
		C	NS
		D	NS
Lauroy et al. [38]	1994	A	9
Boulez and Herriot [10]	1994	NS	NS
Ramos et al. [66]	1994	C	NS
		C	NS
		C	NS
Ngoi et al. [52]	1994	B	NS
Gionnone (p.c.)	1994	C	2
Gould (p.c.)	1994	NS	4
Newman et al. (p.c.)	1994	C	6
Cohen and Wexner [16]	1994	B	3
		B	6
		C	6
		C	9
		C	12
Fingerhut [24]	1995	A	NS
		B	NS
		B	NS
Jacquet et al. [32]	1995	C	1
		B	10
		B	9
Drouard-Passone-Szerzyna (p.c.)	1995	A	9
		B	6
		B	6
		C	5
		C	1
		C	9
		D	2
Ugarte [84]	1995	C	10
Beck (p.c.)	1995	NS	NS
	TOTAL:	A: 4	range (9–26) months
		B: 12	range (2.5–10) months
		C: 20	range (1–12) months
		D: 3	
		NS: 4	

p.c., personal communication; NS, not stated

has been undertaken [33, 88], and those which have occurred remote to the extraction site (Beck, personal communication) [11, 15, 84].

References

1. Alexander RJT, Jaques BC, Mitchell KG (1993) Laparoscopically-assisted colectomy and wound recurrence (letter). Lancet 341:249–250
2. American Society of Colon and Rectal Surgeons (1991) Policy statement. Dis Colon Rectum 34:35A
3. Bacon HE, Khubchandani IT (1964) The rationale of aortoiliopelvic lymphadenectomy and high ligation of the inferior mesenteric artery for carcinoma of the left half of the colon and rectum. Surg Gynecol Obstet 119:503–508
4. Bauer JJ, Harris MT, Gortine SR, Gelert IM, Kreel I (1994) Laparoscopic-assisted intestinal resection for Crohn's disease (abstract). Surg Endosc 8:245
5. Berends FJ, Kazemier G, Bonjer I-U, Lange JF (1994) Subcutaneous metastases after laparoscopic colectomy. Lancet 344:58
6. Beynon J, Davies PW, Billings PJ et al (1989) Perioperative blood transfusion increases the risk of recurrence in colorectal cancer. Dis Colon Rectum 32:975–979
7. Binderow SR, Cohen SM, Wexner SD, Nogueras JJ (1994) Must early post-operative intake be limited to laparoscopy. Dis Colon Rectum 37:584–589
8. Blenkinsopp WK, Stewart-Brown S, Biesovsky L et al (1981) Histopathology reporting in large bowel cancer. J Clin Path 34:509–513
9. Böhm B, Milsom JW, Fazio VW (1994) Postoperative ileus following "open" versus laparoscopic colectomy. Surg Endosc 8:234
10. Boulez J (1994) Multicentric analysis of laparoscopic colorectal surgery in FDCL group: 274 cases. Br J Surg 81[Suppl.]:27
11. Cava A, Rarnon J, Gonzalez-Quintella A, Martin F, Aramburu P (1990) Subcutaneous metastases following laparoscopy in gastric adenocarcinoma. Eur J Surg Oncol 26:63–67
12. Cawthorn SJ, Parums DV (1990) Extent of mesorectal spread and involvement of lateral resection margins as a prognostic factor after surgery for rectal cancer. Lancet 335:1055–1059
13. Chindasub S, Chamtaracharmnong C, Nimitvamit C, Akkaranurukul P, Santitarmmanon B (1994) Laparoscopic abdominoperineal resection. J Laparoendosc Surg 4:17–21
14. Cirocco WC, Schwartzman A, Golub RW (1994) Abdominal wall recurrence after laparoscopic colectomy for colon cancer. Surgery 116:842–846
15. Clair DG, Lautz DB, Brooks DC (1993) Rapid development of umbilical metasteses after laparoscopic cholecystectomy for unsuspected gall bladder carcinoma. Surgery 113:355–358
16. Cohen SM, Schmitt SL, Wexner SD, Lucas FV, Nogueras JJ (1994) Does xylene mesenteric fat clearance improve lymph node harvest after colon resection? Eur J Surg 160:693 –697
17. Cohen SM, Wexner SD (1995) Laparoscopic colorectal surgery: are we being honest with our patients? Dis Colon Rectum 38:723–727
18. Corbitt JD (1992) Preliminary experience with laparoscopic-guided colectomy. Surg Laparosc Endosc 2:79–81
19. Dodson RW, Cullado MJ, Tangen LE et al (1993) Laparoscopic assisted abdominoperineal resection. Contemporary Surgery 42:42–44
20. Dubois F, Icard P, Berthelot G et al (1990) Celioscopic cholecystectomy: preliminary report of 36 cases. Ann Surg 21:60
21. Dunlop MG, Farouk R, Wilson RG, Bartolo DC (1993) Laparoscopic resection rectopexy for rectal prolapse (abstract). Int J Colorectal Dis 8:230
22. Etienne J, Jehaes C, Kartheuser A, de Neve de Roden A (1993) Laparoscopic surgery or benign colorectal disease: a multicenter prospective study (abstract). Br J Surg 80: S45
23. Falk PM, Beart RW, Wexner SD, Thorson AG, Jagelman DG, Lavery IC, Johansen OB, Fitzgibbons RJ Jr (1993) Laparoscopic colectomy: a critical appraisal. Dis Colon Rectum 36:28–34

24. Fingerhut A (1996) Laparoscopic colectomy. The French experience. In: Jager R, Wexner SD (eds) Laparoscopic Colorectal Surgery. Churchill Livingstone-New York, pp 253–257
25. Franklin ME, Ramus R, Rosenthal D, Schuessler W (1993) Laparoscopic colonic procedures. World J Surg 17:51–56
26. Fusco MA, Paluzzi MW (1993) Abdominal wall recurrrence after laparoscopic-assisted colectomy for adenocarcinoma of the colon. Report of a case. Dis Colon Rectum 36:858–861
27. Grinnell RS (1965) Results of ligation of inferior mesenteric artery at the aorta in resections of carcinoma of the descending and sigmoid colon and rectum. Surg Gynecol Obstet 120:1031–1036
28. Guillou PJ, Darzi A, Monson JRT (1993) Experience with laparoscopic colorectal surgery for malignant disease. Surg Endosc 2 [Suppl 1]:43–49
29. Heald RJ, Husband EM, Ryall RDH (1982) The mesorectum in rectal cancer surgery: the clue to pelvic recurrence? Br J Surg 69:613–616
30. Hoffman GC, Baker JW, Fitchett CW, Vansant JH (1994) Laparoscopic assisted colectomy: Initial experience. Ann Surg 219:732–743
31. Hughes ES, McDermott FT, Proliglase Al, Johnson WR (1983) Tumor recurrence in abdominal wall scar after large bowel cancer surgery. Dis Colon Rectum 26:571–572
32. Jacquet P, Averbach AM, Stephens AD, Sugarbaker PH (1995) Cancer recurrence following laparoscopic colectomy. Dis Colon Rectum 38:1110–1114
33. Jacobi C, Keller HW, Sald S (1994) Implantation metastases of unsuspected gall bladder carcinoma after laparoscopy (abstract). Br J Surg 81[Suppl]:82
34. Jacobs M, Verdeja JC, Goldstein HS (1991) Minimally invasive colon resection (laparoscopic colectomy). Surg Laparosc Endosc 1:144–150
35. Joo JS, Agachan F, Wexner SD (1996) Laparoscopic surgery for lower gastrointestinal fistulas (abstract). Surg Endosc 10:238
36. Kockerling F (1996) Laparoscopy alone. Presented at the 5th World Congress of Endoscopic Surgery. Philadelphia, Pennsylvania, March 13–17, 1996
37. Larach SW, Salomon MC, Williamson PR, Goldstein E (1993) Laparoscopic-assisted colectomy: experience during the learning curve. Colo-proctology 1:38–41
38. Lauroy J, Champault G, Risk N, Boutelier P (1994) Metastasic recurrence at the cannula site: should digestive carcinoma still be managed by laparoscopy? (abstract) Br J Surg 81 [Suppl]:31
39. Lazorthes F, Chiotassol P (1986) Stapled colorectal anastomosis: perspective integrity of the anastomosis and risk of postoperative leakage. Int J Colorectal Dis 1:96–98
40. Lointier PH, Lautard M, Massoni C, Ferrier C, Dapoigny M (1993) Laparoscopically assisted subtotal colectomy. J Laparoendosc Surg 3:439–453
41. McDermott JP, Devereaux DA, Caushaj PF (1994) Pitfall of laparoscopic colectomy: an unrecognized synchronous cancer. Dis Colon Rectum 37:602–603
42. McFarlane JK, Ryall RDR, Heald RJ (1992) Total mesorectal excision for rectal cancer. Lancet 341:457–460
43. Miles WE (1908) A method of performing abdominoperineal excision for carcinoma of the rectum and of the terminal portion of the pelvic colon. Lancet II:1812–1813
44. Milsom JW, Lavery IC, Bohm B, Fazio VW (1993) Laparoscopically-assisted ileocolectomy in Crohn's disease. Surg Laparosc Endosc 3:77–80
45. Monson JRT, Darzi A, Carey PD, Guillou PJ (1992) Prospective evaluation of laparoscopic-assisted colectomy in an unselected group of patients. Lancet 340:831–833
46. Montorsi M, Fumagaili U, Rosati R, Bona S, Chella B, Huscher C (1985) Early parietal recurrence of adenocarcinoma of the colon after laparoscopic colectomy. Br J Surg 82:1036–1037
47. Moriya Y, Hojo K, Sawada T et al (1989) Significance of lateral node dissection for advanced rectal carcinoma at or below the peritoneal reflection. Dis Colon Rectum 32:307–315
48. Morgan CN, Griffiths JD (1959) High ligation of the inferior mesenteric artery during operations for carcinoma of the distal colon and rectum. Surg Gynecol Obstet 108:641–650
49. Moynihan BGA (1908) The surgical treatment of cancer of the sigmoid flexure and rectum with special reference to the principles to be observed. Surg Gynecol Obstet 6:463–466

50. Musser DJ, Boorse RC, Madera F, Reed JF III (1994) Laparoscopic colectomy: at what cost? Surg Laparosc Endosc 4:1–5
51. Nduka CC, Monson JRT, Menzies-Gow N, Darzi A (1994) Abdominal wall metastases following laparoscopy. Br J Surg 81:648–652
52. Ngoi SS, Kum CK, Goh PMY et al (1993) Laparoscopic colon resection: the Singapore experience. Presented at the Tripartite Colorectal Surgery Meeting. Sydney, Australia. October 1993
53. Nivatvongs S, Rojanasakul A, Reiman HM et al (1991) The risk of lymph node metastases in colorectal polyps with invasive adenocarcinoma. Dis Colon Rectum 34:323–328
54. Nogueras JJ, Jagelman DG (1993) Principles of surgical resection. Influence of surgical techniques on treatment outcome. Surg Clin N Am 73:103–116
55. Oliveira L, Reissman P, Wexner SD (1996) Laparoscopic creation of stomas (abstract). Surg Endosc 10:209
56. O'Rourke N, Heald RJ (1993) Laparoscopic surgery for colorectal cancer. Br J Surg 80:1229–1230
57. O'Rourke NA, Priq PM, Kelly S, Silora K (1993) Tumor inoculation during laparaoscopy. (Letter). Lancet 342:368
58. Peters WR, Bartels TL (1993) Minimally invasive colectomy: are the potential benefits realized? Dis Colon Rectum 36:751–756
59. Pfeifer J, Wexner SD, Reissman P, Bernstein M, Nogueras JJ, Singh S, Weiss EG (1995) Laparoscopy versus open colon surgery: costs and outcome. Surg Endosc 9:1322–1326
60. Phillips EH, Franklin M, Carroll BJ, Fallas MJ, Ramos R, Rosenthal D (1992) Laparoscopic colectomy. Ann Surg 216:703–707
61. Prasad A, Avery C, Foley RJE (1994) Abdominal wall metastases following laparoscopy. (letter). Br J Surg 81 [Suppl]:31
62. Puente I, Sosa JL, Sleeman D, Desai U, Tranakas N, Hartmann R (1994) Laparoscopic-assisted colorectal surgery. J Laparoendosc Surg 4:1–7
63. Quattlebaum JK Jr, Flanders HD, Usher CH (1993) Laparoscopically-assisted colectomy. Surg Laparosc Endosc 3:81–87
64. Quirke P, Dixon MF (1986) Local recurrence of rectal adenocarcinoma due to inadequate surgical resection. Lancet I:996–998
65. Rajagopal HS, Thorson AG, Sentovitch SM et al (1994) Decade trends in length of post-operative stay following abdominal colectomy (abstract). Dis Colon Rectum 37:26
66. Ramos JM, Gupta S, Anthone GJ, Ortega AE, Simons AJ, Beart RW (1994) Laparoscopy and colon cancer: is the port-site a risk? A preliminary report. Arch Surg 129:897–900
67. Ramos JM, Beart RW, Goes R, Ortega AE, Schlinkert RT (1995) Role of laparoscopy in colorectal surgery. A prospective evaluation of 200 cases. Dis Colon Rectum 38:494–501
68. Reissman P, Teoh TA, Weiss EG, Cohen SM, Nogueras JJ, Wexner SD (1995) Is early oral feeding safe after elective colorectal surgery? Am Surg 222:73–77
69. Reissman P, Cohen SM Weiss EG, Wexner SD (1996) Laparoscopic colorectal surgery: ascending the learning curve. World J Surg 20:277–282
70. Reissman P, Salky B, Pfeifer J, Edye M, Jagelman DG, Wexner SD (1996) Laparoscopy for inflammatory bowel disease. Am J Surg 171:47–51
71. Reissman P, Salky B, Edye M, Jagelman DG, Wexner SD (1996) Laparoscopic surgery in Crohn's: indications and results (abstract). Surg Endosc 10:21 l.I72
72. Reiver D, Kmiot WA, Cohen SM, Weiss EG, Nogueras JJ, Wexner SD (1994) A prospective comparison of laparoscopic procedures in colorectal surgery (abstract). Dis Colon Rectum 37:22
73. Scoggin SD, Frazee RC, Snyder SK, Hendricks JC, Roberts JW, Symmonds RE, Smith RW (1993) Laparoscopic-assisted bowel surgery. Dis Colon Rectum 36:747- 750
74. Senagore AJ, Luchtefeld MA, MacKeigan JM, Mazier WP (1993) Open colectomy versus laparoscopic colectomy: are there differences? Am Surg 59:549–554
75. Sgambati SA, Ballantyne GH (1996) History of minimally invasive colorectal surgery. In: Jager R, Wexner SD (eds) Laparoscopic Colorectal Surgery. Churchill Livingstone, London, pp 13–23
76. Sher ME, Agachan F, Weiss EG, Nogueras JJ, Wexner SD (1996) Laparoscopic surgery for diverticulitis (abstract). Surg Endosc 10:211

77. Sosa JL, Sleeman D, Puente l, McKenney MG, Hartmann R (1994) Laparoscopic assisted colostomy closure after Hartmann's procedure. Dis Colon Rectum 37:149–152
78. Stitz R (1993) Laparoscopic colorectal surgery. Presented at the Tripartite Colorectal Meeting, Sydney, Australia. October 1993
79. Surtees P, Ritchie JK, Phillips RKS (1990) High versus low ligation of the inferior mesenteric artery in rectal cancer. Br J Surg 77:618–621
80. Tate JJT, Kwok S, Dawson JW, Lau WY, Li AKC (1993) Prospective comparison of laparoscopic and conventional anterior resection. Br J Surg 80:1396–1398
81. Teoh TA, Wexner SD (1996) Laparoscopic surgery in colorectal cancer. In: William NS (ed) Colorectal cancer. Churchill Livingstone, London, pp 103–121
82. Trokel MJ, Allendorf JDF, Treat MR et al (1994) lnflammatory response is better preserved after laparoscopy vs laparotomy (abstract). Surg Endosc 8:232
83. Tucker JG, Ambroze WL, Orangio GR, Duncan T, Mason EM, Lucas GW (1994) Laparoscopic-assisted bowel surgery: analysis of 114 cases (abstract). Surg Endosc 8:234
84. Ugarte F (1995) Laparoscopic cholecystectomy port seeding from a colon carcinoma. Am Surg 61:820–821
85. Van Ye, TM, Cattey RP, Henry LG (1994) Laparoscopically-assisted colon resections compare favorably with open technique. Surg Laparosc Endosc 4:25–31
86. Vara-Thorbeck C, Garcia-Cabellero Salvi M, Gutstein D, Toscano R, Gomez A, Vara-Thorbeck R (1994) Indications and advantages of laparoscopy-assisted colon resection for carcinoma in elderly patients. Surg Laparosc Endosc 4:110–118
87. Vayer AJ, Larach SW, Williamson PR et al (1993) Cost effectiveness of laparoscopic colectomy. Dis Colon Rectum 36:34
88. Wade TP, Comitalo JB, Andrus CH, Goodwin MN Jr, Kaminski DL (1994) Laparoscopic cancer surgery: lessons from gall bladder cancer. Surg Endosc 8:698–701
89. Walsh DC, Wattchow DA, Wilson TG (1993) Subcutaneous metastases after laparoscopic resection of malignancy. Aust N Z Surg 63:563–565
90. Weiss EG, Wexner SD (1994) A recommended training schema for laparoscopic surgery. Surg Oncol Clin N Am 3:759–765
91. Wexner SD (1991) Management of the malignant polyp. Seminars Colon Rectal Surg 2:22–27
92. Wexner SD, Cohen SM, Johansen OB, Nogueras JJ, Jagelman DG (1993) Laparoscopic colorectal surgery: a prospective assessment and current perspective. Br J Surg 80:1602–1605
93. Wexner SD, Reissman P (1994) Laparoscopic colorectal surgery: A provocative critique. Int Surg 79:235–239
94. Wexner SD, Cohen SM (1995) Port-site metastases after laparoscopic surgery for cure of malignancy. Br J Surg 82:295–298
95. Wexner SD, Reissman P, Pfeifer J, Bemstein M, Geron N (1996) Laparoscopic colorectal surgery: analysis of 140 patients. Surg Endosc 10:133–136
96. Williams NS, Dixon MF, Johnston D (1983) Reappraisal of the 5 centimeter rule of distal excision for carcinoma of the rectum: a study of distal intramural spread and of patient's survival. Br J Surg 70:150–154
97. Wilson JP, Hoffman GC, Baker JW, Fitchett CW, Vansant JH (1994) Laparoscopic assisted colectomy. Initial experience. Ann Surg 219:732–743
98. Wobbes T, Joosen KHG, Kuypers JHC et al (1989) The effect of packed cells and whole blood transfusions on survival after curative resection for colorectal carcinoma. Dis Colon Rectum 32:743–748
99. Zucker KA, Pitcher DE, Ford RS (1994) Laparoscopic-assisted colon resection. Surg Endosc 8:12–18

Reconstruction

Straight Colorectal and Coloanal Anastomosis

Philip B. Paty

Introduction

Restoration of intestinal continuity and function is an essential element of rectal surgery. For over three decades, the use of anterior resection with rectal reconstruction has been increasing while the use of abdominoperineal resection (APR) has declined [81]. Technical advances in the creation of low anastomoses have contributed significantly to this trend [27, 64]. In most rectal resections, colorectal or coloanal anastomosis can be accomplished rapidly and safely. In cases where reconstruction is not advisable, the barrier is generally oncologic rather than technical. As a result, low anterior resection (LAR) is now the primary surgical treatment for rectal cancer. In some specialty centers, the use of abdominoperineal excision has declined to less than 10% of resections for primary rectal cancer [47].

This chapter addresses the use of straight colorectal and coloanal anasto-mosis in rectal reconstruction, and discusses the conceptual basis, patient selection, operative techniques, and outcomes for colorectal reconstruction.

Rationale for Sphincter Preservation

The widespread use of restorative resections for rectal cancer reflects accep-tance of three principles of sphincter preservation: (1) cancer treatment is not compromised, (2) colorectal anastomoses can be constructed safely and re-liably at any level within the pelvis or anal canal, and (3) anorectal function is acceptable and preferable to a permanent colostomy.

Oncologic Safety

For the vast majority of rectal cancers, preservation of the anal sphincters does not compromise local control or cure. With regard to lateral and proximal clearance, APR and LAR encompass equally the primary sites of regional spread, and multiple retrospective studies show that survival and local control are no different when cancers of equivalent stage and location are treated [53, 62, 85]. The obvious exceptions to this rule are carcinomas arising within or invading the anal canal, which require APR for adequate removal. When performing LAR, obtaining a long (>2 cm) distal mural margin is generally unnecessary and is clearly less important than achieving clear lateral margins and removing the mesorectum as an intact unit. Fewer than 5% of tumors demonstrate any spread within the bowel wall beyond the lowest visible edge of the tumor, and only 2% demonstrate spread greater than 2 cm [9, 84]. Longer distal margins are recommended for bulky or poorly differentiated tumors. Removal of low-lying cancers with low colorectal or coloanal reconstruction provides good treatment results when these principles are respected [12, 67]. Preoperative pelvic irradiation can downstage tumors and may increase the technical ease and oncologic safety of sphincter preservation for low-lying tumors [50, 57, 71].

Reconstructive Safety

The introduction of circular staplers has revolutionized the low pelvic ana-stomosis. Both colorectal and coloanal anastomoses can be performed safely and expeditiously [5, 15]. Mechanical failure of a stapler is rare [10]. In-traoperative complications are few and nearly always operator-dependent [42]. As with hand-sewn anastomoses, the risk of leakage from stapled anastomoses increases with very low reconstructions, but overall clinical leak rates of under 5% have been reported in several series [13, 18, 39, 41]. Staplers have extended the feasibility and safety of restorative resection. Complex methods of distal anastomosis involving disruption of the anal sphincters or pelvic floor have been largely abandoned.

Anorectal Function

Long-term functional results range from excellent to acceptable and are universally preferable to a permanent colostomy [36, 66, 83]. The 10% of cases where function is poor are often associated with technical complications such as anastomotic stricture or leakage with subsequent fibrosis [31, 38]. Most studies have shown that the quality of long-term anorectal function is related to the length of the conserved distal rectum [13, 36, 45]. Anastomoses to the upper and middle rectum can often result in near-normal long-term function. Anastomoses to the anal canal will generally yield complete fecal continence, but problems related to frequency, urgency, and incomplete evacuation are more common [66].

Adequate mobilization of the colon into the pelvis along the curve of the sacrum is essential for preserving continence. The well-mobilized colon follows the curve of the sacrum, reforms the anorectal right angle at the anal hiatus, and is thus configured to flatten rather than evacuate in response to increases in abdominal pressure. This creates a mechanical barrier that is essential for resting continence [75]. Voluntary continence requires preservation of fully innervated anal sphincter muscles.

Although postoperative continence and evacuation may be imperfect, the vast majority of patients are satisfied with their overall anorectal function [66, 83]. Conversions to permanent colostomy are rare.

Principles of Intestinal Healing

Successful healing of suture lines in the large intestine is dependent upon numerous local and systemic factors [74]. In elective operations with a well-prepared colon, most of the important variables are under the control of the surgeon. In experienced hands, anastomotic failure rates are low.

Anastomotic Healing

As in all tissues, optimal healing of rectal anastomoses requires adequate blood supply, avoidance of tension, and absence of excessive inflammation or infection [5]. Anastomotic integrity is initially dependent on sutures or staples. Tensile strength across the anastomosis is acquired by deposition and remodeling of collagen and under ideal conditions reaches 80% of maximum by day 15 [35]. Experiments comparing suture technique – type of suture material, one layer versus two layer, continuous sutures versus running sutures – suggest that tensile strength develops most rapidly in anastomoses constructed with a single layer of continuous, nonabsorbable suture [44, 52]. Stapled colorectal anastomoses constructed with the end-to-end anastomosis (EEA) device have been shown to be stronger at 4 days after operation than sutured anastomoses constructed with a continuous, single-layer nonabsorbable suture [29].

Anastomotic Leak

Anastomotic leakage is the most significant cause of morbidity and mortality following anterior resection [21, 74]. Radiologic leaks can be demonstrated in 5%–35% of colorectal anastomoses [25, 54]. Clinical leak rates are about half the radiologic rate, ranging from 1% to 13% in large series [34, 39, 41, 48]. Prospective studies have revealed that anastomotic leak rates vary among individual surgeons [21, 22]. Many leaks may, therefore, represent technical failures that can be avoided by good surgical judgment and technique.

Direct comparison of handsewn to stapled technique for colorectal anastomoses has been made in five prospective, randomized trials. No difference in radiographic or clinical leak rates has been identified (Table 1). The overall clinical leak rate for both handsewn and stapled anastomoses is approximately 7%. The major risk factor for leakage is the level of the anastomosis within the pelvis. Low, extraperitoneal anastomoses develop leaks much more frequently than high, intraperitoneal anastomoses [13, 19, 21, 28]. Emergency surgery, massive hemorrhage, and infection also increase the risk of leakage [74]. Preoperative radiation delivered using a three- or four-field technique does not appear to increase anastomotic complications [49, 63, 57].

Anastomotic Stenosis

Anastomotic stenosis is usually a complication of low rectal reconstruction, occurring in the distal pelvis or anal canal. In some cases, stenosis is undoubtedly due to technical problems with bowel apposition, but in other cases factors such as bowel ischemia, prolonged fecal diversion, high-dose postoperative radiation therapy, or pelvic sepsis may be the predominant cause. The definition of a stenosis varies among clinical reports, making comparisons difficult. Stapled anastomoses appear to have a slightly higher propensity to

Table 1. Sutured versus stapled colorectal anastomoses in six prospective, randomized trials

Reference	Type of anastomosis	Number of procedures (n)	Radiologic leak (%)	Clinical leak (%)
Brennan et al. (1982) [10]	Sutured	9	11	22
	Stapled	10	10	40
McGinn et al. (1985) [54]	Sutured	60	6.6	3.3
	Stapled	58	24	12
Friend et al. (1990) [22]	Sutured	125	17	8.8
	Stapled	114	13	3.5
Fingerhut et al. (1994) [78]	Sutured	59	10	8.5
	Stapled	54	7.4	3.7
Docherty et al. (1995) [14]	Sutured	113	14	8.8
	Stapled	111	5.2	3.5
Total	Sutured	366	12	6.8
	Stapled	347	12	7.5

develop stenosis than do handsewn anastomoses. Stenoses can be detected endoscopically in approximately 8%–12% of stapled colorectal anastomoses [41, 76]. Clinically significant stenoses causing obstructive symptoms occur in approximately 1%–4% of patients [19]. Most symptomatic stenoses will respond to dilation or time [19, 41]. Reoperation is rarely required [76, 19].

Cancer Recurrence

Cancer cell implantation on a freshly formed anastomosis is believed to be one mechanism of true suture line recurrence. Spillage of intestinal contents from the transected bowel may also seed cancer cells into the pelvis, leading to intrapelvic recurrence. Rectal washouts just prior to transection of the rectum are performed to remove free-floating cancer cells from the rectal lumen and to minimize the risk of cancer cell implantation. Whether cancer cells shed from the tumor actually do implant in this manner is unproven. Tumor cells do adhere more efficiently to multifilament and braided sutures than to monofilament and stainless steel sutures, suggesting a possible physicochemical basis for tumor cell implantation in certain sutured anastomoses [55, 56, 79].

Rectal anastomoses created by circular staplers have been suggested to be at higher risk of local recurrence. However, a careful review of the local recurrences seen in a large prospective rectal cancer trial as well as a thorough review of the published literature found no linkage between anastomotic technique and local recurrence [1, 86]. Recent evidence from a prospective clinical trial suggests that anastomotic leakage may increase the long-term risk of local recurrence and cancer mortality [14].

Patient Selection for Sphincter Preservation

Resection margins are never compromised in order to avoid permanent colostomy. Therefore, the distance of the rectal tumor from the top of the anal canal is the predominant factor determining the feasibility of sphincter preservation. Tumors located at least 1 cm above the anorectal ring are usually suitable. Tumor bulk, extensive extramural disease, narrow pelvic dimensions, prostate enlargement, obesity, or prior pelvic surgery can make reconstruction of low-lying tumors unsafe or technically impossible. Tumor invasion into the anal sphincter muscles or pelvic floor muscles are contraindications to sphincter preservation. Tumor assessment ideally includes digital examination, proctoscopy, computed tomography, and intrarectal ultrasound. For certain patients, sphincter preservation may be technically achievable but unwise. For example, debilitated patients who have impaired sphincter function or who are confined to bed may be better served by a permanent colostomy than by a low reconstruction.

Operative Technique for Sphincter Preservation

Successful colorectal reconstruction begins with optimal cancer resection and treatment. When adequate resection leaves an intact anal sphincter, restoration of intestinal continuity can be accomplished safely in nearly all patients.

Mobilizing the Left Colon

The sigmoid, descending, or transverse colon may be used for anastomosis. However, following high ligation of the inferior mesenteric artery, the blood supply to the sigmoid colon is less reliable than to higher segments [77]. In addition, the sigmoid colon is sometimes unsuitable due to wall thickening, spasm, narrow caliber, or extensive diverticula. In fact, use of the sigmoid colon has been associated with higher leak rates than use of a more proximal segment [37]. Therefore, for most low reconstructions the descending or transverse colon is preferred. The splenic flexure and its mesentery must be taken down by mobilization away from the spleen and the pancreas. The superior rectal artery and vein are divided, the left colic artery is divided near its origin, and the inferior mesenteric vein is divided at the lower border of the pancreas. The length, vascular supply, and viability of the colon are then assessed. The colon and its mesentery are usually divided at the descending sigmoid junction. Arterial pulses should be palpable in the mesentery of the colon. If the arterial supply to the terminal colon through the marginal artery is inadequate, further colon resection is required to prepare the splenic flexure or the transverse colon for anastomosis.

Transecting the Rectum

Sharp dissection under direct vision is essential to achieve adequate lateral clearance, nerve preservation, and optimal hemostasis [16]. For cancers of the mid- and low rectum, the pelvic dissection must be carried down to the anal hiatus. Only after full mobilization of the rectum can the distal margin and the feasibility of sphincter preservation be determined with safety. A distal margin of 2 cm or longer is ideal, but shorter margins may be acceptable for favorable tumors. After rectal washout, the rectum is generally transected from the abdominal approach. The transanal approach may be required for low-lying tumors or when visualization from above is poor due to tumor bulk or pelvic anatomy.

Techniques of Colorectal Anastomosis

A variety of technical options are available for colorectal and coloanal reconstruction (Table 2). Choice of anastomotic technique is dictated by ex-

Table 2. Technical options in colorectal and coloanal anastomosis

Exposure
  Abdominal
  Peranal
  Trans-sacral
  Trans-sphincteric
Conduit
  Sigmoid
  Descending
  Transverse
Anatomy
  Sleeve
  End-to-end
  Side-to-end
  Side-to-side
  J-pouch-to-end
Fixation
  Stapled
    Pursestring
    Double stapled
  Sutured
    Single layer
    Double layer

posure and visibility of the distal rectal stump, the condition and length of the colonic conduit, and the experience and preference of the operating surgeon.

Sutured Colorectal Anastomosis

Handsewn colorectal anastomoses are generally created end-to-end or side-to-end. The suturing technique may be interrupted or continuous, single-layer or double-layer. Two random assigment trials have compared one-layer and two-layer suturing of colorectal anastomoses (Table 3). The trial by Everett [17] suggested an advantage for the one-layer technique in low anastomoses, but this was not confirmed in the trial by Goligher [26], in which a trend toward superiority was seen for the two-layer technique in both high and low anastomoses. These data again suggest that the skill of execution is more important than the particular method. A recent series reports an overall leak rate of 3.4% in 370 patients [48]. Sutured anastomoses are difficult to create in the low pelvis where exposure and visibility are limited. A number of technical variations have been reported to facilitate suturing of low anastomoses [82].

Stapled Colorectal Anastomosis

A circular stapler is preferred for most colorectal anastomoses. In addition to offering speed and ease, staplers allow creation of anastomoses deep in the

Table 3. Randomized trials comparing one layer and two layer suture techniques for colorectal anastomosis

Reference	High anastomosis		Low anastomosis	
	1 layer	2 layer	1 layer	2 layer
Everett (1975) [17]				
Number of procedures (*n*)	29	38	11	14
Radiologic leak	4	6	1	6
Clinical leak	1	1	1	1
Total leaks	5 (17%)	6 (16%)	1 (9%)[a]	7 (50%)[a]
Goligher et al. (1977) [26]				
Number of procedures (*n*)	43	41	26	25
Radiologic leak	15	7	11	6
Clinical leak	1	0	4	4
Total Leaks	16(37%)[b]	7 (17%)[b]	15 (58%)	10 (40%)

1 layer, interrupted sutures; 2 layer, continuous suture + interrupted sutures
[a] $p < 0.05$ (chi square analysis) for 1 layer versus 2 layer
[b] $p = 0.05$ (chi square analysis) for 1 layer versus 2 layer

pelvis that might otherwise require coloanal reconstruction [6, 27]. Pursestring sutures are applied to the distal colon and to the rectal stump, either manually or using pursestring applicators. The circular stapler cuts the two rings of tissue held by the pursestring sutures and creates a double row of staples between the two ends of bowel. The result is an inverted end-to-end anastomosis. The integrity of the anastomosis is checked by air insufflation.

The techniques and pitfalls of circular stapling have been reviewed in detail [69, 28, 19, 41, 59]. A number of maneuvers have been described to facilitate placement of the distal pursestring. Stay sutures, Babcock clamps, adequate light and retraction, and upward pressure on the perineum are helpful. When the rectal stump is short and cannot be visualized from the abdomen, the rectal pursestring can be applied transanally [23].

Improvements in the design of stapling instruments have further enhanced the ease of low reconstructions. A detachable anvil (Premium CEEA, United States Surgical Corporation, Norwalk, Connecticut, USA) allows the both the proximal and distal pursestring sutures to be tied and inspected before the colon is brought into the pelvis. Flatter, thinner anvils (Low Profile Anvil, United States Surgical Corporation, Norwalk, Connecticut, USA) are available that fit more easily into small caliber colons. An anvil that rotates to a horizontal position after firing greatly simplifies extraction of the anvil through the anastomosis and anal canal (Premium Plus CEEA, United States Surgical Corporation, Norwalk, Connecticut, USA).

Outstanding results for stapled rectal anastomoses have been reported in a number of large series (Table 4). Fears of high rates of symptomatic stenoses or local tumor recurrence due to the use of stapling techniques have not been borne out. The added expense of using stapling devices compared to sutures has been estimated to be 5% of the total cost of surgical treatment [80].

Table 4. Clinical results of stapled colorectal anastomoses from selected series

Reference	Number of procedures (n)	Radiologic leak (%)	Clinical leak (%)	Stenosis (%)
Heald and Leicester (1981) [34]	100	17	13	1
Goligher (1982) [24]	101	9	3	5
Leff et al. (1982)[43]	106	ns	8	11
Fegiz et al. (1983) [20]	134	30	16	ns
Kennedy et al. (1983) [39]	236	ns	3	ns
Fazio (1984) [18]	183	6	3	1
Antonsen and Kronberg (1987) [2]	178	ns	15	8
Zannini et al. (1987) [87]	209	ns	9	9
Kyzer and Gordon, (1991) [41]	215	ns	0.4	13
Detry et al. (1995) [13]	605	ns	5	ns

ns, not stated

Double-Stapled Colorectal Anastomosis

Double stapling involves transecting the rectal stump just above a transverse staple line that substitutes for the distal pursestring suture. The circular stapler cuts through the rectal staple line, creating a new double layer of staples between colon and rectum. Since its introduction by Knight and Griffen [40], this technique has been shown to yield excellent clinical results (Table 5). Advantages include elimination of the distal pursestring, less contamination since the rectal stump is never opened, and elimination of the size discrepancy between colon and rectum. Disadvantages include the possibility of rectal tears and/or tumor fragmentation when placing the linear stapler around the rectum. A variation in which the rectal stump is transected between two applications of the linear stapler is known as the "triple staple" technique [61].

Special Techniques for Low Anastomosis

Pull-Through Operations

A variety of operations have been described in which the colon is delivered through the anal canal and then amputated [3, 4, 8]. Anastomotic suturing between the anus and the colon can be done primarily or at a second stage.

Table 5. Clinical results of double stapled colorectal anastomoses

References	Number of procedures (n)	Clinical leak (%)	Stenosis (%)
Griffen et al. (1990) [30]	75	3	3
Moran et al. (1992) [60]	55	9	5
Redmond et al. (1993) [70]	111	3	9
Laxamana et al. (1993) [42]	189	7	ns

ns, not stated

Although good results were reported by selected centers, in most series anastomotic complications were frequent and functional results were marginal to poor. Pull-through procedures have been largely replaced by circular stapling techniques.

Trans-sphincteric and Trans-sacral Procedures

Trans-sphincteric and trans-sacral procedures provide direct exposure to the distal pelvis for anastomotic suturing either by incising the anal sphincters or by removing the coccyx and distal sacrum. Outstanding results have been reported in expert hands [46, 51]. However, because they disrupt the pelvic floor and increase the risk of fecal fistula and incontinence, these procedures are not widely utilized.

Transanal Coloanal Anastomosis

Coloanal anastomosis is used for reconstruction when the distal margin of resection lies within the anal canal and there is no rectal cuff available for intrapelvic anastomosis. Transection of the rectum may be done from the abdominal approach with upward pressure on the perineum or from the anal approach. The peranal coloanal anastomosis described by Parks in 1972 has supplanted nearly all other methods of sutured coloanal reconstruction [64]. The colon is delivered into the anus and is sutured directly to the anal canal at or just above the dentate line. Retraction sutures and a bivalve retractor provide exposure. This technique is widely used for coloanal reconstruction because of its simplicity, primary healing, and avoidance of anorectal eversion. Temporary diversion with either a loop ileostomy or loop colostomy is advocated by most surgeons.

Several variations in surgical technique have been described. The creation of a "sleeve" anastomosis has been advocated for protection against anastomotic dehiscence [73]. However, it is not clear from the literature that a long muscular sleeve actually reduces anastomotic complications, and its use in rectal cancer cases, with potential compromise of the distal resection margin, seems unwarranted. Several series of simple end-to-end coloanal reconstruction have

Table 6. Clinical results of straight coloanal anastomosis

References	Number of procedures (n)	Clinical leak	Gross incontinence	Bowel movements/day	
				Mean	Range
Parks and Percy (1982) [65]	70	3%	1%	ns	
Hautefeuille et al. (1988) [33]	31		3%	2	2–6
Bernard et al. (1989) [7]	38	5%	7%	3.8	ns
Paty et al. (1994b) [68]	81	3%	5%	2	0–10
Cavaliere et al. (1995) [12]	99	10%	18%	3	1–8

reported excellent healing and good function [12, 68]. Moreover, ultralow intersphincteric dissection with removal of the upper internal sphincter followed by end-to-end coloanal reconstruction has been reported with acceptable functional results [11, 72]. Other investigators have advocated total eversion of the anus to facilitate bowel transection and suturing [33].

The oncologic results reported for resection with coloanal reconstruction have been excellent, with local recurrence rates of 5%–10% [12, 65, 67]. Functional results have been reported from several centers (Table 6). Anorectal function is often poor in the first few months after stoma closure. During the first postoperative year, problems with urgency, frequency, and episodic incontinence decrease as the neorectum acquires greater capacity and compliance. In the long term, the vast majority of patients are continent. Stool frequency is variable but acceptable. Approximately 10% of patients have poor function, due either to frequency, gross soilage, or impaired evacuation [68].

Preoperative Radiotherapy and Sphincter Preservation

Preoperative neoadjuvant pelvic irradiation with or without chemotherapy can downstage many rectal cancers and reduce local recurrence rates. Patients with low rectal cancers abutting the anal canal who might otherwise require abdominoperineal resection have been treated with preoperative radiation with the hope of allowing a sphincter-saving resection. In a series of 161 patients from Thomas Jefferson University in Philadelphia, 110 patients with rectal cancers lying 3–6 cm above the dentate line were treated by preoperative radiation and then resection [58]. Only 2% of patients developed anastomotic dehiscence, and only 3% ultimately required permanent colostomy for late anastomotic complications. The 5-year local recurrence rate was 15%. In a similar study from Memorial Sloan-Kettering, 30 patients with distal rectal cancers were selected for preoperative radiation with the goal of avoiding APR [57]. Median distance of the tumor from the anal verge was 4 cm (range 1.5–6 cm). After full dose preoperative pelvic radiation therapy, 29 patients underwent resection, 24 of them (83%) by LAR with coloanal anastomosis. Five patients required APR. One partial anastomotic disruption and two mild anastomotic stenoses were observed. Anorectal function was good or excellent in 77% of patients and acceptable in the remainder. Five patients (17%) developed local recurrence. These studies confirm the safety of preoperative radiation and strongly suggest an improved rate of sphincter preservation for low-lying rectal cancer.

Summary

Successful colorectal or coloanal reconstruction can be accomplished in a large majority of rectal cancer patients. With proper patient selection and meticulous operative technique, restoration of intestinal continuity improves quality of life without compromising cancer treatment.

References

1. Abulafi AM, Williams NS (1994) Local recurrence of colorectal cancer: the problem, mechanisms, management and adjuvant therapy. Br J Surg 81:7–19
2. Antonsen HK, Kronberg O (1987) Early complications after low anterior resection for rectal cancer using the EEA 228 stapling device: a prospective trial. Dis Colon Rectum 30:579–583
3. Babcock WW (1947) Radical single-staged extirpation for cancer of the large bowel with retained functional anus. Surg Gynecol Obstet 85:1–7
4. Bacon HE (1956) Abdomino-perineal proctosigmoidectomy with sphincter preservation: five-year and ten-year survival after "pull-through" operation for cancer of the rectum. J Am Med Assoc 160:628–634
5. Ballantyne GH (1983) Intestinal suturing: review of the experimental foundations for traditional doctrines. Dis Colon Rectum 26:836–843
6. Beart RW Jr, Kelly KA (1981) Randomized prospective evaluation of the EEA stapler for colorectal anastomoses. Am J Surg 141:143–147
7. Bernard D, Morgan S, Tasse D, Wassef R (1989) Preliminary results of coloanal anastomosis. Dis Colon Rectum 32:580–584
8. Black BM, Botham RJ (1957) Combined abdomino-endorectal resection: a critical reappraisal based on 91 cases. Surg Clin N Am 37:989–997
9. Black WA, Waugh JM (1948) The intramural extension of of carcinoma of the descending colon, sigmoid and rectosigmoid: a pathologic study. Surg Gynecol Obstet 87:457–464
10. Brennan SS, Pickford IR, Evans M et al (1982) Staples or sutures for colonic anastomoses–a controlled clinical trial. Br J Surg 69:722–724
11. Castrini G, Papalardo G, Mobarhan S (1985) A new technique for ileo-anal and coloanal anastomosis. Surgery 97:111–116
12. Cavaliere F, Pemberton JH, Cosimelli M, Fazio VW, Beart RW (1995) Coloanal anastomosis for rectal cancer: long-term results at the Mayo and Cleveland Clinics. Dis Colon Rectum 38:807–812
13. Detry RJ, Kartheuser A, Delriviere L, Saba J, Kestens PJ (1995) Use of the circular stapler in 1000 consecutive colorectal anastomoses: experience of one surgical team. Surgery 117:140–145
14. Docherty JG, McGregor JR, Akyol AM, Murray GD, Galloway DJ (1995) Comparison of manually constructed and stapled anastomoses in colorectal surgery. Ann Surg 221:176–184
15. Enker WE, Stearns MW Jr., Janov AJ (1985) Peranal coloanal anastomosis following low anterior resection for rectal carcinoma. Dis Colon Rectum 28:576–581
16. Enker WE (1992) Potency, cure, and local control in the operative treatment of rectal cancer. Arch Surg 127:1396–1401
17. Everett WG (1975) A comparison of one layer and two layer techniques for colorectal anastomosis. Br J Surg 62:135–140
18. Fazio V (1984) Advances in the surgery of rectal carcinoma using the circular stapler. In: Spratt JS (ed) Neoplasms of the colon, rectum, and anus. Saunders, Philadelphia, pp 268–288
19. Fazio V (1988) Cancer of the rectum – sphincter-saving operation: stapling techniques. Surg Clin N Am 68:1367–1382
20. Fegiz G, Angelini L, Bezzi M (1983) Rectal cancer: restorative surgery with the EEA stapling device. Int Surg 68:13–18
21. Fielding LP, Stewart-Brown S, Blesovsky L, Kearney G (1980) Anastomotic integrity after operations for large-bowel cancer: a multicentre study. Br Med J 281:411–414
22. Friend PJ, Scott R, Everett WG, Scott IHK (1990) Stapling or suturing for anastomoses of the left side of the large intestine. Surg Gynecol Obstet 171:373–376
23. Goligher JC (1979) Use of circular stapling gun with peranal insertion of anorectal purse-string suture for construction of very low colorectal or coloanal anastomses. Br J Surg 66:501–504

24. Goligher JC (1982) The use of circular staplers for the construction of colorectal anastomoses after anterior resection. In: Heberer G, Denecke H (eds) Colorectal surgery. Springer, Berlin Heidelberg New York, pp 107–113
25. Goligher JC, Graham NG, Dedombal FT (1970) Anastomotic dehisence after anterior resection of rectum and sigmoid. Br J Surg 57:109–118
26. Goligher JC, Lee PWG, Simpkins KC, Lintott DJ (1977) A controlled comparison of one and two layer techniques of suture for high and low colorectal anastomoses. Br J Surg 64:609–614
27. Goligher JC, Lee PWR, MacFie J, Simpkins KC, Lintott DJ (1979) Experience with the Russian model 249 suture gun for anastomosis of the rectum. Surg Gynecol Obstet 148:516–524
28. Gordon PH, Vasilevsky CA (1984) Experience with stapling in rectal surgery. Surg Clin N Am 64:555–566
29. Greenstein A, Rogers P, Moss G (1978) Doubled fourth-day colorectal anastomotic strength with complete retention of intestinal mature wound collagen and accelerated deposition following full enteral nutrition. Surg Forum 29:78–81
30. Griffen FD, Knight CD, Whitaker JM, Knight CD Jr (1990) The double stapling technique for low anterior resection. Results, modifications, and observations. Ann Surg 211:745–752
31. Hallböök O, Sjödahl R (1996) Anastomotic leakage and functional outcome after anterior resection of the rectum. Br J Surg 83:60–62
33. Hautefeuille P, Valleur P, Perniceni T, Martin B, Galian A, Cherqui D, Hoang C (1988) Functional and oncologic results after coloanal anastomosis for low rectal carcinoma. Ann Surg 207:61–64
34. Heald RJ, Leicester RJ (1981) The low stapled anastomosis. Br J Surg 68:333–337
35. Herrmann JB, Woodward MD, Pulaski J (1964) Healing of colonic anastomoses in the rat. Surg Forum 29:78–81
36. Karanjia ND, Schache DJ, Heald RJ (1992) Function of the distal rectum after low anterior resection for carcinoma. Br J Surg 79:114–116
37. Karanjia ND, Corder AP, Bearn P, Heald RJ (1994) Leakage from stapled low anastomosis after total mesorectal excision for carcinoma of the rectum. Br J Surg 81:1224–1226
38. Keighley MRB, Matheson D (1980) Functional results of rectal excision and endo-anal anastomosis. Br J Surg 67:757–761
39. Kennedy HL, Rothenberger DA, Goldberg SM (1983) Colocolostomy and coloproctostomy utilizing the circular intraluminal stapling devices. Dis Colon Rectum 26:145–148
40. Knight CD, Griffen FD (1980) An improved technique for low anterior resection of the rectum using the EEA stapler. Surgery 88:710–714
41. Kyzer S, Gordon PH (1992) Experience with the use of the circular stapler in rectal surgery. Dis Colon Rectum 35:696–706
42. Laxamana A, Solomon MJ, Cohen Z, Feinberg SM, Stern HS, McLeod RS (1995) Long-term results of anterior resection using the double-stapling technique. Dis Colon Rectum 38:1246–1250
43. Leff EI, Hoexter B, Labow SB, Eisenstatt TE, Rubin RJ, Salvati EP (1982) The EEA stapler in low colorectal anastomoses: initial experience. Dis Colon Rectum 235:704–707
44. Letwin E, Williams HTG (1967) Healing of intestinal anastomoses. Can J Surg 10:109–116
45. Lewis WG, Martin IG, Williamson MER, Stephenson BM, Holdsworth P, Finan PJ, Johnston D (1995) Why do some patients experience poor functional results after anterior resection of the rectum for carcinoma? Dis Colon Rectum 38:259–263
46. Localio SA, Eng K, Coppa GF (1983) Abdominosacral resection for mid-rectal cancer. Ann Surg 198:320–324
47. MacFarlane JK, Ryall RDH, Heald RJ (1993) Mesorectal excision for rectal cancer. Lancet 341:457–460
48. Mann B, Kleinschmidt S, Stremmel W (1996) Prospective study of hand-sutured anastomosis after colorectal resection. Br J Surg 83:29–31
49. Marks G, Mohiuddin M, Goldstein SD (1988) Sphincter preservation for cancer of the distal rectum using high dose preoperative radiation. Int J Radiat Oncol Biol Phys 15:1065–1068

50. Marks G, Mohiuddin M, Mason L, Montori A (1992) High-dose preoperative radiation therapy as the key to extending sphincter-preservation surgery for cancer of the distal rectum. Surg Oncol Clin N Am 1:71–86
51. Mason AY (1970) Surgical access to the rectum: a trans-sphincteric exposure. Proc R Soc Med 63:91–94
52. McAdams AJ, Meikle AG, Taylor JO (1970) One layer or two layer colonic anastomoses. Am J Surg 120:546–550
53. McDermott FT, Hughes ESR, Pihl E, Johnson WR, Price AB (1985) Local recurrence after potentially curative resection for rectal cancer in a series of 1008 patients. Br J Surg 72:34–37
54. McGinn FP, Gartell PC, Clifford PC, Brunton FJ (1985) Staples or sutures for low colorectal anastomoses: a prospective randomized trial. Br J Surg 72:603–605
55. McGregor JR, Galloway DJ, McCulloch P, George WD (1989) Anastomotic suture materials and implantation metastasis: an experimental study. Br J Surg 76:331–334
56. McGregor JR, Galloway DJ, Jarrett F, Brown IL, George WD (1991) Anastomotic suture materials and experimental colorectal carcinogenesis. Dis Colon Rectum 34:987–992
57. Minsky BD, Cohen AM, Enker WE, Paty P (1995) Sphincter preservation with preoperative radiation therapy and coloanal anastomosis. Int J Radiat Oncol Bio Phys 31:553–559
58. Mohiuddin M, Marks GJ (1993) Patterns of recurrence following high-dose preoperative radiation and sphincter preserving surgery for cancer of the rectum. Dis Colon Rectum 36:117–126
59. Moran BJ (1996) Stapling instruments for intestinal anastomosis in colorectal surgery. Br J Surg 83:902–909
60. Moran BJ, Blenkinsop J, Finnis D (1992) Local recurrence after anterior resection for rectal cancer using double stapling technique. Br J Surg 79:836–838
61. Moran BJ, Docherty A, Finnis D (1994) Novel stapling technique to facilitate low anterior resection for rectal cancer. Br J Surg 81:1230
62. Nicholls RJ, Ritchie JK, Wadsworth J et al (1979) Total excision or restorative resection for carcinoma of the middle third of the rectum. Br J Surg 66:625–627
63. Påhlman L, Glimelius B (1990) Pre- or postoperative radiotherapy in rectal and rectosigmoid carcinoma. Report from a randomized multicenter trial. Ann Surg 211:187–195
64. Parks A (1972) Transanal technique in low rectal anastomosis. Proc R Soc Med 65:975–976
65. Parks AG, Percy JP (1982) Resection and sutured colo-anal anastomosis for rectal carcinoma. Br J Surg 69:301–304
66. Paty PB, Cohen AM, Friedlander-Klar H (1993) Long-term functional results of coloanal anastomosis for rectal cancer. Am J Surg (in press)
67. Paty PB, Enker WE, Cohen AM, Lauwers GY (1994a) Treatment of rectal cancer by low anterior resection with coloanal anastomosis. Ann Surg 219:365–373
68. Paty PB, Enker WE, Cohen AM, Minsky BD, Friedlander-Klar H (1994b) Long-term functional results of coloanal anastomosis for rectal cancer. Am J Surg 167:90–95
69. Ravitch MM (1984) Varieties of stapled anastomosis in rectal resection. Surg Clin N Am 64:543–554
70. Redmond HP, Austin OMB, Clery AP, Deasy JM (1993) Safety of double-stapled anastomosis in low anterior resection. Br J Surg 80:924–927
71. Rouanet P, Fabre JM, Dubois JB, Dravet F, Saint Aubert B, Pradel J, Ychou M, Solassol C, Pujol H (1995) Conservative surgery for low rectal carcinoma after high-dose radiation: functional and oncologic results. Ann Surg 221:67–73
72. Schiessel R, Karner-Hanusch J, Herbst F, Teleky B, Wunderlich M (1994) Intersphincteric resection for low rectal tumours. Br J Surg 81:1376–1378
73. Schlum H, Rigler A, Younis N, Peer R (1983) Peranal sleeve anastomosis for low rectal cancer. Israel J Med Sci 19:124–127
74. Schrock TR, Deveney CW, Dunphy JE (1973) Factors contributing to leakage of colonic anastomoses. Ann Surg 177:513–518
75. Shafik A (1987) A concept of the anatomy of the anal sphincter mechanism and the physiology of defecation. Dis Colon Rectum 30:970–982
76. Smith LE (1981) Anastomosis with EEA stapler after anterior colonic resection. Dis Colon Rectum 24:236–242

77. Steward JA, Rankin FW (1933) Blood supply of the large intestine: its surgical considerations. Arch Surg 26:843–848
78. Fingerhut A, Elhadad A, Hay J, Lacaine F, Flamant Y (1994) Infraperitoneal colorectal anastomosis: hand-sewn versus circular staples. A contolled clinical trial. Surgery 116:484–490
79. Uff CR, Yiu CY, Boulos PB, Phillips RKS (1993) Influence of suture physicochemical and surface topographic structure on tumor cell adherence. Dis Colon Rectum 36:850–854
80. West of Scotland and Highland Anastomosis Study Group. (1991) Suturing or stapling in gastrointestinal surgery: a prospective randomized study. Br J Surg 78:337–341
81. Williams NS (1984) The rationale of preservation of the anal sphincter in patients with low rectal cancer. Br J Surg 71:575–581
82. Williams NS (1993) Surgical treatment of rectal cancer. In: Keighley MRB, Williams NS (eds) Surgery of the anus, rectum, and colon. Saunders, London, pp 939–1053
83. Williams NS, Johnston D (1983) The quality of life after rectal excision for low rectal cancer. Br J Surg 70:460–462
84. Williams NS, Dixon MF, Johnston D (1983) Reappraisal of the 5 centimetre rule of distal excision for carcinoma of the rectum: a study of distal intramural spread and of patient's survival. Br J Surg 70:150–154
85. Williams NS, Durdey P, Johnston D (1985) The outcome following sphincter-saving resection and abdominoperineal resection for low rectal cancer. Br J Surg 72:595–598
86. Wolmark N, Gordon PH, Fisher B, Weiand S, Lerner H, Lawrence W, Shibata H (1986) A comparison of stapled and hand-sewn anastomoses in patients undergoing resection of Duke's B and C colorectal cancer: An analysis of disease-free survival and survival from the NSABP prospective trials. Dis Colon Rectum 29:344–350
87. Zannini G, Renda A, Lepore R, Coppola L, Landi R, Dantonio M (1987) Mechanical anterior resection for carcinoma of the mid rectum: long-term results. Int Surg 72:18–19

CHAPTER 22

The Pelvic Pouch

Emmanuel Tiret, Anne Berger, and Rolland Parc

Introduction

Sphincter-saving procedures are now widely accepted in the treatment of rectal carcinoma of the middle and lower thirds of the rectum. The coloanal anastomosis described by Parks in 1972 [8] is the ultimate procedure to preserve the patient's sphincter and hence avoiding a permanent colostomy. However, patients often complain of urgency and increased bowel frequency after a straight coloanal anastomosis. This type of poor functional result may be related to the loss of the rectal reservoir. In an attempt to correct this dysfunction, we have proposed the creation of a neorectum by incorporating a colonic reservoir anastomosed directly to the anal canal [6]. The operative technique used and the results from our series and those from the literature are discussed in this chapter.

Operative Technique

The patient is positioned to allow a combined abdominal and perineal approach. The inferior mesenteric artery is divided at its origin from the aorta or below the left colic artery. The inferior mesenteric vein is divided at the inferior pancreatic border. The rectal dissection is performed according to oncologic principles, and the mesorectum is totally excised down to the levator ani muscles, which are exposed. A clamp is applied below the lower margin of the tumor. Below this clamp, the rectal muscle can be divided circumferentially at the anorectal junction, sparing the mucosa which will be excised later (Fig. 1).

The splenic flexure and the descending colon are mobilized, and the colon is divided proximally at the junction of the sigmoid and descending colon. Its

Fig. 1. A minimum distal margin of 2 cm is needed. If it is possible with this distal margin to preserve a remaining rectal stump of 2 cm, the procedure of choice is a straight colorectal anastomosis. If the remaining rectal stump is less than 2 cm, a coloanal anastomosis is indicated. (Reproduced with permission from [7])

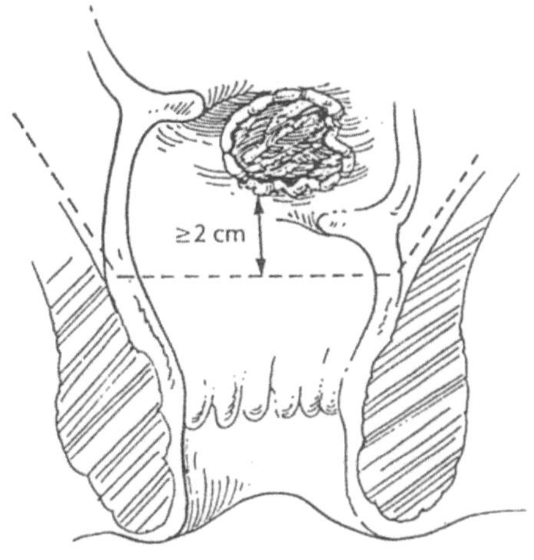

proximal end is closed by a transverse stapler. A J-shaped reservoir of 8 cm is created (Fig. 2). A longitudinal colotomy is performed on the two limbs of the reservoir to insert the limbs of a GIA stapler (Fig. 3). Alternatively, one limb of the GIA stapler can be introduced into the distal colon left open. The colonic pouch is everted to divide the little bridge left over by the stapler. The stab wounds are closed with running 4/0 polyglycolic acid suture. The most distal

Fig. 2. A J-shaped pouch is fashioned using two 8-cm limbs of colon. (Reproduced with permission from [7])

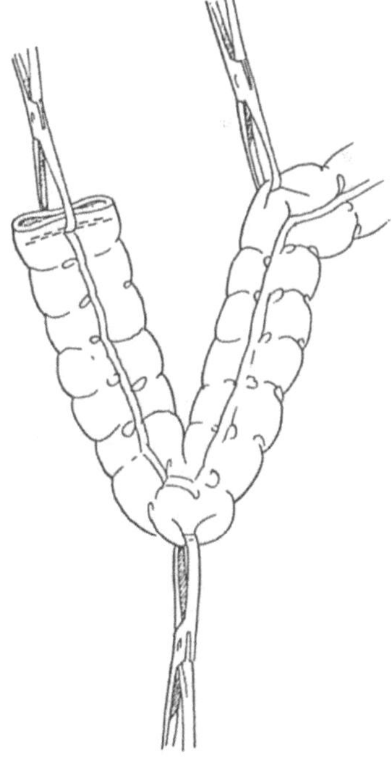

Fig. 3. The limbs of the GIA stapler are inserted by two longitudinal colotomies. (Reproduced with permission from [7])

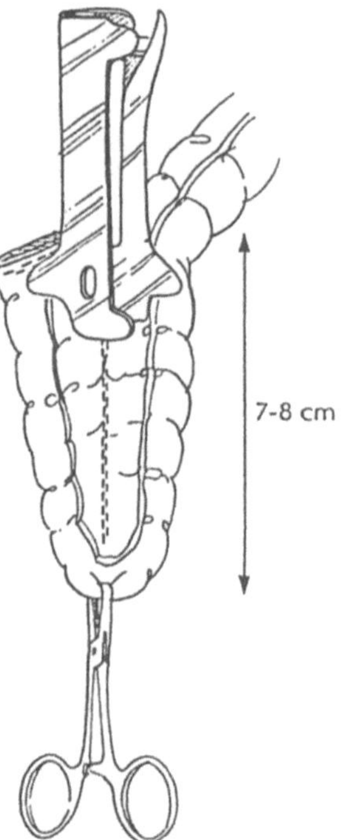

part of the reservoir should descend to the symphysis pubis to ensure that the coloanal anastomosis will be without tension.

From the perineal approach, the rectal stump is irrigated and Gelpi (Aesculap) or Lone Star (Lone Star Medical Products, Houston, TX, USA) retractors are placed on the anal margin. Saline containing lignocaine and adrenaline (1:10 000) is injected into the submucosal plane above the dentate line. A short mucosectomy is made, starting 5 mm above the dentate line up to the superior limit of levator insertion on the anorectal junction, where the rectal muscle had been divided anteriorly. The specimen is removed through the abdomen, and the reservoir brought down to the anus (Fig. 4). It is anchored by three or four stay sutures to the upper end of the sphincter. After opening the apex of the pouch, a coloanal anastomosis is made at the dentate line using interrupted sutures of 4/0 polyglycolic acid (Fig. 5). A Penrose drain is inserted into the reservoir through the anastomosis. Two suction drains are positioned in the pelvis and brought out through lateral abdominal stab wounds. A temporary proximal defunctioning ileostomy or colostomy is constructed and is reversed 8 weeks later.

This technique, including a mucosectomy and a hand-sewn anastomosis, has been routinely used for all eligible patients in our hospital. Alternatively, the distal rectum can be closed at the anorectal junction with a linear stapler (TA 30). The apex of the future reservoir is opened, and a 90 mm GIA stapler is inserted to create the pouch. The head of a 31-mm CEEA stapler is introduced into the reservoir. The coloanal anastomosis is performed mechanically with

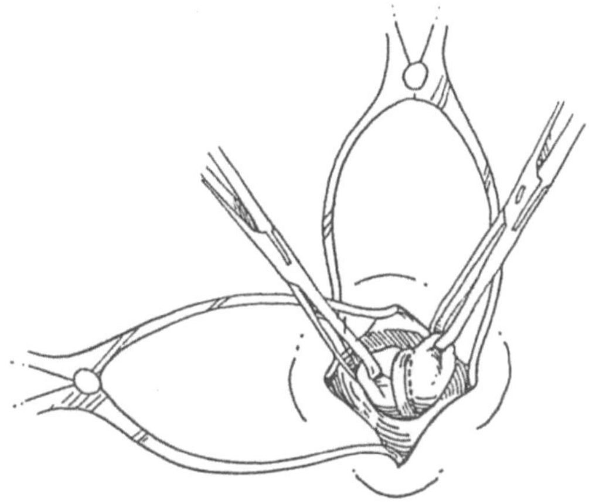

Fig. 4. The apex of the colonic pouch is drawn through the anus with forceps. (Reproduced with permission from [7])

the double stapling technique, which is quicker, and there is no mucosectomy. However, the principal danger is of dividing the distal rectum above the anorectal junction, leaving a short rectal remnant which can in turn lead to some problems with pouch evacuation.

Saint Antoine Hospital Experience

Patients

Two hundred and sixty patients (61% males) underwent a rectal resection with a colonic reservoir and a coloanal anastomosis between 1984 and 1994 at Saint

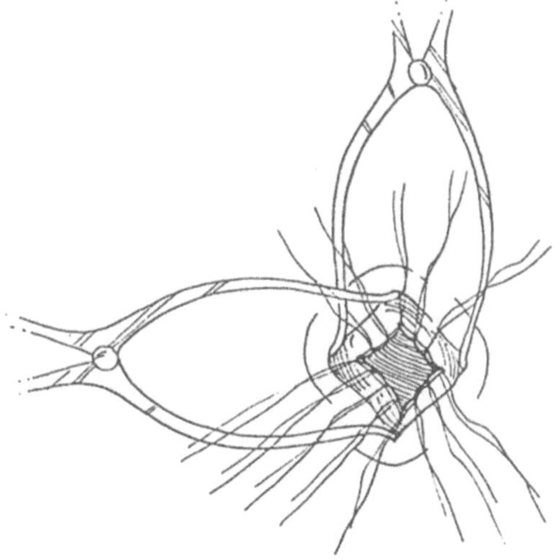

Fig. 5. A coloanal anastomosis is constructed using interrupted absorbable sutures. (Reproduced with permission from [7])

Antoine Hospital, Paris, France. The mean distance from the anorectal junction to the distal edge of the tumor was 3 cm. Twenty seven percent of the tumors were Dukes' A, 30% Dukes' B and 33% Dukes' C. Five percent had distant metastasis (Dukes' D) and 5% had undergone a previous resection (local excision or anterior resection).

The ratio of coloanal anastomosis was evaluated in 1994. One hundred and forty-five patients underwent a curative resection for rectal cancer. Seventy patients (48%) had a colorectal anastomosis, 42 (29%) a coloanal anastomosis with a colonic reservoir, 29 (20%) an abdominoperineal resection, and four (3%) a transanal local excision. A distal margin of at least 2 cm on the fresh specimen, between the lower limit of the tumor and the anorectal junction, was required to make a sphincter-saving procedure. If the distal margin was shorter, an abdominoperineal resection was performed. The choice between a colorectal anastomosis and a coloanal anastomosis with a reservoir depended on the length of the rectal stump above the anorectal junction. A colorectal anastomosis was carried out when it was possible to leave a rectal stump of at least 2 cm. Coloanal anastomosis with a reservoir was preferred in the other patients.

The results of our series of colonic J pouch anastomosis were published in 1992 [1]. The first 162 patients operated between 1984 and 1990 were studied. Postoperative mortality was 0.6% (one myocardial infarction). Five patients (3%) had a pelvic sepsis and/or an anastomotic fistula which healed after spontaneous transanal drainage of the collection. Nine percent of the patients had a surgical complication, requiring a relaparotomy in three cases. No reservoir had to be removed because of a postoperative complication.

Five patients had a surgical complication after closure of the covering colostomy. Three of them had a tear on the anastomosis which was due to digital examination prior to taking down the colostomy. Closure of the colostomy was performed uneventfully a few weeks later.

Functional Results

The patients were prospectively assessed for functional results at 1, 3, 6 and 12 months after the colostomy closure. At 1 month, the mean frequency of bowel movements was 2.7 (range 0.3–9) per 24 h. Daytime continence was perfect in 25% of the patients, and 59% had only minor troubles (imperfect continence to gas, occasional minor leak of mucus or stools). Nightime continence was perfect in 68% of the patients. Discrimination between gas and stools was present in 68% of the patients. Enemas or suppositories were used by 15% to facilitate evacuation. Urgency was experienced by 7% of the patients.

At 6 months, the mean frequency of bowel movements was 2.2 per 24 h (range 0.3–8). Daytime continence was perfect in 44% of the patients, and good in 34%. Nightime continence was perfect in 88% of the patients.

The definitive functional result was ascertained between 6 months and 1 year after stoma closure. At 1 year, the mean frequency of bowel movements was 2.1 per day (range 0.3–8). Daytime continence was perfect in 52% of the patients, while 44% of the patients had minor troubles. Five patients (4%) had frequent major soiling, but three of them had a local recurrence.

Discrimination between gas and stools was present in 95% of the patients. Four percent suffered from urgency. Seventy-seven percent had a normal evacuation and 21% complained of fragmentation. Twenty-five percent needed an enema or a suppository to elicit evacuation.

Oncologic Results

The 100 first patients consecutively operated on between 1984 and 1987 were assessed for oncologic results. All of them were followed for a minimum of 5 years. Twenty nine percent of the tumors were Dukes' A, 30% Dukes' B, 32% Dukes' C, 5% Dukes' D, and 4% unknown. Forty-four patients died during the follow-up period. The crude survival was 59% at 5 years. Thirty-two deaths were cancer related. Twelve patients (12.5%) developed local recurrence at a mean time of 27.6 months (range 6–59 months). Six of these recurrences were isolated, while six had distant metastases. Three of the six patients who had an isolated local recurrence underwent an abdominoperineal (Miles type) operation.

Other Comparative Studies

The benefit of the interposition of a colonic reservoir has been evaluated in six comparative studies. Lazorthes et al. [3] reported a series of 65 coloanal anastomosis. Forty-four patients with a straight coloanal anastomosis were compared retrospectively with 20 patients with a reservoir. The anastomosis was made via a posterior trans-sphincteric approach. Functional results were determined clinically and manometrically.

During the first year, 60% of the patients with a reservoir and 33% of the patients without had one or two stools per day ($p<0,05$). The mean frequency of defecation was 2.4 (SD 1.2) per 24 h versus 3.6 (SD 1.3). After 1 year, 86% of the patients with a reservoir and 33% of the patients without had one or two bowels movements per day ($p<0,01$), showing that reservoir function improved with time. Two out of 20 patients with a pouch had urgency compared with ten out of 42 without.

Nineteen patients without a reservoir were compared manometrically with seven patients with a reservoir. The maximum tolerated volume was 250 ml (SD 51 ml) in the reservoir group versus 191 ml (SD 60 ml). There was also an inverse relationship between the frequency of defecation and the maximum tolerable volume of the neorectum.

Similar conclusions were made by Nicholls et al. [4] who retrospectively compared 15 patients with a reservoir with 13 patients without. Functional result was assessed after a mean period of 47 months (SD 23 months) for the straight coloanal anastomosis versus 7 months (SD 4 months) for the reservoir. Despite this difference in observation time, stool frequency per 24 h was less than two in all patients with a reservoir and above two in 40% of the straight coloanal anastomosis. There was no significant difference in the rate of continence and urgency or the ability to discriminate between gas and stools.

Pelissier et al. [9] compared 36 healthy controls with 33 patients with a reservoir. Patients were evaluated 3 months after colostomy closure and later at 16 months (SD 5.7 months). The authors were unable to demonstrate any significant difference between patients and controls, except for the ability to evacuate which was better in the healthy controls. Only seven patients (21%) were able to evacuate fully during a single defecation at 3 months. This increased to 13 (48.1%) at late evaluation, versus 97% in the control group.

Three prospective randomized studies have compared patients with and without reservoir. The first was reported by Kusunoki et al. in 1991 [2], comparing 28 patients undergoing a colonic J pouch with eight straight coloanal anastomoses. Randomization was stopped because the patients without a reservoir developed more frequent bowel movements and soiling with perineal skin irritation.

Patients were evaluated preoperatively, before colostomy closure, and from 1 month to 2 years after closure. The effectiveness of the reservoir was shown in the markedly decreased frequency of defecation per 24 h and in daytime soiling in the reservoir group in the early period after operation. Frequency of defecation and daytime soiling were inversely correlated with the maximum tolerable volume of the pouch. The maximum tolerable volume of the J pouch increased more quickly and was significantly greater than that of the straight anastomosis at any time.

More recently, Seow-Choen and Goh [10] reported a prospective, randomized study comparing 20 patients with a reservoir with 20 patients without. All anastomoses were performed mechanically (stapling technique). Patients were assessed at 1, 6 and 12 months after ileostomy closure. There was significantly better postoperative anal function in patients with a reservoir. The frequency of motions each day at the three assessment periods was significantly less in those with a reservoir. The advantage of the pouch was confirmed at 12 months after ileostomy closure. All the patients with a pouch reconstruction had normal continence compared with 14 of 20 of those who had a straight anastomosis.

Ortiz et al. [5] randomized 38 consecutive patients in two groups of 19 with or without reservoir. Functional result was assessed at 1 year. Defecation frequency was more than three movements per day in five patients (33.3%) with a reservoir and in 11 (73.3%) of those without, the maximum tolerable volume was significantly greater in patients with a reservoir 335 ml (SD 195) versus 148 ml (SD 38).

Conclusions

The colonic reservoir decreases the frequency of defecation markedly and improves anal function by increasing the maximum tolerable volume of the neorectum. A good functional result can be achieved earlier with a reservoir than with a straight coloanal anastomosis and the difference in favour of the reservoir increases with time. As construction of a reservoir does not increase morbidity, it should be recommended whenever possible.

Results following a colonic reservoir should now be compared prospectively with very low colorectal anastomosis, leaving 3 cm or less of rectal remnant above the anorectal junction. Such a study could definitely answer the question whether a pouch–anal anastomosis is functionally preferable to a straight low colorectal anastomosis.

References

1. Berger A, Tiret E, Parc R, Frileux P, Hannoun L, Nordlinger B, Ratelle R, Simon R (1992) Excision of the rectum with colonic J pouch-anal anastomosis for adenocarcinoma of the low and mid rectum. World J Surg 16:470–477
2. Kusunoki M, Shoji Y, Yanagi H, Hatada T, Fujita S, Sakanone Y, Yamamura T, Utsuno-myia J (1991) Function after anoabdominal rectal resection and colonic J pouch-anal anastomosis. Br J Surg 78:1434–1438
3. Lazorthes F, Fages P, Chiotasso P, Lemozy J, Bloom E (1986) Resection of the rectum with construction of a colonic reservoir and colo-anal anastomosis for carcinoma of the rectum. Br J Surg 73:136–138
4. Nicholls RJ, Lubowski DZ, Donaldson DR (1988) Comparison of colonic reservoir and straight colo-anal reconstruction after rectal excision. Br J Surg 75:318–320
5. Ortiz H, De Miguel M, Armendariz P, Rodiguez J, Choccaro C (1995) Colo-anal anasto-mosis: are functional results better with a pouch? Dis Colon Rectum 38:375–377
6. Parc R, Tiret E, Frileux P, Moszkowski E, Loygue J (1986) Resection and colo-anal ana-stomosis with colonic reservoir for rectal carcinoma. Br J Surg 73:139–141
7. Parc Rf, Berger AM (1992) Coloanal anastomosis. Perspect Colon & Rectal Surg 5(1):99–107
8. Parks AG (1972) Transanal technique in low rectal anastomosis. Proc R Soc Med 65:975–976
9. Pelissier EP, Blum D, Bachour A, Bosset JF (1992) Functional results of colo-anal ana-stomosis with reservoir. Dis Colon Rectum 35:843–846
10. Seow-Choen F, Goh HS (1995) Prospective randomized trial comparing J colonic pouch-anal anastomosis and straight colo-anal anastomosis. Br J Surg 82:608–610

Colonic J-Pouch or Straight Anastomosis in Low Anterior Resection for Rectal Carcinoma?

Rune Sjödahl and Olof Hallböök

Introduction

Modern surgical stapling technique can offer most patients with rectal cancer a sphincter-saving resection. It has been demonstrated recently that continence after anterior resection is related to the length of the residual rectum [12]. Very low anastomoses are, however, common and will be particularly frequent in centers where total mesorectal excision (TME) is accepted as the standard procedure to achieve local radicality. In such operations, the rectum is always transected at the levator plane and the anastomosis constructed to the anal canal or the most distal part of the rectum [13].

Consequences of such a low anastomosis are urgency, frequent bowel movements, and occasional fecal incontinence during the first year, but such problems may persist even longer. They have been described as "the anterior resection syndrome" which can be related to the loss of rectal reservoir function and reduced anal pressure [9, 20, 22]. Such symptoms are particularly common after anastomotic leakage, which is a rather frequent problem as it occurs in 10%–15% of patients undergoing low anterior resection [4, 19]. Improvement of symptoms is associated with an increase in neorectal capacity [16].

Long-term outcome was compared between one group of 19 patients who had symptomatic anastomotic leakage and one group with normal healing, matched according to age, sex, height of anastomosis and follow-up. After a median of 30 months, there was no difference in sphincter function regarding resting and squeeze pressure. Neorectal volume and compliance at sensation of filling, urge to defecate, and maximum tolerated volume were significantly reduced in patients with leakage. The reduction in neorectal reservoir function was reflected in impaired anorectal function measured by a combination of frequency of bowel movements, urgency, incontinence score and bowel emptying [5]. It is thus of utmost importance to avoid anastomotic leakage, not only because of initial morbidity but also with respect to long-term functional results.

One way to improve healing capacity might be to use a side-to-end anastomosis which is well recognized in gastrointestinal surgery, and described by Baker for colorectal anastomosis [1]. A retrospective study of anterior resections showed a leak rate of 4% with a side-to-end anastomosis compared with 23% in the conventional end-to-end anastomosis [23].

One technical modification in order to avoid "the anterior resection syndrome" may be to use the colonic J-shaped pouch as described by Lazorthes and Parc in 1986 [10, 15]. Using this side-to-end anastomotic technique the surgeon may reduce the leak-rate and increase the "neorectal" volume. Although promising this method of reconstruction has not been tested in controlled studies.

Operative Technique of Pouch Construction

After a standardized rectal dissection including TME [8], the rectum is transected at the levator plane, leading to an anastomosis on the top of the anal canal, or approximately 4 cm from the anal verge. The colonic pouch (Fig. 1), about 6 cm in length, is made by folding the colon and creating a side-to-side anastomosis with a stapler introduced through the apex of the pouch. A circular stapler is used for the anastomosis.

The need for a protective stoma is controversial. Some surgeons use it in selected patients if any technical problems are noted when constructing the pouch or anastomosis. They also use it when healing disturbances may be expected or when the patient's general condition is such that an anastomotic leak with pelvic sepsis may be life-threatening. Other surgeons favor a pro-

Fig. 1. Colonic pouch anastomosis

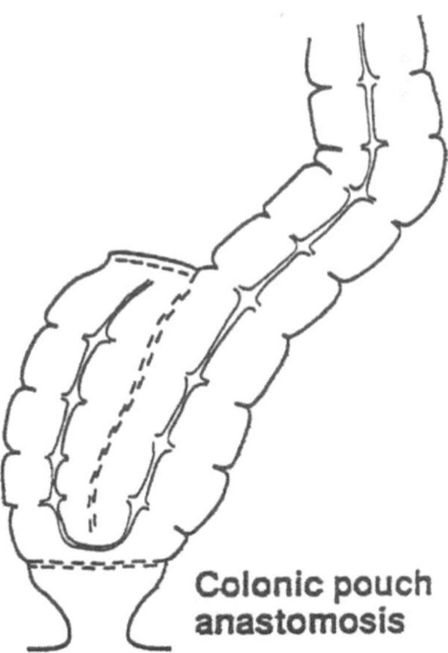

tecting stoma routinely even though they accept that the majority of patients do not need a stoma and that some complications related to the stoma surgery will inevitably occur. The reason for this is that in many hospitals a small number of patients have died because of anastomotic leakage and pelvic sepsis without having a protective stoma. Therefore, we prefer to use a protecting stoma until more knowledge is available regarding how to select those who really need it.

Anastomotic Healing

The rate of anastomotic leakage has been reported to be less than 5% in uncontrolled series of colonic pouch-anal anastomosis [2, 3, 11]. In a controlled trial with colonic pouch-anal anastomosis versus conventional straight anastomosis symptomatic anastomotic leakage was seen in 2% in the pouch group ($n=45$) and in 15% in the group with a conventional straight anastomosis ($n=52$) [7]. Asymptomatic leaks from the blind end of the J-limb have however, been detected in occasional pouch patients.

One reason for the low rate of anastomotic leakage may be that the microcirculation is better preserved at the apex of the pouch than the bowel end in the straight reconstruction. This can be demonstrated by intraoperative laser-Doppler flowmetry. In one investigation, the first recording was done before dissection of the bowel at one point close to the planned bowel end and at another point 8 cm more proximally. A second recording was done at the same sites after dissection and construction of the pouch, but before the anastomosis was completed. Blood flow levels at the site intended for an end-to-end anastomosis were significantly decreased following dissection of the bowel. On the other hand, blood flow levels at the site of the side-to-end anastomosis in pouch patients did not change after dissection and pouch construction. The unaffected blood flow at the site of the anastomosis of the pouch may facilitate and promote anastomotic healing [6].

Another technical factor which may be of importance is the reduced risk of pelvic hematoma due to better filling of the presacral space with the pouch. If such a hematoma becomes infected, it may break through the suture lines in the anastomosis and cause a "secondary" anastomotic leakage. One can also speculate whether the colonic motility may cause different strains on the pouch-anal than on the end-to-end anastomosis.

Bowel Function

In a recent study in which four specialized centers of colorectal surgery participated, 100 patients were randomized to either a straight or a colonic J-pouch anastomosis [7]. Two patients were withdrawn due to inadequate bowel length for pouch construction and one patient at her own request. Thus 97 had surgery within the trial. All patients had a standardized mesorectal excision. A protective stoma was done in 31/52 (59%) of patients with a straight anasto-

Table 1. Postoperative complications after straight or colonic J-pouch reconstruction (no. of patients)

	Straight anastomosis (n=52)	Pouch-anal anastomosis (n=45)
Symptomatic anastomotic leakage	8	1
Staple line haemorrhage	0	0
Bronchopneumonia	3	2
Urinary retention	4	5
Wound infection	4	4
Anastomotic stricture	7	3
Mortality	0	1

mosis and in 32/45 (71%) of those with a colonic pouch (difference not significant). Postoperative complications are shown in Table 1. There was one postoperative death because of hemorrhage and subsequent multiorgan failure (pouch), two early cancer deaths (one pouch, one straight), and one patient declined closure of the loop ileostomy after anastomotic leakage (straight).

After 2 and 12 months postoperatively, 93 and 89 patients, respectively could thus be evaluated. The frequency of bowel movements did not differ preoperatively, but after 2 months the straight group had a threefold increase compared with a pouch group. After 1 year it was twofold and still significantly different from the pouch group. In fact the operation did not change the frequency at all in the pouch patients (Table 2).

An incontinence score from 0–18, where 0 equals no incontinence was used. Table 2 shows that after 2 months the score was fourfold in the straight group compared with that of the pouch group, after 1 year twofold, and the difference was still highly significant. Similar differences were noted regarding the degree of urgency which was evaluated by asking the patients whether they could defer defecation more than 30 min – always (0), often (1), sometimes (2), or never (3). In Table 2, the median values are shown for patients with a pouch and a straight anastomosis at 2 and 12 months [7].

Table 2. Functional results at 2 and 12 months following straight or colonic J-pouch reconstruction (median values)

	Pouch and anastomosis		Straight anastomsis	
	2 months	12 months	2 months	12 months
Bowel motions (24 h)	2.0	2.0	6.4	3.5
Incontinence score	1.5	2.0	7.0	5.0
Degree of urgency	1.0	0	2.0	2.0

In another randomized study frequency of motions per 24 h was two both in the pouch group and straight group with a range of 0.4–4 and 0.5–10, respectively. The urgency did not differ (deferral of less than 15 min; 2/17 and 4/16 in the pouch group and straight anastomosis group, respectively). Normal continence was noticed in all 19 patients with a pouch and in 14/20 with a straight anastomosis [18].

The use of a colonic pouch may, however, have a potential drawback as it can lead to difficult evacuation. Approximately one-quarter of the patients in Parc's original series used medication to empty the pouch [15]. Impaired evacuation has been noted by other investigators [14, 17] and seems to be related to the size of the pouch – the larger the pouch, the more emptying problems [21]. In one of the randomized series [7], there was no statistical difference in the ability to evacuate the bowel but, 10% of the pouch patients regularly used enemas to elicit evacuation after 12 months, and there was a significant decrease within the pouch group in the ability to evacuate between 2 months and 12 months. In another study, constipation was seen in 1/19 and 1/20, respectively and none used an enema [18].

An adaptation period of 1 year is too short to draw firm conclusions about the long-term outcome especially regarding evacuation. In one of our patients with a straight anastomosis, a permanent sigmoidostomy was fashioned after 14 months because of poor bowel function following anastomotic leakage and subsequent stricture formation. In another patient, a colonic pouch was excised after 2 years because of poor function and symptoms of pouchitis. Histopathological examination of the pouch showed chronic inflammation.

Conclusion

It can be concluded that reconstruction with a colonic J-pouch can be done with

- A low incidence of anastomotic leakage
- No increase in frequency of bowel movements
- Almost no problems with urgency and incontinence
- Evacuation problems in 10%–25%

Imperfections of evacuation in some patients require further studies, e.g., regarding the optimal size of the pouch and whether a segment of the sigmoid or descending colon should be used for the pouch. Some patients with rectal cancer have limited life expectancy and should be offered the best functional outcome shortly after the operation. Therefore the colonic J-pouch can be recommended routinely in restorative surgery combined with TME, which at present is the preferred cancer operation for tumors in the lower two-thirds of the rectum.

References

1. Baker JW (1950) Low end-to-side recto-sigmoidal anastomosis: description of the technique. Arch Surg 61:143–157
2. Berger A, Tiret E, Parc R et al (1992) Excision of the rectum with colonic J-pouch anastomosis for adenocarcinoma of the low and midrectum. World J Surg 16:470–477
3. Cohen AM (1993) Colon J-pouch rectal reconstruction after total or subtotal proctectomy. World J Surg 17:267–270
4. Goligher JC, Lee PWR, MacFie J, Lintott DJ (1979) Experience with the Russian model 249 suture gun for anastomosis of the rectum. Surg Gynecol Obstet 148:517–524
5. Hallböök O, Sjödahl R (1996) Anastomotic leakage and the functional outcome after anterior resection of the rectum. Br J Surg 83:60–62
6. Hallböök O, Johansson K, Sjödahl R (1996) Laser-Doppler blood flow measurement in rectal resection for carcinoma – comparison between the straight and colonic J-pouch reconstruction. Br J Surg 83:389–392
7. Hallböök O, Påhlman L, Krog M, Wexner S, Sjödahl R (1996) Randomized comparison of straight and colonic J-pouch anastomosis after anterior resection. Ann Surg 224:58–65
8. Heald RJ, Husband EM, Ryall RDH (1982) The mesorectum in rectal cancer surgery – the clue to pelvic recurrence? Br J Surg 69:613–616
9. Kollmorgen CF, Meagher AP, Wolff BG, Pemberton JH, Martenson JA, Ilstrup DM (1994) The long-term effect of adjuvant postoperative chemoradiotherapy for rectal carcinoma on bowel function. Ann Surg 220:676–682
10. Lazorthes F, Fages P, Chiotasso P, Lemozy J, Bloom E (1986) Resection of the rectum with construction of a colonic reservoir and colo-anal anastomosis for carcinoma of the rectum. Br J Surg 73:136–138
11. Leo E, Belli F, Baldina MT et al (1994) New perspective in the treatment of low rectal cancer: total rectal resection and coloendoanal anastomosis. Dis Colon Rectum 37[Suppl]:s62–s68
12. Lewis WG, Martin IG, Williamson MER, Stephenson BM, Holdsworth PJ, Finan PJ, Johnston D (1995) Why do some patients experience poor functional results after anterior resection of the rectum for carcinoma? Dis Colon Rectum 38:259–263
13. MacFarlane JK, Ryall RD, Heald RJ (1993) Mesorectal excision for rectal cancer. Lancet 341:457–460
14. Nicholls RJ, Lubowski DZ, Donaldson DR (1988) Comparison of colonic reservoir and straight colo-anal reconstruction after rectal excision. Br J Surg 75:318–320
15. Parc R, Tiret E, Frilaux P, Moszkowski E, Loygue J (1986) Resection and coloanal anastomosis with colonic reservoir for rectal carcinoma. Br J Surg 73:139–141
16. Pedersen BK, Huit K, Olsen J, Christiansen J, Jensen P, Mortensen PE (1986) Anorectal function after low anterior resection for carcinoma. Ann Surg 204:133–135
17. Pelissier EP, Blum D, Bachour A, Bosset JF (1992) Functional results of coloanal anastomosis with reservoir. Dis Colon Rectum 35:843–846
18. Seow-Choen F, Goh HS (1995) Prospective randomized trial comparing J colonic pouch-anal anastomosis and straight coloanal reconstruction. Br J Surg 82:608–610
19. Tuson JRD, Everett WG (1990) A retrospective study of anastomotic leaks and strictures after colorectal anastomosis. Int J Colorectal Dis 5:44–48
20. Williams NS, Price R, Johnston D (1980) The long term effect of sphincter preserving operations for rectal carcinoma on function of the anal sphincter in man. Br J Surg 67:203–208
21. Williams NS (1993) New techniques of sphincter saving resection. In: Surgery of the anus, rectum, and colon, vol 2. Saunders, London, pp 1006–1008
22. Williamson MER, Lewis WG, Holdsworth PJ, Filnan PJ, Johnston D (1994) Decrease in the anorectal pressure gradient after low anterior resection of the rectum: a study using continuous ambulatory manometry. Dis Colon Rectum 37:1228–1231
23. Zollinger RM, Sheppard MH (1971) Carcinoma of the rectum and the rectosigmoid. Arch Surg 102:335–338

CHAPTER 24

Role of a Protecting Stoma After Rectal Resection for Cancer

Tracy L. Hull

Introduction

The issue of using a diverting stoma to protect an anastomosis done for rectal cancer is a relatively new dilemma. There has been an evolution in both surgical beliefs and techniques leading to this point. Initially based on the teachings of Miles [15], many believed any rectal cancer necessitated an abdominoperineal resection. This belief was challenged by Dukes [4], who found that almost no cancers in the rectum spread caudad or laterally. Preservation of at least the sphincter mechanism was therefore compatible with cure as long as an acceptable distal margin was obtained. This margin was originally felt to be 5 cm, but this has been scrutinized and in low anastomosis some now accept a 1-cm margin.

The circular stapler has provided a significant technical advance. Before the advent of the circular stapler, all anastomosis were hand sewn and limited at times by a narrow pelvis or short rectal cuff. Most tumors in the lower half to third of the rectum still necessitated an abdominoperineal resection with a permanent colostomy. With mastery of the circular stapler, it is now possible to perform anastomosis just above the anorectal ring. In addition, the technique of end-to-end coloanal anastomosis [19] has allowed a handsewn anastomosis from the transanal approach preserving the sphincter mechanism.

Theoretically, the principle purpose of a stoma is to avoid or decrease the deleterious affects of a leak from the anastomosis, most importantly sepsis and death. Few would argue against a diverting stoma to protect a coloanal anastomosis. Controversy centers around the role of a stoma for a colorectal anastomosis. It is difficult to readily determine the need for fecal diversion after a colorectal anastomosis from reviewing the literature, as few randomized prospective studies exist and the data is confusing. Therefore, this review will provide an overview of the problem of colorectal anastomotic leaks, factors affecting leak rates, pros and cons of using a stoma, and practical suggestions.

Overview of the Problem

The incidence of an anastomotic leak ranges from 0% [12] to 24% [20], although not all leaks are symptomatic. Graffner prospectively performed a gastrograffin enema on all patients on postoperative day 10 and found that 30% had a radiological leak compared to 8% with clinical symptoms of a leak [7]. Similarly, Tuson found that 15.3% of his patients had clinical symptoms consistent with a leak. However, an additional 9% of patients were found to have an asymptomatic (radiological) leak when a gastrograffin enema was performed on postoperative day 9 or 10 [20].

When treating patients, the clinical leak rate is probably the more important consideration. To assess the problem, Table 1 lists the clinical leak rate from several series. The data is divided into anastomosis which are high (above the peritoneal reflection) and low. The data is also divided into those with and without a stoma. Additionally, the mortality rate is listed for those deaths directly related to an anastomotic leak.

Many surgeons hesitate to construct a stoma based on the premise that it may never be closed. When reviewing closure rates for stomas used to protect a

Table 1. Clinical anastomotic leaks for high and low anastomosis

	High				Low			
	Patients (n)	Clinical (n)	leak (%)	Mortality (n)	Patients (n)	Clinical (n)	leak (%)	Mortality (n)
Karanjia [11]								
Stoma	7	0	0	0	118	1	0.8	2
No stoma	25	0	0	0	50	11	22	2
Mealey [14]								
No stoma	40	0	0	0	74	6	8	1
Pakkastie [18]								
Stoma	–	–	–	–	8	1	12.5	
No stoma	74	0	0	0	52	15	28.8	1
Mileski [16]								
No stoma	–	–	–	–	215	11	5.1	4
Fielding [5]								
Stoma	108	11	10	1	214	50	23.3	4
No stoma	1299	67	5	23	407	65	16	10
Graffner [7]								
Stoma	–	–	–	–	25	1	4	0
No stoma	–	–	–	–	25	3	12	0

colorectal anastomosis, the majority of patients will safely have their stoma closed. Karanjia [11] reported on 125 patients who underwent a stoma at the time of anastomosis. Five (4%) were not closed. The complication rate of closure was low; of the 120 closed, seven (6%) developed a fecal fistula which closed spontaneously. Graffner [7] reported that, of 25 patients with a stoma at the time of anastomosis, 23 were closed without complication. Of the remaining two, one developed an anastomotic leak and underwent a Hartman operation and the other patient refused stoma closure. In that same study, of the 25 patients who did not receive a stoma at the time of anastomosis, three underwent a stoma for sepsis and all were uneventfully closed.

Considering other reports of stomas constructed secondary to sepsis from a low anastomosis, Pakkastie's series had 16 out of 60 patients (27%) with an anastomotic leak, and four out of 16 (25%) had a permanent stoma [18]. There were six anastomotic leaks in Mealy's 74 patients, and all received a permanent stoma [14]. Thus the construction of a stoma at the time of anastomosis or for an anastomotic leak does not guarantee that the patient will have a permanent stoma.

Factors Affecting Leak Rate

Certain factors have been found to be associated with a higher rate of anastomotic leak. One such factor is the height of the anastomosis. Colorectal anastomosis can be divided into high and low anastomosis. Low anastomoses are below the peritoneal reflection and are generally less than 7 cm from the anus. Table 1 lists the leak rate with high versus low anastomosis. Low anastomosis have a much higher leakage rate compared to high anastomosis. Pakkastie found the only significant variable for the development of anastomotic leak to be an anastomosis performed less than 7 cm from the anal verge [18]. Tuson also found an increased anastomotic leak rate in low anastomosis [20].

Regarding other variables, Mileski [16] found that diabetes and cardiovascular problems did not increase the chance of an anastomotic leak, but low serum albumin, low hemoglobin, steroid dependence, and the need for perioperative transfusions were associated with an increased incidence. Other variables which have been cited include age [14], anastomosis done by a trainee [20], prolonged preoperative radiotherapy [6], and fecal loading [11].

There is no clear consensus as to whether the type of anastomosis (sutured or handsewn) influences the leak rate. Pakkastie [18] found that his overall leak rate was 12%. When this was divided into sutured versus handsewn anastomosis, 15% of stapled and 3% of sutured had leaks. Tuson found a 24% rate of leak and noted that leaks were more common if sutured [20]. Mileski found a 4% leak rate, with similar leak rates comparing handsewn and stapled anastomosis [16]. Thus the two methods of performing anastomosis probably have similar leak rates.

Surgeon variability may also influence the use of a stoma and leak rate. Fielding [5] conducted a multicenter study and divided the surgeons into groups based on those who use stomas frequently and those who do not. Surgeons who use stomas frequently had a leak rate of 20% with a mortality rate of 7.8%. This was compared to surgeons who rarely used stomas and had a leak rate of 8.4% with a mortality rate of 3.6%. They concluded that all surgeons should know their leak rate and if this drops below 5%, a stoma should only be used in select circumstances. More importantly, the question begs to be asked why surgeons in this study who used stomas more frequently had such higher mortality and leak rates.

The circulation at the proximal end of the bowel has been cited to affect the rate of leakage. When resecting the rectum for cure, the lymphatic drainage bed should be resected; this infers a high ligation of the inferior mesenteric artery. In turn, this can decrease the blood flow to the proximal bowel. Ambrosetti [2] reported a clinical leak rate of only 1% and a radiological leak rate of 1.5%. In 195 out of 200 colorectal anastomoses, the blood supply to both ends of the anastomosis was tested by Doppler ultrasound. If the Doppler signal was consistent with arterial pulsation, the blood supply was considered adequate. In ten patients this signal was absent, and the ends were further resected until the Doppler signal was of arterial pulsation. They feel that this contributed to their low anastomotic leak rate. Similarly, Novell [17] transected the marginal artery at the level of anastomosis and recorded whether blood flow was pulsatile. Nonpulsatile flow was observed in 80 patients. Of these, 15 (19%) developed a leak. This was compared to 195 who had pulsatile blood flow, 18 of which (9%) developed a leak. Additionally, in three patients no blood flow was observed after transecting the marginal artery, and all three developed a leak. They stressed that an absence of pulsatile blood flow did not reliably predict an anastomotic leak. Nevertheless, it appears that pulsatile blood flow will decrease the incidence of an anastomotic leak.

Hallböök [9] used laser Doppler blood flow to assess the microcirculation in bowel used for a colonic J pouch versus a straight colorectal anastomosis. They compared blood flow before dissection and just prior to anastomosis. Flow was unaffected when measured at the side of the bowel as with a colonic J pouch at the curved part of the J. In comparison, flow was significantly decreased at the end of bowel to be used in a straight anastomosis. They concluded that the unaffected blood flow at the site of a colonic J pouch may be favorable in anastomotic healing. However, only one out of 16 (6%) patients had an anastomotic leak in the straight group versus none out of 14 in the pouch group. This may be a pertinent finding, but it did not significantly affect their anastomotic leak rates.

The blood supply to the distal bowel may also be important. This has become apparent when total mesorectal excision (TME) is performed. TME leaves a tube of rectum which relies on blood flow from the pelvic floor. Heald [10] has championed TME, which has heightened the awareness of doing a proper cancer operation which yields a low local recurrence rate (<5%). However, even with his excellent results of low local recurrence, the "refractory problem" of anastomotic leakage has persisted. In one report, the rate was about 9% for clinical leaks and was significantly higher in patients without a diverting stoma [10]. In a recent study by Aitken [1], eight out of 57 patients (14%) had a clinical anastomotic leak after TME. Arbman and coworkers [3] reported an anastomotic leakage of 8%.

Whether TME contributes to leak is a matter of controversy, and no controlled study exists. Recently, Arbman and coworkers [3] from Sweden compared results after rectal cancer surgery before (1984–1986) and after (1990–1992) the introduction of TME. The postoperative clinical anastomotic leak rate and postoperative mortality due to complications showed no differences between the two time periods. Nevertheless, these authors and others [11] argue that a protective stoma is required after TME and a conventional low anastomosis.

In summary, low anastomosis have a higher incidence of leak. Low albumin, low hemiglobin, steroid use, transfusions, limited experience on the part of the surgeon, radiotherapy, and fecal loading may increase the incidence of a leak. The type of anastomosis (handsewn or stapled) is probably not significant. Pulsatile blood flow to the proximal end of the bowel is most likely beneficial. The blood supply to the distal bowel used for the anastomosis must not be compromised.

Pros and Cons of Using a Stoma

Numerous factors have been cited against a diverting stoma. Tuson found that unnecessary colostomies were performed in 19.4% of his patients and that the majority of anastomotic leaks could be managed without a colostomy [20]. Unquestionably, total hospitalization is increased if fecal diversion is used, and stoma closures are not without complication [11], although mortality is rare. Since most of these procedures are done in the elderly, the argument could be made that a stoma robs them of their independence along with adding financial burdens due to the cost of equipment. Additionally, some elderly patients may not have their stoma closed, but, as mentioned earlier, the overwhelming majority do undergo closure. Some feel that mortality and leak rate without a stoma is similar to that in patients who have undergone fecal diversion and that the routine use of stomas should therefore be questioned [14].

Graffner [7] similarly questioned the routine use of stomas. In the only randomized study in the literature, after the tumor was removed and the anastomosis completed, patients were randomized to receive a transverse colostomy. Since they were randomized after the anastomosis, those which were not technically perfect were omitted. There were 25 patients in each group. A gastrograffin enema was done on postoperative day 10. There was a 30% radiological leak rate in both groups. Clinical evidence of a leak was noted in 4% of patients in the colostomy group and in 12% of those without a colostomy. They concluded that a protective colostomy should not be routinely used with a low stapled anastomosis. They felt that, with close observation, the majority of patients can be treated with an emergent colostomy.

Looking at the positive aspects of a diverting stoma, even though there is no evidence that fecal diversion decreases the leak rate, Tuson [20] reported that diverting colostomies mitigate local and systemic effects of a leak. He reported that "conservative management" of leaks in cases with a covering colostomy were successful in most instances (92%). A stoma may also be life-saving, as Fielding found that the death rate was lower after an anastomotic leak with a stoma (9.6%) that without (26.2%) [15]. Goligher sums up the reasoning used by many in support of a diverting stoma: "The main value of (temporary transverse) colostomy at the conclusion of an anterior resection is not so much to prevent dehiscence as to facilitate its management if it should occur" [8].

The choice of stoma for diversion is changing. Initially, a loop colostomy was the stoma of choice. The danger with this type of stoma revolves around potential injury to the marginal artery, leading to ischemia. Additionally, the loop colostomy can be very bulky, leading to pouching difficulties. Consequently, construction of a loop ileostomy is gaining popularity. Both stomas can usually be closed by a local circumferential incision around the stoma. Khoury [13], in his study of 61 patients, found that fecal diversion with a loop ileostomy was the preferred method of diversion. The patients were randomized to receive a loop colostomy or loop ileostomy if diversion was needed. The only statistical difference between the two groups was that ileostomies began to function earlier. The length of hospital stay tended to be longer with colostomies, and ileostomies tended to be closed earlier, but neither reached statistical significance. There was a higher incidence of suture line leaks if a colostomy was used, and the ileostomy was felt to be easier to close (although the time of operation was similar to colostomy closure). They concluded that the loop ileostomy should be constructed rather than a loop colostomy.

Experience of the Cleveland Clinic

At the Cleveland Clinic from 1978 to 1985, there were 744 consecutive colorectal anastomosis studied (The Cleveland Clinic, unpublished data). Nineteen (3%) developed a clinical leak. However, a subgroup of 262 consecutive patients underwent a gastrograffin enema at 10 days postoperatively, with 27 (10%) having radiological evidence of a leak. The anastomosis were divided into high (11–15 cm; $n=354$, 48%), low (6–10 cm; $n=219$, 29%), and very low (<5~cm; $n=171$, 23%) from the dentate line. Temporary colostomies were used in 111 patients (15%), and all were closed by 6 months. In 1985, the colostomy rate decreased to 8.5% after confidence was gained with the circular stapler. Clinical leaks were found in 0.6% of patients with high anastomosis, 3.2% with low anastomosis, and 5.8% with very low anastomosis.

Practical Guidelines

Not all colorectal anastomoses require a diverting stoma, and reliably predicting which anastomosis will leak is unlikely. This was emphasized by Karanjia [11]. In 75 patients, the anastomosis was felt to be perfect and fecal diversion was omitted. However, 15% (11/75) developed symptoms attributed to an anastomotic leak and all occurred in anastomoses less than 6 cm from the anal verge.

Therefore, since predicting which anastomosis will leak is impractical, an attempt should be made to do as much as possible to prevent a leak. Easy steps at the time of operation to promote a technically satisfying anastomosis include a thorough bowel clean out (even if it requires on-table bowel lavage), no anastomotic tension, assessing the marginal artery for pulsatile blood flow, checking the doughnuts after a stapled anastomosis for completeness, instilling air via the anus with saline in the pelvis checking for escape of bubbles, and suture repairing any defect. Use of Doppler ultrasound to assess pulsatile flow should be considered if the equipment is available.

A diverting stoma should be used selectively. I favor a loop ileostomy for the reasons mentioned previously. Most anastomosis above the peritoneal reflection probably do not require fecal diversion unless there is a technical problem with the anastomosis or there are other adverse circumstances. The conditions which favor a stoma with any level of colorectal anastomosis include residual pelvic sepsis, colonic obstruction, malnutrition, immunosuppression, fecal loading, irradiated bowel, contamination, and limited experience of the surgeon.

Overall, it appears that the consequences of a leak are more serious if no stoma was initially constructed. Surgeons are rarely sorry to have constructed a stoma, but more frequently lament on wishing one had been constructed. Consequently, if there is any doubt at the time of initial operation, a diverting stoma should be performed. As pointed out by Fielding [5], the surgeon (not the patient) is probably the single most important factor affecting anastomotic leaks. It is important for the surgeon to use the anastomotic technique he or she is most familiar with, to audit results, and to refine the technique. When trying any new technique (such as TME), a diverting stoma should be considered until experience is gained in the technique.

References

1. Aitken RJ (1996) Mesorectal excision for rectal cancer. Br J Surg 83:214–216
2. Ambrosetti P, Robert J, Mathey P, Rohner A (1994) Left-sided colon and colorectal anastomoses: Doppler ultrasound as an aid to assess bowel vascularization. Int J Colorect Dis 9:211–214
3. Arbman G, Nilsson E, Hallböök O, Sjödahl R (1996) Can total mesorectal excision reduce the local recurrence rate in rectal surgery. Br J Surg 83:375–379
4. Dukes CE (1930) The spread of cancer of the rectum. Br J Surg 17:643
5. Fielding LP, Stewart-Brown S, Hittinger R, Blesovsky L (1984) Covering stoma for elective anterior resection of the rectum: an outmoded operation? Am J Surg 147:524–530
6. Graf W, Glimelius B, Bergstrom R, Påhlman L (1991) Complications after double and single stapling in rectal surgery. Eur J Surg 157:543–547
7. Graffner H, Fredlund P, Olsson S-A Oscarson J, Petersson B-G (1983) Protective colostomy in low anterior resection of the rectum using the EEA stapling instrument. Dis Colon Rectum 26:87–90

8. Goligher JC (1980) Surgery of the anus, rectum, and colon, 4th edn. Bailliere Tindall, London, pp 563–605
9. Hallböök O, Johansson K, Sjödahl R (1996) Laser doppler blood flow measurement in rectal resection for carcinoma – comparison between the straight and colonic J pouch reconstruction. Br J Surg 83:389–392
10. Heald RJ, Karanjia ND (1992) Results of radical surgery for rectal cancer. World J Surg 16:848–857
11. Karanjia ND, Corder AP, Holdsworth PJ, Heald RJ (1991) Risk of peritonitis and fatal septicaemia and the need to defunction the low anastomosis. Br J Surg 78:196–198
12. Kirkegaard P (1978) A new technique for low anterior resection of the rectum: preliminary results with a circular stapling instrument for anastomosis. Dan Med Bull 25:5–7
13. Khoury GA, Lewis MCA, Meleagros L, Lewis AAM (1986) Colostomy or ileostomy after colorectal anastomosis? A randomized trial. Ann R Coll Surg (Engl) 68:5–7
14. Mealy K, Burke P, Hyland J (1992) Anterior resection without a defunctioning colostomy: question of safety. Br J Surg 79:305–307
15. Miles WE (1910) The radical abdominal-perineal operation for cancer of the rectum and of the pelvic colon. Br Med J 2:94.1
16. Mileski WJ, Joe MRJ, Renge RV, Narwold DL (1988) Treatment of anastomotic leakage following low anterior colon resection. Arch Surg 123:968–971
17. Novell JR, Lewis AAM (1990) Preoperative observation of marginal artery bleeding: a predictor of anastomotic leakage. Br J Surg 77:137–138
18. Pakkastie TE, Luukkonen PE, Jarvinen HJ (1994) Anastomotic leakage after anterior resection of the rectum. Eur J Surg 160:293–297
19. Parks AG (1972) Transanal technique in low rectal anastomosis. Proc R Soc Med 65:975–976
20. Tuson JRD, Everett WG (1990) A retrospective study of colostomies, leaks and strictures after colorectal anastomosis. Int J Colorect Dis 5:44–48

Outcome

CHAPTER 25

Functional Results Following Rectal Surgery: A Review

Fabrizio Michelassi and Deborah A. Mhoon

Introduction

The goal of surgical treatment for rectal carcinoma is cure with preservation of
body image and anorectal, urinary, and sexual function. However, this goal
may not be obtainable in all patients and disease recurrence, the need for a
permanent stoma, as well as alterations in anorectal, urinary, and sexual
function may occur. In this chapter we will review the functional results following surgical treatment for rectal adenocarcinoma; we will also report on a
data-gathering protocol which we use at the University of Chicago to help in
the analysis of postoperative function.

Anorectal Function

When a sphincter-saving procedure is performed, anorectal function may be
temporarily or permanently altered. Patients may experience changes in the
degree of continence to flatus, feces, or both; inability or difficulty to evacuate;
changes in the frequency and consistency of bowel movements; and urgency.
Although these changes may be present even after an anterior resection and
low coloproctostomy for a rectal cancer located in the upper third of the
rectum, they are much more frequent and pronounced after a proctectomy and
coloanal anastomosis for a rectal carcinoma located in the middle or lower
third of the rectum. It is common experience that the more extensive is the
proctectomy and the smaller is the residual rectum, the more pronounced are
these changes. As a consequence, patients undergoing a complete proctectomy
with coloanal anastomoses often experience the most dramatic changes in
anorectal function.

Paty and Enker [9] surveyed 81 of 90 eligible patients who were treated with low anterior resection (LAR) and coloanal anastomoses between 1977 and 1990. The median number of bowel movements per day was two (range 0.3 to 15). However, 22% reported four or more bowel movements per day. Fecal incontinence was graded according to the Kirwan scale. Half of the patients (51%) were completely continent; incontinence to flatus without soilage was reported in 21%. Minor leakage described as occasional soiling with liquid stool, occurred in 27% of patients; significant incontinence to solid stool was only reported in 5% of patients. However, these patients posed difficult problems to manage. Overall, 32% of patients used protective pads, at least on a part-time basis.

The inability to defer a bowel movement for at least 10 min was seen in 19% of patients. Multiple evacuations or cluster bowel movements (the need to return to the bathroom multiple times within a short period of time before full evacuation is achieved) was described in 32% of patients. These episodes did not occur on a daily basis but when they occurred, they were disruptive to the patient's daily routine. Fifty-six percent of the patients had good to excellent results. Among the ten patients who experienced poor function, stool frequency was a common occurrence in six patients, and four were enema dependent.

The avoidance of certain foods, namely, salads, vegetables and dairy products, was observed in 56% of patients. Seventeen percent felt that long distance travel was no longer feasible due to their daily bowel habits and 37% required the addition of antimotility drugs, stool softeners, or enemas for regularity. It is not surprising that adjustments in life style were directly related to the degree of functional impairment. Patients with poor results demonstrated a greater incidence of altered life style compared with those who had fewer complaints. However, most problems appeared minor and were well tolerated. Despite some of these inconveniences, patient overall satisfaction with the procedure remained high (74%) and the avoidance of a permanent stoma played a major role in patient approval.

Many authors have attempted to correlate treatment variables with improved or impaired functional outcomes. Lazorthes et al. examined frequency of defecation in 65 patients who underwent an end-to-end (n=45) or a J-pouch (n=20) coloanal anastomosis [6]. Age, sex, and tumor characteristics were similar in both groups of patients. During the first year there was no significant difference in continence rates, but frequency of defecation was lower in patients with a reservoir. There was no significant difference in continence rates. After the first year, 36 patients without a reservoir and 15 patients with a reservoir were available for assessment. Frequency in the reservoir patients still remained lower. There was no difference in continence between the two groups.

Kichoffs et al. [8] also demonstrated reduced stool frequency in patients with a reservoir. All these results support the hypothesis that increased capacity of the neorectum improves functional results after a coloanal anastomoses.

Another treatment variable potentially affecting postoperative functional results may be represented by the use of preoperative or postoperative radiotherapy. Little is known regarding the long-term effects of preoperative radiation therapy on sphincter integrity and function, continence, and urgency. In a phase I/II trial of preoperative radiation therapy and LAR/coloanal anastomosis [7], 22 patients with the diagnosis of invasive, resectable primary adenocarcinoma of the rectum limited to the pelvis received a total of 4680 cGy followed by an additional 360 cGy to the primary tumor. Of the 21 patients who underwent resection 89% reported good to excellent functional results at a median follow-up time of 29 months.

Kollmorgen and associates assessed the long term effect of postoperative radiotherapy in 100 patients with Astler-Coller B2 or C2 lesions of the rectum [5]. Forty-one patients had postoperative chemoradiation and 59 patients did not. To minimize confounding factors, extensive exclusion criteria were used. The two groups of patients were well matched for sex, level of anastomosis, and length of follow-up. The group that received chemoradiation had more bowel movements per day than the group that had surgery only (median 7 vs. 2 bowel movements/day); the former group more often experienced clustering of bowel movements (42% vs. 3%) and night-time movements (39% vs. 17%), wore a protective pad more often (41% vs. 10%), and were more often unable to defer defecation for longer than 15 min (78% vs. 19%). The group that had chemoradiation also had stools of liquid consistency, used antidiarrheal medications, had perineal skin irritation, were unable to differentiate stool from gas, and needed to defecate again within 30 min of a movement significantly more often that the group that did not receive chemoradiation.

Other variables may influence the postoperative functional results: Paty and Enker [9] analyzed the possible correlation between treatment variables and functional outcome. Using multiple linear regression, they found that time since operation had a positive influence in reducing the number of daily bowel movements, while postoperative pelvic radiation therapy significantly correlated with increased frequency. Using multiple logistic regression, use of adjuvant pelvic radiation and male gender significantly correlated with occurrence of bowel movement clustering.

Careful prospective studies will be needed to investigate the role of other possible treatment variables: they include gender of the patient, degree of postoperative anorectal angle, removal or preservation of the anal transitional zone, level of anastomosis (colorectal vs. coloanal).

Urinary Function

The urinary bladder is innervated by the sympathetic and the parasympathetic nerves. Stimulation by the sympathetic nerves contracts the bladder neck, while detrusor muscle contraction is mediated through S2-S4. Injury of S2-S4 causes a neurogenic bladder with decreased sensation and increased capacity. As a consequence, urinary retention and infections are the most common complications following proctectomy. The presence of prostatic hypertrophy and the posterior displacement of the bladder after complete rectal excision in an abdominal perineal resection may add to the postoperative voiding dysfunction. Bladder dysfunction can occur in up to 40% of patients [10] with an increased risk when a wide ileopelvic lymphadenectomy is added to the resection. Hojo et al. [3] performing extended pelvic lymphadenectomy and total resection of the pelvic autonomic nerve system in advanced rectal cancer have reported a decrease in local recurrence and an increase in survival rate. Over the years, Hojo and collaborators have gradually extended the indication for partial nerve preservation, provided the goal of cure was not compromised [4]. Beginning in 1985 complete autonomic nerve preservation (first degree dissection) was attempted in patients with early rectal carcinomas limited to the submucosal layers. When there was suspicion of lateral lymph node involvement along the midrectal artery, the hypogastric nerves were preserved but the hypogastric plexus was sacrificed (second degree dissection). The hypogastric nerves were sacrificed when metastatic involvement of the perirectal lymph nodes or the more proximal lymph nodes along the superior hemorrhoidal artery was suspected (third degree dissection). Selective preservation of the fourth pelvic parasympathetic nerve either unilaterally or bilaterally was performed in patients who required a more extensive ileopelvic lymphadenectomy (fourth degree dissection). Twenty-four patients underwent first degree preservation of the autonomic nerve plexus and six patients, 52 patients, and 16 patients, underwent second, third, fourth degree, respectively. In 36 patients, the pelvic autonomic nerves were completely sacrificed for oncologic reasons (fifth degree dissection).

Most patients with first or second degree dissection of the autonomic pelvic nerves and a sphincter-saving procedure were able to void spontaneously by the twelfth postoperative day (80% and 100%, respectively). The rate of spontaneous voiding by the twelfth post-operative day after a sphincter-saving procedure decreased to 25% and 16%, respectively, after third or fourth degree dissection of the pelvic autonomic nerves. After an abdominal perineal resection, no patient regained spontaneous voiding by the twelfth postoperative day, except 60% of patients who had complete preservation of the pelvic autonomic nerves (first degree dissection). Those patients who underwent a radical pelvic dissection (fifth degree) had severe bladder dysfunction irrespective of whether the procedure was a sphincter-saving procedure or an abdomino-perineal resection. Twenty-one of 36 patients with fifth degree dissection had not recovered bladder sensation by the 60th postoperative day and 28 (78%) were discharged with an indwelling bladder catheter. All but nine patients ultimately recovered the ability to spontaneously void. One patient had to catheterize himself for more than 2 years before recovering the ability to spontaneous voiding.

Preoperative and postoperative assessment of bladder function can be obtained with a cystometrogram. During the filling phase of this test, bladder sensation, compliance and capacity can be measured; during the voiding phase, urine flow and intravescical pressure can be recorded. Injury to the parasympathetic nerves causes varying degrees of atonic, neurogenic bladder, which can be quantitated with a cystometrogram.

Sexual Function

The sympathetic nerves are responsible for contraction of the bladder neck during orgasm and prograde ejaculation in the male and for adequate lubrication of the vagina in the female. Penile erection is achieved by parasympathetic stimulation through S2-S4. As a consequence, injury to the sympathetic nerves is responsible for retrograde ejaculation in the male and diminished vaginal lubrication in the female; injury to the parasympathetic nerves is responsible for impotence in the male patient. The incidence of impotence reported in the literature after a proctectomy is 3.4% for inflammatory bowel disease and 48.6% for cancer [2].

Cavaliere [1], reporting on the sexual function of 302 patients who had undergone a LAR for cancer, found that 60% of male patients were now suffering from retrograde ejaculation. Of 40 patients studied by Williams and Johnston [11], 28 patients had an active sexual life before sphincter-saving procedures and 30% reported impaired function after the procedure. Four complained of total erectile impotence and one had difficulty maintaining an erection. Of the 11 men who were still sexually active, two complained of difficulty in ejaculation. However, of the 20 patients who had been sexually active before abdominoperineal resection 13 patients were inactive afterwards. Eight of the men (47%) had complete impotence and three had difficulty maintaining an erection. Of the five men who reported sexual activity, two were not able to ejaculate. Thus 67% developed some degree of sexual impairment following abdominoperineal resection.

Enker [2] examined the combined roles of autonomic nerve-preserving sidewall dissection (ANP/SWD) in the cure, local control, and in the preservation of sexual potency. The procedure was characterized by truncal nerve preservation within the posterior pelvic compartment with deliberate sacrifice of the inferior hypogastric plexus. Assessment of sexual function was evaluated with respect to the patient's ability to achieve spontaneous erection. Postoperative potency was defined as the ability to achieve a spontaneous erection, to avoid unassisted penetration, and to sustain the erection for the duration of sexual intercourse. Thirty-three (86.7%) of 38 evaluable patients remained potent. Twenty-eight patients (84.8%) retained an erectile capacity of 75%–100%, while five patients (15.2%) retained 50%–75% of their preoperative erectile capacity. All remained capable of unassisted penetration. Five patients became impotent. Twenty-nine patients (87.9%) who remained potent retained normal ejaculations. Five patients had either diminished or absent ejaculation and no patient complained of pain. Two patients complained of decreased sensation soon after surgery, but this symptom disappeared over time.

The only factor which appeared to be significantly correlated with the postoperative sexual outcome of these patients was age at the time of surgery. The mean age of the patients who remained potent was 54.3 years, the mean age of the patients who became impotent was 64 years. Of 24 patients younger than 60, 23 (95.8%) remained potent; of 12 patients aged 60 through 69 years, nine (75%) remained potent; and of two patients 70 years or older, one (50%) remained potent.

In Hojo's series, evaluation of postoperative sexual function demonstrated 12 of 39 (31%) of male patients under 60 years of age eventually recovered erectile function. Preservation of erectile function postoperatively was directly correlated to the degree of preservation of the autonomic pelvic nerves: following a first, second, third, fourth, or fifth degree of nerve preservation the rate of preservation of erectile function was 80%, 100%, 25%, 16%, and 0%, respectively. However, only 6/39 (15%) had normal ejaculatory function after the first postoperative year and most of these patients were in the first degree of nerve dissection.

Following proctectomy for malignant disease, decrease in vaginal lubrication and dyspareunia are the major alterations in female sexual function. When the posterior wall of the vagina is resected because of tumor involvement, a decrease in size of the vaginal canal may interfere with sexual intercourse unless the vaginal canal is reconstructed with a vascularized myocutaneous flap at the time of the abdominoperineal resection.

Measurement of penile tumescence is a reliable method to assess male potency. The test is obtained with a portable device which measures penile circumference and radial rigidity. Spontaneous nocturnal erections or erections following visual stimulation can therefore be recorded and graded. The test is not invasive and the assessment of radial rigidity gives an indirect measurement of axial rigidity and, in turn, of the degree of the erection. To date, there are no tests to assess the ejaculatory function in the male patient and the sexual function in the female patients.

Prospective Assessment of Postoperative Anorectal Function

At the University of Chicago, we have developed a protocol in an effort to systematically collect data on anorectal, sexual, and urinary function that are accurate and free from recollection bias of the patient and subjective bias of the surgeon. The protocol is composed of questionnaires (Appendix I – II) and of a daily diary (Fig. 1).

The questionnaire is aimed at assessing the use of pharmacological aids and diet restrictions to reduce bowel movement frequency, use of enemas to stimulate bowel movements, degree of continence (ability to distinguish flatus from stool and to defer a bowel movement, use of protective pads) and incidence of sexual and urinary complications. The questionnaire also tries to obtain a subjective assessment of the patient's quality of life.

The daily diary is aimed at measuring the timing and consistency of bowel movements, as well as the occurrence, timing, and degree of incontinence. It consists of seven sheets to record oral intake, sleep pattern, bowel activity, and continence daily over one week (Fig. 1a). A 24-h clock allows patients to record the time of each bowel movement and episode of incontinence. Following a detailed legend, patients are able to chart the consistency of each bowel movement and grade the severity of eventual episodes of fecal incontinence (Fig. 1b).

PART II. ASSESSMENT OF BOWEL HABITS

DAY #_1_

Please indicate timing of your main meals and describe what you ate.

Date: _______/_______/_______

Breakfast: ___________ a.m. ____
____

Lunch: ___________ a.m./p.m. ____
____

Dinner ___________ p.m. ____
____

Please indicate the time you went to sleep last night _______________
the time you woke up this morning _______________

a

Using the clock and the symbols in the legend, indicate today's bowel movements and episodes of leakage.

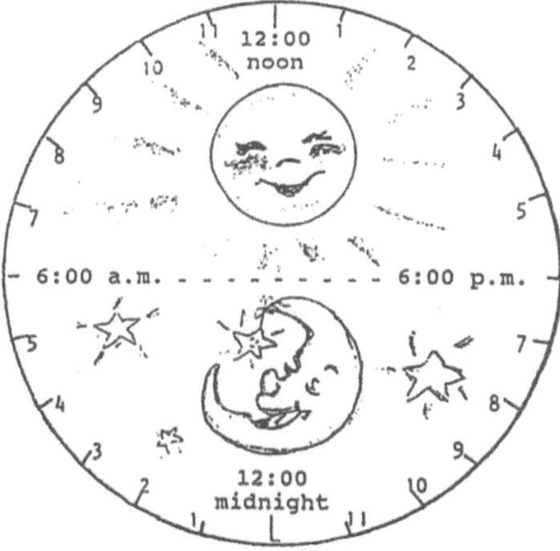

Legend:
B = bowel movement indicate also stool consistency: B_f=formed; B_p=pasty; B_l=liquid
S = Leakage of stool Indicate also seepage entity: S_m=minor seepage requiring cleaning with a tissue or towel; S_x=major seepage, loss of stool

b

Fig. 1a,b. Representation of the protocol mailed to patients at 3, 6, 9, 12, 18, 24 months and yearly thereafter. a Assessment of the patient's diet and sleep pattern. b Assessment of the daily bowel movements

The protocol is mailed to our patients preoperatively at 3, 6, 9, 12, 18, 24 months and yearly after a coloanal procedure or after closure of the temporary stoma. Two to three weeks after receiving the protocol, patients come to our outpatient clinic where the protocol is evaluated. Answers that appear to be unclear or inconsistent with previous answers are clarified; bowel activity and episodes of incontinence are averaged over 7 days and expressed with daytime, night-time, and 24-h mean values. Diet and medications are reviewed, and suggestions are made to improve functional results. A complete physical examination is performed with particular attention given to a digital examination aimed at assessing the status of the coloanal anastomosis and anal canal and sphincter mechanism. This is complemented by a proctosigmoidoscopy or flexible sigmoidoscopy if necessary.

We believe that the protocol avoids physician subjectivity and minimizes patient inaccuracies when evaluating functional outcome. Other methods that rely on physician questioning to gather functional data have several drawbacks. First, frequency and incontinence may vary daily. Asking the patient about bowel function during a physician visit may result in the patient remembering only the most recent frequency or the worse or the best day, which may not be an accurate reflection of average function. In addition, when asked by their surgeon, patients may want to please the surgeon and be hesitant to be completely honest in discussing problems that resulted as a consequence of the surgical procedure.

In conclusion, we believe that this patient-completed protocol is a useful adjunct in the assessment of the functional results in patients after proctectomy. We believe that emphasis on obtaining accurate and reproducible functional assessments after surgery is important for several reasons. First, when counseling patients about their therapeautic options, it is important to present realistic expectations about their functional outcomes. Second, as surgeons, we need a reliable database on which to compare procedures to identify the optimal approach for an individual patient. Third, we need to be able to appreciate subtle differences in functional outcomes as we change the technical aspects of the procedure and try to improve its functional results. Finally, being able to correlate modifications of the procedure and functional outcome enhances our ability to understand the physiology of continence, bladder and sexual function.

Appendix I: Rectal Cancer – Preoperative Questionnaire

Part I. Assessment of Performance Status

A. Anorectal Function

Please answer the following questions as to give us an idea of your baseline bowel habits. If your bowel habits have changed recently because of the rectal cancer, try to remember how your bowel habits were before they changed. If they have not changed, record your bowel habits as they are now:

1. Have your bowel habits changed because of the rectal cancer?
   [ ] No [ ] Yes
   If yes, how?

2. Are you able to differentiate between stool and gas and pass gas without losing stool?
   [ ] Always (everytime)
   [ ] Often (more than half the time)
   [ ] Sometimes (less than half the time)
   [ ] Never
   [ ] Have never tried

3. Do you have pain during a bowel movement?
   [ ] None
   [ ] Occasionally (less than once a month)
   [ ] Sometimes (more than once a month)
   [ ] Often (more than once a week)

4. Do you wear a protective pad during the day?
   [ ] Yes [ ] No

5. Do you wear a protective pad during the night?
   [ ] Yes [ ] No

6. Do you use a protective pad because of:
   Urine incontinence [ ] Yes [ ] No
   Stool incontinence [ ] Yes [ ] No
   Both [ ] Yes [ ] No

7. Do you alter the times that you eat in order to control your bowel pattern?
   [ ] Yes [ ] No
   If "yes" describe

8. How many times do you have to go to the bathroom before you feel as though you're fully evacuated?
   [ ] 1
   [ ] 2–3
   [ ] 4–5
   [ ] 6–8
   [ ] >8

9. Does this happen
   [ ] Always (every day)
   [ ] Often (at least 1/wk)
   [ ] Sometimes (at least 1/month)
   [ ] Never

10. Do you have rectal itching?
   [ ] None
   [ ] Occasionally (less than once a month)
   [ ] Sometimes (more than once a month)

[ ] Often (more than once a week)

11. Do you have rectal bleeding?
    [ ] None
    [ ] Occasionally (less than once a month)
    [ ] Sometimes (more than once a month)
    [ ] Often (more than once a week)

12. Do you use Metamucil or other "fiber" preparations?
    [ ] Always [ ] Often [ ] Sometimes [ ] Never
    If "Always", "Often" or "Sometimes" specify how often and how much
    each day:

13. Do you give yourself enemas to have a bowel movement?
    [ ] Always (every day)
    [ ] Often (at least 1/wk)
    [ ] Sometimes (at least 1/month)
    [ ] Never

14. Do you give yourself suppositories to have a bowel movement?
    [ ] Always (every day)
    [ ] Often (at least 1/wk)
    [ ] Sometimes (at least 1/month)
    [ ] Never

15. Do you alter the times that you eat in order to control your bowel pattern?
    [ ] Yes [ ] No
    If "yes" describe

16. Are you able to delay a bowel movement?
    [ ] Always [ ] Often [ ] Sometimes [ ] Never
    If "Always", "Often" or "Sometimes" for how long can you delay it?

B. Sexual Function

For male patients

1. Are you capable of spontaneous erections?
   [ ] No [ ] Yes

2. Do you need assistance during penetration into the vagina?
   [ ] No [ ] Yes

3. During orgasm, does sperm come out of the penis or is it dry?
   [ ] Sperm [ ] Dry

Use the following for the next three questions:

n/a Not applicable during past 3 months
 0 No reaction
 2 Barely noticeable enlargement

 4 Slight elevation from body
 6 Moderate elevation from body, not enough for penetration
 8 Full but not firm erection; enough for penetration with help
10 Full, firm erection

4. How full and firm are your erections during night time or early morning?
   n/a 1 2 3 4 5 6 7 8 9 10

5. How full and firm are your erections during attempts at penetration?
   n/a 1 2 3 4 5 6 7 8 9 10

6. How full and firm are your erections during intercourse?
   n/a 1 2 3 4 5 6 7 8 9 10

7. How often do you have difficulty getting an erection with a partner?
   [ ] Never
   [ ] Rarely, less than 10% of the time
   [ ] Seldom, less than 25% of the time
   [ ] Sometimes, about 50% of the time
   [ ] Usually, about 75% of the time
   [ ] Nearly always, over 90% of the time
   [ ] Not applicable, no sex in the past 3 months

8. Do you reach orgasm through sexual intercourse?
   [ ] Never
   [ ] Rarely, less than 10% of the time
   [ ] Seldom, less than 25% of the time
   [ ] Sometimes, about 50% of the time
   [ ] Usually, about 75% of the time
   [ ] Nearly always, over 90% of the time
   [ ] Not applicable, no sex in the past 3 months

For female patients

1. Does your vagina usually feel
   [ ] Nicely lubricated
   [ ] Dry
   [ ] With increased secretion

2. How often do you experience pain during sex?
   [ ] Never
   [ ] Rarely, less than 10% of the time
   [ ] Seldom, less than 25% of the time
   [ ] Sometimes, about 50% of the time
   [ ] Usually, about 75% of the time
   [ ] Nearly always, over 90% of the time
   [ ] Not applicable, no sex in the past 3 months

3. How often do you achieve orgasm (climax) during sex with a partner?
   [ ] Never
   [ ] Rarely, less than 10% of the time

[ ] Seldom, less than 25% of the time
[ ] Sometimes, about 50% of the time
[ ] Usually, about 75% of the time
[ ] Nearly always, over 90% of the time
[ ] Not applicable, no sex in the past 3 months

C. Urinary Function

1. Do you lose urine, do you dribble, are you incontinent of urine?
   [ ] Never
   [ ] Rarely, less than 10% of the time
   [ ] Seldom, less than 25% of the time
   [ ] Sometimes, about 50% of the time
   [ ] Usually, about 75% of the time
   [ ] Nearly always, over 90% of the time

2. Do you get up during the night and go to the bathroom to void?
   [ ] No [ ] Yes

3. If yes, how many times?
   1, 2, 3, 4, >5

Appendix II: Rectal Cancer – Post-Operative Questionnaire

Part I. Assessment of Performance Status

A. Anorectal Function

1. How many months since your ostomy closure?

2. Are you able to delay a bowel movement?
   [ ] Always [ ] Often [ ] Sometimes [ ] Never
   If "Always", "Often" or "Sometimes" for how long can you delay it?

3. Do you alter the times that you eat in order to control your bowel pattern?
   [ ] Yes [ ] No
   If "Yes" describe

4. Are you able to differentiate between flatus and gas and pass gas without losing stool?
   [ ] Always [ ] Never
   [ ] Often [ ] Have not tried
   [ ] Sometimes

5. How many times do you have to go to the bathroom before you feel as though you're fully evacuated?
   [ ] 1–3
   [ ] 4–5

    [ ] 6–8
    [ ] >8

6. Does it ever happen that you do not feel fully evacuated?
    [ ] Always
    [ ] Often
    [ ] Sometimes
    [ ] Never

7. Do you have pain during a bowel movement?
    [ ] None
    [ ] Occasionally (less than once a month)
    [ ] Sometimes (more than once a month)
    [ ] Often (more than once a week)

8. Do you wear a protective pad during the day?
    [ ] Yes [ ] No

9. Do you wear a protective pad at night?
    [ ] Yes [ ] No

10. Do you have rectal itching?
    [ ] None
    [ ] Occasionally (less than once a month)
    [ ] Sometimes (more than once a month)
    [ ] Often (more than once a week)

11. Do you have rectal bleeding?
    [ ] None
    [ ] Occasionally (less than once a month)
    [ ] Sometimes (more than once a month)
    [ ] Often (more than once a week)

12. Do you use Metamucil or other "fiber" preparations
    [ ] Always [ ] Often [ ] Sometimes [ ] Never
    If "Always" "Often" or "Sometimes" specify how often and how much
    each day:

13. Do you use any other medication to control your bowel movements?
    [ ] Yes [ ] No
    If "Yes" indicate one(s) and how much:
    [ ] Imodium
    [ ] Lomotil
    [ ] Tincture of opium
    [ ] Questran
    [ ] Other

14. Do you avoid certain foods for fear of watery or increased bowel move-
    ments?
    [ ] Yes [ ] No
    If "Yes", describe

15. Do you have any irritation or rash on the skin around your anus?
    [ ] None
    [ ] Yes, rare (less than once a month)
    [ ] Yes, often (more than once a month)
    [ ] Yes, always (more than once a week)
    Does such irritation or rash require treatment, such as creams or ointments?
    [ ] Yes [ ] No
    If yes, specify

16. Is it necessary for you to perform self digital dilation because of anastomoses or stricture:
    [ ] Yes [ ] No
    If yes, signify how often

17. Do you give yourself daily enemas to aid in evacuation?
    [ ] Yes [ ] No

18. In comparing now to before the first operation please check the following as it applies:
    Increased
    Reduced
    Unchanged

    Social activity/recreation
    [ ] [ ] [ ]
    Physical activity/sports
    [ ] [ ] [ ]
    Travel
    [ ] [ ] [ ]
    Work/school
    [ ] [ ] [ ]
    Sleep/rest
    [ ] [ ] [ ]
    Family activities
    [ ] [ ] [ ]
    Community activities
    [ ] [ ] [ ]
    Household chores
    [ ] [ ] [ ]
    Sense of well-being
    [ ] [ ] [ ]
    Please explain:

19. Do you think your quality of life compared to before the first operation is:
    [ ] Much worse [ ] Worse [ ] Same [ ] Better [ ] Much better

20. Do you think that your quality of life compared to when you had the stoma is:
    [ ] Much worse [ ] Worse [ ] Same [ ] Better [ ] Much better

21. What is your overall satisfaction with the operation?
    [ ] Excellent [ ] Good [ ] Fair [ ] Poor

22. What is your overall adjustment to the new life-style imposed by the operation?
    [ ] Excellent [ ] Good [ ] Fair [ ] Poor

23. Finish this statement: When considering this surgery, I wish I would have known.......

24. Would you recommend this operation to other patients?
    [ ] Yes [ ] No
    If no, specify why:

    Comments:

B. Sexual Function

Please answer if this is the first time you're completing the protocol or if you are having any problems during sexual intercourse:

For female patients only:

Compared to before surgery, is your desire for sexual intercourse:
[ ] Increased [ ] Decreased [ ] Same

Do you have pain during sexual intercourse?
[ ] Yes [ ] No

Did you have pain during sexual intercourse before undergoing the coloanal procedure?
[ ] Yes [ ] No

Did you reach orgasm?
[ ] Yes [ ] No

Did you reach orgasm before undergoing the coloanal procedure?
[ ] Yes [ ] No

For male patients only:

Compared to before surgery, is your desire for sexual intercourse:
[ ] Increased [ ] Decreased [ ] Same

Can you obtain an erection?
[ ] Yes [ ] No

If no, could you before surgery?
[ ] Yes [ ] No

Compared to before surgery, is the erection:
[ ] As strong [ ] Weaker

Do you reach orgasm?
  [ ] Yes [ ] No

During orgasm, does sperm come out of your penis or is it dry?
  [ ] Sperm [ ] Dry

C. Urinary Function

1. Do you lose urine, do you dribble, are you incontinent of urine?
  [ ] Never
  [ ] Rarely, less than 10% of the time
  [ ] Seldom, less than 25% of the time
  [ ] Sometimes, about 50% of the time
  [ ] Usually, about 75% of the time
  [ ] Nearly always, over 90% of the time

2. Do you get up during the night and go to the bathroom to void?
  [ ] No [ ] Yes

3. If yes, how many times?
  1, 2, 3, 4, >5

References

1. Cavaliere A, Bragaglia RB, Manara G, Poggioli G, Gozzetti G (1990) Urogenital dysfunction after abdominoperineal resection for carcinoma of the rectum. Dis Colon Rectum 33:918–922
2. Enker WE (1992) Potency, cure and local control in the operative treatment of rectal cancer. Arch Surg 127:1396–1401
3. Hojo K, Sawada T, Moriya Y (1989) An analysis of survival and voiding, sexual function after wide ileopelvic lymphadenectomy in patients with carcinoma of the rectum, compared with conventional lymphadenectomy. Dis Colon Rectum 32:128–133
4. Hojo K, Vernava III AM, Sugihara K, Katumata K (1991) Preservation of urine voiding and sexual function after rectal cancer surgery. Dis Colon Rectum 34:532–539
5. Kollmorgan CF, Meagher AP, Wolff BG, Pemberton JH, Martenson JA, Illstrup DM (1994) Long term effects of an adjuvant postoperative chemoradiation for rectal carcinoma on bowel function. Ann Surg 220:676–682
6. Lazorthes F, Fages P, Chiotasso P, Lemozy J, Bloom E (1986) Resection of the rectum with construction of a colonic reservoir and colo-anal anastomosis for carcinoma of the rectum. Br J Surg 73:136–141
7. Minsky BD, Cohn AM, Enker WE, Sigurdson E (1992) Phase I/II trial of pre-operative radiation therapy and coloanal anastomosis in distal invasive resectable rectal cancer. Int J Radiat Oncol Biol Phys 23:387–392
8. Nicholls RJ, Lubowski DZ, Donaldson DR (1988) Comparison of colonic reservoir and straight colo-anal reconstruction after rectal excision. Br J Surg 75:318–320
9. Paty PB, Enker WE, Cohen AM, Minsky BD, Friedlander-Klar H (1994) Long-term functional results of coloanal anastomoses for rectal cancer. Am J Surg 167:90–95
10. Schrock TR (1995) Abdominoperineal resection – technique and complications. In: Cohen AM, Winawer SJ (eds) Cancer of the colon, rectum and anus. Mc Graw-Hill, New York, pp 595–604
11. Williams NS, Johnston D (1983) The quality of life after rectal excision for low rectal cancer. Br J Surg 70:460–462

CHAPTER 26

The Effect of Specialization or Organization of Rectal Cancer Surgery

Werner Hohenberger

Introduction

Patients assume that there are no significant differences in the quality of surgery between comparable hospitals. If at all, they may accept some minor differences between individual surgeons with regard to postoperative complications, but they will definitely not accept differences in long-term survival following surgery for cancer.

However, in several institutions internal quality control (i.e., auditing) has revealed such differences do exist. Commonly, quality of surgery is a matter of insider information or of rumours, and opinions and discussions are frequently based more on personal "impression" than on scientific evidence.

There are limited data analyzing the influence of surgeons on short- or long-term outcome after surgery for colorectal cancer. The first study on short-term outcome was published by Fielding and coworkers in 1978 [2]. They documented significant variations in postoperative anastomotic leakage rate and mortality among 21 participating surgeons.

In 1984, Phillips and associates [13] in a multicenter trial examined factors influencing locoregional recurrences after surgery for colorectal cancer. One of the statistically significant parameters was the surgeon. However, the status of the surgeon (consultant versus junior) was not important. Such difference remained even after stratification by sex and Dukes' classification.

More recent studies addressing surgeon variability have been published by Kingston and associates [9], McArdle and coworkers [11] and Möhner and Slisow [12].

Möhner and Slisow [12] measured the influence of regional centralization on survival for rectal cancer patients. They estimated a "centralization index" that gave patient volume in an institution within a specific area relative to the overall number of radical resections of the area population. A low index indicated a small peripheral hospital, a high index a larger center. They concluded that larger centers had a significantly better survival. Hence they argued for centralization of cancer surgery. However, they did not analyze additional factors that might influence survival.

McArdle and Hole [11] analyzed prospectively postoperative complications and long-term survival in patients undergoing surgery for colorectal cancer. The proportion of curative resections, rate of locoregional recurrence, and long-term survival varied between consultant surgeons. They identified the surgeon as an independent risk factor and argued that such operations should only be carried out by surgeons with a special interest in colorectal surgery or surgical oncology.

In contrast, Kingston, Walsh and Jeacock [9] did not find differences in 5-year survival between teaching or nonteaching hospitals in Manchester.

In keeping with the limited information found in the literature, this topic of whether specialization or centralization improve results in certain fields of surgery is frequently discussed among professionals all over the world. On the basis of data available from a German multicenter study on treatment for colorectal cancer, the question raised above will be elucidated and discussed.

German Study Group Colorectal Carcinoma

The prospective multicenter German study was conducted between 1984 and 1992 as a pattern of care study by the German Study Group Colorectal Carcinoma (SGCRC) [4, 5, 10]. Seven German hospitals participated (five university, two municipal). The spectrum of surgical activities within these seven surgical departments varied to some extent. All participating surgeons practised "general surgery" and all covered the entire field of gastrointestinal surgery, some having a particular interest in colorectal surgery. Nearly all were routinely involved in endocrine surgery, commonly that of the thyroid. Some practised vascular and/or thoracic surgery (cardiac surgery excluded) and very few were also engaged with orthopedic surgery, although to a limited extent.

Before the study started, the standards of the operations to be performed were demonstrated by one of the study group chairmen. For rectal cancer surgery, the standard in our department is as follows:

- Complete mobilization of the left colon to the middle part of transverse colon
- Central ligation of the inferior mesenteric vein and artery
- Preservation of the autonomic nerves
- Margin of clearance of 5 cm of the tubular rectum and the corresponding mesorectum for tumors of the upper third of rectum
- Complete sharp mesorectal excision for tumors of the lower two third of rectum

At that time major emphasis was put on the distal margin of clearance [6, 7]. During the recruitment period, the use of circular stapler was gradually introduced, and when the study was closed, 68% of all anastomoses were performed by stapling techniques [10]. If hand-sewn anastomosis was performed, most surgeons intentionally left some perirectal tissue at the distal stump of the rectum to secure blood supply to the rectum distally to the rectal transection line (Fig. 1). With the introduction of circular staplers, however, the mesorectum [3, Chap. 15] was removed completely as a "clean" distal rectum facilitated application of the suture clamp. Thus when the study started, the mesorectum was removed primarily for technical reasons, thus adding more radicality as a consequence. The oncologic importance of complete mesorectal excision was not completely understood at that time.

Patients and Methods

In the SGCRC study, data were collected from 1101 unselected patients treated for invasive solitary rectal carcinoma between 1984 and 1986. The median age was 64.0 years, the sex ratio (males/females) was 919/482 (1.9:1). The resectability rate was 94.0% (1036/1101). A total of 871 patients underwent a resection for cure (R0) (79.1% of all patients or 84.1% of patients with a resected tumor). 752 out of the R0 patients (86.3%) were treated by surgery alone. The number of patients included from the seven participating departments were 401, 311, 148, 77, 68, 63 and 33, respectively.

The patients were followed up until death or for at least 5 years. At the termination of the study the vital status was unknown in 16 (1.5%), and the tumor status unknown in 22 patients (2%). Observed 5-year survival rates were

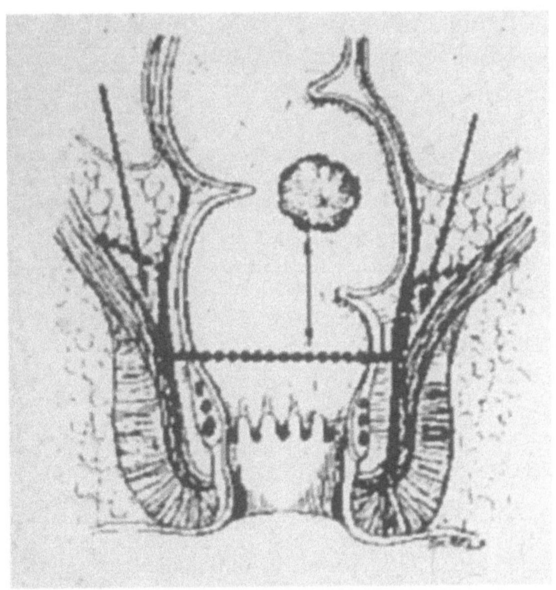

Fig. 1. In previous years, part of the distal mesorectum was intentionally left behind to preserve blood supply to the rectal stump. The potential risk of recurrences from lymph node metastases and other tumor deposits left behind was not realized

calculated according to the Kaplan–Meier method with death from any cause as event. For multivariate analyses of the data, logistic regression techniques were used. For further details on patients and methods, see [10, 5, 4].

Interinstitutional Variability

All Patients

Table 1 shows the 5-year survival rates for all 1101 patients as well as for patients with tumor resection classified according to the UICC R classification [14]. The observed overall 5-year survival rate was 45.3 % but varied between institutions from 30% to 50%. Similar interinstitutional variations could also be observed for patients according to tumor resection group (any R, 31%–53%; R0, 37%–64%; and R 1/2, 0%–13%.

Patients with R0 Resection

For more specific analyses of prognostic factors after R0 resection, a homogenous group of patients was selected by excluding patients with any of the following features (some patients fulfilled more than one exclusion criterion):

- Carcinoma in familial adenomatous polyposis (one patient)
- Carcinoma in ulcerative colitis (three patients)
- Treatment by procedures other than anterior resection and abdominoperineal excision (68 patients)
- Distant metastases (22 patients)
- Postoperative death (25 patients)
- Local tumor status not specified (15 patients)

Table 1. Observed 5-year survival rates in all patients with solitary rectal carcinoma

Patient groups	No. of patients	5-year survival rates (%)	
		Total[a]	Individual departments[b]
Total	1101	45.3 (42.2–48.4)	50–46–46–45–44–36–30–36–30
Tumor resection			
any R	1036	48.0 (44.8–51.2)	53–51–49–48–37–31
R0	871	55.3 (51.8–58.8)	64–58–54–54–53–44–37
R1,2	165	9.8 (4.8–14.8)	13–10–9–0–0

[a]With 95% confidence interval in parentheses.
[b]Only figures for departments with more than ten patients in the respective patient group.

This left 744 patients for analysis. Table 2 shows the observed 5-year survival rate in relation to tumor stage. Considerable interinstitutional variations could be observed in all stages: stage I, 75%–91%; stage II, 44%–79%; and stage III, 10%–57%. The variability was more pronounced with more advanced stages. Locoregional recurrence was observed in 161 (21.6%) of the 744 patients (Table 3). Again a considerable interinstitutional variability was noted especially in stage III tumors: stage I, 3%–14%; stage II, 9%–42%; and stage III, 14%–55%. In a multivariate analysis (Table 4) locoregional recurrence was the most important factor influencing survival. Stage, grade, intraoperative tumor spillage, and department also had a significant impact on survival.

Intersurgeon Variability

To analyze intersurgeon variability data from three departments out of the seven, more than 100 patients were analyzed. A subgroup of 603 patients was selected to enable homogeneity, and the selection criteria were:

- No distant metastasis (M0)
- Treatment by anterior resection (418 patients; 69.3%) or abdominoperineal excision (185 patients; 30.7%)
- No residual tumor (R0)

Nine patients were excluded (three with multiple synchronous colorectal carcinoma, six dying postoperatively). The remaining 594 patients, corresponding to 67% of all 887 R0 patients, were operated on by 43 surgeons, 14 of whom performed more than 15 operations each during the recruitment period (16, 16, 19, 19, 20, 22, 23, 23, 24, 27, 38, 45, 51, 111 respectively). Twenty-nine other surgeons had done fewer (under 15) operations and were categorized as surgeons with low volume. The frequency of locoregional recurrence for each

Table 2. Observed 5-year survival for patients with rectal carcinoma without distant metastases and resected for cure (M0, R0) related to tumor stage (UICC staging system) [14]

Tumor stage	No. of patients	5-Year survival rates (%)	
		Total[a]	Individual departments[b]
Stage I	193	78.7 (72.6–84.8)	91–79–77–76–75
Stage II	234	64.1 (57.6–70.6)	79–58–55–44
Stage III	317	40.9 (35.3–46.5)	57–54–50–46–44–31–10
Total	744	58.3 (54.6–62.0)	69–61–61–54–54–45–45

[a]With 95% confidence interval in parentheses.
[b]Only figures for departments with more than ten patients in the respective groups.

Table 3. Rectal carcinoma: frequency of locoregional recurrence after resection for cure (M0, R0) related to tumor stage (UICC staging system) [14]

Tumor stage	Total		Frequency of locoregional recurrence (%): figures for the individual departments[a]
	n	%	
Stage I	18/193	9.3	3–8–9–12–14
Stage II	41/234	17.9	9–14–19–33–42
Stage III	101/317	31.9	14–14–31–38–42–44–55
Total	161/744	21.6	10–15–20–22–25–31–37

[a]Only figures for departments with more than ten patients in the respective patient group.

of the 14 surgeons ranged from 4% to 54%, with a mean for all of 19.7% (117/594).

There were also striking differences between departments. In two (Departments A and B) the frequency of locoregional recurrence was about the same for each surgeon (Fig. 2). In the third department (Department C) the locoregional recurrence rate showed a significant variability between surgeons.

In a multivariate analysis (Table 5) it was found that the frequency of locoregional recurrence (Fig. 2) was determined not only by tumor-related factors but also by department and individual surgeon. The low frequency of locoregional recurrence experienced by some surgeons cannot be explained by a different stage distribution, because the proportion of stage III cases for these surgeons was nearly identical to the respective figure for the other surgeons (45% versus 42%).

Table 4. Analysis of independent prognostic factors after curative resection (M0, R0) for solitary rectal carcinoma (logistic regression analysis)

Variable	Odds ratio	95% Confidence interval	*p* value
Locoregional recurrence			
No	1.00		
Yes	12.09	7.17–20.38	0.0001
Stage			
III	1.00		
II	0.47	0.31–0.71	0.0003
I	0.25	0.16–0.41	0.0001
Histological			
Low grade	1.00		
High grade	2.19	1.40–3.43	0.0006
Intraoperative tumor spillage			
No	1.00		
Yes	2.16	1.24–3.78	0.0069
Department			
B-G	1.00		
A	0.61	0.40–0.92	0.0182

Study end-point was observed 5-year survival.

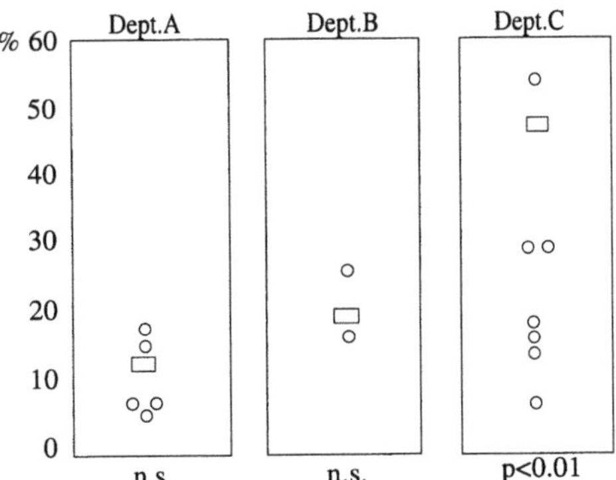

Fig. 2. Locoregional recurrence rate in relation to departments and surgeons. *Circles* indicate the recurrence rate for surgeons who performed more than 15 operations. The *rectangle* shows the results in the group of surgeons with low number of operations (15 or less operations)

Table 5. Factors influencing locoregional recurrence after resection for cure (R0): results of multiple logistic regression analysis (n=594)

Variable	Odds ratio	95% Confidence interval	p value
Stage (TNM)			
I	0.47	0.23–0.98	0.0452
II	1.00		
III	2.83	1.68–4.79	0.0001
Tumour site			
Upper third	0.43	0.24–0.77	0.0043
Middle/lower			
Third	1.00		
Local spillage of tumour cells			
No	0.28	0.15–0.52	0.0001
Yes	1.00		
Department			
A	0.31	0.18–0.54	0.0001
B, C	1.00		
Surgeon			
1, 3–14	1.00		
LF[a]	1.71	1.02–2.86	0.0433
2	4.32	1.69–11.97	0.0023

The grade of differentiation was not significant. Surgical procedure was low anterior resection versus abdominoperineal resection.
[a]LF, low frequency: group of 29 surgeons with low volume of operations (15 or less).

Figure 3 gives the correlation between the locoregional recurrence rates and 5-year survival. The Spearman rank-correlation analysis gave a highly statistical significance with rs=0.733 ($p < 0.005$). This indicates that surgeons with low recurrence rates have high survival rates and vice versa. This finding

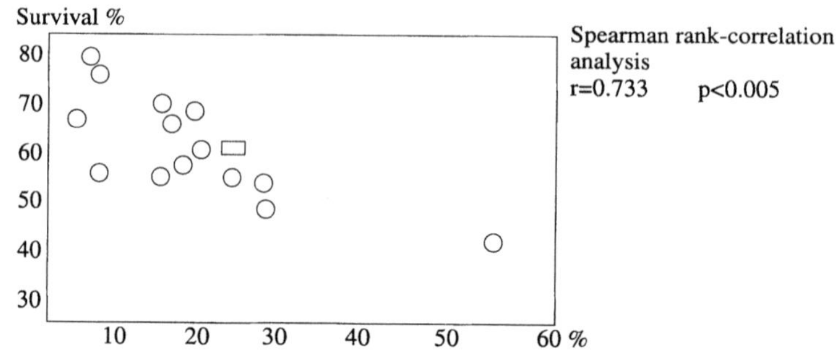

Fig. 3. Correlation between locoregional recurrence rate and observed 5-year survival. *Circles* indicate the recurrence rate for surgeons who performed more than 15 operations. The *rectangle* shows the results in the group of surgeons with low number of operations (15 or less operations)

explains the wide intersurgeon variability with respect to 5-year survival rates (Fig. 4).

General Comments

The data presented here demonstrate the influence of institutions and individual surgeons within these departments on long-term results after radical operation for rectal cancer. In univariate analysis, the observed 5-year survival rate within the institutions differed significantly. The differences were more

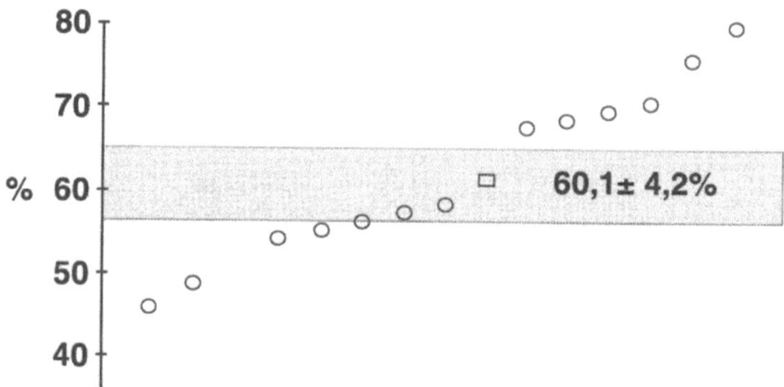

Fig. 4. Observed 5-year survival rates related to individual surgeons. *Circles* indicate the recurrence rate for surgeons who performed more than 15 operations. The *rectangle* shows the results in the group of surgeons with low number of operations (15 or less operations)

pronounced with more advanced stages of the tumor. Long-term survival correlated significantly with the rate of locoregional recurrence.

Locoregional recurrence seems to be the most important problem following rectal cancer surgery, as its occurrence is the key factor determining success or failure, particularly with regard to long-term survival. In univariate analysis, the rate of locoregional recurrence varied significantly between the participating centers, and these differences were more pronounced in stage III than in stage II tumors. For patients who developed a locoregional recurrence during follow-up, the institution was the most important prognostic factor.

Years ago, Hohenberger and Hermanek [6] pointed out and stressed the influence of locoregional recurrence on final outcome. In R0 resection and irrespective of any other parameter, the 5-year survival for patients who did not develop locoregional recurrence was 85%±5%. In patients with recurrence, survival was markedly reduced to 23%±10%.

The present study confirmed the correlation between locoregional recurrence and survival, and documented the influence of individual surgeons on locoregional recurrence. In Department A, all surgeons had a rate of locoregional recurrences of less than 18%. Even the less experienced surgeons (fewer than 15 operations performed) were within this range. In Department B, the results were also at an acceptable level (17%–23%). In Department C, however, there was a remarkable difference between individual surgeons, ranging from 8% to 55%. In multivariate analysis of 5-year survival rates, the most detrimental prognostic factor was the presence of locoregional recurrence.

These findings give substantial support to the notion that the differences within the participating centers and individual surgeons do result from differing surgical techniques and standards. What seem to be the critical steps in rectal cancer surgery, especially in patients with cancer of the middle and lower rectum, that may influence successful surgery?

1. Heald [3] focused on the interest and expertise of surgeons on total mesorectal excision (TME) without damaging the "holy plane". The excision must be performed by sharp dissection, to avoid tears in the dissection line. There is no place for blunt pelvic dissection for rectal cancer [1].
2. Avoidance of tears of the specimen, especially in tumors invading the peritoneal reflection anteriorly is critical, as is avoidance of incisions of tumors at any site, even in men with a narrow pelvis and large tumor.
3. Another critical point is the decision between sphincter preservation or excision for small tumors in the lower third of the rectum. A detailed preoperative evaluation, including endosonography, is important to select the best procedure at an early stage of the operation.
4. En bloc excision including organs that are attached to the tumor is important. These attachments may be due to adhesions from inflammation, but also to true tumor invasion. If the surgeon in the evaluation tries to separate the layers, almost none of these patients will survive, even if the pathologist confirms true tumor invasion and the surgeon includes all organs involved in a second step, finally achieving a R0 resection [8].

5. Furthermore, a distant margin of clearance is essential. From earlier studies, we conclude that for tumors of the upper rectal third, TME is not necessary. However, a resection margin of 5 cm of the mesorectum measured on the fresh unstretched specimen is required, and it has to include not only the intestinal wall but also the mesorectum without coning. For tumors of the middle and lower third treated with TME, a distal margin of 1 cm may be sufficient, at least for low-grade carcinomas.

The prevention of locoregional recurrence will evidently increase long-term survival for patients with rectal cancer. The question is whether only highly specialized surgeons are able to achieve such a high standard of low recurrence rates. Furthermore, is centralization the solution or what is the influence of organization and quality management?

Almost none of the surgeons involved in this study practiced colorectal surgery exclusively. All of them were "general surgeons", mainly involved in gastrointestinal surgery and with a special interest in colorectal surgery. On the other hand, all participating departments are referral centers. Furthermore, colorectal cancer is the most frequently resected tumor in all major surgical departments in Germany. So, centralization and specialization may certainly to some extent positively influence the quality following surgery for rectal carcinoma.

Centralization is commonly associated with better quality. We know, however, that there are some surgeons, who are able to maintain a high standard even if they move to peripheral institutions with a lower patient volume. It is obvious that such surgeons need an ongoing surgical practice with a specific procedure. The amount of practice needed differs among surgeons. This study reveals that even in large surgical centers there are experienced surgeons who do not reach the level of others. So, centralization per se does not guarantee high quality.

In this context, the influence of experience has to be discussed. Surgeons with an outstanding experience in a specific field may achieve the best results. But even young, less experienced surgeons are able to perform operations to a set standard early in their career. The fact that even young surgeons in training can achieve high-quality results and that in a single department the "quality figures" of all surgeons working there may be close, immediately directs our attention to the possible influence of organization.

Modern terms, commonly encountered in such discussions are "quality control" and "quality management". An integrated part of such mechanisms is to define a standard. Frequently one will hear surgeons claim that they perform the identical procedure although results vary. However, if one looks behind such statements and into an operating theater, one may eventually realise that differences exist, i.e., between the arguments used and technical steps of specific procedures. This may not only be true for comparison between different institutions, but also between surgeons within a department. Only by ensuring quality control and the transformation of a set standard to the procedure actually performed will the set standard be reached. An important control mechanism is the work performed by the pathologists in examining the specimen, inspecting the resection lines carefully, reporting on the margin of clearance, and controlling the completeness of the mesorectal excision. Another measure of quality is the number of lymph nodes removed.

Within a department, there must be a named person responsible for auditing the surgical standard. Both the surgeon and the pathologist must document all relevant data including complications and analysis of long-term results.

In summary, specialization, centralization, and personal experience influence the quality of rectal cancer surgery. More important seem to be organization, quality management, and the surgeon's interest.

Acknowledgement. The author wishes to express his gratitude to Prof. Dr. Dr. h.c. Paul Hermanek for allowing use of data from the German Prospective Multicenter Study of the Study Group Colorectal Carcinoma (SGCRC) in this publication.

References

1. Cohen AM (1991) Surgical considerations in patients with cancer of the colon and rectum. Semin Oncol 18:381–387
2. Fielding LP, Stewart-Brown S, Dudley HAF (1978) Surgeon-related variables and the clinical trial. Lancet II:778–779
3. Heald RJ (1988) The "Holy Plane" of rectal surgery. J R Soc Med 81:503–508
4. Hermanek P, Wiebeit H, Staimmer D, Riedi St and the German Study Group Colo-Rectal Carcinoma (SGCRC) (1995) Prognostic factors of rectum carcinoma. Experience of the German Multicentre Study SGCRC. Tumori 81[Suppl]:60–64
5. Hermanek P Jr, Wiebelt H, Riedi St, Staimmer D, Hermanek P and the Colorectal Carcinoma Study Group (SGKRK) (1994) Langzeitergebnisse der chirurgischen Therapie des Colonkarzinoms. Ergebnisse der Studiengruppe Kolorektales Karzinom (SGKRK). Chirurg 65:387–297
6. Hohenberger W, Hermanek P (1989) Weite des aboralen Sicherheitsabstandes bei anteriorer Rektumresektion. In: Gall FP, Zirngibl H, Hermanek P (eds) Das kolorektale Karzinom. Kontroverse Fragen, neue Ergebnisse. Zukschwerdt, Munich, pp 161–174
7. Hohenberger W, Hermanek P Jr, Hermanek P, Gall FP (1992) Decision making in curative rectum carcinoma surgery. Onkologie 15:209–220
8. Hohenberger W, Thom N, Hermanek P, Gall FP (1992) Pelvine multiviszerale Resektion aus der Sicht der Chirurgie. Langenbecks Arch Chir Suppl. (Kongressbericht):83–88
9. Kingston RD, Walsh S, Jeacock J (1992) Colorectal surgeons in district general hospitals produce similar survival outcomes to their teaching hospital colleagues: review of 5-year survival in Manchester. J R Coll Surg Edinb 37:235–237
10. Kessler H, Hermanek Jr P, Wiebeit H (1993) Operative mortality in carcinoma of the rectum. Results of the German Multicentre Study. Int J Colorect Dis 8:158–166
11. McArdle CS, Hole D (1991) Impact of variability among surgeons on postoperative morbidity and mortality and ultimate survival. Br Med J 307:1501–1505
12. Möhner M, Slisow W (1990) Untersuchung zum Einfluss der regional zentralisierten Behandlung auf die Überlebenschancen beim Rektumkarzinom in der DDR. Zbl Chir 115:801–812
13. Phillips RKS, Hittinger R, Blesovsky L, Fry JS, Fielding LP (1984) Local recurrence following curative surgery for large bowel cancer: l. The overall picture. Br J Surg 71:12–16
14. UICC (1992) TNM classification of malignant tumors. Hermanek P, Sobin LH (eds) 4th edn, 2nd revision. Springer, Berlin, Heidelberg, New York

CHAPTER 27

Surgery for Rectal Cancer:
The Relationship Between Treatment Volume and Results

Lars Påhlman

Introduction

Two important factors must be considered when the relationship between treatment volume and results is discussed in rectal cancer surgery; the volume required during the training period to attain the appropriate technical skill, and the volume needed to maintain and also improve the technical ability.

During the training period when the young surgeons start to experience the difficulty of rectal cancer surgery, it is important that they have the opportunity to see numerous procedures. Therefore training should be at a centre where rectal cancer surgery is commonly undertaken, and where more than one experienced surgeon can assist regularly.

Secondly, when the surgeon has the technical ability and knows how to operate and starts to perform the procedure as the principal operator the main question arises about volume. How many procedures should be done yearly to assure that quality is maintained, and what numbers give the opportunity for further training with a realistic chance of improving surgery? Such questions are difficult to answer. I will argue that the whole team has to be well-trained in order to achieve exellent results.

The wide difference in postoperative mortality and local recurrence rates noticed in the literature indicates that training is important. Does this imply that treatment volume must be high? Other related questions can be raised such as: Is low volume equivalent to a small hospital? Does low volume imply inferior organization? Or is the difference a matter of inherently "bad" or "good" surgeons or perhaps badly or well-trained surgeons? This review will discuss the relationship between treatment volume and results, i.e. postoperative mortality and morbidity, long-term survival and local recurrence rate after potentially curative rectal cancer surgery.

Postoperative Mortality

In a study from the Royal Infirmary, Glasgow, comprising 645 sequentially operated patients with colorectal cancer during 1974–1979, the overall postoperative mortality rate after surgery for colorectal cancer differed from 8%–30% when the results from 13 consultant surgeons were compared [9]. Among patients operated on for cure, the corresponding difference in postoperative mortality between the "best" and the "worst" results was 0%–20%.

Interpretation of such data is difficult as patient selection can differ enormously. Some surgeons may have operated on more emergency cases or patients with a more advanced Dukes' stage. The degree of tumour differentiation may differ, and patients are not equal with respect to concomitant diseases. A multivariate analysis with postoperative mortality as the dependent variable was undertaken in order to elucidate the effect of age, emergency surgery, cardiac or respiratory diseases, local spread, Dukes' stage and degree of differentiation. The adjusted relative hazard ratio which express the variation between surgeons varied from 0.56–2.03. Importantly and, as illustrated in Fig. 1, there is no data indicating that surgeons with a high case load during the study period had better outcome, i.e. postoperative mortality, than surgeons who had operated on fewer patients. Thus the hypothesis that volume is important was refuted.

Similar figures have been found in a Swedish county when postoperative mortality was studied in three different hospitals of varying size and with a different infrastructure [6]. In a district general hospital, the postoperative mortality for rectal cancer was 3%. In one of the small community hospitals mortality was 0% compared with 13% in the other small community hospital. The number of patients operated on in the period 1989–1990 was 33, 29, and 24 patients, respectively.

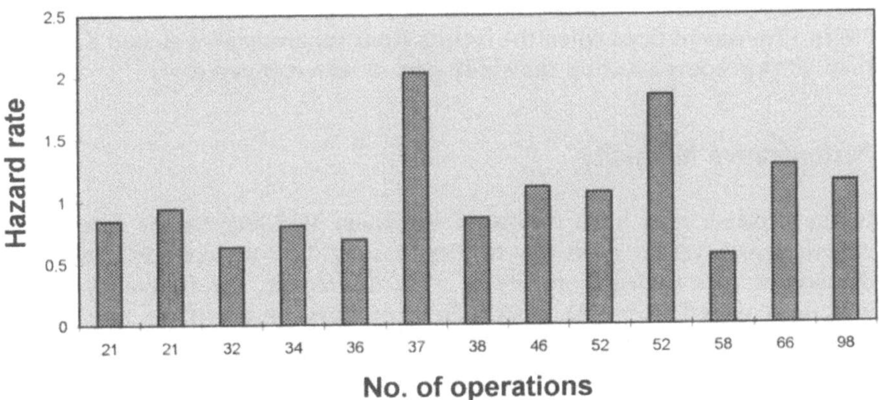

Fig. 1. The adjusted relative hazard ratio according to the number of operations performed (data from McArdle and Hole [9])

These data suggest that a good organisation with well-trained colorectal surgeons can reduce postoperative mortality as demonstrated for the district general hospital. At the community hospital with the highest mortality (13%) rectal cancer surgery was performed by nearly all consultants, irrespective of training and interest. It is interesting that the last group of surgeons have decided on the basis of this study to reorganize rectal cancer surgery so that only one or two consultants will be responsible for the treatment of rectal cancer.

In the Swedish Rectal Cancer Trial, where almost 1200 patients were recruited during 1987–1990, the postoperative mortality ranged from 0%–25% among participating hospitals [14]. In this trial, preoperative radiotherapy was tested against surgery alone in a randomized fasion. There was no indication that radiotherapy had any impact on postoperative mortality. However, a tendency was observed to the effect that there was a higher mortality rate in hospitals which performed only few rectal resections during the study period (less than ten) than in those which operated on more rectal cancer patients.

In rectal cancer surgery it is not only the operation and the surgeon that are crucial. Even the postoperative period is critical, and a well-organized team is important to ensure that patients with postoperative complications can be evaluated by experienced professionals, and action can be taken as soon as problems occur.

In a part of the Uppsala region, all rectal cancer patients operated on with rectal resection (abdominoperineal resection or low anterior resection) during 1987, were reviewed retrospectively [11]. A total of 21 procedures were performed at the university hospital, 43 at two different district general hospitals and 64 at eight different community hospitals. The postoperative mortality at the university hospital was 0%, at the district general hospitals 5%, and at the community hospitals 3%. Some of the community hospitals had high mortality rates, which again indicates that the entire treatment structure of patient care must be optimal.

In an unpublished Scottish trial, the outcome after surgery for colorectal cancer was explored. A wide difference in postoperative mortality ranging from 0% to 17% was noticed when the results from surgeons who all had done more than 20 procedures during the study period was compared [5].

Postoperative Morbidity

In the Scottish trial from the Royal Infirmary in Glasgow, the frequency of wound sepsis varied from 6% to 35% among 13 surgeons [9]. The wound dehiscence rate varied from 0% to 11%. Moreover, the frequency of chest infections varied from 6% to 24% between surgeons, and the rate of intra-abdominal abcesses from 0% to 10%. These figures represent suggestive evidence that the surgeon is probably the most important factor in the treatment of patients with colorectal cancer.

In the study from the Jönköping county in Sweden, the frequency of wound infections noticed between the three different hospitals was 1%, 5% and 14%

respectively, and the rate of abdominal abscesses demonstrated at surgery 3%, 6%, and 5% [6]. The number of anastomotic leaks was 0%, 2%, and 4% between the hospitals, where the district general hospital had better results than two community hospitals.

In the Uppsala region where the results after rectal cancer treatment in the university hospital were compared with those from two district general hospitals and eight community hospitals, the anastomotic leak rate in 1987 following sphincter saving surgery was 13%, 17% and 15%, in the three hospital groups respectively [10]. Allthough the rates are identical, a significant difference between the hospitals was noticed. At the university hospital total mesorectal excision (TME) with very low anastomosis was done routinely. This was not the case in the other hospitals, indicating that the leak rate in the smaller hospitals was rather high. A total of 89% of the patients at the university hospital underwent a sphincter-saving resection compared with 52% at the district general hospitals, and 42% at the community hospitals. Such figures illustrate the fact that although results appear identical, patient and treatment characteristics influence outcome. We also know from other studies that if very low anastomoses are performed, the leak rate will increase [7].

Local Recurrence Rate

There is evidence from the literature that a reduction in local recurrence rate will increase survival [8]. This has been nicely shown by Professor Hermanek in Erlangen where the results of rectal cancer surgery were compared among eight different surgeons in Germany (Chap. 26). Figure 2 summarizes their data and demonstrates the obvious correlation with an increasing survival rate if the rate of local recurrence decreases.

Figures from the Royal Infirmary in Glasgow demonstrate a wide difference between surgeons with respect to local recurrence rate which varies from 0% to

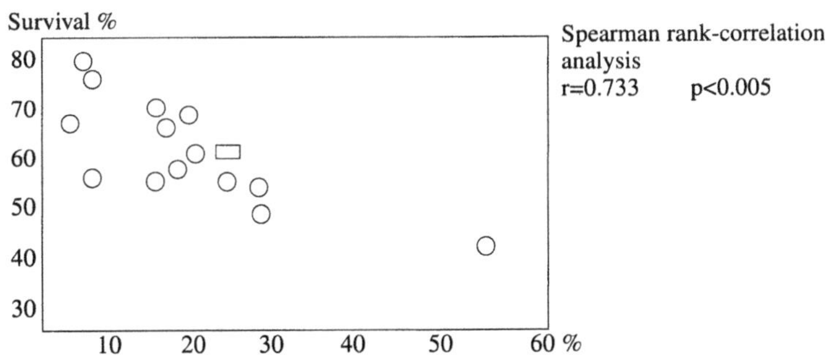

Fig. 2. Relationship between survival and local recurrence rate after rectal cancer surgery. (Figure from Chap. 26)

21% [9]. Similar differences were found in a later Scottish trial in which local recurrence rates ranged from 8% to 38% [5]. In the large bowel cancer project originating from St. Mary's Hospital, London, the local recurrence rate in patients undergoing curative surgery for a rectal cancer was compared among 20 consultants who treated more than 30 patients during the study period (range 31–101 patients). Three surgeons reported less than 5% local recurrences, seven surgeons 5%–10%, three surgeons 10%–15%, six surgeons 15%–20%, and one surgeon more than 20% local recurrences [13]. The variability among surgeons is apparently wide. In the latter series, as in most others, the interpretation of the data is that volume per se is of relatively limited importance while the outcome of surgery depends more on the quality of the surgeon.

In the Swedish Rectal Cancer Trial, the local recurrence rate differed from less than 5% to more than 30% in the hospitals recruiting patients to the trial [15]. These figures have not been analysed with respect to surgeon volume. However, it was evident that the recurrence rate varied within the same range when failure rates from one university hospital were compared with those from other university hospitals. The same variation was also noticed between different district general and community hospitals. This indicates that both the small and larger teaching hospitals showed similarly "good" or "bad" figures. If surgery is organized in an optimal way, the local recurrence rate is low if well-trained colorectal surgeons perform most rectal cancer operations, irrespective of the size of the hospital.

In the Jönköping county, the local recurrence rate at both the district general hospitals where two well-trained colorectal surgeons performed all rectal cancer operations was 6% compared with failure rates of 14% and 21% at two community hospitals with less subspecialisation. In the community hospitals, rectal cancer surgery was performed by several surgeons not specifically trained in colorectal cancer surgery [6].

In the Uppsala region in 1987, the local recurrence rate at the university hospital was less than 5% compared with 17% at the district general hospitals, and 20% at the community hospitals [11]. The interesting finding in this retrospective study are the good results found at some community hospitals with less than 10% local recurrence rate. This suggests that good organization with well-trained and interested surgeons can improve results despite low volume.

The results following rectal cancer surgery at the university hospital in Uppsala improved substantially after a reorganisation in the early 1980s. Before 1980, all general surgeons operated on patients with rectal cancer. The local recurrence rate at that time was 50% [12]. At the beginning of the 1980s, rectal cancer surgery was concentrated to one unit with well-trained and interested surgeons, and at the same time the TME technique was also adopted. Since 1985, the local recurrence rate has been less than 5% (L. Påhlman, unpublished data).

Similar improvements in local recurrence rate have been noticed in other hospitals in Sweden where the TME technique was adopted. In Motala, a relatively small community hospital, the local recurrence rate since 1990 has been less than 5% (E. Nilsson, unpublished data) and in the Linköping area, the local recurrence rate was reduced from 18% in the mid 1980s to less than 5% after 1990 [1].

The reduction in the local recurrence rate at the university hospital in Uppsala has also had an impact on survival. The overall national survival figures for patients with rectal cancer have been slightly improved during each successive 5-year period over the last 30 years in Sweden [3]. When different areas in Sweden are compared, the figures and trend are similar. However, from 1985–1990 the survival figures in Uppsala, an area where TME surgery was introduced early, the 5-year survival figures improved approximately 17% compared with the overall national figures of Sweden. This is highly suggestive of the notion that good surgical technique is of importance [2]. It must be added, however, that radiotherapy was used in Uppsala during the same period, which also might have an impact on survival.

Long-Term Survival

As stated above the effects of local recurrence on survival are probably of significant importance. Data presented by Mr. R.J. Heald [4, 8] and Prof. Hohenbergen (Chap. 26) indicate that survival will improve if local recurrence rate decreases. In the Royal Infirmary, Glasgow, 10-year survival differed between surgeons, ranging from 20% to 63% [9]. This is a further argument for the notion that good surgery most probably improves long time survival. The 2-year survival in Jönköping county was 73% at a district general hospital compared with 67% and 58% at the two community hospitals [6]. The community hospital reporting the highest local recurrence rate (21%) had the worst survival figure (58%), a strong argument for emphasising the importance of a low local recurrence rate.

Conclusion

It is evident from the data presented in this review that surgery is less than optimal as performed by some surgeons or in some hospitals. It is, therefore, important to give surgeons the opportunity to undergo training and to adopt new and improved techniques. It is more difficult to find good arguments which support the hypothesis that treatment volume per se is an important factor. Rather, it appears that the relationship between treatment volume and results is more a consequence of bad organization or badly trained surgeons than volume itself.

How often must an operation be done to maintain quality once you have learned the procedure? Such data are not easily found in the literature. Probably it must be done so frequently that it is possible to evaluate morbidity and results yearly in terms of proportions, preferably also with fairly low confidence limits. However, in colorectal units where pelvic surgery for other indications than rectal cancer is common, the opportunity for training should be better.

We know the "best" results. It is important to reproduce them and to argue for a quality standard set by many surgeons worldwide [10]. The only way to reach such aims is to have a prospective registration and to introduce regular audit.

References

1. Arbman G, Hilsson E, Hallböök O, Sjödahl R (1996) Local recurrence following total mesorectal excision for rectal cancer. Br J Surg 83:375–379
2. Dahlberg M, Påhlman L, Bergström R, Glimelius B (1996) Improved survival in patients with rectal cancer: a population based register study (manuscript)
3. Enblad P, Adami H-O, Bergström R, Glimelius B, Tusemo U-B, Påhlman L (1988) Improved survival in cancer of the colon and rectum? Study of 61,769 cases diagnosed in Sweden in 1960–81. JNCI 80:586–594
4. Heald RJ, Husband EM, Ryall RDH (1982) The mesorectum in rectal cancer surgery – the clue to pelvic recurrence? Br J Surg 69:613–616
5. Galloway DJ, McGregor JR, Walsh PV, Bell A, Sugden BA, Docherty JG (1994) Surgeon related variability in colorectal cancer recurrence. International Soceity of University Colon and Rectal Surgeons, XVth biennial congress, Singapore, meeting abstract
6. Järhult J, Mikkelsen I, Thulin A (1995) Kolorektal cancerkirurgi utanför regionsjukhusen – Goda resultat, men intern specialisering önskvärd. Läkartidningen (Swe) 92:2325–2328
7. Karanjia MD, Corder AP, Bearn P, Heald RJ (1994) Leakage from stapled low anastomosis after total mesorectal excision for carcinoma of the rectum. Br J Surg 81:1224–1226
8. MacFarlane JK, Ryall RD, Heald RJ (1993) Mesorectal excision for rectal cancer. Lancet 341:457–460
9. McArdle CS, Hole D (1991) Impact of variability among surgeons on postoperative morbidity and mortality and ultimate survival. BMJ 302:1501–1505
10. McCall JL, Cox MR, Wattchow DA (1995) Analysis of local recurrence rates after surgery alone for rectal cancer. Int J Colorect Dis 10:126–132
11. Påhlman L (1993) Kvalitetsutredning om rektalcancerkirurgi – Ökad specialisering nödvändig. Läkartidningen (Swe) 90:2853–2855
12. Påhlman L, Glimelius B (1984) Local recurrences after surgical treatment for rectal carcinoma. Acta Chir Scand 150:331–335
13. Phillips RKS, Hittinger R, Blesovsky L, Fry JS, Fielding LP (1984) Local recurrence following 'curative' surgery for large bowel cancer: II. The rectum and rectosigmoid. Br J Surg 71:17–20
14. Swedish Rectal Cancer Trial (1993) An initial report from a Swedish multicentre study examining the role of preoperative irradiation in the treatment of patients with resectable rectal carcinoma. Br J Surg 80:1333–1336
15. Swedish Rectal Cancer Trial (1996) Local recurrence rate in a randomized multicentre trial of preoperative radiotherapy compared to surgery alone in resectable rectal carcinoma. Eur J Surg (in press)

The Role of Adjuvant Treatment if Surgery Is Optimal

CHAPTER 28

Role of Radiotherapy in Addition to Optimal Surgery

Bengt Glimelius

Introduction

Surgery has been the standard primary treatment for rectal cancer, with overall survival rates below 50% after 5 years and with little improvement in recent years [9]. In these patients, peri-operative radiotherapy has been extensively investigated and used in order to decrease an often unacceptably high local recurrence rate. Since a local recurrence of a rectal carcinoma is often extremely disabling, a gain in local pelvic control represents in itself an important achievement of an additional treatment, even if survival is not substantially improved.

The rationale for combining surgery and radiation is that surgery removes the bulk of the tumour tissue, whereas radiotherapy kills peripheral tumour cells where they are few in a well-vascularized area. Surgery sometimes has to leave peripherally located tumour cells to preserve essential normal tissue. The major cause of pelvic failure is lateral spread of microscopic foci of tumour cells that are not removed at surgery [1, 31]. Surgical techniques aimed at removing this lateral spread have also resulted in apparently lower local recurrence rates [21, 27].

This chapter presents the collected experience from *controlled clinical trials* to date and discusses the potential value of peri-operative radiotherapy in rectal cancer even in instances where surgery is "optimal".

Radiation Dose–Effect Relations

Dose and Fractionation

The effects of irradiation in terms of local tumour control and acute and late damage of normal tissue depend not only on the total dose, but also on the dose delivered in each fraction and the total treatment time.

Several attempts have been made to estimate the biological effect of various radiation schedules. In this review, the linear-quadratic (LQ) time formula [13] is used to transform the effects of different radiation schedules into the effects achieved when a conventional fractionation of 2 Gy daily, 10 Gy/week is used.

To achieve a high probability (90% or more) of eradicating subclinical disease from an adenocarcinoma in a surgically undisturbed area, it is necessary to deliver a dose in the order of 50 Gy [7, 11]. This dose (50 Gy in 25 fractions over 5 weeks) gives an LQ time of 43 Gy with an α/β of 10 Gy for both acute responding tissues and tumours. The repair rate (γ/α) is then assumed to be 0.6 Gy/day, and the time before proliferation starts (t_k) to be 7 days [13, 14, 43].

In order to reduce treatment duration, i.e. to shorten the time period between start of radiotherapy and surgery, it is necessary to give either multiple fractions per day or higher doses per fraction.

A dose of 5.0 Gy daily has been used in several preoperative trials as a suitable alternative both for the patient and the surgeon (see below). Using the coefficients selected above, the acute effects of a total dose of 25 Gy in five 5-Gy fractions in 5 days correspond approximately to a dose of 42 Gy in 21 2-Gy fractions in 29 days. With higher doses per fraction, the therapeutic range shrinks due to an increase in the risk of late toxicity [12]. The LQ times for acute effects for the various regimens used in controlled clinical trials are found in Table 1. Since the size of each radiation fraction (1.75–5 Gy) and the time between the first and the last fraction (1–40 days) vary considerably between the trials, the LQ times give a better estimate of the relative efficacy of the radiation given in the different trials than the total doses do.

Radiotherapy Before or After Surgery?

The rationale for additional radiotherapy in patients with an operable rectal carcinoma is to kill proliferating tumour cells not removed by surgery. It is reasonable to suspect fewer such cells before than after surgery due to tumour cell proliferation. For the same cure rate, the efficacy of the radiotherapy must thus be higher after surgery than before in terms of residual tumour cell proportion. Much evidence also indicates that, for a similar result, a higher dose is required post- than preoperatively. The assumption of a greater dose efficacy of preoperative compared to postoperative radiotherapy has not been tested and confirmed in controlled studies, with the exception of one study discussed below.

Table 1. Pelvic recurrence after surgery or a combination of surgery and radiotherapy (RT) in rectal carcinoma

Study	Irradiation dose (Gy)	Fractions (n)	LQ time	Surgery alone			Surgery and RT			p value[a]	Reduction in local failure rates (%)
				Local recurrences (n)	Total (n)	(%)	Local recurrences (n)	Total (n)	(%)		
Preoperative											
Toronto	5	1	7.5	–	c	–	–	–	–	–	–
MRC1	5	1	7.5	–	d	–	–	–	–	–	0
	20	10	20.4	–	d	–	–	–	–	–	0
St Marks	15	3	22.5	51	210[e]	24	31	185	17	*	29
VASOG II	31.5	18	26.8	–c	–	–	–	–	–	–	–
Bergen	31.5	18	26.8	31	131	24	24	138	17	NS	29
VASOG I	25	10	27.5	32	87[f]	37	27	93	22	NS	22
North-West[b]	20	4	30.0	46	126	37	17	133	13	**	65
EORTC	34.5	15	35.2	49	175	28	24	166	14	**	50
MRC2[b]	40	20	36.0	65	140	46	50	139	36	*	22
Stockholm	25	5	37.5	120	425	28	61	424	14	**	50
SRCT	25	5	37.5	131	557	24	51	553	9	**	63
Postoperative											
Odense	50	25	35.4	57	250	23	46	244	19	NS	17
MRC3	40	20	36.0	79	235	34	48	234	21	**	38
GITSG	40	48	36.0	27	106	25	15	96	16	NS	36
NSABP	46.5	26	39.3	45	184	24	30	184	16	NS	33
EORTC	46	23	40.8	30	88	34	25	84	30	NS	13
Rotterdam	50	25	43.8	28	84	33	21	88	24	NS	41
Preoperative versus postoperative											
Uppsala											
Preoperative RT	25.5	5	38.0	–	–	–	27	209	13	–	–
Postoperative RT	60	30	46.9	–	–	–	45	204	22	*	–

LQ, linear-quadratic. [a]NS=p>0.05. [b]Only tethered tumours. [c]Not reported. [d]Only actuarial data reported, with no difference between groups. [e]Outpatient attenders only reported. [f]Autopsy series only reported. *p<0.05. **p<0.01.

The main reason for choosing postoperative irradiation in rectal cancer is that patients with a high probability of cure by surgery alone, i.e. those with a tumour in Dukes' stage A, can be excluded. In addition, patients in whom generalized disease is found at surgery can be excluded.

Combination with Chemotherapy

The purpose of combining radiotherapy and chemotherapy is to achieve a better tumour effect without simultaneously increasing normal tissue reactions. True clinical synergism has not been shown, and knowledge of how to combine the two modalities is limited [25, 44]. An increased frequency of severe adverse effects has also been seen with several drug–radiation combinations [44].

Review of Radiotherapy Trials in Rectal Carcinoma

Local Recurrence Rates After Surgery Alone

It is known that variables such as patient selection, skill and endurance of the surgeon, follow-up routines and definitions of radicality and local failure influence local recurrence rates. These variables can explain the substantial variations reported in the literature, from <10% to 65% [20, 21, 27, 33, 34].

In published controlled trials with adjuvant radiotherapy (pre- or postoperatively), the local recurrence rate in the surgery alone group has always exceeded 20% (average, 27%; range, 23%–46%, see Table 1). Thus the knowledge of how much additional radiotherapy reduces local recurrence rates is based upon studies where the average local recurrence rates at the participating hospitals are between 25% and 30%. Within all series, the recurrence rates are higher when the tumour has penetrated the bowel wall and/or has given lymph node metastases (i.e. Dukes' stages B and C).

Local Recurrence Rates After Additional Radiotherapy

In trials employing low radiation doses, one should probably not expect significant effects in the light of the dose–response relationship. This notion is supported by several early trials [8, 22, 37, 38]. Local failure rates were, however, not properly analyzed in some of these studies (Table 1). A comparison with later trials, where higher doses have been used, can thus not always be properly made.

As presented in Table 1, all controlled trials with *preoperative* radiation for which appropriate data are available have reported a lower local failure rate in the irradiated group of patients than in the non-irradiated group ([18, 19, 23, 29, 39, 41]; MRC Trial Office 1995, personal communication). The difference is statistically significant in six of the eight trials. With radiotherapy delivered *postoperatively*, a reduction in local recurrence rates is also observed, but statistical significance is only reached in one out of six trials ([3, 10, 17, 42]; MRC Trial Office 1995, personal communication; EORTC Trial Office 1995, personal communication). The relative reduction in local failure rates is usually higher in the preoperative trials (range, 22%–65%) than in the postoperative trials (range, 13%–41%) in spite of the fact that higher doses were used postoperatively (corresponding to LQ times between 35.4 and 43.8 Gy) than preoperatively (LQ times between 22.5 and 37.5 Gy in trials adequately reported).

The results from the trials thus indicate that preoperative irradiation is more efficient in reducing local recurrence rate than postoperative irradiation. Lower local failure rates were also seen after preoperative than after postoperative radiotherapy in the only trial directly comparing the two approaches [35]. A similar finding was seen even when a higher dose was used postoperatively than preoperatively (Table 1).

Survival After Additional Radiotherapy

In 20%–50% of the patients with recurrent disease, a local recurrence is the only residual tumour. Thus, in theory at least, preoperative radiotherapy should improve survival if the follow-up period is sufficiently long. In a meta-analysis including all controlled trials published up to 1984, a marginal positive effect on 5-year survival of 4.3% was demonstrated [5]. Recent trials prescribing higher radiation doses and with a more pronounced reduction in local failure rates were not included in this meta-analysis.

The survival curves in two preoperative trials deviate with increasing follow-up time, but the differences do not reach statistical significance [18, 29]. In the preoperative Stockholm trial [39], no effect on survival was seen except when the survival data are corrected for postoperative deaths (see below). In patients randomized to either preoperative radiotherapy or to surgery alone in the Stockholm area between 1987 and 1993 (between 1987 and February 1990, the patients participated in the Swedish Rectal Cancer Trial), a statistically significant survival benefit of radiotherapy was observed [6]. In these patients, no increase in postoperative mortality was seen (see below). Finally, in the Swedish Rectal Cancer Trial, a significantly improved overall 5-year survival was seen in irradiated patients (58%) compared to non-irradiated patients (48%; $p=0.004$; SRCT Office 1995, personal communication).

None of the trials using postoperative radiotherapy alone has demonstrated any impact on survival. Two trials have, however, demonstrated a survival benefit when postoperative radiotherapy was combined with chemotherapy [10, 17], but not when radiotherapy was given alone (Table 2). Since another trial found that chemotherapy in addition to radiotherapy improved survival [24], it is likely that the chemotherapy rather than the postoperative radiotherapy is responsible for the improvement.

A consensus conference sponsored by NIH discussed adjuvant treatment in rectal cancer and recommended that patients with Dukes' B and C tumours

Table 2. Pelvic recurrence and overall 5-year survival after surgery and postoperative radiotherapy, chemotherapy or both

Study	Additional treatment	Total no. of patients	Local recurrences		Five-year survival (%)	p value
			(n)	(%)		
GITSG	None	14	58	24	43	-
	Chemotherapy	13	48	27	56	NS
	Radiotherapy	10	50	20	52	NS
	Chemotherapy + radiotherapy	5	46	11	59	*
NSABP	None	45	184	24	43	-
	Radiotherapy	30	184	16	41	NS
	Chemotherapy	40	187	21	53	*
NCCTG	Radiotherapy	25	100	25	47	-
	Chemotherapy + radiotherapy	14	104	14	58	*

NS=$p > 0.05$.
*$p < 0.05$.

should receive adjuvant treatment with postoperative radiotherapy (45–55 Gy in 5–6 weeks) together with chemotherapy, i.e. 5-fluorouracil (5-FU) and se-mustine (me-CCNU). The conclusion was mainly based on the results of three trials in the United States (Table 2). Updated results from these studies were reviewed in a clinical announcement by the NCI [30]. It was stated once more that postoperative radiotherapy and chemotherapy should be the standard treatment for Duke's B and C rectal cancer. A subsequent trial indicated that the addition of me-CCNU to 5-FU is not required [32]. In this trial, it was also seen that continuous 5-FU infusion was more effective than bolus 5-FU during radiotherapy.

Acute/Subacute Toxicity from Additional Radiotherapy

Before it is possible to evaluate the advantages and disadvantages of different treatment approaches, adverse effects and costs of additional treatments must also be known.

Preoperative radiotherapy may influence postoperative morbidity and mortality. An increased frequency of perineal wound sepsis after abdomino-perineal resection was found in some trials [36, 39, 40]. In these trials, the hospital stay was usually slightly longer, about 3–5 days on average, in pre-operatively irradiated patients. The anastomotic integrity after a low anterior resection does not seem to be influenced by preoperative radiotherapy [18, 19, 36, 39, 40].

Both compliance and acute tolerability have usually been better after pre-operative than postoperative radiotherapy. Between 12% and 27% of the pa-tients did not receive the planned postoperative dose [3, 10, 17, 42], whereas this occurred in less than 10% in the groups of patients randomized to preoperative radiotherapy [8, 18, 19, 22, 23, 29, 39, 41]. This difference in acute toxicity was also seen in the single trial directly comparing preoperative with postoperative radiotherapy [36].

A higher postoperative mortality was found in patients receiving radiotherapy in two reports [19, 39]. This was observed in patients older than 75 years and in those with metastatic disease at surgery. The causes of death were not obviously related to irradiation, but rather to infection and cardiovascular causes. In these trials radiotherapy was given with anterior–posterior beams, and a large volume of the body thus received the same dose as the tumour target. In the Uppsala trial [35], the same target dose was used as in the Stockholm trial [39], but the irradiation technique (three beams) spared parts of the pelvis and abdomen other than the clinical target volume containing the tumour cells. No effect on postoperative mortality was observed, even though there was no age limit in this trial [36]. High-dose preoperative radiotherapy can thus be delivered without increasing postoperative mortality. It is expected that a large tissue volume, irradiated to a high dose, should be deleterious, at least in elderly patients. This conclusion is supported by results from the Swedish rectal cancer trial with 1168 patients, in which no effect on postoperative mortality was observed in patients treated with three or four beams [40].

Acute neurogenic pain a few hours after irradiation of the lower lumbar region was reported in one of the trials using 5-Gy fractions preoperatively [35]. Pain was usually of short duration in the few patients affected, but remained for several months in some. Subacute neurogenic symptoms and signs have developed in some of the affected patients, leading to inability to walk in a few. When the entire experience in Uppsala from 1979 to 1994 was reviewed, it was found that 19 out of 550 patients (4%) treated with 5×5 (or 5.1×5) Gy within prospective protocols had reported pain.

In six patients (1%), the pain lasted more than a few days, and in four of them subacute neurogenic symptoms developed. The pain was more common in women than in men and appears to occur more often in diabetic patients and in patients with previous neurologic disorders. An extensive re-evaluation of the treatment did not disclose any technical or human error, and the genesis of this acute adverse effect is still unknown [16]. The observation of this rare complication probably caused by an effect on the nerves in the lower lumbar region does, however, point to the need for correct radiation technique with appropriate clinical target volumes and screening of tissue which has a minimal risk of harbouring tumour cells.

Late Radiation-Associated Toxicity

Several studies report late morbidity in the form of intestinal obstruction after postoperative radiotherapy [2, 28]. The frequency of obstruction and/or late diarrhoea, suggesting bowel damage, has been related to the volume of small bowel included in the radiation-treated volume [26]. In this report, radiotherapy with beams extending high up in the abdomen was reported to cause small-bowel intestinal obstruction in 30%–40% of patients, compared to 5%–10% when only the dorsal pelvic cavity was included. In the Uppsala trial, all patients with a follow-up period between 5 and 10 years were re-examined with respect to late adverse effects of radiation. Those given preoperative radiotherapy did not differ with respect to bowel obstruction or other possible late adverse effects from those given surgery alone [15]. In patients irradiated postoperatively, a higher late morbidity was found even when a technique that largely avoided irradiation of extended small-bowel volumes was used. This could have been anticipated, since the postoperative dose was higher than the preoperative one.

Conclusions

Until more efficient chemotherapy regimens are available, radiation therapy should be included in rectal cancer treatment, primarily since it reduces the local failure rate. Contrary to the opinion held in the United States [30], we believe that radiotherapy is more effective given preoperatively. Preoperative radiotherapy also improves survival, although the magnitude of the survival benefit still does not allow firm conclusions about whether the survival improvement is an additional reason for recommending radiotherapy as an adjunct to surgery.

Using a preoperative approach, there is, however, concern about irradiating patients with a Dukes' stage A lesion and those with metastatic disease disclosed at surgery. Dukes' A lesions can now be identified with intraluminal ultrasonography before surgery [4] and thus be spared radiotherapy. This, however, requires that surgery is properly performed so that local failures are kept at a very low level. In the trials reporting a reduced local recurrence rate related to Dukes' stage, this also applies to Dukes' stage A, and to the same extent as to Dukes' stages B and C [39, 41]. In the latter two trials, non-irradiated Dukes' stage A patients had an unacceptably high local failure rate of 14% and 11%, respectively, compared to 5% and 3% among irradiated patients.

We believe that the proportional reduction in local recurrence rate after preoperative radiotherapy might be at least as high following "optimized" surgery, as advocated by Heald and Ryall [21], as it is when combined with "standard" surgery. It is anticipated that the local failure rate then will be very low (perhaps 0%–3%). However, this has not been formally tested in a randomized trial. When the local failure rate without radiotherapy is 6%–7%, overtreatment is substantial. Radiotherapy must therefore be safe, both in the short and long term. The dose must also be sufficiently high (>40 Gy when given in 2-Gy fractions, or comparable doses using other fractionation schedules).

Therefore, radiotherapy must be given with techniques that exclude volumes not at risk for tumour cells. All treatment modalities should be used in an optimal way so that the severely disabling condition of a local pelvic recurrence of a rectal cancer can be entirely eliminated.

References

1. Adam IJ, Mohamdee MO, Martin IG, Scott N, Finan PJ, Johnston D, Dixon MF, Quirke P (1994) Role of circumferential margin involvement in the local recurrence of rectal cancer. Lancet 344:707–711
2. Balslev I, Pedersen M, Teglbjaerg PS, Hanberg-Sørensen F, Bone J, Jacobsen NO, Overgaard J, Sell A, Bertelsen K, Hage E, Hansen L, Kronborg O, Høstrup H, Nørgaard-Pedersen B (1986) Postoperative radiotherapy in Dukes B and C carcinoma of rectum and rectosigmoid. Cancer 58:22–28
3. Bentzen SM, Balslev I, Pedersen M, Teglbjaerg PS, Hanberg-Sørensen F, Bone J, Jacobsen NO, Sell A, Overgaard J, Bertelsen K, Hage E, Fenger C, Kronborg O, Hansen L, Høstrup H, Nørgaard-Pedersen B (1992) Time to loco-regional recurrence after resection of Dukes' B and C colorectal cancer with or without adjuvant postoperative radiotherapy. A multivariate regression analysis. Br J Cancer 65:102–107
4. Beynon J, Mortensen NJ McC, Foy DMA, Channer JL, Virjee J, Goddard P (1986) Preoperative assessment of local invasion in rectal cancer: digital examination, endoluminal sonography or computed tomography? Br J Surg 73:1015–1017
5. Buyse M, Zeleniuch-Jacquotte A, Chalmers TC (1988) Adjuvant therapy of colorectal cancer. Why we still don't know. JAMA 259:3571–3578
6. Cedermark B, Stockholm Colo-Rectal Cancer Study Group (1994) The Stockholm II trial on preoperative short term radiotherapy in operable rectal carcinoma. A prospective randomized trial. ASCO 13:577 (abstr)
7. Denham JW (1986) The radiation dose-response relationship for control of primary breast cancer. Radiother Oncol 7:107–123
8. Duncan W, Smith AN, Freedman LS, Alderson MR, Arnott SJ, Bleehen NM (1984) The evaluation of low dose pre-operative X-ray therapy in the management of operable rectal cancer, results of a randomly controlled trial. Br J Surg 71:21–25
9. Enblad P, Adami H-O, Bergström R, Glimelius B, Krusemo UB, Påhlman L (1988) Improved survival of patients with cancers of the colon and rectum? J Natl Cancer Inst 80:586–597
10. Fisher B, Wolmark N, Rockette H, Redmond C, Deutsch M, Wickerman DL, Fisher ER, Caplan R, Jones J, Lerner H, Gordon P, Feldman M, Cruz A, Legault-Poisson S, Wewxler M, Laurence W, Robidoux A (1988) Postoperative adjuvant chemotherapy or radiation therapy for rectal cancer: results from NSABP Protocol R-01. J Natl Cancer Inst 80:21–29
11. Fletcher GH (1984) Subclinical disease. Cancer 53:1274–1284
12. Fletcher GH (1991) Hypofractionation: lessons from complications. Radiother Oncol 20:10–15
13. Fowler JF (1989) The linear-quadratic formula and progress in fractionated radiotherapy. Br J Radiol 62:679–694
14. Fowler JF (1990) How worthwile are short schedules in radiotherapy? A series of exploratory calculations. Radiother Oncol 8:165–181
15. Frykholm G, Glimelius B, Påhlman L (1993) Pre- and postoperative irradiation in adenocarcinoma of the rectum: final treatment results of a randomized trial and an evaluation of late secondary effects. Dis Colon Rectum 36:564–572
16. Frykholm-Jansson G, Sintorn K, Montelius A, Påhlman L, Glimelius B (1995) Acute lumbosacral plexopathy after preoperative radiotherapy in rectal carcinoma. Radiother Oncol 38:121–130
17. Gastrointestinal Tumor Study Group (1985) Prolongation of the disease-free interval in surgically treated rectal carcinoma. N Engl J Med 312:1464–1472
18. Gérard A, Buyse M, Nordlinger B, Loygue J, Pène F, Kempf P, Bosset JF, Gignoux M, Arnand JP, Desaive C, Duez N (1988) Preoperative radiotherapy as adjuvant treatment in rectal cancer. Ann Surg 208:606–614
19. Goldberg PA, Nicholls RJ, Porter NH, Love S, Grimsey JE (1994) Long-term results of a randomised trial of short-course low-dose adjuvant pre-operative radiotherapy for rectal cancer: reduction in local treatment failure. Eur J Cancer 30A:1602–1606

20. Gunderson L, Sosin H (1974) Areas of failure found at reoperation (second or sympto-
    matic look) following "curative surgery" for adenocarcinoma of the rectum. Cancer
    34:1278–1292
21. Heald RJ, Ryall RDH (1986) Recurrence and survival after total mesorectal excision for
    rectal cancer. Lancet I:1479–1482
22. Higgins G, Humphery E, Dwight R, Roswit B, Lee L, Keehn R (1986) Preoperative radiation
    and surgery for cancer of the rectum. VASOG trial II. Cancer 58:352–359
23. Horn A, Halvorsen JF, Dahl O (1990) Preoperative radiotherapy in operable rectal cancer.
    Dis Colon Rectum 33:823–838
24. Krook JE, Moertel CG, Gunderson LL, Wieand HS, Collins RT, Beart RW, Kubista TP,
    Poon MA, Meyers WC, Maillard JA, Twito DI, Morton RF, Veeder MH, Witzig TE, Cha S,
    Vidyarthi SC (1991) Effective surgical adjuvant therapy for high-risk rectal cancer. N Engl
    J Med 324:709–715
25. Lawrence TS, Davis MA, Maybaum J (1994) Dependence of 5-fluorouracil-mediated
    radiosensitization on DNA-directed effects. Int J Radiat Oncol Biol Phys 29:519–523
26. Letschert JGJ, Lebesque JV, de Boer RW, Hart AAM, Bartelink H (1990) Dose-volume
    correlation in radiation-induced late small-bowel complications: a clinical study. Radio-
    ther Oncol 18:307–320
27. MacFarlane JK, Ryall RDH, Heald RJ (1993) Mesorectal excision for rectal cancer. Lancet
    341:457–460
28. Mak AC, Rich TA, Schultheiss TE, Kavanagh B, Ota DM, Romsdahl MM (1994) Late
    complications of postoperative radiation therapy for cancer of the rectum and recto-
    sigmoid. Int J Radiat Oncol Biol Phys 28:597–603
29. Marsh PJ, James RD, Schofield PF (1994) Adjuvant preoperative radiotherapy for locally
    advanced rectal carcinoma. Results of a prospective, randomized trial. Dis Colon Rectum
    37:1205–1214
30. NCI (1991) Clinical announcement. Adjuvant therapy of rectal cancer, 14:e mars
31. Ny IOL, Luk ISC, Yuen ST, Lau PWK, Pritchett CJ, Ny M, Poon GP, Ho J (1993) Surgical
    lateral clearence in resected rectal carcinomas, a multivariate analysis of clin-
    icopathological features. Cancer 71:1972–1976
32. O'Connell MJ, Martenson JA, Wieand HS, Krook JE, MacDonald JS, Haller DG, Mayer RJ,
    Gunderson LL, Rich TA (1994) Improving adjuvant therapy for rectal cancer by combining
    protracted infusion fluorouracil with radiation therapy after curative surgery. N Engl J
    Med 331:502–507
33. Phillips RKS, Hittinger R, Blesovsky L, Fry JS, Fielding LP (1984) Local recurrence fol-
    lowing "curative" surgery for large bowel cancer: I. The overall picture. Br J Surg 71:12–16
34. Påhlman L, Glimelius B (1984) Local recurrences after surgical treatment for rectal car-
    cinoma. Acta Chir Scand 150:331–335
35. Påhlman L, Glimelius B (1990) Pre- and postoperative radiotherapy in rectal carcinoma:
    report from a randomized multicenter trial. Ann Surg 211:187–195
36. Påhlman L, Glimelius B, Graffman S (1985) Pre- versus postoperative radiotherapy in
    rectal carcinoma: an interim report from a randomized multicentre trial. Br J Surg 72:961–
    966
37. Rider WD, Palmer JA, Mahoney LJ, Robertson CT (1977) Preoperative irradiation in
    operable cancer of the rectum: report of the Toronto trial. Can J Surg 20:335–338
38. Roswit B, Higgins G, Keehn R (1975) Preoperative irradiation for carcinoma of the rectum
    and rectosigmoid colon: report of a National Veterans Administration randomized study.
    Cancer 35:1597–1602
39. Stockholm Rectal Cancer Study Group (1990) Preoperative short-term radiation therapy in
    operable rectal carcinoma. A prospective randomized trial. Cancer 66:49–55
40. Swedish Rectal Cancer Trial (1993) Initial report from a Swedish multicentre study ex-
    amining the role of preoperative irradiation in the treatment of patients with resectable
    rectal carcinoma. Br J Surg 80:1333–1336
41. Swedish Rectal Cancer Trial (1995) Local recurrence rate in a randomized multicentre trial
    of preoperative radiotherapy compared to surgery alone in resectable rectal carcinoma.
    Eur J Surg 162:397–402

42. Treurniet-Donker AD, van Putten WLJ, Wereldsma JCJ, Bruggink EDM, Hoogenraad WJ, Roukema JA, Snijders-Keilholz A, Meijer WS, Meerwaldt JH, Wijnmaalen AJ, Wiggers T (1991) Postoperative radiation therapy for rectal cancer. Cancer 67:2042–2048
43. Withers HR, Taylor JMG, Maciejewski B (1988) The hazard of accelerated tumor clonogen repopulation during radiotherapy. Acta Oncol 27:131–146
44. von der Maase H (1986) Experimental studies on interactions of radiation and cancer chemotherapeutic drugs in normal tissues and a solid tumour. Radiother Oncol 7:47–68

CHAPTER 29

Adjuvant Therapy for Rectal Cancers when Surgical Therapy Is Optimal

Bernard Levin

Introduction

As surgical techniques have improved and evolved, medical and radiation oncologists have been challenged to improve on the results achieved by surgical extirpation of cancers of the colon and rectum. Adjuvant therapy administered preoperatively, intraoperatively, or postoperatively has been the subject of many studies. The significance of such research is related to the serious health consequences of large bowel cancer. The annual incidence worldwide of this malignancy is approximately 575 000 [43]. In developed countries, the incidence of colorectal cancer increases with age from eight per 100 000 for 40-year-old individuals to approximately 500 per 100 000 for a cohort of 80-year-old persons.

As the proportion of aged in the population of western countries increases, the absolute number of cases of rectal cancer will also increase, unless primary and secondary prevention measures prove more successful. An issue for discussion is therefore the role of adjuvant therapy in the presence of optimal surgical therapy, particularly in communities where adjuvant therapy is not yet widely used. In attempting to answer this, it is important to understand the current status of adjuvant therapy.

Biology of Rectal Cancer

Relapse of tumor regionally or systemically following curative resection of rectal cancer is potentially life-threatening. The principal risk factors for relapse are the depth of intramural and extramural invasion and the presence of regional lymph node metastases [19, 33, 46]. Quirke et al. [41] have demonstrated that local recurrence is related to incomplete circumferential clearance. In one series, they showed that 20 of 52 patients (38%) with rectal cancer had tumor at the lateral resection margin. In over half of these cases, the surgeon believed a curative resection had been performed.

Reports of local recurrence range from 4% to 30% [8, 22, 41] and some authors have pleaded for a standardized method of reporting so as to enable accurate comparisons to be made between series. For example, it is recommended by Marsh et al. [27] that "local recurrence after operation for rectal carcinoma be defined as any detectable local disease at follow-up, occurring either alone or in conjunction with generalized recurrence, in patients who have undergone resection. A rate should be given both for all patients and for those operated on for cure but not for the latter group alone as this could introduce bias."

The point of view that surgical techniques for rectal cancer have achieved maximum effectiveness has prompted trials in the USA of preoperative and postoperative adjuvant therapy [36]. However, if it could be conclusively shown by prospective randomized studies that a local recurrence rate as low as 4% as reported by Heald and colleagues [26] and others [28] could be achieved outside of a few selected centers, recommendations in the USA for the use of adjuvant therapy [36] would require re-evaluation. Published data from both Europe and the USA suggest that the rate of local recurrence following rectal cancer surgery is substantial.

The rates of pelvic and systemic recurrence can be ascertained from those patients in the surgical control groups in prospective adjuvant therapy trials. For example, the European Organization for Research and Treatment of Cancer (EORTC) reported a 35% actuarial local recurrence rate [17]. A substantial number of patients who develop pelvic recurrences also have concomitant or subsequent distant metastases. In the study by Gerard [17], the sites of first recurrence in patients followed for an average of 3 years were in the pelvis alone in 13%, at distant sites alone in 10%, and both local recurrence and systemic metastases were found in 13%. In the Gastrointestinal Tumor Study Group Trial, the first recurrence was in the pelvis only in 21% and at distant sites in 31%. In contrast, in a reoperative series, although 64% had pelvic failure as a component of their disease recurrence, 36% in the series also developed distant metastases [20].

The interpretation of local failure rates in rectal cancer is complex due to reported variables such as whether the diagnosis is made by clinical, surgical or autopsy criteria; first or cumulative site of failure; sole or component of failure. Irrespective of the success of local control measures, it is likely that systemic spread will require appropriate systemic therapy.

Pharmacological Background of Adjuvant Therapy

5-Fluorouracil and Levamisole

In Stage III colon cancer, an intergroup trial compared postoperative levamisole, 5-fluorouracil (FU) plus levamisole and surgery alone in patients with Dukes' stage B2 and C colon adenocarcinoma. 5-FU/levamisole improved the recurrence-free survival and overall survival significantly in 971 patients with Dukes' stage C colon cancer. The recurrence rate was reduced at all sites but most strikingly for tumor sites outside the abdominal cavity [31]. In a subsequent update the earlier results were confirmed [32]. 5-FU/levamisole reduced the recurrence rate by 39% ($p<0.0001$). The observed recurrence rate for patients with surgical resection only, levamisole, or 5-FU/levamisole was 53% versus 52% versus 37%, respectively. The cancer-related death rate was reduced by 32% ($p<0.004$) (surgery only 45%, levamisole 44%, 5-FU/levamisole 33%). Unfortunately, a comparison with 5-FU alone was not performed.

The mechanism of action of levamisole in this combination is unknown although recent evidence suggests that levamisole augments the effect of 5-FU on the stabilization (reduced degradation) of human leukocyte antigen (HLA) class I mRNAs and furthermore enhances the accumulation of these stabilized mRNAs by increasing their rate of transcription [1].

Levamisole is now being incorporated into combination treatment programs which include 5-FU and Leucovorin.

5-FU and Leucovorin

Two major mechanisms of cytotoxicity are associated with 5-FU administration, one directed at DNA and the other at RNA. Inhibition of DNA synthesis by 5-FU results from its incorporation into deoxyribonucleotide derivatives. 5-Flurodeoxyuridine monophosphate (5-FdUMP) is an inhibitor of thymidylate synthase. Binding to the enzyme is enhanced considerably by the sequential binding of 5,10-methylene tetrahydrofolate to form a stable ternary complex. The extent to which thymidylate synthase is inhibited is dependent upon the availability of reduced folate [3]. This can be provided by exogenous Leucovorin (5-formyltetrahydrofolate).

The combination of Leucovorin and 5-FU has been evaluated in numerous trials in patients with metastatic disease. Despite some variability in study results, it is generally considered that a greater percentage of patients respond to 5-FU plus Leucovorin and this effect is accompanied by a small survival benefit [2, 40].

5-FU and Leucovorin have been evaluated as adjuvant treatment and preliminary results from four prospective randomized trials indicate that this combination is effective (Table 1). In a randomized trial of patients with resected Dukes' stage B and C colon cancer, 5-FU and Leucovorin produced an improvement in disease-free (73% vs 64%; $p<0.001$) and 3-year overall survival (84% vs 77%; $p=0.003$) rates compared with the combination of 5 FU, semustine and vincristine [48].

Table 1. Randomized studies assessing 5-fluorouracil and leucovorin as postoperative therapy for colorectal cancer (modified from [14])

Reporting group	No. of patients	Median follow-up	Disease-free survival (%)		Overall survival (%)	
			5-FU/LCV	Control	5-FU/LCV	Control
NSABP [48]	1081	48 months	73*	64[a]	84*	77
Intergroup [37]	309	42 months	77*	64	75	71
Italian/Canadian [10]	1493	37 months	72*	63	83*	78
Francini et al. [12]	239	4.5 years	74*	59	79*	65

NSABP National Surgical Adjuvant Breast Bowel Project; 5-FU, 5-fluorouracil; LCV, Leucovorin.
*Refers to statistically significant benefit for the treatment cohort versus control patients.
[a]Control group received semustine, vincristine, and 5-fluorouracil (MOF).

An Intergroup Study randomized 309 patients with resected Dukes' stages B_2 and C cancers to 5-FU plus low-dose Leucovorin (20 mg/m2) for 6 months or to an observation arm. After a median follow-up of 3.5 years, a significant reduction in disease relapse was noted for the treatment arm (77% vs 64%; $p<0.001$). It is not clear whether a statistically significant decrease in overall survival will be observed with a more extended follow-up period [37].

Recently, European and Canadian investigators randomized approximately 1500 patients with resected Dukes' stages B2 and C colorectal cancers to receive either postoperative 5-FU and high-dose Leucovorin (200 mg/m2) for 6 months or no additional therapy. After a median follow-up of 37 months, treated patients experienced a significant improvement in disease-free survival (72% vs 63%; $p<0.001$) and overall survival (83% vs 78%; $p=0.03$) [10].

In an Italian trial, investigators randomized 239 patients with Dukes' stages B2 and C colon cancers to receive either postoperative 5-FU and Leucovorin or no additional therapy. After a median follow-up of 4.5 years, in Dukes' C patients, the estimated 5-year survival rate was 69% in the adjuvant arm and 43% in the control arm ($p=0.0025$) [12]. An oral fluoropyrimidine formulation [39] has demonstrated activity comparable to 5-FU plus Leucovorin in patients with advanced colorectal cancer and may be appropriate for adjuvant therapy.

Preoperative Radiation Therapy and Chemoradiation

The rationale for combining radiation and chemotherapy is that randomized controlled studies of preoperative and postoperative radiation therapy alone have not demonstrated an increase in overall survival [5]. Of the eight modern randomized trials of preoperative radiation therapy, two show a statistically significant difference in local recurrence rates.

The first is that of the EORTC [18], in which there was a 12% decrease in local failure for the patients who received 3450 cGY (34% vs 22%; $p<0.05$) [7]. The Stockholm trial also showed a significant difference in disease-free survival (70% vs 59%; $p=0.05$ [45]. Concern over the design of the trials of preoperative radiation therapy has not diminished the significance of the conclusion that preoperative irradiation alone does not enhance overall survival [13], leading to attempts to enhance radiation therapy by co-administering 5-FU.

Chemoradiation. In vitro and in vivo evidence exists of 5-FU sensitization of radiation therapy [6, 30, 35]. In vitro studies have shown that 5-FU produces its cytotoxic effects both by inhibiting the synthesis of DNA and by altering the processing and tumors of RNA. Radiation enhancement of the action of 5-FU could be due to potentiation of these effects or inhibition of repair of sublethal radiation injury or by other effects on the cell cycle.

At The University of Texas M.D. Anderson Cancer Center, Rich and colleagues have demonstrated preoperative chemoradiation for advanced primary and recurrent rectal cancer to be highly effective in controlling pelvic cancer [29]. Subsequently, preoperative chemoradiation therapy using infusional 5-FU (300 mg/m^2) by continuous intravenous infusion over 120 h/week was administered to 77 patients with clinically stage T3 rectal cancer confirmed by endorectal ultrasonography in 85% of patients (44).

Surgery was performed approximately 6 weeks after the completion of chemoradiation therapy and included 25 abdomino-perineal resections and 52 anal-sphincter-preserving procedures. Posttreatment tumor stages were T1-2, N0 in 35%, T3 in 25% and T1-3, N1 in 11%; 29% had no evidence of cancer. Overall pelvic control was obtained in 99%. The actual survival rate was 83% at 3 years. Acute, preoperative and late complications were not more numerous or more severe with chemoradiation therapy than with radiation therapy alone; the combination regimen resulted in a significant reduction in rates of local recurrence, distant metastasis, cancer-related deaths and all deaths.

The EORTC has reported the only phase III trial of preoperative chemoradiation in clinically resectable rectal cancer [4]. Local control was identical for the two groups at 85% after 5 years. However, survival was worse in patients who received preoperative chemoradiation than in those who received preoperative radiation alone (46% vs 59%; $p=0.06$) due to a disproportionate number of perioperative and intercurrent deaths. The study has been criticized on the grounds of a suboptimal total dose and delivery of radiation and chemotherapy [13].

Postoperative Combined Modality Therapy

Postoperative trials allow for selection of those whose surgical and pathologic staging has placed them at high risk of recurrence. The results of four published trials are summarized in Table 2.

Two randomized trials (GITSG [15, 25] and Mayo Clinic/NCCTG [9]) have demonstrated a decrease in local recurrence and an improvement in disease-free and overall survival following administration of postoperative irradiation and chemotherapy for patients with resected high-risk rectal cancer. Although initial studies incorporated semustine, a leukemogen, subsequent studies have shown that this compound is not a necessary component of combined mo-

Table 2. Randomized, controlled trials of postoperative adjuvant therapy for rectal cancer (modified from [14])

Group	No. of patients	Regimen	5-year disease-free survival (%)	5-year overall survival (%)
GITSG [15]	227	Observation	47	43
		Radiation therapy	55	56
		5-FU/semustine	55	52
		5-FU/semustine/ radiation therapy	71[*]	59[*]
NSABP [48]	555	Observation	30	43
		Radiation therapy	33	41
		MOF	42[a]	53[a]
NCCTG [9]	240	Radiation therapy	42	47
		5-FU/semustine/ radiation therapy	63*	58*
GITSG [16]	210	5-FU/semustine/ radiation therapy	54[b]	66[b]
		5-FU/radiation therapy	68[b]	75[b]
Intergroup [37]	660	PVI 5-FU/radiation therapy	63[b]	70[b]
		Bolus 5-FU/radiation therapy	53[b]	60[b]

5-FU, 5-fluorouracil; GITSG, Gastrointestinal Tumor Group Study; NSABP, National Surgical Adjuvant Breast and Bowel Program; MOF, semustine (methyl-CCNU), vincristine, and 5-fluorouracil; NCCTG, North Central Cancer Treatment Group; PVI, protracted venous infusion.
[*]Refers to statistically significant benefit for treatment cohort versus control cohort.
[a]Treatment advantage was observed only in men over 65 years of age.
[b]Four-year data.

dality therapy (Table 2) [16]. While the first NSABP study [11] initially failed to show a benefit for combined modality therapy (Table 2), a more recent study from the NSABP showed benefit for combined modality treatment [42]. An Intergroup study [38] compared protracted infusion 5-FU with bolus 5-FU during radiation therapy. As indicated in Table 2, infusional 5-FU was associated with improved relapse free and overall survival.

Current Trials. A current Intergroup trial will define further in the postoperative setting, the role of continuous infusion 5-FU, 5-FU and Leucovorin as well as levamisole when combined with radiation therapy. Other trials in the USA are comparing preoperative versus postoperative chemoradiation therapy in patients with Dukes' stage B2 and C rectal cancers.

Biomarkers

Even in the face of optimal surgical therapy it may be particularly useful to identify individuals at especially high rate of pelvic recurrence or distant spread. Although still under investigation, DNA ploidy [34], tumor proliferation (by Ki-67, proliferating cell nuclear antigen, PCNA, determination) [47] and molecular genetic techniques (allelic loss, p53 mutations) [21, 23] have been reported to have prognostic significance in colorectal cancer. Immunohistochemical quantitation of thymidylate synthase has been used to evaluate likelihood of response to adjuvant therapy in rectal cancer [24].

Conclusions

Despite optimal surgical techniques, the issue which cannot be influenced in a major way is that of systemic spread. Systemic therapy or combined chemoradiation may still be required. However, a definitive demonstration of the benefits of such therapy in the face of optimal surgical technique will require appropriately designed prospective trials. Measures to be evaluated include local recurrence, distant spread as well as duration and quality of survival.

The concept of introducing a standardized surgical technique into a specific population (e.g., Norway) to be followed later by prospective clinical trials of adjuvant therapy, seems feasible and appropriate. Standardization of reporting surgical and pathological outcome data will be an important first step in this process.

References

1. AbdAlla EE, Blair GE, Jones RA et al (1995) Mechanism of synergy of levamisole and fluorouracil: induction of human leukocyte antigen class I in a colorectal cancer cell line. J Natl Cancer Inst 87:489–496
2. Advanced colorectal cancer meta analysis project (ACCNAP) (1992) Modulation of fluorouracil by leucovorin in patients with advanced colorectal cancer: evidence in terms of response rate. J Clin Oncol 10:896–903
3. Berger SH, Hakala MT (1984) Relationship of dUMP and free FdUMP pools to inhibition of thymidylate synthase by 5-fluorouracil. Mol Pharmacol 25:305–309
4. Boulis-Wassif S, Gerard A, Loygue J et al (1984) Final results of a randomized trial on the treatment of rectal cancer with preoperative radiotherapy alone or in combination with 5-fluorouracil, followed by radical surgery. Cancer 53:1811–1818
5. Buyse M, Zeleniuch-Jacquole A, Chalmes TC (1988) Adjuvant therapy of colorectal cancer: why we still don't know. JAMA 259:3571–3578
6. Byfield JE, Calabro-Jones P, Klisah I et al (1982) Pharmacologic requirements for obtaining sensitization of human tumor cells in vitro to combined 5-fluorouracil and radiation. Int J Radiat Oncol Biol Phys 8:1923–1933
7. Cohen AM, Minsky BD, Friedman (1993) In: De Vita V Jr, Hellman S, Rosenberg SJB (eds) Cancer: principles and practice of oncology, 4th edn. Lippincott, Philadelphia
8. DeAzevedo J, Dozois RR, Gunderson LL (1992) Locally recurrent rectal cancer: surgical strategy. World J Surg 16:490–494
9. Douglass HO Jr, Moertel CG, Mayer RJ et al (1986) Survival after post-operative combination treatment of rectal cancer. N Engl J Med 315:1294–1295
10. Erlichman C, Marsoni S, Seitz J et al (1994) Event free and overall survival is increased by FUFA in resected B and C colon cancer: a prospective pooled analysis of 3 randomized trials. Proc Am Soc Clin Oncol 13:A562

11. Fisher B, Wolmark N, Rockette H et al (1988) Postoperative adjuvant chemotherapy or radiation therapy for rectal cancer. Results from NSABP protocol R-01. J Natl Cancer Inst 80:21–29
12. Francini G, Petrioli R, Lorenzini L et al (1995) Folinic acid and 5-fluorouracil as adjuvant chemotherapy in colon cancer. Gastroenterology 106:899–906
13. Freedman GM, Coia LR (1995) Adjuvant and neoadjuvant treatment of rectal cancer. Semin Oncol 22:611–624
14. Fuchs CS, Mayer RJ (1995) Adjuvant chemotherapy for colon and rectal cancer. Semin Oncol 22:472–487
15. Gastrointestinal Tumor Study Group (1985) Prolongation of the disease-free interval in surgically treated rectal carcinoma. N Engl J Med 312:1465–1472
16. Gastrointestinal Study Group (1992) Radiation therapy and fluorouracil with or without semustine for the surgical adjuvant treatment of patients with adenocarcinoma of the rectum. J Clin Oncol 10:549–557
17. Gerard A, Berrod JL, Pene F, Loygue J, Langier A et al (1985) Interim analysis of a phase III study on preoperative radiation therapy in resectable rectal carcinoma. Cancer 55:2373–2379
18. Gerard A, Buyse M, Nordlinger B et al (1988) Preoperative radiotherapy as adjuvant treatment in rectal cancer. Final results of a randomized study of the European Organization for Research and Treatment of Cancer (EORTC). Ann Surg 208:606–614
19. Grotz RL, Pemberton JH, Gunderson LL (1994) Treatment results with radical surgery. In: Cohen AM, Winawer SJ, Friedman MA, Gunderson LL (eds) Cancer of the colon, rectum and anus, McGraw-Hill, New York, pp 605–614
20. Gunderson LL, Sosin H (1974) Areas of failure found at operation (second or symptomatic look) following curative surgery for adenocarcinoma of the rectum: clinicopathologic correlation and implications for adjuvant therapy. Cancer 34:1278–1292
21. Harnelin R, Laurent-Puig P, Olschwang S et al (1994) Association of p53 mutations with short survival in colorectal cancer. Gastroenterology 106:28–42
22. Heald RJ, Karanjia ND (1992) Results of radical surgery for rectal cancer. World J Surg 16:848–857
23. Jen J, Kim H, Piantodosi S, Liu ZF, Levitt RC et al (1994) Allelic loss of chromosome 18q and prognosis in colorectal cancer. N Engl J Med 331:213–221
24. Johnston PG, Fisher ER, Rockette HE et al (1994) The role of thymidylate synthase in prognosis and outcome of adjuvant therapy in patients with rectal cancer. J Clin Oncol 12:2640–2647
25. Krook JE, Moertel CG, Gunderson LL et al (1991) Effective surgical adjuvant therapy for high-risk rectal carcinoma. N Engl J Med 324:709–715
26. MacFarlane JK, Ryall RDH, Heald RJ (1993) Mesorectal excision for rectal cancer. Lancet 341:457–460
27. Marsh PJ, James RD, Schofeld PF (1995) Definition of local recurrence after surgery for rectal carcinoma. Br J Surg 82:465–468
28. Mcall JL, Cox MR, Wattchow D (1995) Analysis of recurrence rates after surgery alone for rectal cancer. Int J Colorect Dis 10:126–132
29. Minsky BD, Cohen AM, Enker WE et al (1994) Pre-operative 5-FU, low dose leucovorin and concurrent radiation therapy for rectal cancer. Cancer 73:273–278
30. Moertel CG, Childs D, Reitemeier R et al (1969) Combined 5-fluorouracil and supervoltage therapy of locally unresectable gastrointestinal cancer. Lancet II:865–867
31. Moertel CG, Fleming RT, MacDonald JS et al (1990) Levamisole and fluorouracil for adjuvant therapy of resected colon carcinoma. N Engl J Med 322:352–358
32. Moertel C, Fleming T, MacDonald J et al (1995) Fluorouracil plus levamisole is effective adjuvant therapy after resection of Stage II colon carcinoma: a final report. Ann Intern Med 122:321–326
33. Moossa AR, Ree PC, Marks JE et al (1975) Factors influencing local recurrence after abdomino-perineal resection for cancer of the rectum and rectosigmoid. Br J Surg 62:727–730
34. Moran RM, Rothenberger DA, Gallo RA et al (1992) A predictive model for distant metastases in rectal cancer using DNA ploidy studies. Am J Surg 163:599–601

35. Myers CE (1981) The pharmacology of the fluoropyrimidines. Pharmacol Rev 33:1–15
36. NIH Consensus Conference (1990) Adjuvant therapy for patients with colorectal cancer. JAMA 1444–1450
37. O'Connell MJ, Maillard J, MacDonald J et al (1993) An intergroup trial of intensive course 5-FU and low dose leucovorin as surgical adjuvant therapy for high risk colon cancer. Proc Am Soc Clin Oncol 12:552 (abstr)
38. O'Connell MJ, Martenson JA, Wieand HS et al (1994) Improving adjuvant therapy for rectal cancer by combining protracted-infusion fluorouracil with radiation therapy after curative surgery. N Engl J Med 331:502–507
39. Pazdur R, Lassere Y, Rhodes V, Ajani JA, Sugarman et al (1994) Phase II trial of UFT plus oral leucovorin: an effective oral regimen in the treatment of metastatic colorectal carcinoma. J Clin Oncol 11:2296–2300
40. Poon MA, O'Connell MJ, Wieand HS et al (1991) Biochemical modulation of fluorouracil with leucovorin: confirmatory evidence of improved therapeutic efficacy in advanced colorectal cancer. J Clin Oncol 9:1067–1972
41. Quirke P, Dudley P, Dixon MF et al (1986) Local recurrence of rectal adenocarcinoma due to inadequate surgical resection. Histopathological study of lateral tumor spread and surgical excision. Lancet II:996–999
42. Rockette H, Deutsch M, Petrelli N et al (1994) Effect of combined postoperative radiation therapy when used with adjuvant chemotherapy in Dukes' B and C rectal cancer: results from NSABP R-02 (abstr). Proc Am Soc Clin Oncol 13:193
43. Schottenfeld D (1995) Epidemiology (adenocarcinoma of the colon and rectum). In: Cohen AM, Winawer SJ (eds) Cancer of the colon, rectum and anus. McGraw-Hill, New York, pp 7–10
44. Shumate CR, Rich TA, Skibber JM, Ajani JA, Ota DM (1993) Pre-operative chemotherapy and radiation therapy for locally advanced primary and recurrent rectal carcinoma: a report of surgical morbidity. Cancer 71:3690–3696
45. Stockholm Rectal Cancer Study Group (1990) Preoperative short-term preoperative radiation therapy in operable rectal cancer. A randomized trial. Cancer 66:49–55
46. Welch JP, Donaldson GA (1979) The clinical correlation of an autopsy study of recurrent colorectal cancer. Ann Surg 189:496–502
47. Willett CG, Warland G, Coen J et al (1995) Rectal cancer: the influence of tumor proliferation on response to pre-operative irradiation. Int J Radiat Oncol Biol Phys 32:57–61
48. Wolmark N (1993) The benefit of leucovorin-modulated fluorouracil as postoperative adjuvant therapy for primary colon cancer: results from National Surgical Adjuvant Breast and Bowel Project Protocol C-03. J Clin Oncol 11:1879–1887

The Role of Adjuvant Treatment if Surgery Is Optimal: A Clinical Epidemiologist's View

Olof Nyrén and Paul Blomqvist

Introduction

In clinical epidemiology, modern statistical and epidemiological methods are used to answer questions that arise in clinical practice. The study designs can be either observational or experimental. With its roots in analytical epidemiology which is based mainly on observational methods, clinical epidemiology has inherited its mother discipline's concern with methodological issues. Special attention is paid to threats to the external and internal validity of the studies. Particularly, clinical epidemiology regularly uses methods developed to accommodate the influence of confounding factors and other cofactors which cannot be controlled by the investigator.

Given the complexities associated with the evaluation of adjuvant therapy for rectal cancer, it seems therefore relevant for clinical epidemiologists to comment on methodological aspects of such studies. In this chapter, we will address a few questions related to the design of studies of adjuvant therapy. Thus, our intentions are neither to discuss state of the art in colorectal adjuvant therapy, nor to contribute with ideas regarding new therapeutic modifications. Instead, we will focus on how to best evaluate adjuvant therapy in clinical trials, with special emphasis on the case where surgery has been optimized.

A Common Cancer Form

Rectal cancer is an important public health concern. In Sweden, rectal cancer is the sixth most common malignancy in men, afflicting approximately 900 annually (the age-adjusted incidence rate in 1991 was 20.5 per 10^5 per year) [6].

Also in women, rectal cancer ranks number 6 among all cancers, with 800 new cases annually (the age-adjusted incidence was 14.4 per 10^5 per year in 1991). The incidence has increased over the past decades with an annual change of about 0.7% [6]. In the United States, the estimated number of new cases in 1993 was 43 000 [4].

Although it has been repeatedly stated that the prognosis of rectal cancer has remained virtually unchanged [27], survival has, in fact, improved slowly. In Sweden, the 1-year crude survival among all patients diagnosed with rectal cancer, computed with the life-table method [10], has increased from 62% in men diagnosed in 1961–1963 to 74% in men diagnosed during 1987–1989 and from 65% to 78% in women [18]. Relative 1-year survival, defined as crude survival divided by the expected survival (based on the survival experience in the demographically corresponding background population) [11], increased from 65% to 79% in men and from 68% to 81% in women. The improvement in survival did not occur exclusively during the first year of follow-up, which indicates that postoperative mortality was not the only reason for the improvement. The crude and relative 5-year survival in Swedish men with rectal cancer increased from 26% and 34% to 36% and 45%, respectively. The corresponding increase in crude and relative survival among women was from 34% and 42% to 43% and 53%, respectively [18].

These data are in accordance with American national end result statistics, which showed that the overall 5-year survival among men and women was 35% [28]. In a French study, it was shown that the improvement in rectal cancer prognosis was essentially confined to patients with Dukes' stage C at surgery [24], indicating that a shift in stage distribution is unlikely to explain the development, and that improved treatment may have had a significant impact. Still, however, approximately half of the patients succumb to their disease within 5 years.

What Are the Relevant Endpoints?

According to the recommendations by the 1990 National Institutes of Health Consensus Conference on adjuvant treatment of colorectal cancer [20] the efficacy should be evaluated by the following three independent primary endpoints: (i) incidence of pelvic recurrence; (ii) disease-free survival (time to any relapse); and (iii) overall survival. All endpoints are highly relevant, not the least the first one; the symptoms caused by a pelvic recurrence can induce considerable morbidity, and it is often refractory to conventional management with surgery or radiation therapy [3, 16, 19]. The pelvic recurrence rate is generally given as the percentage who have experienced that endpoint at 1, 5, or 10 years after the operation, but sometimes the time base is less clear. Also, survival is commonly expressed as the proportion still alive at fixed follow-up times. These data are conceptually easy to understand and are suitable for comparisons between studies. The dynamics over time, however, are less well expressed, and no account is taken of patients who did not reach these observation points. Thus, considerable improvement of the short-term survival among those surviving less than 5 years may be overlooked if only 5- or 10-year survival is computed.

The solution is the construction of survival curves (also named 'actuarial', 'product-limit', or 'Kaplan-Meier' curves) [22], which has become the most common way of describing the time-to-event. The treatment groups are usually compared using the log-rank test [26]. Stratified analyses [33] and multivariate regression techniques are now widely used to adjust for the influence of prognostic factors. The latter techniques include simple linear logistic regression without consideration to the time aspect [8] and modeling that accounts for survival time, e.g., the proportional hazards regression model of Cox [9].

In order to control for the influence of prognostic factors, these factors must be measured reliably and without systematic errors. This may not always be accomplished. Of particular concern is preoperative adjuvant therapy, which may have the potential of down-staging the tumor selectively in the treatment arm. The introduction of biased measurements of prognosis in the multivariate models may distort the results. Although short-term radiation followed by surgery shortly thereafter will rarely cause any down-staging, it may sometimes be more appropriate to use the results of preoperative diagnostic imaging – which has a similar chance of ascertaining the true stage in both treated patients and untreated controls – as the stage variable in the multivariate model. The introduction of increasingly sophisticated techniques (e.g., endorectal ultrasound, magnetic resonance tomography, or radiolabeled monoclonal antibodies) will hopefully lead to more reliable preoperative staging in future trials.

One of the most difficult questions related to the choice of endpoints is how to deal with deaths from competing causes. In the age groups afflicted by rectal cancer, a sizable proportion of the patients are expected to die within a 5- or 10-year period due to causes unrelated to rectal cancer. This proportion may vary considerably between different populations. Clearly, this reduces the value of crude survival statistics. Therefore, many investigators exclude deaths in which the cancer in question was not known to be present at time of death, to calculate 'disease-specific survival'.

However, in some instances, it may not be possible to establish the exact cause of death, for instance if an autopsy was not carried out. In other instances seemingly cancer-unrelated deaths may still be linked to the cancer or its treatment, e.g., suicide and secondary cancers. In the Stockholm I trial of preoperative short term radiotherapy, an excess of postoperative deaths was observed in the radiation therapy arm, but the causes of deaths were mainly cardiovascular and thromboembolic [7]. Similar observations were made among patients treated with a two-portal radiation technique in a another recent Swedish multicenter trial [35]. Which deaths should be excluded in such situation, and which should not?

To avoid these intricate questions, one may choose to compute the relative survival rate [11], which is the survival rate adjusted for normal life expectancy. This rate provides the answer to the question: "What is the survival rate so far as cancer is concerned?" It is defined as the ratio of the observed survival rate for the group of patients under consideration to the expected. The expected survival rate is derived from a group which is similar to the patient group in all possible factors affecting survival except for the cancer. Usually, investigators use the general population with the same age and sex distribution as the study group.

Although various methods for regression analysis of relative survival rates have been described, according to which the disease-specific hazard rate is either proportional or additive to the hazard rate in the general population [1, 17], there are no commercially available software packages specially designed for such analyses. Further methodological development is highly desirable. The use of relative survival ought to be encouraged in future studies.

For clinical decision-making, physicians need to have data on short- and long-term adverse events and on quality-of-life aspects. For health policy decisions, monetary costs, and cost-benefit deliberations are of paramount importance. Unfortunately, costs in the form of health care expenditure, absenteeism, and impaired quality of life are less well documented in the studies reported so far. Assessments of these aspects should be included in future protocols, with due consideration to the limitations of subjective quality-of-life data in unblinded studies.

Which Results Can Be Expected from Optimized Surgery?

The overall 5-year survival after surgery for cure (without adjuvant treatment) varies by approximately 20% (40%–60%) in the literature. This variation is likely to be explained by differences in stage distribution since the prognosis is dependent on the stage. The reports of local recurrence rates, on the other hand, vary considerably more, between 4 and 50%. The lowest local recurrence rate was reported from a UK district hospital [25], where total mesorectal excision (TME), performed essentially by one very experienced surgeon, gave a recurrence rate of one fifth of that observed in previous large trials [13–15]. Also, the overall recurrence rate was approximately one third of that in other studies with surgery alone.

Although different surgical techniques have not been tested in randomized trials, and although subtle favorable patient characteristics and possible up-staging by the meticulous dissection may explain some of the superiority of MacFarlane et al. [12, 25], their and other reports [5, 32] indicate that improvements of the surgical results can be achieved.

What is a realistic estimate of what can be achieved in routine care with many surgeons involved? Most likely, the results will not be as outstanding as those described by MacFarlane and coworkers [25]. A likely scenario is local recurrence rates of 10%–15% and overall recurrence rates of 30%–40%.

Who Is Expected To Benefit from Adjuvant Therapy?

The selection of appropriate candidates for adjuvant therapy is likely to be of importance for the net benefit. Although some patients with stage I cancers do, in fact, develop local or general recurrences which are ultimately fatal [31], their life expectancy is only moderately reduced. In view of the risk of treatment-related death [7], it is uncertain if the net effect of adjuvant therapy is positive in this category.

Therefore, postoperative adjuvant therapy programs have generally been limited to cancers of Dukes' stage B_2 and C categories. However, modifications of the mode of delivery of radiotherapy may greatly reduce the risk of treatment-related morbidity and mortality [35, 36] thereby possibly shifting the risk-benefit relationship in a more favorable direction. This is particularly relevant since Cedermark et al. [7] noted a reduction of local recurrences in all Dukes' stages after preoperative short-term radiotherapy. Regardless of tumor stage, it seems well-advised to exclude patients above the age of 75 or 80 years, in whom the gain is expected to be small due to the short life expectancy. Elderly patients have also less tolerance to radiation [7].

Which Type of Adjuvant Protocol?

Generally speaking, radiotherapy reduces mainly local recurrences, whereas chemotherapy is more effective against distant recurrence. The more demanding – and expensive – but also more selective postoperative combination therapy (radiation and chemotherapy) has been shown repeatedly to improve local control and survival in TNM stage II and III rectal cancer [14, 15, 23]. This led the National Institutes of Health Consensus Development Conference to recommend that the latter approach should be followed in clinical practice [2]. Although recent data seem to indicate that preoperative radiation alone, in fact, may also increase survival [36], it appears that a combination therapy protocol is needed in order to make any important difference if surgery is optimized to attain a local recurrence rate of 10%–15% without adjuvant therapy. Whether it should be given preoperatively or postoperatively, or both, is out of the scope of this chapter.

What Is the Appropriate Comparison?

As a general rule, it is recommended that treatment schedules to be compared in a randomized clinical trial be as different as is ethically acceptable in order to give maximum chance of ascertaining the effect of the new treatment [33]. Thus, it seems advisable to compare an adjuvant treatment schedule against surgery alone. Given the recommendations by the National Institutes of Health Consensus Development Conference [2], this may be considered unethical. Although there are no data after 1990, it appears that the routine use of adjuvant therapy in rectal cancer has not yet become prevailing practice in Europe. In a Swedish study outside academic hospitals [21] 14% of the patients were given preoperative radiation therapy, and in a French population-based study [24] approximately 30% of the patients received adjuvant radiotherapy. In light of this, and the expected good results of optimized surgery, one is inclined to endorse surgery alone as the reference, provided that measures are taken to maintain the highest surgical standards.

What Sample Size Is Required?

Some previous studies have ended up with inconclusive results merely because the investigators made unrealistic assumptions regarding the expected benefits of the new treatment (i.e., they dimensioned the studies after what they considered a clinically useful benefit, not after what was a realistic expectation of the treatment effect). This leads us to the question what is a clinically useful benefit.

Since every additional patient cured, and every local recurrence avoided is an unquestionable benefit – on the condition that these benefits are not outweighed by important losses in quality of life – the question boils down to what is justifiable in terms of resource requirements to obtain the benefits foreseen. If the treatment is unduly expensive and the expected benefit will be limited to such a marginal proportion that the clinical implementation of the treatment schedule is unrealistic, then a trial should not be carried out. It may be advisable to make some preliminary cost-benefit calculations when a new study is considered.

In the following example, a rough estimation is made of the costs and benefits of the implementation of a postoperative combination therapy schedule recently proposed and tested by O'Connell et al. [30]. Costing was based on charges from one university hospital 1994, in turn derived from cost accounting on typical admissions.

National data on admissions in 1993 were obtained from the Swedish National Board of Health and Welfare. Effects, i.e., overall survival rate and rate of recurrence, were estimated from relevant clinical trials [14, 15, 30].

To compute the baseline costs, it was estimated that for a typical patient, the care consists of one admission with operation and two visits the first year, and then at least one consultation per year during the following 4 years. Patients not surviving require an additional admission and on average 30 days of palliative care.

Costs incurred during years 1 through 5 were discounted to the base year at 5% interest rate. Overall mortality was estimated at 10% annually. The program cost was calculated from a base of 1800 new cases diagnosed in Sweden in 1992.

With these assumptions, the total 5-year cost for the program with no adjuvant therapy was estimated at 216.7 million SEK (30.7 million USD), with two thirds incurred during the base year.

Those considered for adjuvant therapy were patients under the age of 70 years, operated for cure, and with TNM stage II and III tumors (34% of the incident cases). The major effect was assumed to be a 10% increased crude survival and a reduction in local recurrence incidence by 50%. With these assumptions, the total 5-year cost for a program including adjuvant therapy in selected cases was 280.1 million SEK (39.7 million USD).

Table 1. Number of patients required in each of two treatment arms in order to statistically ascertain various degrees of improvement in prognosis, by expected failure rate (significance level 5%; power 80%, two-tailed test)

Failure occurring in	Reduction of hazard rate (%)					
	10%	20%	30%	40%	50%	60%
15%	11540	3153	1533	933	640	480
50%	3462	946	460	280	192	144

Thus, compared to the regimen with surgery alone, costs increased by 29%. The total number of years survived during the 5 years only increased from 8100 with surgery to 8640 with the adjuvant schedule. The marginal cost per extra life year saved thus was 117 400 SEK (16600 USD), a cost that could realistically be borne by an affluent Western society.

Given that a trial is at all meaningful, what sample size is required? If a life-table approach is chosen, with comparison of two survival distributions, the number of patients required is dependent on the number of failures observed. Table 1 shows the number of patients required in each treatment arm in order to ascertain the effect of an intervention. The table has two rows: one for failures that are expected to occur in 15% of the control patients (local recurrences within 5 years), and the second row is for failures that are expected to occur in 50% of the control patients (death within 5 years). We specified the risk of erroneously rejecting a null hypothesis that is really true (α) at 5% and the risk of erroneously failing to reject a null hypothesis that is, in fact, false (β) at 20% (two-tailed test).

It is seen from the table that it takes 1533 patients in each treatment arm in order to ascertain a 30% reduction in recurrence rate (from 15% to 10.5%), while it takes 946 patients in each treatment arm to ascertain a 20% reduction in mortality (from 50% to 40%). Although such a study is a major undertaking, it lies within the bounds of what is feasible.

Can Observational Studies Contribute?

Observational studies can sometimes offer a powerful and cost-effective alternative to intervention studies. The former studies usually circumvent the ethical dilemmas associated with random assignment of possibly lifesaving treatments which at the same time may be potentially hazardous. The main drawback is of course confounding. With modern multivariate statistical methods, however, it is often possible to control for effects of the irrelevant factors that otherwise invalidate non-experimental studies, on condition that these factors have been properly measured. Computerized health care registers offer opportunities for accrual of large numbers of cases with the studied outcome, as well as for the identification of suitable control subjects. One example of such an approach is the application of a case-control methodology to study the impact of sigmoidoscopic screening on colon cancer mortality [29, 34].

Could a similar approach also be used in the evaluation of adjuvant therapy of rectal cancer? The answer is basically no. Firstly, the study base is not easily defined. The target population is all rectal cancer patients who have undergone surgery for cure. Information about whether or not operations are for cure is generally not obtainable through health care registers.

Therefore, to define the study base from which the controls are to be drawn, one needs to review virtually all case records of operated incident cases in the study area. Since the relevant outcomes in rectal cancer (local or general recurrence, or death) are fairly common, prospective studies are comparably efficient. Hence, the cost-effectiveness advantage of a case-control approach is less apparent, particularly in light of the work needed to define the study base.

Moreover, retrospective staging of the tumors may not be feasible. Variations in surgical techniques between hospitals with a special interest in rectal cancer surgery (hospitals that are also most likely to use adjuvant therapy) and hospitals with less specialization may systematically bias the staging of patients from specialized centers towards higher stages (i.e., more lymph nodes in the specimens). Also, preoperative radiotherapy has the potential of down-staging the tumors. Therefore, confounding by stage is likely to be a major problem. From an internal validity perspective, we argue for randomized clinical trials.

Conclusion

Controlled clinical trials remain the only valid way of evaluating the effect of new adjuvant therapies. During the past decade, it has been clearly demonstrated that adjuvant treatment has the potential of improving not only prognosis in terms of local recurrence, but also in terms of overall survival. Expected improvements in the surgical technique are likely to entail considerably lower rates of local and general recurrence in future trials, compared to the trials published to date. This constitutes a special challenge to surgeons and oncologists, since the number of patients required in a trial will increase accordingly. However, with the establishment of large collaborative groups, such studies remain feasible.

References

1. Andersen PK, Borch-Jensen K, Deckert T, Green A, Hougaard P, Keiding N, Kreiner S (1985) A Cox regression model for the relative mortality and its application to diabetes mellitus survival data. Biometrics 41:921–932
2. Anonymous (1990) Adjuvant therapy for patients with colon and rectal cancer. JAMA 264:1444–1450
3. Beart RW, Martin JK, Gundersen LL (1986) Management of recurrent rectal cancer. Mayo Clin Proc 61:826–836
4. Boring CC, Squires TS, Tong T (1993) Cancer statistics, 1993. CA Cancer J Clin 43:7–26

5. Buhre LMD, Mulder NH, de Ruiter AJ, van Loon AJ, Verschueren RCJ (1994) Effect of extent of anterior resection and sex on disease-free survival and recurrence in patients with rectal cancer. Br J Surg 81:1227–1229
6. Center for Epidemiology, National Board of Health and Welfare (1994) Cancer Incidence in Sweden 1991. Fritzes, Stockholm
7. Cedermark B, Johansson H, Rutqvist LE, Wilking N (1995) The Stockholm I trial of preoperative short term radiotherapy in operable rectal carcinoma. Cancer 75:2269–2275
8. Cox DR (1958) The regression analysis of binary sequences. J R Statist Soc Series B 20:215–242
9. Cox DR (1972) Regression models and life tables. J R Statist Soc Series B 34:187–202
10. Cutler SJ, Ederer F (1958) Maximum utilization of the life table method in analyzing survival. J Cron Dis 8:699–712
11. Ederer F, Axtell LM, Cutler SJ (1961) The relative survival rate: a statistical methodology. NCI Monograph No 6:101–121
12. Fielding LP (1993) Mesorectal excision for rectal cancer. Lancet 341:471–472
13. Fisher B, Wolmark N, Rockette H, Redmond C, Deutsch M, Wickerham DL et al (1988) Postoperative adjuvant chemotherapy or radiation therapy for rectal cancer: Results from NSABP protocol R-01. J Natl Cancer Inst 80:21–29
14. Gastrointestinal Tumor Study Group (1985) Prolongation of the disease-free interval in surgically treated rectal carcinoma. N Engl J Med 312:1465–1472
15. Gastrointestinal Tumor Study Group (1986) Survival after postoperative combination treatment of rectal cancer. N Engl J Med 315:1294–1295
16. Gilbert SG (1978) Symptomatic local tumor failure following abdominoperineal resection. Int J Radiol Oncol Biol Phys 4:801–807
17. Hakulinen T, Tenkanen L (1987) Regression analysis of relative survival rates. Appl Statist 36:309–317
18. Holm L-E, Rosén M, Ericsson J, Stenbeck M, Barlow L (1995) Digestive organs. Acta Oncol Suppl 4:11–37
19. Holm T, Cedermark B, Rutqvist L-E (1994) Local recurrence of rectal adenocarcinoma after 'curative' surgery with and without preoperative radiotherapy. Br J Surg 81:452–455
20. Jacobs-Perkins A (1990) Consensus developed for colon/rectal cancer. J Natl Cancer Inst 82:820
21. Järhult J, Mikkelsen I, Thulin A (1995) Kolorektal cancerkirurgi utanför regionsjukhusen. Läkartidningen 92:2325–2328
22. Kaplan EL, Meier P (1958) Nonparametric estimation from incomplete observations. J Am Statist Ass 53:457–481
23. Krook JE, Moertel CG, Gunderson LL, Wieand HS, Collins RT, Beart RW et al (1991) Effective surgical adjuvant therapy for high-risk rectal carcinoma. N Engl J Med 324:709–715
24. Launoy G, Gignoux M, Pottier D, Lefort F, Soumrany A, Maurel J, Beck A (1993) Prognosis of rectal cancer in France. Eur J Cancer 29A:263–266
25. MacFarlane JK, Ryall RDH, Heald RJ (1993) Mesorectal excision for rectal cancer. Lancet 341:457–460
26. Mantel N (1966) Evaluation of survival data and two new rank order statistics arising in its consideration. Cancer Chemother Rep 50:163–170
27. Moertel CG (1992) Accomplishments in surgical adjuvant therapy for large bowel cancer. Cancer 70 (supplement September 1):1364–1371
28. Myers MH, Ries LA (1989) Cancer patient survival rates: SEER program results for 10 year follow-up. CA Cancer J Clin 39:21–32
29. Newcomb PA, Norfleet RG, Storer BE, Surawicz TS, Marcus PM (1992) Screening sigmoidoscopy and colorectal cancer mortality. J Natl Cancer Inst 84:1572–1575
30. O'Connell MJ, Martenson JA, Wieand HS, Krook JE, Macdonald JS, Haller DG, Mayer RJ et al (1994) Improving adjuvant therapy for rectal cancer by combining protracted-infusion fluorouracil with radiation therapy after curative surgery. N Engl J Med 331:502–507
31. Papillon J (1994) Surgical adjuvant therapy for rectal cancer: Present options. Dis Colon Rectum 37:144–148

32. Paty PB, Enker WE, Cohen AM, Lauwers GY (1994) Treatment of rectal cancer by low anterior resection with coloanal anastomosis. Ann Surg 219:365–373
33. Peto R, Pike MC, Armitage P, Breslow NE, Cox DR, Howard SV, Mantel N et al (1976) Design and analysis of randomized clinical trials requiring prolonged observation of each patient. I. Introduction and design. Br J Cancer 34:585–612
34. Selby JV, Friedman GD, Quesenberry CP, Weiss NS (1992) A case-control study of screening sigmoidoscopy and mortality from colorectal cancer. N Engl J Med 326:653–657
35. Swedish Rectal Cancer Trial (1993) Initial report from a Swedish multicentre study examining the role of preoperative irradiation in the treatment of patients with resectable rectal carcinoma. Br J Surg 80:1333–1336
36. The Stockholm Colorectal Cancer Study Group (1994) The Stockholm II trial of high dose preoperative radiotherapy in operable rectal cancer. Proc ASCO 577 (abstract)

International Standardization and Research Strategies

International Standardization and Documentation of the Treatment of Rectal Cancer

Odd Søreide, Jarle Norstein, L. Peter Fielding, and William Silen

Introduction

Rectal cancer is a major killer. Commonly reported 5-year survival figures for unselected patients irrespective of stage of the disease and treatment range around 50%. This is, however, relative survival to normal population deaths. If we look at the death rate as a proportion of all patients who present with the disease, the crude 5-year survival drops to around 35% [62, 73].

The cause of death in these patients is largely related to the malignancy. The natural history of the disease demonstrate three distinctive areas leading to death (Fig. 1): (1) that related to advanced disease at presentation; (2) that dealing with the development of distant metastatic disease following potentially curative surgery; and (3) that related to locally occurring recurrent disease.

To improve treatment results all three phases of this natural history must be considered: (1) early detection by screening; (2) systemic adjuvant chemotherapy; and (3) surgical technique and local adjuvant treatments. However, the first two strategies have only led to a marginal improvement in overall results. This review is dedicated to a consideration of the third phase of

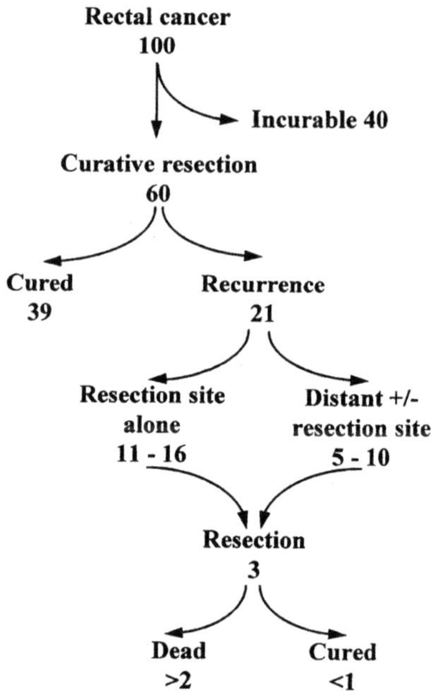

Fig. 1. Schematic outline of the natural history of rectal cancer. The figures are mainly based on data published by Nelson [74, 75]

rectal cancer natural history, namely local tumour recurrence and its prevention.

The exact incidence of such recurence is difficult to determine because of the variation in the populations described in the literature and mandates a careful review of the various causes of such local recurrence. Irrespective of the exact incidence it is clear that the majority of local recurrences are apparent within the first year after resection of primary tumour (45%–74% first year) and more than 2/3 occur by the end of the second year (67%–95% second year) (referenced by [38]).

In the past 50 years, the principle of surgical treatment for tumours with curative intent has been the "en bloc" resection. While this principle is generally adhered to by most surgeons in dealing with colonic cancer, the tenets of the en bloc resection are, for a variety of reasons, more likely to be violated when dealing with rectal cancer.

First, the detailed embryology and anatomy in the pelvis is less well understood than that of the intra-abdominal colon. Secondly, the technical points associated with resection in the pelvis are substantially more complicated because of the proximity of other organs in the same area (e.g. ureter, bladder, uterus, prostate and seminal vesicles or posterior wall of the vagina). Thirdly, the confined pelvic space makes dissection difficult, especially in men.

The Large Bowel Cancer Project in Britain, first published in 1978 [29], demonstrated unequivocally that there are surgeon-related variances in outcome. Not only were these differences seen for postoperative mortality but also for local tumour recurrence. Some 13 years later McArdle and colleagues [65] confirmed this surgeon variability in a focused analysis of surgery for colorectal cancer in Scotland.

In order to assess accurately the reasons for the large variation in the outcomes of the treatment of rectal cancer and to institute appropriate measures for improvement, it appears mandatory that a concerted effort be made to standardize treatments and data gathering methods.

Background – The International Documentation System

An International Working Party Report to the World Congress of Gastroenterology, Sydney 1990, concluded that there is not only a need to define the terminology to describe the full anatomical extent of colorectal cancer (i.e. staging), but also that there are several additional features which have prognostic importance [30]. In their final report, the Working Party identified those features of clinical and histopathological analysis which should also be recorded in all cases of large bowel cancer and suggested an International Documentation System (IDS) for colorectal cancer.

The IDS divides all clinical and pathologic features into three subsections (Table 1):

- Basic information
- Variables of proven prognostic significance, and

Table 1. International Documentation System (IDS) for colorectal cancer (CRC) proposed in a Working Party Report to the World Congresses of Gastroenterology, Sydney 1990 (reproduced from [30] with permission)

Information type	Clinical features	Pathology features
Basic information	Country Hospital (name/code) Patient identification Patient race Past tumour history	Number of primary tumours Tumour measurements Appearance of serosal surface Associated pathology Tumour type
Variables of proven prognostic significance	Surgeon (name/code) Patient gender and age Presentation Anatomic extent of tumour Residual tumour	Extent of direct spread Regional nodal status Local residual tumour Distant metastasis status Venous involvement Histology of infiltrating margin Tumour grade
Information of probable prognostic significance	Preoperative treatment Anatomical site of primary Tumour mobility Technique of tumour mobilization Tumour perforation Surgical procedure Resection of distant metastasis Postoperative treatments	Tumour perforation Inflammatory cell infiltrate Lymphoid aggregates

– Information of probable prognostic significance

The IDS, therefore, represents a "minimal basis data set" for documentation upon which new factors of prognostic significance can be added. An important objective for the Working Group was also to establish an internationally acceptable language by which the variables (or features) in the IDS should be described. The documentation details are given in Appendices A and B.

The Working Party conclusions will form the basis for the documentation recommendations given in this chapter. However, since the Working Party report in 1990, evidence has now accumulated that issues not specifically discussed in that report, particularly details of surgical technique, are prognostically important. The type of surgery is clearly related to local failure rate (Chap. 3), and thus, the need for standardization of surgical technique and the methods for accurate documentation of this surgery require specific review and nomenclature.

Documentation Details

Clinical Documentation

Presentation

Mode of presentation is of potential prognostic importance. Most patients seen in clinical practice have symptomatic tumours and nearly all multivariate analyses to date have included only symptomatic patients. We, however, foresee that an increasing proportion of patients will be identified by screening or surveillance programs. An example of the latter is Hereditary Non-Polyposis Colorectal Cancer (HNPCC) where asymptomatic family members of the index patient are approached and evaluated.

Patients identified as part of a screening or surveillance program are found at a less advanced tumour stage [101, 102]. The apparent prolonged survival which may be observed in these asymptomatic patients may partly be explained by "lead time bias" which results from the difference in time between the detection of disease by screening and the onset of symptoms. Thus, whether the screen-detected cancers have an intrinsically improved survival beyond that of the "lead time" is not yet not known and hence the need for this aspect of documentation.

Symptomatic individuals presenting as an emergency must be identified. Bowel obstruction or perforation occurs in 6% of patients with rectal cancer (national data from Finland [64]) and are independent adverse prognostic factors. The definition of terms used here is not clear. In line with the Working Party Report an *emergency presentation is defined as the need for urgent surgery within 48 h of admission.* Furthermore, there is no established definition of "bowel obstruction" to categorize its severity. The arbitrary classification used here is based on the assumption that the physiological impacts of obstruction are related to the clinical spectrum categorized in Appendix A.

Perforation refers either to a local abscess originating as a result of penetration of the tumour or a defect giving rise to faecal peritonitis. Occasionally the normal bowel proximal to the obstructive lesion may perforate. Common to all such patients, however, is the poor prognosis.

Feinstein pointed out 30 years ago that "symptoms" provide important prognostic information [25]. He later documented that this is a universal phenomenon found in a variety of tumours including cancer of the rectum [27]. These symptoms can be classified as *primary*, i.e. related to the tumour at its primary site or to inflammation surrounding the tumour; none of the symptoms per se implies dissemination of the tumour; *systemic*, i.e. those occurring in the body as a whole without requiring anatomical dissemination from the tumour's primary site; the systemic symptoms do not per se imply that the tumour has spread beyond that primary site; and *distant (metastatic)*, i.e. effects of the cancer if extended beyond its primary locus when accompanied by appropriate documentation of distant spread; these symptoms imply per se that the cancer has spread beyond its primary locus. The taxonomy of symptoms is given in Table 2.

Table 2. Taxonomy of clinical symptoms as suggested by Feinstein, Schimpff and Hull [27]

Primary symptoms	Systemic symptoms	Distant (metastatic) symptoms
Rectal bleeding	Persistent anorexia	Jaundice, ascites
Bloody stool	Major weight loss (> 10% or more of customary weight or an absolute loss of 4.5 kg for women and 9 kg for men)	Enlarged, hard nodular liver
Other persistent changes in the size, texture, colour or odour of stools	Persistent fatigue or weakness	Hard non-hepatic intra-abdominal masses
Persistent recent changes in the defecatory process (constipation, diarrhoea)	Persistent pain in the back or hip without evidence of bony metastasis or of an explanatory lesion	Hard masses palpable at body surfaces in skin or lymph nodes
Increased or irregular frequency of bowel movements	Persistent nausea and vomiting	Pain in the back or other bones (with X-ray evidence of metastasis)
Difficult, painful, urgent or incontinent defecation	"Obstipation" (i.e. absence of customary bowel movements for at least 3 days) or other clinical evidence of intestinal obstruction	Other appropriate symptoms (with associated radiographic or endoscopic evidence of metastasis)
Feeling of incomplete evacuation or sensation of a rectal mass		

In a recent paper, Feinstein has argued strongly for incorporation of such patient-based variables to produce an improved clinical system of classification and staging of malignant tumours [82]. Others have emphasized that this process of clinimetrics [26], in which clinical phenomena are measured through observations made by patients and clinicians, can produce useful rating scales or other taxonomies reflecting the biological behaviour of tumours. Thus clinimetrics is relevant to the subject of prognostic factors in patients with rectal cancers.

Performance Status and Comorbidity

A patient with cancer may exhibit functional effects which can be classified as *performance status* or *physical capacity* [59]. The prognostic impact of the Karnofsky Performance Status (or similar systems) is well documented [59, 60]. Feinstein has demonstrated that functional incapacity can be incorporated into TNM staging to give additional prognostic information [82]. Another important point is that a patient's performance status frequently affects not only his or her prognosis but also the choice of individual treatment [27]. Several such systems of classification have been published, but the most widely used is that of the American Society of Anaesthesiologists (Appendix A).

Patient Investigation

General

Every department engaged in cancer management has established formal preinvestigation protocols or more informal "house rules" for preoperative assessment of colorectal cancer such as that published by the United Kingdom Coordinating Committee for Cancer Research (UKCCCR) [99]. In rectal cancer, preoperative investigation is carried out in order to:

1. Ascertain distant tumour spread (M-status), as this is required for tumour staging (see later) and may influence treatment strategy (palliative resection, stoma or no treatment)
2. Identification of factors that will determine treatment strategy such as:
   - Synchronous colonic cancer, which occurs in about 5% of patients and will dictate extent of resection,
   - Colonic polyps, which may affect extent of resection and follow-up (interval and type),
   - Hepatic lesions; potential for hepatic resection (the method chosen for investigation will substantially affect the number of patients identified to harbour hepatic metastases),
   - Assessment of involvement of adjacent organs in patients with fixed lesion.

The minimal investigative protocol should therefore include colonoscopy (or double contrast barium enema), liver ultrasonography and chest X-ray. If follow-up of patients is undertaken (see later) preoperative carcinoembryonic antigen (CEA) should be added.

Tumour Mobility

Assessment of tumour mobility by preoperative palpation has prognostic importance and should be categorized as *freely mobile* (confined within the bowel wall), *tethered* (extended through the wall and partially fixed) *or fixed* (fixed to an adjacent structure and immobile). The usefulness of such clinical staging is discussed by Hildebrandt and Feifel (Chap. 6). Although clinical examination cannot differentiate between fixation due to malignant spread from that associated with dense inflammatory reaction surrounding the tumour, a negative effect on prognosis is observed [12, 22, 57].

The presence of fixation of a tumour to surrounding structures brings into play considerations of preoperative radiation to diminish the bulk and attachment of the tumour with a view to improving local tumour control (Chap. 28).

Rectal and Pelvic Imaging

Endorectal ultrasound (EUS) is currently the best method of preoperative staging of the local lesion and regional lymph nodes. EUS has an accuracy of around 85% for depth of invasion (compared with histology) and 75%–80% for predicting lymph node metastases (Chap. 6).

At present no data have been accrued to demonstrate that an accurate preoperative staging of rectal cancer has altered patient survival or increased local control. If we accept the notion that the treatment of rectal cancer should be standardized and not individualized (see later) it may be argued that EUS is not required in routine operations for rectal cancer.

Except for research purposes, use of EUS should currently be limited to:

- Evaluation of patients for potential local treatment (tumour size < 3 cm, T1-2 tumour, no nodal metastasis, well or moderately differentiated histology)
- Evaluation of patients with tethered or fixed lesions
- As a stratification tool in adjuvant studies, particularly because radiation is not required in Dukes' A (TNM T1-2, N0, M0) lesions.

Ground Rules for Surgical Technique

Definition of Terms – Anatomy of the Rectum

The anatomist's definition of the rectum is where the taeniae coli fuse to form a continuous longitudinal muscle coat. The Japanese "General Rules for Clinical and Pathological Studies on Cancer of the Colon, Rectum and Anus" [54] define rectum as "portion (of large bowel) from level of promontorium to upper edge of puborectalis muscle".

Surgeons also vary in their definitions. The "rectum" may vary from < 12 cm from the anal verge to "below the promontory on barium enema". Some national cancer registries record all distal large bowel tumours below 20 cm as "rectal" (Norwegian Cancer Registry); other authors refer to rectal cancer as those tumours found at or below the peritoneal reflection. A problem with the latter definition is that the peritoneum covers the rectum obliquely.

We recommend that a rectal lesion should be related to its distance from the *anal verge* by proctoscopy and not the dentate line and that the height of the tumour should refer to its lower edge as seen at endoscopy.

The rectum should be defined anatomically as the distal large bowel commencing opposite the sacral promontory and ending at the upper border of the anal canal. When measured from below with a rigid sigmoidoscope, the upper limit is 16 cm from the anal verge. If the lower margin of a tumour lies within 16 cm of the anal verge it is defined as a rectal tumour. A tumour is considered rectal if any part is located at least partly within the supply of the superior rectal artery. Tumours are classified as rectosigmoid when differentiation between rectum and sigmoid according to the above rule is not possible [30, 46].

Recording the height of the tumour in all patients will avoid confusion related to anatomical description and will facilitate subdivision of lesions into those occurring in the upper rectum (12–16 cm from anal verge), middle rectum (6–11 cm from anal verge), and lower rectum (< 6 cm from anal verge).

Optimal Resection Technique: General Methods

The review by McCall and Wattchow (Chap. 3) demonstrates that the surgical approach now known as total mesorectal excision (TME), a technical modification introduced by Heald [43], gives the lowest recurrence rates. In 13 studies published to date, a local failure rate of < 10% has been achieved in all but three in which the failure rate was 19%, 13% and 11%.

The TME technique specifically addresses the problem of local recurrence after rectal cancer surgery. Reviews have clearly shown that local recurrence rates after "standard" operations range from 20% to 30% and are clearly stage dependent (Chap. 3). In 50%–80% of such patients, the local recurrence is the solitary site of failure [1, 80]. Local failure occurs in the mesorectum, i.e. the block of fatty tissue surrounding the rectal bowel wall. The area of failure is commonly within or contiguous with the operative site, i.e. the area where the surgeon has dissected. This contrasts with the fact that isolated intramural recurrence in the bowel at the anastomotic site in the absence of any extramural recurrence is an infrequent finding. The length of bowel resected distal to tumour is of minor or no importance in influencing the incidence of local recurrence [68].

The mesorectum is contained within the posterior pelvic visceral compartment and is separated from the surrounding pelvic structures by an embryologically determined well defined plane [42]. Dissection along these well-defined anatomical planes assures TME as demonstrated by Takahashi (see Fig. 4 in Chap. 13). The mesorectum contains a rich complement of lymphatic tissue. Spread from the rectal cancer occurs in an orderly fashion from the primary through these mesorectal lymphatics (as pointed out by Gabriel, Dukes and Bussey more than 60 years ago [34]), and then extends in an upward and lateral direction [50, 70]. Distal lymphatic spread, on the other hand, is very rare (Chap. 13).

A "standard" rectal resection described in so many textbooks [35, 105] differs in several aspects from TME which have been discussed in a recent review [95]:

- Standard surgery commonly employs blunt pelvic dissection by the insertion of the surgeon's hand into the loose areolar tissue plane between the meso-rectum and the sacral promontory. As pointed out by Havenga and coworkers (Chap. 10), the hand will be directed directly into the mesorectum by the rectosacral ligament and thus across the commonest field of spread. TME is carried out by sharp dissection under direct vision along the delicately shiny surface of the mesorectum.
- TME focuses on circumferential dissection to remove the mesorectum enveloped in its covering. Most conventional operations have been concerned with distal bowel margin only.
- The TME technique is also based on a clear anatomical understanding of the so-called "lateral ligaments", surgically developed structures which in fact are the anchoring points of the mesorectum to the pelvic autonomic nerve plexuses (Chaps. 8–10). A recent study documents that there are no circumscribed structures that can be defined as the lateral ligament [42]. Most surgical textbooks recommend that "the ligaments are then clamped, divided and ligated" [35]. Such an approach will invariably damage the tangentially running autonomic nerve plexuses on which sexual and bladder function depend and may also damage mesorectal integrity.
- Many who advocate "standard resection" hold the opinion that abdominoperineal resection (APR) is "the gold standard by which all other operations must be judged, not only for carcinomas of the distal third of the rectum but for all bulky tumours of the middle third as well" [72]. Proponents of TME focus on restorative rectal resections, and they may even accept a bowel resection margin of 1 cm [58].
- It appears that results from TME alone are substantially superior to the best reported from conventional surgery plus radiotherapy or combination chemoradiotherapy [66].

It may seem to the observant reader that two strong proponents for optimal surgery and TME differ in their operative strategy as to the planes of pelvic dissection (Chaps. 15, 16; [23]). Heald argues for dissection along the *visceral* pelvic fascia whereas Enker is a proponent for dissection along the *parietal* fascia. The plane of dissection is particularly relevant to how the inferior hypogastric nerve plexus is handled (Chap. 10). While slight differences in approach may exist, Enker has pointed out that the distinctions between the two may only be a matter of semantics. Enker and Heald both agree that the focal issue is how to capture all mesorectal disease while simultaneously reducing the operative morbidity, i.e. related to autonomic nerve damage.

It is clear that the results of the differing resection techniques have prognostic importance in determining local failure rate and survival. Thus the IDS should be amended (Appendix A) to included TME *and* conventional resection. Furthermore, if a TME has been attempted, it must fulfil specific criteria of which the circumferential integrity of the mesorectum by its smooth surface appears to be the most important (see "Standards for Specimen Evaluation"). Table 3 gives a suggested operative report listing.

The question whether or not the entire mesorectum, particularly the distal mesorectal "tail", needs to be removed in all patients during a rectal resection is disputed. Some experts who otherwise have adopted the principles of TME do not routinely remove the entire mesorectum in "high" anterior rectal resections (Chap. 16; [3]). Still their local recurrence rates are among the best in the world.

This apparent contradiction can be explained by the pattern of lymph node spread within the mesorectum. Although mesorectal spread is found in up to

Table 3. Suggested operative report listing

Findings	Above or below peritoneal reflection; tumour orientation Liver assessment (including intraoperative ultrasonography) Krukenberg tumour pT4 category (tumour attached to a contiguous organ but without tumour on the surface, or tumour which is apparent on the surface of the specimen) Peritoneal dissemination Synchronous lesion
Operative details	Degree of nerve preservation (Chap. 17) Synchronous resection Type of resection (HAR, LAR, PME, TME, APR, APR + TME, Hartman) Removal of other organs (resection en block +/-) Type of lymph node dissection [apical, lateral (iliac and/or obturator node)] "High tie" (IMV flush with the aorta, preservation of left colic artery) Breaching of mesorectal surface Rectal or tumour perforation during dissection Macroscopic tumour left after resection (biopsy +/-) Level and type of anastomosis (straight, pouch, staples, handsewn) Complete doughnuts (+/-), reinforcing sutures? Testing the competence of the anastomosis Permanent or covering stoma (colon or ileum) Cancerocidal washout (pelvis and or intraluminal) Omentopexy (+/-) Drains (+/-) Blood loss and amount of transfusion

HAR, high anterior resection; PME, partial mesorectal excision; LAR, low anterior resection; APR, abdominoperineal resection; TME, total mesorectal excision; IMV, inferior mesenteric vein.

30% of patients, downward lymph node spread from the tumour is found in less than 5% and seems to occur in patients whose proximal lymphatic channels are occluded by tumour [37] and is a marker of poor patient prognosis [90]. However, where distal lymph node spread occurs, it is usually found within 3 cm of the luminal tumour [8] although discontinuous mesorectal deposits up to 4 cm below the main tumour mass have been noted [43]. In Morikawa and coworkers' study, the lymph node metastasis rates distal to the tumour was 6.4% between 2 and 4 cm and 0% more than 4 cm [70].

Thus, full mesorectal excision can be extended 3 cm beyond the caudal edge of the tumour when a transection of the mesorectum can be carried out safely so long as the transection occurs radially at 90° to the rectal wall. Therefore, tumours of the upper rectum (> 8 cm) may be suitable for this type of partial mesorectal excision (PME) and should be documented both in the operative report (Table 2) and in reporting by pathologists (Appendix B).

Aitken carried out this form of PME in 64 patients with rectal cancer for tumour above 7–8 cm from the anal verge with only one local recurrence [3]. The follow-up time was, however, short in his study, and we feel that more studies are required before PME should be accepted as standard treatment. The trend towards ultralow resections with bowel margins 2 cm or less in length [58] should not have the consequence that surgeons compromise in their effort to remove an adequate length of mesorectum. For most patients this implies TME.

«Coning» Prevention

A cone (Greek *kōnos*; Latin *conus*) is defined in Dorlands Illustrated Medical Dictionary as "A solid figure or body with a circular base tapering to a point". The term was coined in this setting by Anderberg and associates [5]. Coning of the specimen during rectal tumour resection means that the surgeon during dissection enters and transects the mesorectum in a tapering fashion toward the rectal wall which will be used for anastomosis, or to the levator muscles during APR (creating an inverted cone, i.e. with its base oriented superiorly). The manual dissection method described in so many textbooks where the surgeon's hand will be directed by the rectosacral «ligament» directly into the mesorectum inevitably produces this effect on the surgical specimen and should be avoided (Chap. 5).

After "conventional" resection the mesorectum is the most common site of cancer persistence and hence tumour recurrence derived from lymph nodes found superiorly and laterally to the tumour [50, 70]. In patients with lymph node metastasis 50%–60% of nodes containing tumour are less than 6 mm in size and are therefore not palpable during surgery. Complete resection of the mesorectum, the key element of TME, therefore reduces the risk of local tumour recurrence (Chap. 5; [84]).

Low Anterior Versus Abdominoperineal Resection

Some will argue that abdominoperineal resection (APR) is the "gold standard" in rectal cancer surgery. McCall and Wattchow (Chap. 3) challenge this view by stating that APR gives higher local failure rates than low anterior resection (LAR). We believe that the misconception can be traced to the textbook published by Miles in 1923, where he described a cylindrical field of spread beyond the levator ani muscles, even to the ischiorectal fossa (see Fig. 1A in Chap. 15). This apparent radicality was his justification for advocating APR [69]. A recent review concludes that for tumours of similar pathological characteristics, APR does not offer significant advantages over LAR [100].

Low-lying lesions pose specific problems (reviewed in Chap. 3). Inadvertent tumour perforation occurs more frequently during APR and the large surgical wound may increase the risk for tumour implantation. Lateral lymph node involvement is also more common with distal third lesions leading to higher local recurrence rate (Chap. 13).

The considerations given above relates to "conventional" APR using the manual dissection technique. We will argue that the logical next step is to combine TME *and* APR as practised by Cawthorn and coworkers [16], Dixon et al. [21], Enker and associates [24], and MacFarlane, Ryall and Heald [66].

Heald has been able to perform sphincter-saving surgery (LAR) in 89% of 394 consecutive patients undergoing radical surgery (Chap. 15). Sphincter-saving surgery should be considered the "gold standard" of rectal cancer surgery, although there are tumours which will need APR.

Proximal Level of Dissection/Resection

Many authors argue that ligation of the inferior mesenteric artery (IMA) should be flush with the aorta to remove the few lymph node that may remain with a more distal ligation, while others preserve the left colic artery. A review [10], a comparative but non-randomized study [81] and a recent study [19] all conclude that the level of ligation does not influence survival or the anastomotic leak rate. It should be noted however that all studies on this topic are based on "standard or conventional" surgery.

Metastasis to lymph nodes at the origin of IMA (lymph node station 253 in the Japanese terminology [54]) occur in only 2% of rectal cancer patients with Dukes' C lesions (Chap. 12). Moreover a "high tie" flush with the aorta may damage the sympathetic nervous trunks.

Clear recommendations as to level of dissection can at this stage not be given. It is important though that the "apical node" is marked clearly on the specimen, and that the pathologist comments specifically on the status of nodes along major named vascular trunks; in rectal cancer that means along the superior rectal, left colic (if applicable) and IMAs (Appendix B).

The mesocolon is transected radially to the planned point of division of the bowel. There is no documentation that the level of proximal bowel transection has any relationship to outcome measures, as long as the length allows an anastomosis to be constructed without tension and adequate circulation.

In 1954, Cole and associates started to ligate the vascular pedicle before mobilizing the cancer-bearing segment [18]. This approach became known as the "no touch technique" and was popularized by Turnbull [97]. Although the theoretical value of early ligation seems reasonable, a later prospective randomized study (on colon cancer) has failed to demonstrate any benefit apart from the finding that liver metastases appeared later, particularly where there was evidence of blood vessel invasion in the resected specimen [56]. No study on rectal cancer only exists.

Lateral Node Dissection

Operations which extend beyond the mesorectum into the lateral pelvic tissues and remove lymph node along the iliac and obturator vessels are characterized as lateral node dissection or extended pelvic lymphadenectomy (EPL) (Chap. 18). These nodes lie external to the parietal pelvic fascia and are not removed during standard LAR or APR, nor during TME. Normally less than 1% of the lymphatic drainage from the middle and upper rectum goes to the lateral pelvic lymph node (if we accept the method used for investigation used by the authors) [8]. The frequency distribution of cancer spread to these nodes, in particular to lymph nodes along the common iliac artery (lymph node station 273), internal iliac (lymph node station 272) and obturator fossa and artery (lymph node station 282) is given by Takahashi (Chap. 13) and Moriya (Chap. 12). Further, a historical perspective and discussion on its current role has been published by Harnsberger and coworkers [41].

The frequency of lateral nodal involvement is less than 15% but varies according to level of tumour (higher with low tumours; Chap. 13) and tumour stage (see Table 1 in Chap. 18). The lateral nodes may be involved in up to one third of patients who have positive apical lymph nodes. Commonly, lateral lymph nodes are associated with rectal cancers that are extraperitoneal, transmural (T4 tumours) and which contain mesorectal lymph node metastases. It has never been shown convincingly that the local recurrence rate or survival is improved with these extensive procedures (Chap. 18); no randomized study to study its effectiveness has ever been carried out. Whether lateral lymph node spread is a sign of regional or systemic disease is unclear; both local recurrence rate increases and survival decreases with involved lateral lymph nodes.

Moreira and coworkers have in the only comparative study published to date assessed the role of lateral lymph node dissection in 95 patients and compared the results with those of 83 patients who had resection without lateral dissection [71]. Although the local recurrence rate differed (7% after lateral dissection versus 16% without), the overall recurrence rate (local and distant) and 5-year survival were not significantly different. Recurrence, metastasis and survival were related more to venous or neural invasion and tumour spread than to node dissection. Moreira et al. concluded that it is unlikely that EPL will provide significant benefit to the patients with low rectal cancer.

The data and considerations given above are the reasons that Japanese surgeons have failed to convince Western collegues that EPL should be routinely used. The major objections are related to the high incidence of urinary and sexual dysfunction resulting from autonomic nerve damage (Chap. 18). The rate of autonomic nerve dysfunction after standard surgery is also high (15%–50% for impotence [23]), and greater efforts to preserve nerve supply must be a future goal, which will be aided by the careful dissection methods associated with TME described above.

Perioperative Measures – Cancerocidal Washout

The concept of implantation of tumour cells as one of many causes of local tumour recurrence originates from the observation by Patel, Tovee and Langer [79] that perforation of the tumour during dissection increases local recurrence rates significantly. Exfoliated and viable tumour cells can also be found in the bowel lumen (see review by Abulafi and Williams [1]). Thus the practice of cancerocidal washout, particularly of the bowel lumen before the anastomosis is made, has become popular, although some question its routine use (Chap. 16). Therefore, no clear recommendations can be given based on trial evidence.

Anastomotic Technique

Type of Reconstruction (Manual Versus Stapled). There is no one standard method of reconstruction of bowel continuity after rectal resection. Manual anastomosis, either in one or two layers, appears to have higher leakage rates than stapled anastomosis in retrospective studies [100]. However, when more recent prospective trials are examined, there does not seem to be any significant differences in leak rates [4]. The stapler has the considerable advantage that an anastomosis can be constructed at a much lower level than is feasible by hand. Optimal surgery using the TME technique necessitates stapled anastomosis either by the conventional end-to-end circular stapler or by the double-stapling technique [104].

Some authors have claimed that a stapled anastomosis gives a higher incidence of local recurrence, but a recent review does not support this view [1]. Therefore, the reconstruction technique chosen must must be recorded and leak rates should be monitored.

The biofragmentable ring introduced by Hardy and associates in 1984 [40] for sutureless intestinal anastomosis has never gained popularity. This ring cannot be used in the low rectum.

Straight Anastomosis Versus Colonic Pouch. The loss of rectal reservoir and the reduced resting anal pressure after a rectal resection and reconstruction leads to poor bowel function [98]. Construction of a "neorectum" using a colonic pouch has been used to improve bowel function [9]. A pouch could also have the advantage that the leak rate is lower.

The experience with the J-pouch reconstruction is still limited and recommendations as to safety and end-results can not be given as yet. The rectal "stump" must be kept short (< 2 cm) if a pouch is added (Chap. 22). A recent study claims other potential advantages with the pouch technique. Blood flow (measured by the Laser Doppler flowmetry) was reported to be better at the site of the pouch used for anastomosis than that of cut end of left colon used for an end-to-end anastomosis [39]. The conclusions drawn by the authors are, however, not well supported by their data and further studies are awaited. TME may partially devascularize the anorectal stump during dissection of the distal tail as there are no anastomosing branches between the superior and inferior rectal arteries in the posterior part of the rectum [7]. Whether a colonic pouch and a coloanal anastomosis are safer than the straight anasomosis and will reduce the anastomotic dehiscence rate remains to be proven.

Protecting Stoma

The need for a covering colostomy after rectal reconstruction is a debatable issue (Chap. 24). Only one controlled study has attempted to examine this problem in a systematic way in elective low colorectal anastomosis [36]. Stomas provided no benefit in this study, and were also found to be of questionable value even for the small number of patients in whom leakage was suspected.

Heald has argued consistently that TME gives relatively high (>10%) anastomotic leakage rate, particularly in anastomosis below 6 cm [44]. Comparative data to support this observation are however not available. Arbman and coworkers have compared the frequency of complications before and after introduction of TME; anastomotic leak rate and total frequency of complications were similar [6]. Data from Norway may on the other hand suggest that TME in the introductory phase of this technique increases leak rate (Norwegian Rectal Cancer Study Group, personal communication).

In view of the complexity and multifactorial nature of the problem, we believe that it is unlikely that a randomized trial will ever be carried out. On the basis of the data presented by Hull (Chap. 24), we may draw the following conclusions:

1. Reliably predicting which anastomosis will leak is unlikely
2. A diverting stoma is not required in all patients and should be used selectively. The following conditions that may favor a stoma are:
   - Technical problems with the anastomosis (including incomplete doughnuts)
   - Anastomotic tension
   - Colonic obstruction or faecal loading
   - Low anastomosis (lower third)
   - Introduction of new technique such as TME (although a recent study does not find increased leak rate with TME [6])

- Adverse patient factors (malnutrition, immunosuppresion, pelvic contamination or sepsis).

The choice of stoma – loop colostomy or loop ileostomy – is debated. In a randomized study, Khoury and coworkers [61] concluded that loop ileostomy was the preferred method but this conclusion is not convincingly supported by their data. We need more studies on this topic, including cost-effectiveness and quality-of-life evaluations.

Standards for Specimen Evaluation

The anatomical extent of tumour is the most powerful predictor of outcome and should therefore be described in detail [27]. The International Comprehensive Anatomical Terminology (ICAT) documentation system recommended by the Working Party is given in Appendix B [30].

Pathologic examination should document that TME has actually been performed by systematic examination of the lateral or circumferential resection margin (CRM). The ICAT categorization and quality control of TME require therefore that pathologic examination is standardized. There is currently one method recommended for macroscopic description, sectioning (including inking), lymph node harvest, description of circumferential margin and microscopy which can be used both routinely and for research. This method is based on transverse whole-mount sectioning of the specimen. Quizilbash [86], and later Chan, Boey and Wong [17], Quirke and coworkers [84, 85], Cawthorn et al. [16] and Ng and associates [76] all open the fresh specimen along the antimesenteric border and pin the specimen to a cork board. After fixation, the specimen is sliced serially and transversely at 5–8 mm intervals and mea-

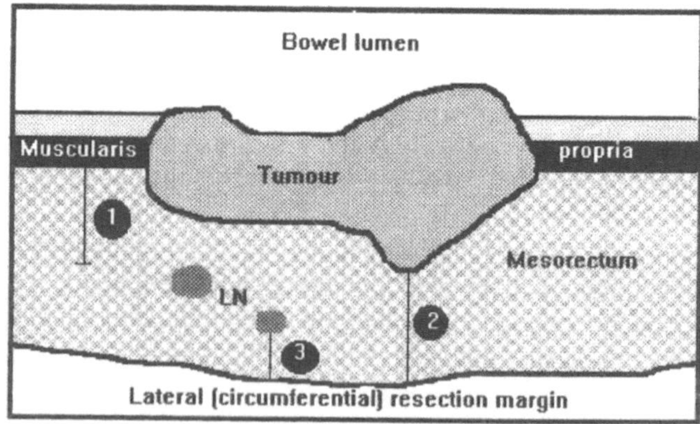

Fig. 2. Schematic display of serial slices for macroscopic examination of rectal cancer as recommended by Quirke (Chap. 5). Measurements showing maximal spread are: *1.* distance from muscularis propria to outermost limit of tumour; *2.* distance from tumour edge to circumferential margin; and *3.* distance from a satellite tumour or involved lymph node to circumferential margin

surements as to tumour penetration are made (Fig. 2). Lymph nodes are harvested and CRM is examined systematically. Multiple blocks are sampled and routinely processed for H&E staining with emphasis on CRM involvement. A similar system has been described in the USA [45].

Of particular importance are the measurements made on the specimen (Fig. 2). Extent of tumour spread through the bowel wall (in millimetres) is an independent prognostic factor after conventional surgery; the deeper the tumour penetrates, the higher the CRM involvement rate and the poorer the survival [2, 16, 55].

Quirke and coworkers have demonstrated that CRM involvement, defined as tumour 1 mm or less from the circumferential margin, predicts local recurrence with an accuracy of 85% [84]. While the predictive importance of CRM involvement for local recurrence has been confirmed by Adam et al. [2], Cawthorn and associates [16] could not demonstrate such association. These apparently contradictory findings are most probably explained by the very low local recurrence rate (8%) in the study by Cawthorn et al., where TME was routinely used [16].

Three points appear important:

1. The circumferential margin should be well described. In a TME resection this margin appears smooth. Irregularity is highly suggestive of breaching of the mesorectum (Chap. 5);
2. The depth of tumour penetration should be measured (see above); and
3. The maximum number of lymph nodes present must be examined in order to produce a more reliable TNM classification. A minimum of 12 nodes is necessary for adequate staging [46]. As documented 15 years ago, the mean number of lymph node harvest per hospital varies considerably, from 1.0 (SD 1.6) to 11.2 (SD 5.8) [11]. Therefore, the number of involved lymph nodes should be compared with the total number present. Thus N staging should be given as pN0 (0/15) or pN1 (2/19).

Staging and Matrix for Staging System Conversion

General

Staging is defined as the assessment and description of the anatomical extent of cancer at certain time points in its natural history, as a rule at diagnosis or first treatment. Hermanek has reviewed the currently used staging systems of which UICC TNM staging now should be the preferred (Chap. 4). Table 4 gives the data elements which are required for TNM staging and also gives the matrix – originally published by the Working Group [30] – for conversion of the TNM system to the other currently used staging systems.

Table 4. International Comprehensive Anatomical Terminology (ICAT) for colorectal cancer and matrix for staging system conversion (reproduced from [30] with permission)

Line Feature	pTNM	Line	pTNM Stage	pTNM Line	ACPS Stage	ACPS Line	Concord Hospital Stage	Concord Hospital Line	Dukes and Bussey 1958 Stage	Dukes and Bussey 1958 Line	Astler-Coller Stage	Astler-Coller Line	Japanese Research Society Stage	Japanese Research Society Line
Microscopic description of tumour depth			0	3	0	3	A-1	3	A	4,5	A	3	I	3–5
1. Primary tumour cannot be assessed	pTX	1		12		12		12		12		12		12
2. No evidence of primary tumour	pT0	2		15,16		15,16		15,16		15,16		15,16		15,16
3. Carcinoma in situ; severe dysplasia	pTis	3		18,19		18,19		18,19		18,19		18,19		18,19
4. Tumour invades submucosa	pT1	4		22		22		22						22
5. Tumour invades muscularis propria	pT2	5				25		25	B	6–8	B-1	4,5		
6. Tumour invades through muscularis	pT3	6	I	4,5						12		12	II	6,8
propria into the subserosal	pT4	7,8		12	A	4,5	A-2	4		15,16		15,16		12
connective tissue or non-				15,16		12		12		18,19		18,19		15,16
peritonealized pericolic														
or perirectal tissue	pNX	9		18,19		15,16		15,16						18,19
7. Tumour directly invades	pN0	12		22		18,19		18,19	C-1	4–8	B-2	6–8		22
other organs or structures	pN1	13,15,16,18,19				22		22		13,14		12		
8. Tumour to and invading	pN2	14,15,16,18,19	II	6–8		25		25		15–17		15,16	III	7 or 4–8
free (serosal)														
surface of the specimen	pN3	17,20		12						18,19		18,19		12 13,14
				15,16	B	6–8	A-3	5						15,16 15,16
Regional lymph node status	(p)MX	21		18,19		12		12	C-2	4–8	C-1	4,5		18,19 18,19
9. Cannot be assessed	(p)M0	22		22		15,16		15,16		13,14		13,14		22 22
10. Number of lymph nodes examined	(p)M1	23				18,19		18,19		15–17		15–17		

Item													
11. Number of nodes positive for tumour			III	1–8		22		22	20		18–20	IV	4–8
12. Line 11=0	RX	24		13,14		25	25						13,14
13. Line 11=1–3 positive nodes	R0	25		15–17						C-2	6–8		17
14. Line 11=>3 positive nodes	R1/R2	26–28		18–20	C	1–8	B-1	6,7			13,14		20
				22		13,14		12			15–17		22
						15–17		15,16			18–20		
Status of nodes on vascular trunk													
15. Not recorded			IV	1–8		18–20		18,19					
16. Negative for tumour				9,12–14		22		22				V	1–8
17. Positive for tumour				15–17		25		25					9,12–14
				18–20									15–17
Apical node status													
				23	D	1–8	B-2	8					18–20
18. Not recorded						9,12–14		12					23
19. Negative for tumour						15–17		15,16					
20. Positive for tumour						18–20		18,19					
						23		22					
						24–28		25					
Distant metastasis: status before definitive treatment													
21. Cannot be assessed							C-1	1–8					
22. None								13,14					
23. Present								15–17					
								18,19					
								22					
								25					
Residual tumour: status after definitive treatment													
24. Cannot be assessed							C-2	1–8					
25. None								13,14					

Table 4 (*Contd.*)

Line	Feature	pTNM Line	pTNM Stage	pTNM Line	ACPS Stage	ACPS Line	Concord Hospital Stage	Concord Hospital Line	Dukes and Bussey 1958 Stage	Dukes and Bussey 1958 Line	Astler-Coller Stage	Astler-Coller Line	Japanese Research Society Stage	Japanese Research Society Line
26.	Locally in line of bowel resection only (shown histologically)							15–17						
27.	Distant only (histologically or clinically)							20						
28.	Both local and distant							22						
								25						
							D-1	1–8						
								9,12–14						
								15–17						
								18–20						
								22						
								26						
							D-2	1–8						
								9,12–14						
								15–17						
								18–20						
								23						
								24–28						

Notes

[1] All data are of proven prognostic significance.

[2] Distant metastasis (Lines 21–23) is not considered in Dukes-Bussey and Astler-Coller system.

[3] Residual tumour status (lines 24–26) is considered in ACPS stage and Concord Hospital System only. It may be recorded in the TNM system by the additional R classification.

The Imperfection of Staging

Survival rates (cancer-specific) in Dukes' A tumours may vary from as low as 77% [75] to as high as 98% [20]. Similarly wide variation is also seen in Dukes' B lesions, while in Dukes' C cancer variation is less. Local recurrence is also found in patients with Dukes' A lesions (Norwegian Cancer Registry, personal communication) even though we should not expect local recurrence in these patients.

The varying rates reflect not only differences in surgical technique but also the imperfection of staging. The pN staging differs; the more sensitive the method of lymph node detection, the more reliable is the staging. For instance, Hida and coworkers found that the average number of lymph nodes in the mesorectum was 21 when a conventional manual method was used for examination of the specimen. This increased to 73 when a clearing method was used [50]. Reliable staging improves the results in the individual stages. This phenomenon – known as the "Will Rogers phenomenon" or "stage migration" [28] – has also been described for rectal cancer [48]. Mesorectal excision and standardized evaluation of the specimen will ensure a more complete lymph node dissection and therefore a more correct pN staging.

One advantage of the Japanese type of radical surgery is that staging is probably as accurate as it is currently possible to achieve.

Residual Tumour Status

The Working Party [30] considered that information on the presence of residual tumour at the time of definitive treatment should be recorded in every case and have included these features in the proposed International Comprehensive Anatomical Terminology (ICAT). This R classification which addresses the residual tumour problem is defined as:

Rx Macroscopic residual tumour cannot be assessed
R0 No residual tumour
R1 Microscopic residual tumour
R2 Macroscopic residual tumour

For rectal cancer an R0 resection will imply that the mesorectum is excised, that there is no tumour at the circumferential resection margin nor in the bowel resection line [47].

Currently the R staging is optional in the TNM system. This issue will probably be addressed in the forthcoming 1997 TNM revision. Item 20 in Appendix B gives an alternative R classification.

On the basis of the pTNM and R classification, the Working Party [30] has defined an "incurable" tumour as:

Those neoplasms with distant metastases (histologically proven, or with convincing clinical evidence) and those with tumour demonstrable histologically in a line of resection (almost always in a lateral (or deep) resection margin (i.e. *the CRM*) (the text in italics added by the authors).

It should be noted that using this definition, adjacent organ invasion does not qualify a tumour for the "incurable" classification.

Japanese Versus Western Type Rectal Resection

From the descriptions given it is apparent that rectal cancer surgery can be divided into three categories:

1. Conventional rectal resection (HAR, LAR, APR) the resection technique practised by most surgeons, particularly in the Western hemisphere. It is characterized by unintentional breaching of the meso-rectum, in particular at the circumferential margin (see "Standards for Specimen Evaluation" and Chap. 5) and gives the highest local recurrence rates (Chap. 3). It may damage the pelvic autonomic nerves by clamping of the "lateral ligament".
2. TME focuses on the importance of circumferential sharp dissection in anatomical layers (Chap. 15). The mesorectum is respected and autonomic pelvic nerves are preserved. This is in principle the technique used by Enker (Chap. 16). However TME could be a part of HAR, LAR or APR if the surgeon choose to do so.
3. Japanese type resections include TME (or PME) as an integral part. This is apparent when the dissection described by Takahashi (Chap. 13) and Moriya (Chap. 17) is evaluated. In addition, extramesenteric lymph node dissection of the iliac and/or obturator nodes (lateral nodes) are commonly carried out especially for "low" Dukes' B (T3, N0, M0) and C (T_{any}, N1-2, M0) cancers. Occasionally block dissection of the retroperitoneum between the ureters and laying bare the vena cava and aorta (from above the IMA) is added. The pelvic autonomic nerves are often dissected and partially resected (Chaps. 13, 17).

Japanese surgeons tend to tailor their operation to the individual. Preoperative assessment of tumour invasion of the rectal wall (T stage) and identification of lymph node metastases by EUS are therefore necessary in their practice and will guide therapy more than in the Western world (Chaps. 13, 17).

Outcome Analysis

Immediate Results

The literature abounds with outcome measures after rectal cancer surgery. A common problem is the subjectivity of the elements incorporated in many. Table 5 gives the immediate outcome measures that we recommend to be recorded in all rectal cancer patients.

Table 5. Suggested immediate outcome parameters to be recorded in all patients with a (colo)rectal malignancy

---

Mortality (30 day figures or in-hospital if LOS > 30 days)
Morbidity
    Major leaks (pelvic sepsis)
    Minor (radiological) leaks
    Bleeding requiring transfusion (volume)
    Small-bowel obstruction
    Wound infection/dehiscence (abdominal and perineal)
    Stoma-related complications
    Medical (general) complications (lungs, renal, DVT/PE,
    cardiac, neurological)
    Voiding (transurethral or suprapubic catheterization,
    intermittent catheterization, catheter   removed)
Length of stay (LOS)
    Post-operative
    ICU days
Reoperations (reasons)

LOS, length of stay; DVT/PE, deep vein thrombosis, pulmonary embolism; ICU, intensive care unit.

Late Follow-Up Information

The Working Party [30] has suggested that follow-up information should be kept simple except in studies in which specific aims are being assessed. Such basic follow-up information is given in Table 6. Follow-up data elements must however be defined.

Table 6. Basic follow-up information as proposed by the Working Party [30]

Date of last follow-up
Last follow-up status
    Alive
    Deceased with unknown colorectal carcinoma status
    Deceased with colorectal carcinoma (recurrence)
    Deceased with other causes
    Lost to follow-up (censored)
Condition at last follow-up (if alive)
    No tumour recurrence
    Local recurrence only
    Distant metastases only
    Both local and distant recurrence
Additional treatment (type and start date)
    Radiation (adjuvant or therapeutic)
    Chemotherapy (adjuvant or therapeutic)
Identification of new primary (site and date of diagnosis)
    Colorectal
    Other

Date at which each of these features were "suspected" or "proven" (cytology, histology or unequivocal clinical evidence) should be recorded.

Definition of Recurrence

There are wide variations in local recurrence rates depending on the definition of local recurrence employed and the subgroup studied, i.e. rates can vary by manipulation of inclusion criteria [67]. Furthermore, the level of reported recurrence rates depends on the completeness of follow-up and the accuracy of diagnosis of recurrent disease (tissue verification, imaging, endoscopy and/or clinically). A Swedish study has also shown that the incidence of local recurrence is probably underestimated in the absence of routine autopsy [15].

We suggest that recurrence is defined as:

Local recurrence: Evidence of recurrent disease within the pelvis after a R0-resection, including recurrence at the site of anastomosis and perineal wound.

Distant recurrence: Evidence of disease outside the pelvis after a R0-resection, including metastasis in aortic and/or inguinal lymph nodes.

Recurrence rates should be given in the following categories as proposed by Abulafi and Williams [1] and the Stockholm Rectal Cancer Group [51]:

1. Local recurrence occurring in isolation
2. Distant recurrence alone
3. Local plus distant recurrence
4. Total local recurrence rate (1 + 3).

A particular problem arises when adjuvant radiation therapy is added, as radiotherapy gives a significant reduction in local recurrence rates, particularly if a standard rectal cancer resection has been performed (Chap. 28). Thus any study using adjuvant radiotherapy should report local recurrence within *and* outside the radiation field separately [67].

Functional Consequences

Functional consequences of rectal cancer surgery are rarely considered in clinical studies, and routine collection of such data is probably not feasible unless done in specific studies. There are many problems in designing good trials to include parameters of patient function from which indices can be used for assessment of postoperative status.

Furthermore, the functional results after treatment must be evaluated in light of preoperative performance; sexual and urinary functions illustrate this point. For example in men changes in voiding postoperatively is often due to benign prostatic hypertrophy which may have been subclinical prior to surgery. Function is not only related to surgery but also to several other factors (Table 7) and thus a cautious approach to functional evaluation seems warranted. The data acquisition model described by Michelassi (Chap. 25) is simple and interesting and should be further evaluated in carefully designed

Table 7. Factors which will influence functional results after rectal cancer surgery

Age, gender, number of births
Preoperative function
Relation to anal transitional zone
Intraoperative dilatation of anal sphincter
Degree of pelvic autonomic nerve preservation
    Total autonomic nerve preservation
    Partial preservation of pelvic nerves
    No nerve preservation
Proximal colon (length)
Level of anastomosis (centimetres from anal verge)
Type of reconstruction (straight or pouch)
Occurrence of anastomotic dehiscence
Anastomotic stricture
Recidual tumour status or recurrence
Pre- and/or postoperative chemotherapy and/or radiation
Length of follow-up

Table 8. Data elements to describe functional consequences and status after rectal cancer surgery

Genito-urinary
    Voiding; need for long-term urinary catheter
    Incontinence (urge or stress)
    Impotence and impaired ejaculation
    Female sexual disturbances
Ano-rectal
    Continence (to flatus and faeces)
    Urgency
    Nocturnal control
    Anastomotic stricture

studies addressing this issue. Both genitourinary and anorectal consequences should be considered. Relevant data elements are outlined in Table 8.

Guidelines for Management

Guidelines for Adjuvant Therapy

Pre- and/or Postoperative Radiation/Chemotherapy

It is beyond the scope of this chapter to review extensively the complex and often conflicting literature on this subject. Some controversies most often discussed are related to:

1. The question of single or combined modality adjuvants;
2. Should adjuvants be given pre- or postoperatively?
3. Selection criteria;
4. Dose/time/volume considerations of radiotherapy; and
5. Effect on local tumour control and survival.

The major problem in absolutely all studies on adjuvant therapy is that the surgery has not been standardized or optimized, nor have instruments for quality control of surgery been used. Therefore in a new era of "optimal surgery" where we should expect local recurrence rates to be around 10% or less after surgery alone (figures which never have been achieved by *any* of the no-adjuvant treatment arms in published randomized clinical trials) the place for adjuvant radiation and chemotherapy must be redefined.

Glimelius (Chap. 28), Levin (Chap. 29) and Nyren (Chap. 30) have all discussed the role of adjuvant treatment in the light of optimal surgery. They all conclude that we need new randomized clinical trials. Currently there is one ongoing study in Holland comparing TME with or without preoperative radiotherapy (Study no. CKVO 95–04; University Hospital, Leiden). Enker and co-workers (Chap. 16) have also outlined possible areas where adjuvant treatment strategies should be considered and investigated.

Perioperative Measures – Intra-Portal 5FU

Based on the fact that two-thirds of patients with recurrent *colorectal* cancer have liver metastases and that many (up to one-third) appear to have isolated hepatic metastases at autopsy have led to trials addressing whether intraportal regional therapy might improve results. So far ten studies on adjuvant cytotoxic portal vein infusion in primary colorectal cancer have been published. A meta-analysis suggests that a reduction in risk of death can be expected, but the benefit appears to be limited to node-positive patients [83].

However, analysis of failure patterns in two studies suggest that the benefit – if any – may be due more to a systemic effect than to the regional one [31, 103]. In support of this is the fact that the published results of both adjuvant systemic chemotherapy for 6–12 months and portal vein infusion for 1 week are roughly comparable with an approximate 5% improvement in absolute survival at 3 years [96]. However, this is a complex subject which requires more study because if 1 week of intraportal treatment is equivalent to 12 months of postoperative peripheral treatment, the intraportal route might offer certain advantages. A potential effect will probably disappear if rectal cancer is studied separately, as the dominating failure pattern after rectal cancer resection is that of local recurrence.

Guidelines for Follow-Up

Routine follow-up of patients may have three purposes; (1) For the surgeon to monitor the results after rectal cancer surgery focusing mainly on the important outcome measures of local recurrence and survival; (2) early detection of recurrent disease and the selection of those patients who might benefit from treatment (radiation, chemotherapy, surgery); and (3) detection of independent colonic neoplasms.

Whereas most will agree that auditing of personal or hospital series is required as a quality control instrument (Chap. 27), the value of long-term routine follow-up incorporating laboratory tests, imaging and endoscopy remains controversial. The benefit for *patient groups* is, at best, marginal (Fig. 1). In fact the average percentage of the total colorectal cancer population benefited by postoperative screening, by being rendered disease free through second-look surgery, is 0.7% (range 0.2%–1.7%) [75].

An international symposium concerning management of recurrent colorectal cancer demonstrated that experts have differing views on whether survival could be increased and whether follow-up is cost-effective [94]. The lack of professional consensus is still apparent nearly 10 years later. A recent meta-analysis concluded that although more operations with curative intent were performed in the intense follow-up group and more metachronous tumours were found, the total number of operations for recurrences and curative operations for metachronous tumours did not differ between the follow-up and no follow-up groups. More importantly, 5-year survival did not differ [13]. This study also demonstrated that CEA should be included in the follow-up program if such was instituted.

Recently a randomized clinical trial has been published in which intense follow-up (clinical examination, endoscopy, computed tomography of pelvis after APR, chest X-ray, liver function tests, CEA and occult faecal blood) was compared with no follow-up [77]. The design of this study appears however not optimal, and the possibility of a type II error exists. The follow-up period was from 5.5 to 8.8 years. Intense follow-up did not prolong survival. The same conclusion will probably emerge after analysis of a randomized study carried out in Fynen, Denmark (Ole Kronborg, data presented at the EuroSurgery meeting, Barcelona 1995). The design of this study has been published [63] and follow-up is now more than 10 years.

In contrast to such evidence, it is a well-documented fact that a "potentially curative" surgical resection of a recurrence both locally [88] and hepatic [96] gives a survival benefit for the individual patient.

Because of the individual versus population controversy and the lack of well-designed controlled studies, it is impossible to formulate general guidelines as to "optimal follow-up". The new prospective studies should be tailored to the problem in question; rectal cancer with its dominant problem of local recurrence should probably be followed differently from colonic cancer where distant spread prevails.

The design of future studies should allow the following questions to be answered:

1. Is detection of a recurrence a consequence of the follow-up program itself, or did patients already have symptoms that warranted investigations?
2. Can patients be identified and undergo potentially curative treament at a presymptomatic stage?
3. What are the therapeutic consequences and does additional treatment (surgery or other) prolong survival?

Politics of Change

The strong evidence of differences in outcome related to surgical technique and surgeon variability can no longer be ignored. Arguments are still voiced that there are simply no data to allow objective comparison between "conventional or standard" and more optimal approaches [89]. The question may however be raised whether comparative studies, preferably in the randomized clinical trial format, can be carried out.

We argue that the question of optimal surgery for rectal cancer is an issue of surgical proficiency and not suitable nor appropriate for the randomized clinical trial format. Silen, commenting on the paper by MacFarlane et al [66], agrees and argues that it is unlikely that a proper randomized clinical trial comparing "conventional or standard" surgery with "optimal" (TME) surgery will ever be carried out because the the key variable – the surgeon – can never be adequately controlled [91]. The ethics of such studies must also be raised; the most debated issue is the possible exploitation of experimental subjects in the pursuit of medical knowledge [87] in the context of learning the proficient use of a surgical technique which conforms to the tenets of the "en bloc" surgical resection of tumours.

It was concluded at a recent international meeting in Oslo, Norway (June 1995) that the "best" surgical technique was that of TME [33]. How can we develop a strategy for implementing this technique in routine surgery nationally and internationally? The following three areas appear important.

Standards for Clinical Documentation

Auditing of results on hospital, regional or preferably national levels should be carried out with feed-back to individual hospitals and surgeons. Such systems have been introduced in Sweden and Norway where all patients are accounted for to minimize the problem of selection bias. The National Cancer Data Base [93] run by the American College of Surgeons may also offer opportunity for all patients to be recorded. Data-base registries can be established on a permanent basis such as the cancer registries of Norway and Sweden, or ad hoc as the German Study Group Colorectal Carcinoma (Chap. 26).

Such registries must record a Minimal Basis Data Set such as the IDS described here (Table 1 and Appendices A and B) to allow accumulation of relevant data.

Joint regional or national efforts will also allow prognostic factor development much earlier than that of individual surgeons and institutions. As an example, in Norway there are around 1000 new patients with rectal cancer per year, but no single institution treats more than 50 patients annually, many less than ten. Tissue and blood sample banking may add powerful research tools to such data bases.

Standardization of Training for Surgeons and Pathologists

The organization of rectal cancer treatment and surgery is probably more important than number of cases treated (Chaps. 26, 27). Therefore surgeons and pathologists should be trained adequately so that they can master the technical modifications of TME. In Norway, rectal cancer surgery has been removed from the training curriculum of the general surgeon. For surgeons in training such procedures are reserved for those specializing in "gastro-intestinal surgery", a formal 3-year training period after being certified as "general surgeon". Rectal cancer surgery is also being concentrated in fewer hands with some hospitals referring their patients to institutions with higher volume and a more comprehensive infrastructure.

For the practising surgeon, specific training schemes must be organized. In Norway and Sweden, surgical work-shops based on live video demonstrations of operations performed by experts, and even hands-on experience assisting such experts have been organized, the main aim being to update and qualify "certified TME surgeons". Heald has described his experience from 16 teaching workshops in 13 cities in Scandinavia, and TME workshops on similar lines have also been established in the UK by the Royal College of Surgeons of England [44].

For pathologists, seminars have been arranged in Norway and the Netherlands with leading international experts as instructors (Quirke), and instruction videos have been produced and distributed.

In Norway a national group (Norwegian Rectal Cancer Group) under the auspices of the Norwegian Gastrointestinal Cancer Group (NGICG) – a multidiciplinary body – has been established, with a base currently within the Norwegian Cancer Registry. This group will have the responsibility of implementing TME nationally, to audit results and to give regular feedback to the participating institutions. The link to the Cancer Registry ensures that all patients can be accounted for. The group will also arrange meetings where results will be shared and specific problems addressed, for instance those related to anastomotic dehiscence. When the data base is operating effectively, specific studies will be initiated.

Medicopolitical Climate for Change

Professional Responsibility

The surgical community must now accept that there are hard data to support the notion that surgeons applying similar treatment principles can consistently achieve the same low failure rates.

We must train surgeons adequately so that they can master the technical modifications of TME. Concentration of rectal cancer surgery in fewer hands such as described from Scandinavia should be accepted as an important step to achieve high quality of patient care. For those in practice, specific training schemes must be organized.

Standardization of the describtion and reporting should be implemented. Auditing of results at hospital, regional and national levels should be organized. Studies on adjuvant therapy should not be carried out unless surgery is standardized and quality control measures implemented.

Role of Academic Institutions

The "academic surgeon" must take the responsibility for being the driving force to promote change. In principle, there are two strategies which can be applied; a centripetal referral of patients to large teaching institutions, or a centrifugal spread of knowledge from the academic institutions to hospitals with an adequate volume of patients.

We will argue strongly for the latter; the centrifugal spread of knowledge recognizes the practicalities of patient care, especially when geographic distances are large, and the need for large community hospitals to maintain their overall competence. Data from the USA also support this view; 60% of patients with rectal cancer are treated in community hospitals and 51% are treated by surgery alone [93]. Thus to achieve improvements in rectal cancer surgery we must focus more on spread of knowledge. Data from Sweden (Chap. 26) clearly demonstrate that excellent results can be obtained in medium-sized hospitals with a relatively low treatment volume if training has been adequate even though relatively few rectal cancer operations are carried out by a single surgeon.

Academic surgeons who criticize the TME results [53] should recognize that many clinical problems can be evaluated only by using observational epidemiological methods although this approach may be more susceptible to bias. The scientific basis for this argument can be found in the recently published paper by Solomon and McLeod [92]. Analytic studies have been the major thrust in population epidemiology, but their role in clinical epidemiology has been dampened somewhat because of the stance taken by some that only randomized clinical trials are valuable in evaluating clinical practice. We argue strongly in favour of observational methodology in the research area of rectal cancer surgical proficiency and find additional support for this view in a recently published review by Hu and coworkers [52].

This approach can be complemented by the randomized clinical trial format for clearly defined treatment method comparisons which will help the documentation process necessary for future physician-related variance analyses.

Thus, focus on the quality of surgery and standardization of technical methods and documentation systems will lead to quality improvement. The involvement of large group of surgeons in these clinical studies are mandatory and will, by diffusion of knowledge within these groups, lead to better clinical results.

Appendix A

Modified International Documentation System (IDS) (additions and modifications marked in boldface; reproduced from Fielding et al. [30] with permission)

Clinical features – Pretreatment

Item		Alternative first level	Alternative second level
#	Name		

Basic patient information

1.	Country	–	
2.	Hospital (Name/code)	–	
3.	Patient identification (Name/code)	–	
4.	Race	– African – Asian – Other	
5.	Past history	– Colorectal carcinoma – Other malignant tumour	– No/Yes – No/Yes

Data of proven prognostic significance

6.	Surgeon identification (Name/code)	–	
7.	Gender	– Male/Female	
8.	Date of birth	– Day/month/year	
9.	Clinical presentation	– Asymptomatic	– Population screening program – Early detection/surveillance program – Coincidental finding during investigation of another disease
		– Symptomatic elective – Symptomatic obstruction	– To solids only – To solids and gas – To solids and gas plus systemic effects
		– Symptomatic perforation (± obstruction)	
9b.	**Comorbid disease class (ASA grade)**	**– Healthy patient with a localized pathologic process** **– Patient with severe disease limiting activity, not incapacitating** **– Patient with incapacitating systemic disease** **– Moribund patient**	

Data of probable prognostic significance

10.	Preoperative treatment	– Radiotherapy	– No/Yes
		– Chemotherapy local	– No/Yes
		– Chemotherapy systemic	– No/Yes
11.	Anatomical site of tumour	– Appendix	
		– Cecum	
		– Ascending colon	
		– Hepatic flexure	
		– Transverse colon	
		– Splenic flexure	
		– Descending colon	
		– Sigmoid colon	
		– Rectum	__cm from anal verge
		– Colon NOS	

Clinical features – Post-treatment

Item # Name	Alternative first level	Alternative second level

Data of proven prognostic significance

12.	Definitive treatment start date	– Day/month/year	
13.	Timing of surgery	– Elective	
		– Urgent (< 48 h)	
		– Emergency (< 6 h)	
14.	Site of distant metastasis	– Cannot be assessed (**Mx**)	
		– No tumour spread seen (**M0**)	
		– Within abdomen (**M1**)	– Distant nodes
			– Liver
			– Peritoneum
			– Other
		– Outside abdomen (M1)	– Lung
			– Bone
			– Brain
			– Other
15.	Liver status	– Right lobe deposits	– Numbers 0, 1, 2, 3, 4, 5+
		– Left lobe deposits	– Numbers 0, 1, 2, 3, 4, 5+
16.	Liver tumour burden	– 0%	
		– $< 25\%$	
		– 25%–50%	
		– 51%–75%	
		– $> 75\%$	
17.	Residual tumour	– None	
		– Locally contiguous with original bowel resection only	
		– Distant metastasis only	
		– Both local and distant tumour	

Data of probable prognostic significance

18.	Tumour mobility at surgery	– Mobile – Tethered – Fixed	
19.	Technique of tumour mobilization	– Conventional – Turnbull "no-touch"	
20.	Tumour perforated	– None – Spontaneous – Iatrogenic	
21.	Type of procedure	– Non-resecting surgery	– Laparotomy – stoma only – Laparotomy – bypass only
		– Local therapy – Limited resection – Radical resection	

22. Name of procedure

- Electrocoagulation
- Laser ablation
- Cryotherapy
- Endoscopic polypectomy
- Submucous excision
- Disc excision
- Segmental excision
- Right hemicolectomy
- Transverse colectomy
- Right and transverse colectomy
- Left colectomy
- Left and transverse colectomy
- Sigmoid colectomy
- High anterior resection (HAR)[1]
- Low anterior resection (LAR)
- Total mesorectal excision (TME)
- Partial mesorectal excison (PME)[2]
- Abdomino-perineal excision (**standard**)
- **Abdomino-perineal excision + TME**
- Subtotal colectomy
- Total colectomy
- Proctocolectomy
- Pelvic exenteration

22b. Laparoscopically assisted   – **No/Yes**

Specify:________________

If [no]– **Unclear anatomy**
    – **Perforation**
    – **Bleeding**
    – **Other**

If [yes] –
Intraoperative complications
    – **None**
    – **Bleeding**
    – **Perforation**
    – **Contamination**

Violation of cancer principles
    – **No/Yes**

23.	Adjacent organs resected	– Not applicable	
		– En-bloc	Specify:___________
		– Separated	Specify:___________
24.	Liver or other metastasis resection (synchronous)	– No/Yes	
24b.	**Clinical evidence of residual tumour after definitive treatment**[3]	**– Cannot be assessed (Rx)** **– None (R0)** **– Microscopic residual tumour (R1)** **– Microscopic residual tumour (R2)**	
25.	Postoperative Rx	– Radiotherapy	– No/Yes
		– Chemotherapy local	– No/Yes
		– Chemotherapy systemic	– No/Yes

[1]Anastomosis above peritoneal reflection.
[2]Distal mesorectum transected (see text).
[3]Current TNM system (Chap. 4).

Appendix B

Pathology features (reproduced from Fielding et al. [30] with permission; additions and modifications marked in boldface)

Item # Name	Alternative first level	Alternative second level
Basic patient information		
1. Number of primary carcinomas of the colon and rectum	Give number	
2. Measurements at tumour site	– Bowel wall transverse measurement – Max. tumour size – transverse – longitudinal – thickness – Distal clearance margin (bowel)	___cm ___cm ___cm Fresh specimen ___cm Fixed specimen ___cm
3. Serosal surface involved (macroscopically)	– No/Yes	
4. Associated pathology	– None – Ulcerative colitis – Crohn's disease – Familial adenomatosis – Radiation colitis – Schistosomiasis	

<table>
<tr><td></td><td></td><td>– Contiguous adenoma with cancer
– Separate adenoma</td><td>– No/Yes
– None
– Give number</td></tr>
<tr><td>5.</td><td>Tumour type</td><td>– Adenocarcinoma
– Mucinous adenocarcinoma
– Signet ring cell carcinoma
– Undifferentiated
– Other</td><td></td></tr>
</table>

Data of proven prognostic significance

<table>
<tr><td>6.</td><td>Microscopic description of tumour depth</td><td>– Primary tumour cannot be assessed (**pTx**)
– No evidence of primary tumour (**pT0**)
– Severe dysplasia, carcinoma in situ (**pTis**)
– Tumour invades submucosa (**pT1**)
– Tumour invades muscularis propria (**pT2**)
– Tumour invades through muscularis propria into the subserosal connective tissue or non-peritonealized pericolic or perirectal tissue (**pT3**)
– Tumour invades directly into other organs or structures (**pT4a**)
– Tumour to and invading free (serosal) surface (**pT4b**)</td><td></td></tr>
<tr><td>7.</td><td>Regional lymph node status</td><td>– Regional lymph nodes cannot be assessed (pNx)
– Number of regional lymph nodes examined
– Number involved with tumour</td><td>

– Give number

– **pN1**: 1–3 positive nodes
– **pN2**: >3 positive nodes</td></tr>
<tr><td>8.</td><td>Status of nodes along major named vascular trunk</td><td>– Not recorded
– Negative for tumour
– Positive for tumour (**pN3**)</td><td></td></tr>
<tr><td>9.</td><td>Apical node status</td><td>– Not recorded
– Negative for tumour
– Positive for tumour (**pN3**)</td><td></td></tr>
<tr><td>10.</td><td>Tumour transected shown histologically</td><td>– Cannot be assessed
– None
– Proximal line of resection (**R1**)
– Circumferential margin (**R1**)
– Distal line of resection (**R1**)</td><td>

– No/Yes
– No/Yes
– No/Yes</td></tr>
<tr><td>11.</td><td>Proven distant metastases</td><td>– No/Yes
– The presence of distant metastases cannot be assessed (**pMx**)
– No distant metastases (**pM0**)
– Distant metastases shown histologically (**pM1**)
– Distant metastases shown clinically only (**M1**) and (**R2**)</td><td></td></tr>
<tr><td>12.</td><td>Histology in line of resection of excised distant metastasis</td><td>– No metastasis excised
– No tumour in line of resection
– Tumour in line of resection</td><td></td></tr>
</table>

13.	Venous involvement	– Not specified
		– Negative for tumour
		– Intramural veins positive
		– Extramural veins positive
		– Both intra- and extramural veins positive
14.	Histologic pattern of infiltrating margin	– Not recorded
		– Expanding (well-circumscribed)
		– Diffusely infiltrating
15.	Tumour grade	– Well-differentiated
		– Moderately differentiated
		– Poorly differentiated or undifferentiated
		– Grade cannot be assessed

Data of probable prognostic significance

16.	Tumour perforation	– Not specified
		– None
		– Spontaneous
		– Surgically induced
17.	Involvement of distal "doughnut" tissue	– Not applicable
		– No tumour
		– Tumour present
18.	Mixed inflammatory cell infiltrate	– Not specified
		– Not conspicuous
		– Conspicuous
19.	Lymphoid aggregates	– Not specified
		– None
		– Present

Residual tumour status

20.	**Residual tumour status after definitive treatment**	**– Cannot be assessed**
		– None
		– Local tumour in resection line of bowel only (shown histologically)
		– Local tumour in circumferential resection margin
		– Distant metastases only (shown histologically or clinically)
		– Both local residual tumour and distant metastases

References

1. Abulafi AM, Williams NS (1994) Local recurrence of colorectal cancer: the problem, mechanisms, management and adjuvant therapy. Br J Surg 81:7–19
2. Adam IJ, Mohamdee MO, Martin IG, Scott N, Finan PJ, Johnston D, Dixon MF, Quirke P (1994) Role of circumferential margin involvement in the local recurrence of rectal cancer. Lancet 344:707–711
3. Aitken RJ (1996) Mesorectal excision for rectal cancer. Br J Surg 83:214–216
4. Akyol AM, McGregor JR, Galloway OJ, Murray G, Georg WD (1991) Recurrence of colorectal cancer after sutured and stapled large bowel anastomosis. Br J Surg 78:1297–1300

5. Anderberg B, Enblad P, Sjødahl R, Wetterfors D (1983) Recurrent rectal carcinoma after anterior resection and rectal stapling. Br J Surg 71:98–100

6. Arbman G, Nilsson E, Hallbook O, Sjødahl R (1996) Can total mesorectal excision reduce the local recurrence rate in rectal surgery? Br J Surg 83:375–379

7. Ayoul SF (1978) Arterial blood supply of the human rectum. Acta Anat 100:317–327

8. Bartholdson L, Hultborn A, Hulten L, Roos B, Rosencrantz M, Ahren C (1972) Lymph drainage from the upper and middle third of the rectum as demonstrated by Au. Acta Radiol Ther 16:352–360

9. Berger A, Tiret E, Parc R, Frileux P, Hannoun L, Nordlinger B, Ratelle R, Simon R (1992) Excision of the rectum with colonic J-pouch anal anastomosis for adenocarcinoma of the low and mid rectum. World J Surg 16:470–477

10. Bland KI, Polk HC (1983) Therapeutic measures applied for the curative and palliative control of colorectal carcinoma. Surg Ann 15:123–161

11. Blenkinsopp WK, Stewart-Brown S, Blesovsky L, Kearney G, Fielding LP (1981) Histopathology reporting in large bowel cancer. J Clin Pathol 34:509–513

12. Bonfanti G, Rozzetti F, Doci R, Battici F, Marolda R, Bignami P, Gennari L (1982) Results of extended surgery for cancer of the rectum and sigmoid. Br J Surg 69:305–307

13. Bruinvels DJ, Stiggelbout AM, Kievet J et al (1994) Follow-up of patients with colorectal cancer, a meta-analysis. Ann Surg 219:174–182

14. Burke HB, Henson DE (1993) Criteria for prognostic factors and for an enhanced prognostic system. Cancer 72:3131–3135

15. Carlsson U, Larson A, Ekelund G (1987) Recurrence rates after curative surgery for rectal carcinoma, with special reference to their accuracy. Dis Colon Rectum 30:431–434

16. Cawthorn SJ, Parums DV, Gibbs NM, A'Hern RP, Caffarey SM, Broughton CIM, Marks CG (1990) Extent of mesorectal spread and involvement of lateral resection margin as prognostic factors after surgery for rectal cancer. Lancet 335:1055–1059

17. Chan KW, Boey J, Wong SKC (1985) A method of reporting radial invasion and surgical clearance of rectal carcinoma. Histopathology 9:1319–1327

18. Cole WH, Packard D, Southwick HW (1954) Carcinoma of colon with special reference to to prevention of recurrence. JAMA 155:1549–1553

19. Corder AP, Karanjia ND, Williams JD, Heald RJ (1992) Flush aortic tie versus selective preservation of the ascending left colic artery in low anterior resection for rectal carcinoma. Br J Surg 79:680–682

20. Davis NE, Evans EB, Cohen JR, Theile DE, Job DM (1987) Colorectal cancer: a large unselected Australian series. Aust NZ J Surg 57:153–159

21. Dixon AR, Maxwell WA, Thornton Holmes J (1991) Carcinoma of the rectum: a 10-year experience. Br J Surg 78:308–311

22. Durdey P, Williams NS (1984) The effect of malignant and inflammatory fixation of rectal carcinoma on prognosis after rectal excision. Br J Surg 71:787–790

23. Enker WE (1992) Potency, cure, and local control in the operative treatment of rectal cancer. Arch Surg 127:1396–1402

24. Enker WE, Thaler HT, Cramer ML, Polyak T (1995) Total mesorectal excision in the operative treatment of carcinoma of the rectum. J Am Coll Surg 181:335–346

25. Feinstein AR (1966) Symptoms as an index of the biological behaviour and prognosis in human cancer. Nature 209:241–245

26. Feinstein AR (1987) Clinimetrics. Yale University Press, New Haven

27. Feinstein AR, Schimpf CR, Hull EW (1975) A reappraisal of staging and therapy for patients with cancer of the rectum. Arch Intern Med 135:1441–1453

28. Feinstein AR, Sosis DM, Wells CK (1985) The Will-Rogers phenomenon: stage migration and new diagnostic techniques as a source of misleading statistics for survival in cancer. N Engl J Med 312:1604–1608

29. Fielding LP, Stewart-Brown S, Dudley HAF (1978) Surgeon-related variables and the clinical trial. Lancet 2:778–779

30. Fielding LP, Arsenault PA, Chapuis PH, Dent O, Gathright B, Hardcastle JD, Hermanek P, Jass JR, Newland RC (1991) Clinicopathological staging for colorectal cancer: an international documentation system (IDS) and an international comprehensive anatomical terminology (ICAT). J Gastroenterol Hepatol 6:325–344

31. Fielding LP, Hittinger R, Grace RH, Fry JS (1992) Randomized controlled trial of adjuvant chemotherapy by portal-vein perfusion after curative resection for colorectal carcinoma. Lancet 340:502–506
32. Fielding LP, Henson DE (1993) Multiple prognostic factors and outcome analysis in patients with cancer. Communication from the American Joint Committee on Cancer. Cancer 71:2426–2429
33. Fielding LP (1995) Optimising surgical treatment of rectal cancer. (Meeting report). Lancet 346:113
34. Gabriel WB, Dukes C, Bussey HJ (1935) Lymphatic spread in cancer of the rectum. Br J Surg 23:395–413
35. Gordon PH (1995) Radical surgery – low anterior resection (chap. 61). In: Cohen AM, Winaver SJ, Friedman MA, Gundersson LL (eds) Cancer of the colon, rectum and anus. McGraw-Hill, New York, pp 571–588
36. Graffner H, Fredlund P, Olsen S-A, Oscarson J, Petersson B-G (1983) Protective colostomy in low anterior resection of the rectum using the EEA stapling instrument. A randomized study. Dis Colon Rectum 26:87–90
37. Grinell RS (1966) Lymphatic block with atypical and retrograde lymphatic metastasis and spread in carcinoma of the colon and rectum. Ann Surg 163:272–280
38. Grotz RL, Pemberton JH, Gunderson LL (1995) Treatment results with radical surgery. In: Cohen AM, Winaver SJ, Friedman MA, Gundersson LL (eds) Cancer of the colon, rectum and anus. McGraw-Hill, New York, pp 605–613
39. Hallbook O, Johansson K, Sjödahl R (1996) Laser Doppler blood flow measurement in rectal resection for carcinoma – comparison between the straight and colonic J pouch reconstruction. Br J Surg 83:389–392
40. Hardy Jr TG, Pace WG, Maney JW, Katz AR, Kaganov AL (1985) A biofragmentable ring for sutureless bowel anastomosis. Dis Colon Rectum 28:484–490
41. Harnsberger JR, Vernava III AM, Longo WE (1994) Radical abdominopelvic lymphadenectomy: historic perspective and current role in the surgical management of rectal cancer. Dis Colon Rectum 37:73–87
42. Havenga K, DeRuiter MC, Enker WE, Welwaart K (1996) Anatomical basis of autonomic nerve-preserving total mesorectal excision for rectal cancer. Br J Surg 83:384–388
43. Heald RJ, Husband EM, Ryall RDH (1982) The mesorectum in rectal cancer surgery – the clue to pelvic recurrence? Br J Surg 69:613–616
44. Heald RJ (1995) Total mesorectal excision is optimal surgery for rectal cancer: a Scandinavian consensus. (Leading article). Br J Surg 82:1297–1299
45. Henson DE, Hutter RVP, Sobin LH, Bowman HE (1994) for the members of the Cancer Committee, College of American Pathologists, and the Task Force for Protocols on the Examination of Specimens from Patients with Colorectal Cancer. Protocol for the examination of specimens removed from patients with colorectal carcinoma. Arch Pathol Labor Med 118:122–125
46. Hermanek P, Henson DE, Hutter RVP, Sobin LH (editors) (1993) UICC TNM Supplement 1993: a commentary on uniform use. Springer, Berlin Heidelberg New York
47. Hermanek P, Wittekind Ch (1994) Diagnostic seminar: The pathologist and the R classification. Path Res Pract 190:115–123
48. Hermanek P (1995) pTNM and residual tumor classifications: problems of assessment and prognostic significance. World J Surg 19:184–190
49. Hermanek P, Gospodarowicz MK, Henson DE, Hutter RPV, Sobin LH (1995) Prognostic factors in cancer. Springer, Berlin Heidelberg New York, pp 64–79
50. Hida J, Mori N, Kubo R, Matsuda T, Morikawa E, Kitaoka M, Sindoh K, Yasutomi M (1994) Metastasis from carcinoma of the colon and rectum detected in small lymph nodes by the clearing method. J Am Coll Surg 178:223–228
51. Holm T, Cedermark B, Rutquist L-E (1994) Local recurrence of rectal adenocarcinoma after "curative" surgery with and without preoperative radiotherapy. Br J Surg 81:452–455
52. Hu X, Wright JG, McLeod RS, Lossing A, Walters BC (1996) Observational studies as alternatives to randomized clinical trials in surgical clinical research. Surgery 119:473–475

53. Isbister WH (1990) Basingstoke revisited. Aust NZ J Surg 60:243–246
54. Japanese Research Society for Cancer of the Colon and Rectum (1983) General rules for clinical and pathological studies on cancer of the colon, rectum and anus. Jpn J Surg 13:557–573
55. Jass JR, Love SB, Northover JMA (1987) A new prognostic classification of rectal cancer. Lancet I:1303–1306
56. Jeekel J (1987) Can radical surgery improve survival in colorectal cancer? World J Surg 11:412–417
57. Jensen HE, Balslev I, Nielson J (1970) Extensive surgery in the treatment of carcinoma of the rectum. Acta Chir Scand 136:431–434
58. Karanjia ND, Schache DJ, North WRS, Heald RJ (1990) "Close shave" in anterior resection. Br J Surg 77:510–512
59. Karnofsky DA, Abelman WH, Craver LF, Burchenal JH (1948) The use of nitrogen mustard in the palliative treatment of carcinoma with particular reference to bronchogenic carcinoma. Cancer 1:634–669
60. Karnofsky DA, Burchenal JH (1949) The clinical evaluation of chemotherapeutic agents in cancer. In: Macleod CM (ed) Chemotherapy of cancer. Columbia University Press, New York, pp 191–205
61. Khoury GA, Lewis MCA, Meleagros L, Lewis AAM (1986) Colostomy or ileostomy after colorectal anastomosis? a randomized study. Ann Roy Coll Surg Engl 68:5–7
62. King's Fund Forum (1990) Cancer of the colon and rectum. Br J Surg 77:1063–1065
63. Kronborg O, Fenger C, Deichgraber E, Hansen L (1988) Follow-up after radical surgery for colorectal cancer: design of a randomized study. Scand J Gastroenterol 149 (Suppl):159–162
64. Kyllonen LEJ, Husa AI (1986) Carcinoma of the rectum in Finland – changes in two decades. An epidemiological and clinical study. Acta Chir Scand 152:749–762
65. McArdle CS, Hole D (1991) Impact of variability among surgeons on postoperative morbidity and mortality and ultimate survival. Br Med J 302:1501–1505
66. MacFarlane JK, Ryall RDH, Heald RJ (1993) Mesorectal excision for rectal cancer. Lancet 1:457–460
67. Marsh PJ, James RD, Schofield PF (1995) Definition of local recurrence after surgery for rectal carcinoma. Br J Surg 82:465–468
68. McDermott FT, Hughes ESR, Pihl E, Johnson WR, Price AB (1985) Local recurrence after potentially curative resection for rectal cancer in a series of 1008 patients. Br J Surg 72:34–37
69. Miles E (1923) Cancer of the rectum. Harrison and Sons, London
70. Morikawa E, Yasutani M, Shindov K, Matsuda T, Mori N, Hida J, Kubo R, Kitaoka M, Nakamura M, Fujimoto K, Inufusa H, Hatta M, Izumoto G (1994) Distribution of metastatic lymph nodes in colorectal cancer by the modified clearing method. Dis Colon Rectum 37:219–223
71. Moreira LF, Hizuta A, Iwagaki H, Tanaka N, Orita K (1994) Lateral lymph node dissection for rectal carcinoma below the peritoneal reflection. Br J Surg 81:293–296
72. Murray JJ, Veidenheimer MC (1993) Abdomino-perineal excision of the rectum. In: Fielding LP, Goldberg SM (eds) Surgery of the colon, rectum and anus. Rob and Smith's Operative Surgery. Chapman and Hall, London
73. Myers MH, Ries LA (1989) Cancer patient survival rates: SEER program results for 10 year follow-up. CA Cancer J Clin 39:21–32
74. Nelson RL (1993) The decision to treat patients with recurrent colorectal cancer. Cancer 71:4298–4301
75. Nelson RL (1995) Postoperative evaluation of patients with colorectal cancer. Semin Oncol 22:488–493
76. Ng IOL, Luk ISC, Yuen ST, Lau PWK, Pritchett CJ, Ng M, Poon GP, Ho J (1993) Surgical lateral clearance in resected rectal carcinomas. A multivariate analysis of clinicopathologic features. Cancer 71:1972–1976
77. Ohlsson B, Breland U, Ekberg H, Graffner H, Tranberg K-G (1995) Follow-up after curative surgery for colorectal carcinoma. Randomized comparison with no follow-up. Dis Colon Rectum 38:619–626

78. Patel SC, Tovee EB, Langer B (1976) Twenty-five years of experience with radical surgery of carcinoma of the extraperitoneal rectum. Br J Surg 63:384–388
79. Patel SC, Tovee EB, Langer B (1977) Twenty-five years' experience with radical surgical treatment of carcinoma of the extraperitoneal rectum. Surgery 82:460–465
80. Pearlman NW (1995) Surgery for pelvic recurrence. In: Cohen AM, Winaver SJ, Friedman MA, Gundersson LL (eds) Cancer of the colon, rectum and anus. McGraw-Hill, New York
81. Pezim ME, Nicholls RJ (1984) Survival after high or low ligation of the inferior mesenteric artery during curative surgery for rectal cancer. Ann Surg 200:729–733
82. Piccirillo JF, Feinstein AR (1996) Clinical symptoms and comorbidity: significance for the prognostic classification of cancer. Cancer 77:834–842
83. Piedbois P, Buyse M, Gray R et al (1995) Portal vein infusion is an effective adjuvant treatment for patients with colorectal cancer. Proceedings of the American Society of Clinical Oncology 14:192
84. Quirke P, Dixon MF, Durdey P, Williams NS (1986) Local recurrence of rectal adenocarcinoma due to inadequate surgical resection. Histopathology study of lateral tumour spread and surgical excision. Lancet II:996–999
85. Quirke P, Dixon MF (1988) The prediction of local recurrence in rectal adenocarcinoma by histopathology examination. Int J Colorect Dis 3:127–131
86. Quizilbash AH (1982) Pathologic studies in colorectal cancer. A guide to surgical pathology examination of colorectal specimens and review of features of prognostic significance. In: Sommers SC, Rosen PP (eds) Pathology annual, vol 17. Appleton-Century-Crofts, New York, pp 1–46
87. Rosner F (1987) The ethics of randomized clinical trials. Am J Med 82:283–290
88. Sagar PM, Pemberton JH (1996) Surgical management of locally recurrent rectal cancer (review). Br J Surg 83:293–304
89. Scholefield JH, Northover JMA (1995) Surgical management of rectal cancer. Br J Surg 82:745–748
90. Scott N, Jackson P, Al-Jaberi T, Dixon MF, Quirke P, Finan PJ (1995) Total mesorectal excision and local recurrence: a study of tumour spread in the mesorectum distal to rectal cancer. Br J Surg 82:1031–1033
91. Silen W (1993) Mesorectal excision for rectal cancer (letter). Lancet 341:1279–1280
92. Solomon MJ, McLeod RS (1995) Should we be performing more randomized controlled trials evaluating surgical operations? Surgery 118:459–467
93. Steele GD (1994) The National Cancer Data Base Report on colorectal cancer. Cancer 74:1979–1989
94. Sugerbaker P, Attiyeh FF, Killingback M, Oates GD, Schofield PF, Staab HJ, Steele G Jr, Sugerbaker PH (1986) The management of recurrent colorectal cancer (symposium). Int J Colorect Dis 1:133–151
95. Søreide O, Norstein J (1996) Local recurrence after rectal cancer surgery – a strategy for change. J Am Coll Surg (in press)
96. Taylor I (1996) Liver metastases from colorectal cancer: lessons from past and present clinical studies (review). Br J Surg 83:456–460
97. Turnbull RB Jr, Kyle K, Watson FR, Spratt J (1967) Cancer of the colon: influence of the no-touch isolation technic on survival rates. Ann Surg 166:420–427
98. Williams NS, Price R, Johnston D (1980) The long-tem effect of sphincter-preserving operations for rectal carcinoma on function of the anal sphincter in man. Br J Surg 67:203–208
99. Williams NS, Jass JR, Hardcastle DJD (1988) Clinicopathological assessment and staging of colorectal cancer. Br J Surg 75:649–652
100. Williams NS (1993) Surgical treatment of rectal cancer. In: Keighley MRB, Williams N (eds) Surgery of the anus, rectum and colon (chap. 31) Saunders, London, pp 939–1053
101. Winawer SJ, Andrews M, Flehinger B, Sherlock P, Schottenfield D, Miller DG (1980) Progress report on controlled trial of fecal occult blood testing for the detection of colorectal neoplasia. Cancer 45:2959–2964
102. Winawer SJ, Schottenfeld D, Flehinger BJ (1991) Colorectal cancer screening. J Natl Cancer Inst 83:243–253

103. Wolmark N, Rockette H, Wickerham DL et al (1990) Adjuvant therapy of Dukes's A, B and C adenocarcinoma of the colon with portal-vein fluorouracil infusion: preliminary results of national surgical adjuvant breast and bowel project protocol C-02. J Clin Oncol 8:1466–1475
104. Yule AG, Fiddian RV (1983) "Two gun" surgery – low anterior resection of the rectum avoiding the anorectal purse string suture. Br J Surg 70:100–115
105. Zollinger Jr RM, Zollinger RM (1993) Atlas of surgical operations. 7th edn. McGraw-Hill, New York

Subject Index

Springer-Verlag
and the Environment

We at Springer-Verlag firmly believe that an international science publisher has a special obligation to the environment, and our corporate policies consistently reflect this conviction.

We also expect our business partners – paper mills, printers, packaging manufacturers, etc. – to commit themselves to using environmentally friendly materials and production processes.

The paper in this book is made from low- or no-chlorine pulp and is acid free, in conformance with international standards for paper permanency.

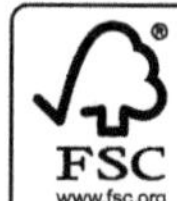